Handbuch der experimentellen Pharmakologie

Handbook of Experimental Pharmacology

Heffter-Heubner New Series

Herausgegeben von / Edited by

O. Eichler
Heidelberg

A. Farah
Syracuse, N. Y.

H. Herken
Berlin

A. D. Welch
New Haven, Conn.

Vol. XX/1

Springer-Verlag Berlin Heidelberg GmbH 1966

Pharmacology of Fluoridcs

Part 1

Contributors

E. W. Alther · R. E. Banks · F. Brudevold · J. W. Clayton jr.

H. Goldwhite · J. C. Krantz jr. · R. L. Metcalf

F. L. M. Pattison · R. A. Peters · F. G. Rudo · J. L. Shupe

F. A. Smith · M. D. Thomas · J. A. Weatherell

Sub-Editor

Frank A. Smith

With 155 Figures

Springer-Verlag Berlin Heidclberg GmbH 1966

Originally published by Springer-Verlag Berlin Heidelberg New York 1966
Softcover reprint of the hardcover 1st edition 1966

Library of Congress Catalog Card Number AGR 25—699

ISBN 978-3-662-23198-2 ISBN 978-3-662-25198-0 (eBook)
DOI 10.1007/978-3-662-25198-0

Title No. 5729

Preface

One might well ask why another volume dealing with biological aspects of compounds of fluorine should be offered to the scientific community, already burdened with a literature too massive to be comfortably ingested. Prior to World War II this question simply did not arise: there was not sufficient interest or literature in the field to warrant anything beyond the classical monograph published by KAJ ROHOLM in 1937[1].

ROHOLM'S work was directed chiefly toward a better understanding of the effects of fluorides on the general health of workers in the cyrolite industry. However, with the demonstration that water-borne fluoride was a causative agent of both mottled enamel and increased resistance to dental caries, the groundwork was laid in the 1930's and early 1940's for a greatly increased interest in the biological effects of fluorides in human beings. During this time and earlier for that matter, work also had been going steadily ahead in the less spectacular area of effects produced in poultry and livestock when fluorine-containing rock phosphate was incorporated in the ration, and when pasture land was contaminated with fluorides released during the large-scale conversion of rock phosphate to fertilizer and phosphoric acid. These latter aspects of the problem had led to the development of a respectable literature in plant physiology, dealing with the effects of fluoride on vegetation. Much of the work in this period, especially that dealing with dental health and with chronic experimental poisoning in animals, was reviewed by EICHLER in 1950, in an earlier volume of this Handbuch[2].

As a result of research initiated during World War II, the commercial uses of fluorine and fluorides increased rapidly and enormously, and this growth has been sustained in the post-war years. For example, in 1963 the yearly consumption of hydrogen fluoride was estimated to be 215,000 short tons, of which production of aluminum fluoride, fluorocarbons, uranium and synthetic cyrolite consumed 30, 31, 10 and 12%, respectively. In addition to these industries, a partial list of the processes or industries wherein inorganic fluorides are used includes production of steel, chemical cleaning, as catalysts, electrotinning of steel, as a laundry sour, in acidizing oil wells, beryllium production, electropolishing, as an abrasive and as an electrolyte.

After World War II, and as a result of research initiated in those days, great interest arose in the potentialities of organic compounds of fluorine. In the popular press, these were identified with the rodenticide known as 1080, or sodium fluoroacetate, and with the "nerve gases" such as DFP, or diisopropyl fluorophosphate. Less well appreciated is the fact that organic fluorine compounds, *e.g.* fluorocarbons, are used in very considerable amounts in aerosol propellents, hydraulic fluids, in fire extinguishing systems, as refrigerants, and in plastics.

---

[1] ROHOLM, K. (1937): Fluorine intoxication. A clinical-hygienic study with a review of the literature and some experimental investigations. H. K. Lewis and Co., London. 364 p. See also ROHOLM, K. (1938): Handbuch der experimentellen Pharmakologie. Siebenter Band. Fluor und Fluorverbindungen. Springer-Verlag. Berlin p. 1—62.

[2] EICHLER, O. (1950): Chronic poisoning by fluorides, p. 1032—1107, *In* Handbuch der experimentellen Pharmakologie. Zehnter Band, Die Pharmakologie anorganischer Anionen. Springer-Verlag, Berlin, Göttingen, Heidelberg.

Finally, there is a continuing scientific interest in the development of new pharmacological agents containing fluorine. Fluorine-containing steroids, anesthetic agents and anti-cancer drugs come immediately to mind.

Historically then, interest in the biological effects of fluorides came about initially in relation to water fluoridation programs and atmospheric contamination problems. After World War II interest was augmented by the industrial growth of both inorganic and organic fluorine compounds.

One is tempted to suspect at times that the rapidly expanding literature in the field reflects a feeling that fluorine and fluorides have suddenly become more toxic than they used to be. Obviously, such is not the case. What has come about however, is an appreciable increase in the hazard associated with these materials. That is to say, the possibility of encountering the characteristic toxic effects of these materials *under the conditions of their use* has been increased, because the variety, amounts, and ways of usage have increased so tremendously.

This distinction between hazard and toxicity is often lost sight of. It is the increased hazards of fluoride which have led to the burgeoning literature in the field of biological effects of fluorides. This volume is an attempt to evaluate and bring together in one place at least a portion of the extensive and widespread literature dealing with certain of these aspects.

A succeeding volume is intended to deal in a similar fashion with other equally important areas.

Rochester, N. Y. 18. April 1965 FRANK A. SMITH

Contributors

ERNEST W. ALTHER, Dr., Cantonal Agricultural College, Flawil, St. Gallen/Schweiz.

R. E. BANKS, Professor Dr., Faculty of Technology, University of Manchester, Manchester/England.

FINN BRUDEVOLD, Dr., Professor Forsyth Dental Infirmary, 140 The Fenway, Boston 15, Massachusetts/USA.

J. WESLEY CLAYTON JR., Dr., Haskell Laboratory for Toxicology and Industrial Medicine, E. I. du Pont de Nemours and Co., Wilmington, Delaware/USA.

H. GOLDWHITE, Professor Dr., Faculty of Technology, University of Manchester, Manchester/England. *Present Address:* Department of Chemistry, California State College at Los Angeles, Los Angeles, California/USA.

JOHN C. KRANTZ JR., Professor Dr., Department of Pharmacology, University of Maryland School of Medicine, Baltimore, Maryland/USA.

R. L. METCALF, Professor, Dr., Department of Entomology, University of California, Riverside, California/USA.

F. L. M. PATTISON, Professor Dr., Department of Chemistry, University of Western Ontario, London, Ontario/Canada.

SIR RUDOLPH A. PETERS, Professor Dr., Department of Biochemistry, Tennis Court Road, Cambridge/England.

FRIEDA G. RUDO, Professor Dr., Department of Pharmacology, University of Maryland School of Medicine, Baltimore, Maryland/USA.

JAMES L. SHUPE, Dr., Formerly Professor of Veterinary Science, Utah State University. *Present Address:* Research Veterinarian Animal Disease and Parasite Research Division, U.S. Agricultural Research Service, Logan, Utah 84321/USA.

FRANK A. SMITH, Professor Dr., University of Rochester, School of Medicine and Dentistry, Department of Radiation Biology and Biophysics, Rochester 20, New York/USA.

MOYER D. THOMAS, Professor Dr., Air Pollution Research Center, University of California, Riverside, California/USA.

JOHN A. WEATHERELL, Professor Dr., Biological Research Unit, School of Dentistry, University of Leeds, Blundell Street, Leeds 1/England.

Contents

Chapter 1: Fluorine Chemistry

By R. E. BANKS and H. GOLDWHITE

Chapter 4: The Role of Fluorides in Tooth Chemistry and in the Prevention of Dental Caries

By F. Brudevold

Chapter 5: The Effects of Fluoride on Plants

By M. D. Thomas and E. W. Alther

Chapter 7: Fluorine-Containing Insecticides

By R. L. METCALF

Chapter 9: The Mammalian Toxicology of Organic Compounds Containing Fluorine

By J. W. Clayton jr.

Chapter 1

Fluorine Chemistry

By

R. E. Banks and H. Goldwhite[1]

With 2 Figures

I. Introduction

Fluorine is a common element; in the combined state it constitutes about 0.065% by weight of the earth's crust, and is more abundant than chlorine. Despite this fact, the chemistry of fluorine has been studied in detail only during the past two decades.

The science of fluorine chemistry began with investigations of the reaction between fluorspar (calcium fluoride) and sulphuric acid by Marggraf (1768) and by Scheele (1771). The latter maintained that an acid ("Flussäure") which was combined with lime in fluorspar was liberated in the reaction, but its exact nature remained undiscovered since the primary product, hydrogen fluoride, attacked the glass apparatus used and became contaminated with fluorosilicic acid. The position was clarified in 1809 when Gay-Lussac and Thénard distilled fluorspar with sulphuric acid in lead or silver apparatus and obtained almost pure hydrogen fluoride. Shortly afterwards (1813) Ampère suggested to Davy that the acid from fluorspar and sulphuric acid was analogous to the acid containing hydrogen and chlorine; the acceptance of this view led to attempts to isolate the new element fluorine with the result that knowledge of inorganic fluorides began to accumulate.

During the next seventy years many eminent chemists, including Davy, Faraday, Frémy, Gore, and Knox, failed in their attempts to isolate fluorine. Finally, on June 26th., 1886, Moissan succeeded; he electrolysed hydrogen fluoride containing potassium fluoride in a platinum cell and liberated gaseous fluorine for the first time.

Progress in the study of fluorine chemistry was not accelerated by Moissan's discovery. Fluorine was found to react with considerable violence with many materials, and this, coupled with the hazards of working with hydrogen fluoride and the experimental difficulties involved in the generation of fluorine discouraged investigators. Only Moissan and a few other pioneers continued to prepare and study fluorine, and no significant progress in the application of the element to chemical synthesis was made for nearly fifty years.

Most important advances were made during this period, however, by Swarts, a contemporary of Moissan. Starting in 1891, he laid the foundation of modern organic fluorine chemistry by developing general methods of preparation of organic fluoro-compounds by the technique of halogen-exchange between organic chlorides, bromides, or iodides and inorganic fluorides, notably antimony trifluoride. This

[1] Present address: Department of Chemistry, California State College at Los Angeles.

work led to the introduction of dichlorodifluoromethane (CF_2Cl_2, *Freon 12*[1]) by MIDGLEY and HENNE in 1930 as an inert non-toxic refrigerant which had such outstanding advantages over other refrigerants that it rapidly became a major industrial chemical. Since anhydrous hydrogen fluoride was required for the preparation of dichlorodifluoromethane, it became available commercially for the first time and was soon employed as a catalyst in alkylation processes for the production of gasolines.

The early 1930's also saw a revival of interest in elementary fluorine. The work of RUFF on the preparation and properties of the highly reactive halogen fluorides, and of BOCKEMÜLLER and of BIGELOW on the direct fluorination of organic compounds merits attention; but special significance attaches to the studies of SIMONS and BLOCK (1937) on the direct action of fluorine on heated carbon in the presence of a mercury catalyst since they obtained evidence that a series of fluorocarbons, both acyclic (C_nF_{2n+2}) and cyclic (C_nF_{2n}), analogous to the familiar hydrocarbon series existed. These fluorocarbons were remarkable for their high chemical and thermal stability, properties which stem from the high carbon-fluorine bond dissociation energy and from the steric shielding effect and high electronegativity of the fluorine atoms. Finally, before this most important decade in the history of fluorine chemistry drew to a close, it was reported that chlorotrifluoroethylene ($CF_2{=}CFCl$) and tetrafluoroethylene ($CF_2{=}CF_2$) can be polymerised to give materials (Kel-F[2] and Teflon[1], respectively) of outstanding stability.

The stage was now set for the tremendous advances in fluorine chemistry brought about by the demand during the Second World War for materials capable of use as buffer gases, coolants, lubricants, and sealants in industrial plants handling corrosive uranium hexafluoride. This demand led to the commercial development of processes for the manufacture of fluorocarbons, polytetrafluoroethylene, and polychlorotrifluoroethylene, and the production of elementary fluorine on an industrial scale. When the restrictions on these wartime developments were lifted, it was clear that fluorine chemistry was firmly established as a branch of chemical science with immense potential industrial application.

Since the war, a combination of academic and industrial interests has led to the growth of fluorine chemistry into a vast subject. The object of this chapter is to provide a guide to present-day knowledge of the subject and its applications. More detailed information can be obtained from the textbooks and reviews listed at the end of this chapter.

II. Inorganic fluorine chemistry

A. Elementary fluorine

1. Occurrence

(FINGER 1961)

Fluorine does not occur in the free state in nature, but in combination with other elements is widely distributed in the mineral kingdom; it lies thirteenth in the table of element abundances. The most important mineral containing fluorine is fluorspar, calcium fluoride, and at the present time this is the ultimate source of almost all other fluorine compounds.

---

[1] Trade-name, E. I. du Pont de Nemours, U.S.A.
[2] Trade-name, Minnesota Mining and Manufacturing Co., U.S.A.

2. Preparation

(Rudge 1962)

Fluorine cannot be liberated from fluorides by chemical methods since it is the most powerful oxidising agent known, and it is still prepared by Moissan's electrolytic method. The most widely used procedure is to electrolyse a mixture of potassium fluoride and hydrogen fluoride, of approximate composition $KF \cdot 2\,HF$, in a mild steel cell, fitted with special carbon anodes, at 70—100°. The fluorine generated is contaminated with hydrogen fluoride which is removed by cooling and by passage of the gas over sodium fluoride.

3. Physical properties of fluorine and their effect on its chemistry

(Leech 1956; Sharpe 1957)

The physical properties of fluorine are listed in Table 1. Those properties which have a special bearing on the chemistry of fluorine and its compounds are discussed briefly below.

a) Isotopes of fluorine

The isotope ^{19}F is found exclusively in nature. Other isotopes can be prepared by nuclear reactions but they all have short half-lives. The longest lived is ^{18}F and its half-life of 1.87 hours is too short to enable it to be used widely as a tracer in the study of reactions of fluorine compounds.

Table 1. *Physical properties of fluorine*

Atomic number	9		
Atomic weight (^{12}C = 12.0000)	18.9984	Critical temperature	—129°
Boiling point	—187.9°	Critical pressure	55 atm.
Freezing point	—217.9°	Dielectric constant	1.56/—184°
Colour	pale yellow		
Latent ht. of fusion	372 cal. mol^{-1}	Covalent radius of atom	0.71 Å
Latent heat of vaporization	1600 cal. mol^{-1}	Dissociation energy of molecule	38 kcal
Trouton constant	18.8 e.u.	Standard entropy of molecular fluorine	48.6 cal. mol.$^{-1}$ deg.$^{-1}$
Specific gravity of liquid	1.11 at b. pt.	Standard entropy of atomic fluorine	37.9 cal. g atom^{-1} deg.$^{-1}$
Surface tension of liquid	14.6 dyne/cm at —216°		
First ionization potential	401 kcal/g atom; 17.4 eV	Electron affinity	84 kcal/g atom; 3.74 eV
Electronegativity (Pauling's scale)	4.0	Nuclear spin quantum no.	$^1/_2$
		Nuclear magnetic moment	2.625 nuclear magnetons

b) Covalent radius

This is much smaller for fluorine (0.71 Å) than for the other halogens, and the volume of a covalently bonded fluorine atom is only about one third of that of a similar chlorine atom. Steric repulsions between adjacent fluorine atoms are consequently much smaller than those between other adjacent halogens, and polyfluoro-compounds are often much more stable than corresponding polychloro-compounds. In particular fluorine forms a series of fluorocarbons analogous to the hydrocarbons (covalent radius of hydrogen is 0.34 Å) but few chlorocarbons are known.

c) Dissociation energy

Fluorine has a relatively low dissociation energy (38 kcal) compared with chlorine (57 kcal) or even bromine (46 kcal). This fact, combined with the fact that bonds between fluorine and other elements are usually strong, explains why fluorine reacts with so much vigour with most elements.

d) Ionisation potential

The energy required for the reaction $F(g) \rightarrow F^+(g) + e$ is 401 kcal/g atom. The standard heat of formation of the gaseous F^+ ion is 420 kcal/g ion, an extremely high value compared with those of other positive halogen ions (Cl^+, 327 kcal/g ion; Br^+, 301 kcal/g ion; I^+, 268 kcal/g ion), which means that fluoronium ions, even in a solvated form, are very unlikely to be formed in a chemical reaction.

e) Entropy

The standard entropies of molecular fluorine (48.6 e.u.) and atomic fluorine (37.9 e.u.) are similar to those of molecular chlorine (53.3 e.u.) and atomic chlorine (39.5 e.u.), and, in fact, to those of bromine and iodine as well. Consequently differences between fluorine and the other halogens arise from differences in heat effects (heats of reaction, bond strengths) and not in entropy effects.

f) Electronegativity

Fluorine is easily the most electronegative of the elements, that is, i tpowerfully attracts electrons to itself. This property is manifested in, for instance, the high acid strength of trifluoroacetic acid, CF_3CO_2H, and the lack of basicity of perfluoro-amines, *e.g.*, tristrifluoromethylamine, $(CF_3)_3N$.

g) Nuclear magnetic properties

Fluorine, ^{19}F, has a nuclear spin quantum number $^1/_2$ and is detectable by n.m.r. techniques. The high abundance (100%) of the ^{19}F isotope and its high nuclear magnetic moment make the n.m.r. method a very suitable one for structural work on fluorine compounds, and for the detection and estimation of fluorine (see p. 44).

4. Chemical properties of fluorine

(LEECH 1956)

At appropriate temperatures, fluorine, the most reactive of the elements, attacks all the other elements, with the exceptions of oxygen and nitrogen, to form fluorides. Perhaps the most remarkable demonstration of the extreme oxidising power of fluorine has been the recent preparation of xenon tetrafluoride from the elements at red heat. Fortunately, a fluoride film coherent enough to prevent further attack is formed when fluorine contacts massive mild steel, copper, nickel, and Monel so that these materials can be used to handle fluorine at ordinary temperatures. In the absence of hydrogen fluoride, fluorine is without effect on glass at ordinary temperatures.

5. Valency of fluorine and bonding in fluorine compounds

Fluorine has the electronic configuration $1s^2\,2s^2\,2p^5$; the filled valency shell is $2s^2\,2p^6$, and since the energy separation between these levels and the $3s$, $3p$, and $3d$ levels is very great fluorine should be exclusively univalent. *No compound is known in which fluorine exhibits a valency greater than one,* and this distinguishes fluorine from the other halogens which do have variable valencies.

Fluorine can form both covalent and electrovalent bonds with other elements, and since it is the most electronegative element the former are strongly polar. However, although fluorine is electron-withdrawing in this way, it can also act as an electron donor by mesomeric interaction of its unshared electron-pairs with an unsaturated system.

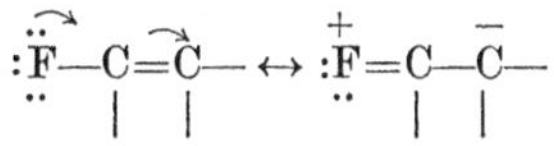

Fluorine is the most effective of the halogens in this type of back-coordination.

The small size of the covalently bound fluorine atom and its high electronegativity allow it to participate in hydrogen bonding; in fact some of the most striking of all hydrogen bonding phenomena occur with fluorides. The great stability of the ion HF_2^-, in which the hydrogen lies equidistant from the two fluorines, and the high boiling point of hydrogen fluoride in relation to the other hydrogen halides are two examples.

6. The fluoride ion

(SHARPE 1957) (see Table 2)

Table 2. *Properties of the fluoride ion*

Ionic radius	1.36 Å
Heat of hydration	123 kcal/g ion
Entropy of hydration . .	—29 e.u.
Standard potential for the $^1/_2F_2/F^-$ aq. electrode .	+2.8 v.

a) Ionic radius

The fluoride ion (r = 1.36 Å) has an ionic radius very similar to that of the oxide ion (r = 1.40 Å) and consequently oxides and fluorides of similar formula type, *e.g.*, MgO and NaF, frequently have similar structures. Since the fluoride ion is much smaller than the chloride ion (r = 1.81 Å), fluorides and chlorides of the same metal usually have quite different structures.

b) Heat and entropy of hydration

The entropy of hydration of fluoride ion is not too different from that of chloride ion. The heat of hydration of fluoride ion is, however, about 32 kcal greater than that of chloride ion. This extra heat must be balanced against the difficulty of hydrating the small fluoride ion when assessing the possibility of hydrating an ionic fluoride. Many fluorides do not form hydrates and, in general, fluorides and chlorides of the same metal do not form similar hydrates, *e.g.*,

CaF_2, anhydrous	$CaCl_2$, several hydrates
$KF \cdot 2\,H_2O$	KCl, anhydrous
NaF, anhydrous	$NaCl \cdot 2\,H_2O$

7. Standard potential of fluorine-fluoride ion electrode

This is extremely high (+ 2.8 v, *cf.* + 1.36 v for chlorine) and accords with the observation that fluorine is the most powerful of oxidising agents. Since no other redox potential approaches this value it is clear that free fluorine cannot be produced by chemical oxidation of fluoride ions or by electrolysis of solutions containing any negative ion other than fluoride.

8. Hydrogen fluoride

(Leech 1956; Rudge 1962)

This compound is one of the most interesting of all inorganic fluorine compounds and, since it is the intermediate in the manufacture of most other fluorine compounds from fluorspar, it warrants detailed description.

a) Preparation and handling

Hydrogen fluoride is prepared industrially by treating calcium fluoride with concentrated sulphuric acid:

$$CaF_2 + H_2SO_4 \rightarrow CaSO_4 + 2\,HF$$

The volatile hydrogen fluoride, b.p. 19.5°, is condensed and purified by distillation. Hydrogen fluoride can be conveniently prepared on a laboratory scale by heating dry potassium bifluoride, KHF_2.

Since hydrogen fluoride containing even traces of moisture rapidly attacks glass, it is usually manipulated in metal or plastic apparatus. The anhydrous gas, and aqueous hydrofluoric acid of strength $> 70\,\%$, can be stored in mild steel; weaker acid can be manipulated in lead apparatus if fluorosilicic acid is absent, but is more conveniently used in polyethylene.

Hydrogen fluoride produces very painful and dangerous burns if it comes into contact with the skin, and these must receive immediate medical attention.

b) Properties of anhydrous hydrogen fluoride

(see Table 3)

Anhydrous hydrogen fluoride is highly associated in the liquid state, as indicated by its relatively high boiling point and Trouton constant (*cf.* HCl, b.p. —85°; H_2O, Trouton constant 26.0). This association persists in the vapour phase, and vapour pressure measurements at the boiling point suggest that the mean degree of association at 1 atm. pressure corresponds to $(HF)_{3\cdot45}$. However, at 80°/1 atm. the vapour is essentially monomeric. Electron diffraction measurements on gaseous hydrogen fluoride confirm this picture, and the molecules are held together by hydrogen bonds in the form shown below.

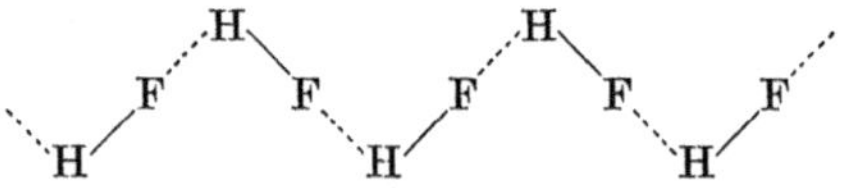

Table 3. *Physical properties of hydrogen fluoride*

Boiling point	19.5°	Specific gravity of liquid	0.988 at 13.6°
Freezing point	—83°	Dielectric constant	83.6 at 0°
Latent ht. of fusion	1094 cal. mol^{-1}	Dipole moment (gas at low pressure)	1.91 D
Latent ht. of vaporization to saturated vapour	1780 cal. mol^{-1}	Conductivity (probably some water still present)	1.4×10^{-6} ohm^{-1} at —15°
Trouton constant	26.6 e. u.		

Liquid hydrogen fluoride has the high dielectric constant of 83.6 at 0°. This is very similar to the dielectric constant of water (87.9 at 0°) and, like water, hydrogen fluoride is an excellent solvent. It exceeds water as an ionizing solvent; even very weakly basic substances, for instance alcohols and ketones, dissolve in it to give conducting solutions. Liquid hydrogen fluoride must therefore be regarded as an extremely strong acid, capable of protonating even extremely non-basic compounds. The type of equilibria established in liquid hydrogen fluoride are probably as follows:

$$2\,HF + ROH \rightleftharpoons R\overset{+}{O}H_2 + HF_2^- \quad \text{for alcohols}$$

$$2\,HF + R_2C{=}O \rightleftharpoons R_2\overset{+}{C}OH + HF_2^- \quad \text{for ketones}$$

$$2\,HF + HNO_3 \rightleftharpoons H_2\overset{+}{N}O_3 + HF_2^- \quad \text{for nitric acid}$$

The behaviour of inorganic substances in anhydrous hydrogen fluoride is difficult to generalize. A few metallic fluorides (alkali metals, Ag, Tl, Ba, NH_4) are soluble and behave as strong electrolytes. When other metal salts are dissolved, the following type of equilibrium is established:

$$M^+A^- + HF \rightleftharpoons M^+F^- + HA$$

When A^- is chloride, bromide, iodide, cyanide, or azide, the corresponding acid is insoluble in hydrogen fluoride and is expelled; thus the salt is converted into the fluoride. When A^- is an oxyanion, it may be protonated by the hydrogen fluoride (see HNO_3 above) or it may react to give a fluorinated compound. Thus sulphates give fluorosulphonic acid:

$$SO_4^{2-} + 7\,HF \rightarrow HSO_3F + H_3O^+ + 3\,HF_2^-$$

Salts of a few very strong acids, *e.g.*, perchloric acid and fluoroboric acid, dissolve in hydrogen fluoride to give their own anions.

c) Aqueous hydrogen fluoride

In dilute aqueous solution hydrogen fluoride is a weak acid; in $M/10$ solution it is about 10% ionised. A simple thermodynamic argument shows that the weakness of aqueous hydrogen fluoride as an acid, compared with the other hydrogen halides, must be attributed to the high bond strength in hydrogen fluoride (bond energies: HF, 135; HCl, 103; HBr, 87; HI, 71 kcal). In more concentrated solutions (5—15 M), ionisation into H_3O^+ and the complex anions HF_2^-, $H_2F_3^-$, $H_3F_4^-$ takes place, and hydrogen fluoride becomes a strong acid.

The most familiar property of aqueous hydrogen fluoride is its ability to dissolve glass. This is, of course, no indication of its acid strength, but simply the result of its facile reaction with silica and silicates:

$$4\,HF + SiO_2 \rightarrow SiF_4 + 2\,H_2O$$

B. Inorganic fluorides

1. Some general considerations

It will already be obvious that inorganic fluorides are frequently quite different from corresponding chlorides, bromides, and iodides. Ionic fluorides are usually higher melting and higher boiling than the corresponding other halides. This is a consequence of the small size of the fluoride ion which leads to more energy being needed to separate the ions in the crystal.

This high energy of separation might be expected to lead to low solubilities of fluorides in water. This is often the case; however solubility is determined not only by this high lattice energy but also by the high heat of hydration of fluoride ion, and actual solubilities are hard to predict. Thus lithium and sodium fluorides are much less soluble than the chlorides; but for potassium and rubidium the situation is reversed. Silver(I) fluoride is very soluble, in contrast to the other silver halides.

Covalent fluorides often have much lower melting and boiling points than corresponding covalent chlorides and bromides. It is inferred from this that intermolecular association is low in the fluorides. The high polarity of the covalent bonds formed by fluorine leads to high dipole-dipole repulsions between adjacent molecules and thus lowers intermolecular attraction due to van der Waals forces.

Fluorine compounds often show very high covalencies — much higher than corresponding chlorides (compare SF_6 and the highest chloride of sulphur, the unstable SCl_4; IF_7 and ICl_3). This can be attributed in part to the small size of covalently bonded fluorine, but energy considerations are also important. Consideration of a simple thermodynamic cycle shows that the low dissociation energy of fluorine compared with chlorine means that many fluorine compounds will be much more exothermic than the corresponding chlorine compounds.

Many of the covalent non-metal fluorides, *e.g.*, CF_4 and other fluorocarbons, NF_3, SF_6, are extremely stable compounds which resist attack by a wide variety of reagents. It should be pointed out that this stability is not thermodynamic. For instance, the hydrolyses of the compounds CF_4 and SF_6, which do not proceed at all under normal conditions, would be strongly exothermic:

$$CF_4(g) + 2\,H_2O(g) \rightarrow CO_2(g) + 4\,HF(g) \qquad \Delta G^0 = -36\text{ kcal}$$

$$SF_6(g) + 3\,H_2O(g) \rightarrow SO_3(g) + 6\,HF(g) \qquad \Delta G^0 = -72\text{ kcal}$$

These reactions must therefore have very high energies of activation, and it is perhaps because a water molecule cannot co-ordinate on to a combined fluorine atom (which has no orbitals of sufficiently low energy available to accept electrons from the water molecule) that these compounds resist hydrolysis.

Three general features are prominent in the chemistry of the metal fluorides. First, the highest oxidation states reached in their salts by many metals are observed in the fluorides (*e.g.*, Ag in AgF_2, Co in CoF_3, Rh in RhF_4). Second, many fluorides of high oxidation state are much more salt-like than corresponding chlorides (*cf.* AuF_3 and $AuCl_3$, PbF_4 and $PbCl_4$). Third, the small size of fluoride ion, leading to high lattice energies, means that many complex ions containing fluorine are stable.

2. General methods of preparation of inorganic fluorides

Specific methods will be mentioned below under individual compounds but there are a number of general methods which cover a wide range of preparations.

a) General methods

α) Use of aqueous hydrogen fluoride. Fluorides which are not extensively hydrolysed in solution can be prepared by reactions of conventional type (carried out, of course, in platinum or plastic vessels if HF is used) in aqueous solution, *e.g.*,

$$Ag_2CO_3 + 2\,HF \rightarrow 2\,AgF + H_2O + CO_2\uparrow$$

$$BaCl_2 + 2\,NaF \rightarrow BaF_2\downarrow + 2\,NaCl$$

$$Bi_2O_3 + 6\,HF \rightarrow 2\,BiF_3 + 3\,H_2O$$

β) Use of anhydrous hydrogen fluoride. This is useful if the required fluoride is susceptible to hydrolysis, or forms a stable hydrate. Frequently metal chlorides give metal fluorides under these conditions, *e.g.*,

$$TiCl_4 + 4\,HF \rightarrow TiF_4 + 4\,HCl$$

$$CrCl_3 + 3\,HF \rightarrow CrF_3 + 3\,HCl$$

γ) Use of antimony trifluoride (promoted by antimony pentachloride). Many covalent chlorides can be converted into fluorides with this reagent (which is also widely used in making organic fluorine compounds), *e.g.*,

$$BCl_3 \xrightarrow{SbF_3} BF_3$$

$$SiCl_4 \xrightarrow{SbF_3} SiF_4$$

δ) Use of elementary fluorine. Most non-metals and metals, and many of their compounds, give fluorides by direct fluorination, *e.g.*,

$$S \xrightarrow{F_2} SF_6$$

$$Ta_2O_5 \xrightarrow{F_2} TaF_5$$

$$W \xrightarrow{F_2} WF_6$$

ε) Use of halogen fluorides. Simple and complex fluorides are prepared by the use of bromine trifluoride, chlorine trifluoride, or other halogen fluorides, *e.g.*,

$$3\,UF_4 + 2\,ClF_3 \longrightarrow 3\,UF_6 + Cl_2$$

$$Pt \xrightarrow{BrF_3} PtF_4 \cdot 2\,BrF_3 \xrightarrow{Heat} PtF_4 + 2\,BrF_3$$

$$K_2PtCl_4 \xrightarrow{BrF_3} K_2PtF_6$$

b) Group I fluorides, MF (M = Li, Na, K, Rb, Cs)

The alkali metal fluorides can be made from carbonates or hydroxides and aqueous hydrogen fluoride. Since, with the exception of lithium fluoride, they all form acid fluorides the proportion of acid and base used must be carefully controlled.

The alkali metal fluorides are typical salts; they are high-melting and high boiling compounds and, with the exception of lithium fluoride, fairly water soluble. They all crystallize in the face-centered cubic system.

Sodium, potassium, rubidium, and caesium all give acid fluorides of the type MHF_2. In addition, potassium forms a number of more complex acid fluorides.

c) Group II fluorides, MF_2 (M = Be, Mg, Ca, Sr, Ba)

With the exception of beryllium fluoride the Group II fluorides form a fairly uniform group. They are all sparingly soluble in water and can be prepared by precipitation methods.

Beryllium fluoride is usually prepared by thermal decomposition of ammonium fluoroberyllate:

$$Be(OH)_2 \xrightarrow{\text{Fuse, } NH_4HF_2} (NH_4)_2BeF_4 \xrightarrow{900^\circ} BeF_2$$

It is soluble in water and considerably hydrolysed. It melts at 800° and (a point of contrast with the other beryllium halides) the fused salt is a conductor of electricity. Beryllium fluoride is an intermediate in the production of metallic beryllium; on being heated with magnesium at high temperatures it is reduced to the metal.

d) Group III fluorides, MF_3 (M = B, Al, Ga, In, Tl)

Boron trifluoride is a gas at room temperature (b.p. —101°) and is clearly a covalent compound. It can be prepared by heating boron trioxide with calcium fluoride or a fluoroborate and concentrated sulphuric acid. The gas produced is either stored under pressure or converted to a complex, *e.g.*, an etherate, for use as a catalyst. The coordinate unsaturation of boron trifluoride — it forms complexes with an extremely wide range of donors including amines, ethers, aldehydes and ketones — explains its remarkable catalytic activity, and it is widely used to promote organic reactions (*e.g.*, esterification, isomerization of olefins, polymerization of olefins, and Friedel-Crafts acylation and alkylation).

Boron trifluoride also combines with fluoride ion to give the very stable complex ion BF_4^-, fluoroborate (SHARP 1960). Fluoroboric acid or its salts are more conveniently prepared by dissolving boric acid in concentrated hydrofluoric acid, or by allowing acid fluorides to react with boric acid; *e.g.*,

$$H_3BO_3 + 2\ NH_4HF_2 \rightarrow NH_4BF_4 + NH_3 + 3\ H_2O$$

Fluoroboric acid is a strong acid in aqueous solution; the free acid is not known but the aqueous solution and salts have uses in electroplating and also in the preparation of aromatic organic fluorides.

In contrast to boron trifluoride, aluminium, gallium and indium fluorides are all high-melting and only slightly soluble ionic solids. Thallic fluoride, TlF_3, prepared by the action of fluorine on thallic oxide, is relatively low melting and is rapidly decomposed by water, yielding thallic oxide. Thallous fluoride, TlF, obtained from the oxide or carbonate and aqueous hydrogen fluoride, is very water soluble.

Aluminium, gallium, and indium all form complex fluoroanions, of which the best known is hexafluoroaluminate, AlF_6^{3-}. The sodium salt, Na_3AlF_6, is cryolite, the flux used in the refining of aluminium; it occurs naturally and is also made industrially by treating a solution of sodium aluminate (alumina in sodium hydroxide) with ammonium fluoride.

e) Group IV fluorides (C, Si, Ge, Sn, Pb)

In this group a clear transition from covalent fluorides for the lighter members to ionic fluorides for the heavier members is apparent.

α) Carbon. Carbon is unique among the elements in the variety of fluorides it forms. The detailed chemistry of these fluorocarbons is discussed in the organic section of this chapter, but a few general remarks about the carbon fluorides are in place here. The bond between carbon and fluorine is a very strong one (107 kcal; *cf.* C—Cl bond strength, 66 kcal) but the stability of the fluorocarbons cannot be attributed solely to this fact. As was pointed out earlier, fluorocarbons are not, *thermodynamically*, especially stable to hydrolysis, for instance, and reasons for their stability must be sought in high energies of activation for their reactions. These can be attributed partly to steric factors, the fluorine atoms shielding the carbon atoms from attack, and partly to the inability of an attacking reagent to coordinate to fluorine.

β) Silicon. Fluorides of silicon are far fewer in number than those of carbon. They are hydrolysed easily, the initial stage in hydrolysis presumably being coordination of water with silicon, which has available *d*-orbitals. Silicon tetrafluoride (b.p. —96°) can be prepared by heating a mixture of silica and a metal fluoride with concentrated sulphuric acid. It is obtained on a relatively large scale during acid treatment of phosphatic rocks, which frequently contain a small percentage of fluoride, and is regarded principally as a nuisance in this process. It is washed out of the waste gases by water, which hydrolyses it to silica and fluorosilicic acid:

$$3\ SiF_4 + 2\ H_2O \rightarrow SiO_2 + 2\ H_2SiF_6$$

consequently, large amounts of this acid and its salts are available. It has achieved little commercial importance as yet, but processes to recover fluorine from it in an economically more useful form are under development. The only higher fluoride of silicon known is Si_2F_6, obtained by reaction of the corresponding chloride with zinc fluoride.

γ) Germanium, tin and lead. The remaining elements of the group form both di- and tetra-fluorides. Germanium difluoride is an unstable white solid prepared by heating germanium with the tetrafluoride; little is known about it. The tetrafluoride is very like silicon tetrafluoride; it is a gas, easily hydrolysed, and forms complex fluorogermanates very like the fluorosilicates.

Tin difluoride (stannous fluoride) is a soluble crystalline solid made by dissolving the metal or stannous hydroxide in aqueous hydrogen fluoride. Stannic fluoride, formed by direct fluorination of tin, is a salt-like crystalline solid. It is much less easily hydrolysed than the corresponding chloride. Many hexafluorostannates, containing the SnF_6^{2-} ion, have been prepared.

Lead difluoride (plumbous fluoride) is salt-like (m.p. 818°) and can be hydrolysed by steam, though it is only slowly hydrolysed by cold water. Lead also forms a fairly insoluble chlorofluoride, PbClF, which is used in the determination of fluorine.

The action of fluorine on lead difluoride gives the reactive lead tetrafluoride. This is a fairly high-melting solid which is rapidly hydrolysed. Stable complex fluoroplumbates are known.

f) Group V fluorides (N, P, As, Sb, Bi)

In this group trifluorides of all the elements, and pentafluorides of all except nitrogen, are known. In addition, various oxyfluorides have been prepared.

α) Nitrogen. (HOFFMAN and NEVILLE 1962). The chemistry of the fluorides of nitrogen is currently being investigated in some detail. Obscurities and uncertainties in older work are being cleared up, and some remarkable new compounds and reactions are being discovered. The inert nitrogen trifluoride (b.p. —129°) is produced best by electrolysis of molten ammonium bifluoride. It is a colourless non-explosive gas which is not hydrolysed by acids or alkalis. It does react, however, with heated metals, *e.g.*, copper, to give tetrafluorohydrazine, $F_2N—NF_2$, a relatively inert gas (b.p. —73°) which readily dissociates reversibly into nitrogen difluoride radicals on being heated or irradiated:

$$N_2F_4 \rightleftharpoons 2\,NF_2\cdot$$

A by-product in the production of nitrogen trifluoride by electrolysis is difluorodiazine, N_2F_2, which exists in both the *cis*- and *trans*-forms (b.p. —106° and —111°, respectively). A further fluoride of nitrogen is the highly explosive fluorine azide, N_3F, (b.p. —82°), produced by the action of fluorine on hydrazoic acid.

Difluoroamine, NHF_2, (b.p. —24°), is best produced by the reduction of tetrafluorohydrazine with a mercaptan or thiophenol; it reacts with boron trichloride to give chlorodifluoroamine, NF_2Cl (b.p. —67°). The preparation of monofluoroamine, NH_2F, has been claimed a number of times but the existence of this compound is still somewhat doubtful.

A number of oxyfluorides of nitrogen are known. Nitrosyl fluoride, NOF, (b.p. —60°), prepared from nitrosyl chloride and silver(I) fluoride, and nitryl fluoride, NO_2F (b.p. —72°), prepared by reaction of fluorine with N_2O_4, resemble the corresponding chlorides. The action of fluorine on nitric acid gives the highly explosive fluorine nitrate, NO_3F (b.p. —46°).

β) Phosphorus. (GEORGE 1960; PAYNE 1961). Phosphorus trifluoride, PF_3 (b.p. —101°), and phosphorus pentafluoride, PF_5 (b.p. —75°), can be prepared by fluorination of the corresponding chlorides with arsenic trifluoride. Mixed halides of phosphorus are also known.

Phosphorus oxyfluoride, POF_3, a readily hydrolysed gas, b.p. —39°, can be obtained by treatment of the corresponding chloride with zinc fluoride. Hydrolysis of this oxyfluoride with base yields difluorophosphoric acid, HPO_2F_2, which cannot be isolated. Monofluorophosphoric acid, an oily liquid which cannot be distilled without decomposition, can be obtained by reaction of phosphoric acid and concentrated hydrofluoric acid:

$$H_3PO_4 + HF \rightarrow H_2PO_3F + H_2O$$

The dialkyl esters of this acid are remarkably potent anticholinesterases and were developed as potential chemical warfare agents (SAUNDERS 1961). Salts of hexafluorophosphoric acid, HPF_6, can be prepared from phosphorus pentachloride and an excess of a metal fluoride; these are quite stable and are not attacked by base. The free acid is a strong one in aqueous solutions but cannot be isolated.

γ) Arsenic, antimony, and bismuth (GEORGE 1960; PAYNE 1961). Treatment of the oxides of these elements with hydrogen fluoride gives, in each case, the trifluoride. Arsenic trifluoride, AsF_3 (b.p. 57°) is a readily hydrolysed liquid which has been used in the preparation of other inorganic fluorides. Antimony trifluoride (m.p. 292°) is a relatively volatile solid which sublimes at about 320°. It is an extremely useful fluorinating agent for organic chloro-compounds and is widely used in preparing organic fluorine compounds (see p. 26). Bismuth trifluoride (m.p. 725°) is an ionic solid; the metallic character of bismuth is evident here.

Arsenic pentafluoride (b.p. —53°), obtained from the trifluoride and antimony pentafluoride, is a reactive gas which is easily hydrolysed. Antimony pentafluoride itself (b.p. 150°) is made by the action of hydrogen fluoride on the pentachloride; it is a good fluorinating agent used mainly in organic chemistry. The mixed chlorofluoride, SbF_3Cl_2, prepared by the action of chlorine on antimony trifluoride, is also much used in preparing organic fluorine compounds. Bismuth pentafluoride, BiF_5 (b.p. 230°), is prepared by reaction of the trifluoride with fluorine under vigorous conditions. The three pentafluorides of this sub-group all give complex fluoroanions: AsF_6^-, SbF_6^-, BiF_6^-.

Not many oxyfluorides of these elements are known. Arsenic oxyfluoride, $AsOF_3$ (b.p. 26°), is made by reaction of fluorine with a mixture of arsenic trichloride and arsenic trioxide. A bismuth oxyfluoride, BiOF, has also been claimed.

g) Group VI fluorides (O, S, Se, Te)

α) Oxygen. (GEORGE 1960). Three fluorides of oxygen have been well established. The best known is oxygen difluoride, OF_2 (b.p. —145°), produced in the reaction of fluorine with aqueous sodium hydroxide. This gas is slowly hydrolysed in water at room temperature. It is a powerful oxidising agent but it does require a high activation energy for reaction with, for example, hydrogen, methane, or carbon monoxide.

Oxygen monofluoride, O_2F_2 (b.p. —57°), is produced by the action of an electrical discharge on an oxygen-fluorine mixture at —180°. It is a red liquid which decomposes at its boiling point to its constituent elements. Ozone fluoride, O_3F_2, (b.p. —157°), is obtained by the action of ultraviolet light on a mixture of liquid oxygen and liquid fluorine. It is a strong oxidising agent, reacting vigorously at —183° with phosphorus, charcoal, bromine, iodine, *etc.* It decomposes at its boiling point into oxygen and oxygen monofluoride.

Fluorine forms no oxy-acids.

***β*) Sulphur.** (Cady 1960; Roberts 1961). When sulphur burns in fluorine all three well-authenticated sulphur fluorides, SF_4, SF_6, and S_2F_{10}, are formed. The lower fluorides of sulphur which have been claimed (S_2F_2, SF_2) have not been satisfactorily characterized.

Sulphur hexafluoride, SF_6 (sublimes —65°), is prepared by burning sulphur in fluorine and washing the product with aqueous alkali to remove the other fluorides produced. It is non-toxic and chemically very inert. It is used as a dielectric in high-voltage equipment.

Sulphur tetrafluoride, SF_4 (b.p. —40°), was originally isolated as a product from the reaction of sulphur with fluorine at —75°. Much improved methods are now available including the action of halogen fluorides on sulphur, and the reaction between sulphur dichloride and sodium fluoride in acetonitrile at 70—80°:

$$3\,SCl_2 + 4\,NaF \rightarrow SF_4 + S_2Cl_2 + 4\,NaCl$$

Sulphur tetrafluoride is a very reactive gas; it is rapidly hydrolysed to thionyl fluoride, SOF_2, and oxidised in the presence of dinitrogen tetroxide to thionyl tetrafluoride, SOF_4.

The most interesting properties of sulphur tetrafluoride are connected with its fluorinating ability. Its reactions with hydroxyl and carbonyl groups are discussed in the organic section (see p. 27), but it is also potentially a useful inorganic fluorinating agent, and a number of its reactions have been described, *e.g.*,

$$SF_4 + SnS_2 \rightarrow SnF_4 + 3\,S$$

$$MoO_3 + 3\,SF_4 \rightarrow MoF_6 + 3\,SOF_2$$

Sulphur tetrafluoride reacts with chlorine monofluoride or trifluoride to give the interesting sulphur chloride pentafluoride, SF_5Cl (b.p. —21°). This easily hydrolysed gas is an oxidising agent and behaves as if it were polarized in the direction $\overset{\delta-}{SF_5}$—$\overset{\delta+}{Cl}$. In the gas-phase, it adds to olefinic double bonds to give organic compounds containing the stable SF_5 group, *e.g.*,

$$SF_5Cl + CH_2{=}CH_2 \rightarrow SF_5CH_2CH_2Cl$$

Disulphur decafluoride, S_2F_{10} (b.p. 29°), a toxic by-product of the direct fluorination of sulphur, is best prepared by photochemical reduction of SF_5Cl with hydrogen:

$$2\,SF_5Cl + H_2 \rightarrow S_2F_{10} + 2\,HCl$$

It decomposes rapidly at 200° into sulphur tetrafluoride and sulphur hexafluoride.

Many oxyfluorides of sulphur are known; their properties are summarized in Table 4 below. In addition, mixed oxyhalides, *e.g.*, SOFCl, SO_2FBr, are known.

Derivatives of two oxy-acids of sulphur which contain fluorine are known. Fluorosulphurous acid itself is unknown but its salts are prepared by reaction of alkali-metal fluorides with sulphur dioxide:

$$KF + SO_2 \rightleftharpoons KSO_2F$$

The fluorosulphites dissociate on being heated alone. They are, nevertheless, useful mild fluorinating agents and have been used to prepare acyl fluorides and phosphonitrilic fluorides from corresponding chlorides.

Fluorosulphuric acid, HSO_3F (b.p. 163°), is a strong monobasic acid, prepared by combination of sulphur trioxide with hydrogen fluoride. It is very water soluble and is to some extent hydrolysed in solution. Metal fluorosulphates are typical salts,

Table 4. *Oxyfluorides of sulphur*

Compound	b. p. (°C)	Preparation	Remarks
SOF_2, thionyl fluoride	—44	$SOCl_2 + SbF_3$	Like $SOCl_2$ but less reactive
SO_2F_2, sulphuryl fluoride . . .	—55	$SO_2 + F_2$	Relatively inert; only slowly hydrolysed
SOF_4, thionyl tetrafluoride . . .	—49	$SF_4 + O_2 + N_2O_4$	Hydrolyses readily
$O(SO_2F)_2$, pyrosulphuryl fluoride	51	$SO_3 + SbF_5$	Slowly hydrolysed to HSO_3F
$O_2(SO_2F)_2$, peroxydisulphuryl difluoride	67	$F_2 + SO_3$	Quite stable; hydrolysed by hot water
$FSO_2OSO_2OSO_2F$, trisulphuryl fluoride	120	$SO_2 + O_2(SO_2F)_2$	Fairly stable, easily hydrolysed
FSO_2OF, fluorine fluorosulphate	—31	$F_2 + SO_2/AgF_2$	Very reactive and explosive
SF_5OF, pentafluorosulphur hypofluorite	—35	$SOF_2 + F_2/AgF_2$	Very reactive. Oxidising agt.
SF_5OSF_5, bis-pentafluorosulphur oxide	31	$SF_5Cl + O_2$, photochemically	Inert
$SF_5O_2SF_5$, bis-pentafluorosulphur peroxide	49	$SF_5Cl + O_2$, photochemically	Stable to alkali; reacts vigorously with organic materials

which are hydrolysed in aqueous solution. A number of fluorosulphates of non-metals are also known.

γ) Selenium and tellurium (George 1960). Tetrafluorides and hexafluorides of both elements are known, in addition to a number of oxyhalides. The hexafluorides SeF_6 (sublimes —47°) and TeF_6 (sublimes —39°) are produced by burning the elements in fluorine. They are much more reactive than sulphur hexafluoride and, at high temperatures, selenium hexafluoride is a fluorinating agent; it is hydrolysed by alcoholic alkali. Tellurium hexafluoride is hydrolysed quite rapidly by water.

Selenium tetrafluoride, SeF_4 (b.p. 106°), is prepared by low-temperature fluorination of selenium. It is a reactive compound, easily hydrolysed, and a vigorous fluorinating agent. Tellurium tetrafluoride, TeF_4 (m.p. 130°), is made by reduction of the hexafluoride with tellurium. It is also a reactive compound, attacking glass at 200° and platinum at 300°.

The highly toxic ditellurium decafluoride, Te_2F_{10} (b.p. 53°), prepared in the fluorination of TeO_2/Te mixtures, is more reactive than the sulphur analogue and attacks mercury at its boiling point.

h) Group VII fluorides (Cl, Br, I) (interhalogen compounds)

(Musgrave 1960; Wiebenga et al. 1961)

The known halogen fluorides are listed below with their boiling points. They are all produced by direct combination of the elements in appropriate ratios.

ClF (—101°)	ClF_3 (12°)		
BrF (20°)	BrF_3 (126°)	BrF_5 (41°)	
		IF_5 (101°)	IF_7 (sublimes, 4°)

All the halogen fluorides are very reactive compounds, and with most metals and non-metals act as fluorinating agents with almost as much vigour as fluorine itself. The convenient physical properties of compounds like chlorine trifluoride and bromine trifluoride make them easier to handle than gaseous fluorine; consequently, chlorine trifluoride has been used in the atomic energy field to prepare uranium hexafluoride.

Liquid bromine trifluoride and iodine pentafluoride have a definite, though low, conductivity in the pure state, and are believed to be ionized:

$$2\,BrF_3 \rightleftharpoons BrF_2^+ + BrF_4^-$$
$$2\,IF_5 \rightleftharpoons IF_4^+ + IF_6^-$$

A considerable acid-base chemistry has been developed in these media, and complexes containing the above ions have been prepared, *e.g.*, $BrF_2^+SbF_6^-$, $K^+BrF_4^-$, $K^+IF_6^-$.

It is pertinent to note here the polyhalide anions. In addition to those based on the halogen fluorides, just mentioned, one or two others containing fluorine, including $IBrF^-$, have been described but, in general, polyhalide anions containing fluorine are rare.

A number of oxyfluorides of the halogens are known. Reaction of halogen oxides with fluorine is a general method of preparation:

$$2\,ClO_2 + F_2 \rightarrow 2\,ClO_2F$$
$$2\,BrO_2 + F_2 \rightarrow 2\,BrO_2F$$
$$2\,I_2O_5 + 2\,F_2 \rightarrow 4\,IO_2F + O_2$$
$$2\,HIO_4 + 2\,F_2 \rightarrow 2\,IO_3F + 2\,HF + O_2$$

However the most studied of these compounds, perchloryl fluoride, ClO_3F (b.p. —47°), is easily obtained by the reaction between a perchlorate and fluorosulphuric acid. It is stable to aqueous alkali, and acts as an oxidising agent. Its interesting reactions with compounds containing activated methylene groups are described later (see p. 29).

i) Fluorides of the transition metals

(Katz and Sheft 1960; Peacock 1960; Sharpe 1960)

This subject is so large that it can only be briefly outlined here. The many oxidation states of these metals and the ease with which they form complexes mean that an extremely large number of their fluorides, oxyfluorides, and fluorocomplexes are known, and research in this area is adding to the number rapidly. Table 5 gives the known binary fluorides of the transition metals (including the lanthanides and actinides).

In general, transition metal fluorides of higher oxidation states are prepared by the action of fluorine or halogen fluorides on the metal or on its compounds of lower oxidation state. Fluorides of lower oxidation states are often made by reducing those of higher oxidation states with hydrogen, metals, *etc.*

Few generalizations can be made about transition metal fluorides. Fluorination tends to bring out high (but not necessarily the highest possible) oxidation states. For a metal having a range of fluorides those of lower oxidation state tend to be salt-like; the higher fluorides are frequently volatile. The higher fluorides are usually very susceptible to hydrolysis.

To illustrate some of the interest and complexity of this particular topic the fluorides, oxyfluorides, and complex fluorides of the elements cobalt and uranium will be considered in some detail. These elements have been chosen because of their intrinsic interest and because cobaltic fluoride is used in preparing fluorinated organic compounds (see p. 20) while the fluorides of uranium are used in refining the metal and in separating the fissile isotope ^{235}U.

Table 5. *Transition metal fluorides*

ScF_3	TiF_3	VF_3	CrF_2	MnF_2	FeF_2	CoF_2	NiF_2	CuF_2	ZnF_2
	TiF_4	VF_4	CrF_3	MnF_3	FeF_3	CoF_3			
		VF_5	CrF_4	MnF_4					
			CrF_5						
YF_3	ZrF_4	NbF_3	MoF_3	TcF_6	RuF_3	RhF_3	PdF_2	AgF	CdF_2
			MoF_4			RhF_4	PdF_3	AgF_2	
		NbF_5	MoF_5		RuF_5				
			MoF_6						
LaF_3	HfF_4	TaF_3				IrF_3	PtF_4	AuF_3	Hg_2F_2
			WF_4	ReF_4	OsF_4	IrF_4	PtF_5		HgF_2
		TaF_5		ReF_5	OsF_5		PtF_6		
			WF_6	ReF_6	OsF_6	IrF_6			
AcF_3				ReF_7					

Lanthanides (Ce, Pr, Nd, Pm, Sm, Eu, Gd, Tb, Dy, Ho, Er, Tm, Yb, Ln)
All trifluorides MF_3 and, in addition, EuF_2, SmF_2
CeF_4, TbF_4

Acitinides

ThF_4	PaF_4	UF_3	NpF_3	PuF_3	AmF_3	CmF_3
	PaF_5	UF_4	NpF_4	PuF_4	AmF_4	CmF_4
		UF_5				
		UF_6	NpF_6	PuF_6		
		U_2F_9				
		U_4F_{17}		Pu_4F_{17}		

α) Cobalt. Two fluorides of cobalt are known. Cobaltous fluoride, CoF_2, prepared by the action of hydrogen fluoride on anhydrous cobaltous chloride is a pink solid, stable to water and only slightly soluble. When its aqueous solution is treated with potassium fluoride $KCoF_3$ is formed. K_2CoF_4 can be obtained from a KF/CoF_2 melt.

Cobaltic fluoride, CoF_3, a powerful fluorinating agent for organic compounds, is prepared by the action of fluorine on cobaltous fluoride at 160—250°. It is a buff powder, instantly hydrolysed by water or moist air, which is thermally quite stable and does not give free fluorine when it is heated. Cobaltic fluoride forms a variety of complexes; reaction with potassium fluoride in anhydrous hydrogen fluoride gives the blue compound K_3CoF_6, while ammonia gives the amine $CoF_3 \cdot 3\,NH_3$. A hydrate of empirical formula $CoF_3 \cdot 3.5\,H_2O$ is obtained by electrolytic oxidation of hydrated cobaltous fluoride suspended in hydrogen fluoride; it is probably the hydrated complex $(CoF_3 \cdot 3\,H_2O)\ 0.5\,H_2O$.

β) Uranium. Uranium forms a tri-, tetra-, penta-, and hexa-fluoride and, in addition, remarkable mixed-valency fluorides, *e.g.* U_2F_9,U_4F_{17}, the structures of which are uncertain. Of these compound sthe tetra- and hexa-fluorides have been studied most fully.

Uranium tetrafluoride is generally made by the action of hydrogen fluoride on uranium dioxide at 550°:

$$UO_2 + 4\,HF \rightarrow UF_4 + 2\,H_2O$$

It is a green solid (m.p. 960°), insoluble in water, and can be reduced to the trifluoride, UF_3, with hydrogen. Reaction with magnesium gives metallic uranium, and this method is used commercially. The tetrafluoride forms a range of complexes when it is melted with alkali-metal fluorides, *e.g.*, Na_2UF_6, K_3UF_7.

Uranium hexafluoride, UF_6, is prepared from the tetrafluoride by fluorination with fluorine or chlorine trifluoride. It is a colourless solid which sublimes without melting at 56° and 1 atmosphere pressure; because of its volatility it is used in the gaseous diffusion process for the concentration of the ^{235}U isotope. It is an extremely reactive compound, rapidly hydrolysed, and a powerful oxidising and fluorinating agent. A number of complex fluorides have been made from the hexafluoride and alkali-metal fluorides, *e.g.*, Na_3UF_9, Rb_2UF_8, but little is known of their chemistry.

The stable uranyl cation, UO_2^{2+}, forms a fluoride salt, UO_2F_2, which may be formally regarded as an oxyfluoride and this, in turn, forms complex oxyfluorides such as $K_3UO_2F_5$.

j) Fluorides of the rare gases

(Bartlett 1962; Claasen et al. 1962; Holloway and Peacock 1962; Weeks et al. 1962)

The most remarkable demonstration of the extreme oxidising power of fluorine and its compounds has been the recent preparation of the first true compounds of the rare gases. Xenon is oxidised by the vapour of platinum hexafluoride to give the orange-yellow solid xenon hexafluoroplatinate(V):

$$Xe + PtF_6 \rightarrow Xe^+ [PtF_6]^-$$

Reaction between xenon and fluorine at 400° in a nickel vessel gives xenon tetrafluoride, XeF_4, a stable colourless crystalline solid, which dissolves in water to give a solution containing a xenon compound whose nature has not yet been established.

A photochemically-induced reaction between xenon and fluorine at room temperature gives xenon difluoride, XeF_2, another crystalline solid.

III. Organic fluorine chemistry

The relatively small size of the univalent fluorine atom and the high strength of the C-F bond make it theoretically possible to progressively substitute fluorine for hydrogen in any of the vast number of hydrocarbons and their derivatives. Such an exercise has obvious practical limits, but already several thousand organic compounds containing fluorine are known and there is every reason to expect that this number will continue to increase steadily.

A. Methods for the introduction of fluorine into organic compounds

Only two organic fluorine compounds have been found in nature in appreciable amounts, *viz.*, monofluoroacetic acid, CH_2FCO_2H, the toxic principle of the deadly poisonous South African plant *Dichapetalum cymosum* ("gifblaar") and of *Acacia georginae* ("gidyea") of Australia, and ω-fluorooleic acid,

$$CH_2F(CH_2)_7CH{=}CH(CH_2)_7CO_2H,$$

a toxic compound occurring in the shrub *Dichapetalum toxicarium* ("ratsbane") which grows in Sierra Leone. These two compounds have no value as basic starting materials for the preparation of organic fluorides. Traces of fluoropalmitic acid have also been found associated with the fluorooleic acid.

Fluorine is introduced into organic structures by synthesis involving inorganic fluorinating agents. These can be divided into two groups according to their activity and hence the degree of control which can be exercised over them: (I) fluorine, high-valency fluorides of certain metals, *e.g.*, CoF_3, AgF_2, and halogen fluorides, *e.g.*, ClF_3, BrF_3; (II) hydrogen fluoride and derived compounds, *e.g.*, KF,

SbF_3, SF_4. Group (I) consists of vigorous fluorinating agents which, in general, are capable of substituting all hydrogen and functional groups in organic substrates by fluorine and are thus used to prepare saturated *fluorocarbons*, *i.e.*, compounds containing only carbon and fluorine, *e.g.*,

perfluoro-n-heptane, $CF_3CF_2CF_2CF_2CF_2CF_2CF_3$

perfluoro(methylcyclohexane), 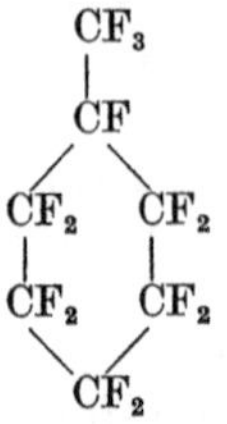

With care, it is possible in certain cases to restrict the amount of fluorine introduced by these agents and thus obtain polyfluorinated products containing some hydrogen, *hydrofluorocarbons*, or a functional group, *fluorocarbon derivatives*, *e.g.*,

1*H*, 3*H*-decafluorocyclohexane, 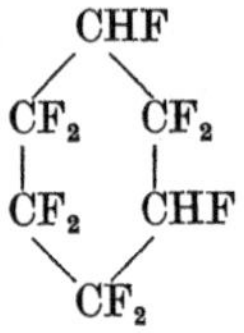

hexafluoroacetone, 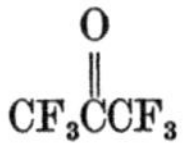

The most important method of preparation of fluorocarbon derivatives direct from hydrocarbon derivatives, however, is electrochemical fluorination, which will be discussed under category (I). Use of the mild fluorinating agents in Group (II) allows fluorine to be introduced at selected sites in organic molecules; these agents do not normally replace hydrogen by fluorine.

1. Fluorinating agents based on elementary fluorine

a) Elementary fluorine

(TEDDER 1961)

It is generally accepted that direct fluorination of hydrocarbons proceeds initially by a simple free-radical chain mechanism of familiar type:

$$F_2 \longrightarrow 2\,F\cdot$$

$$F\cdot + RH \longrightarrow HF + R\cdot \xrightarrow{F_2} RF + F\cdot \xrightarrow{RH} HF + R\cdot \xrightarrow{F_2} \textit{etc.}$$

(where RH = hydrocarbon)

and the ease of chain initiation results from the small bond dissociation energy of fluorine [D(F—F) = 38 kcal/mole; *cf.* D(Cl—Cl) = 57 kcal/mole] and the low activation energies required for abstraction of hydrogen from hydrocarbons by fluorine atoms. The violence of fluorination reactions stems from the immense heat liberated, which, unless rapidly dissipated, causes extensive fragmentation of the carbon skeleton to occur.

$$>CH— + F_2 \rightarrow >CF— + HF \qquad \Delta H \approx -103 \text{ kcal}$$

(*cf.* ΔH for chlorination $\approx$ —23 kcal)

$$>C{=}C< + F_2 \rightarrow >CF—CF< \qquad \Delta H \approx -107 \text{ kcal}$$

(*cf.* ΔH for chlorination $\approx$ —33 kcal)

The most successful and widely-used method of direct fluorination of organic compounds is the *vapour-phase method*, in which both reactants are diluted with nitrogen and allowed to meet in a heated metal tube packed with metal gauze, turnings, or shot. This method was developed during the Second World War for the production of fluorocarbons from hydrocarbons, but was subsequently abandoned in favour of the "metallic fluoride process" (see below) and has been used since only in academic studies on the fluorination of different types of organic compound. Attention has been turned recently to the development of vapour-phase reactors fitted with reactant inlet jets of special design which promote mild fluorination.

Details of some typical vapour-phase fluorinations are given in Table 6; where yields of products are not quoted, they are poor (1—15 %) and cannot be estimated with any accuracy. Low yields result from the inability to prevent skeletal fission and from the difficulties encountered in the separation of complex reaction products.

It is fair to advise that direct fluorination as a method of preparation of organic fluorides should be avoided whenever possible.

Table 6. *Direct vapour-phase fluorination* of organic compounds*

Starting material	Reactor type/temp. (°C)	Products (yield %)
C_2H_6	unpacked[1]/64	C_2F_6 (96)
n-C_7H_{16}	packed[2]/135	n-C_7F_{16} (62)
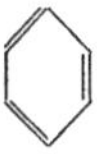	packed[2]/265	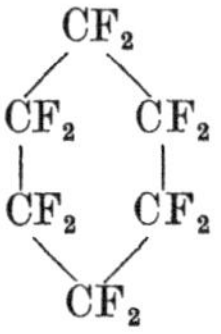 (58)
CH_3OH	packed[2]/160—180	CF_3OF(50), CF_4, COF_2, F_2O
CH_3SH	packed[2]/200	CF_3SF_5(10), $CSHF_7$, CF_4, SF_6
CH_3COCH_3	packed[3]/60—100	CF_3COCF_3, CH_2FCOCH_3, CF_3COF, $(COF)_2$, CF_4, COF_2
HCN	unpacked[1]/150	CF_3NF_2(60[4]), $(CF_3)_2NF$(6[4]), CF_4(23[4])
CH_3NH_2	packed[3]/100	CF_3NF_2, $C_2F_5NF_2$, $(CF_3)_2NF$
$HCON(CH_3)_2$	packed[3]/275	$(CF_3)_2NF$(38), $(CF_3)_3N$, $(CF_3)_2NN(CF_3)_2$
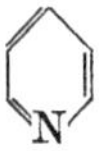	packed[5]/280	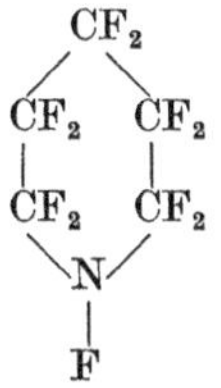 (0.3), C_5F_{12}
CS_2	packed[6]/48	CF_3SF_5, CF_3SF_3, $SF_5CF_2SF_5$, $SF_5CF_2SF_3$, CSF_2, CF_4, SF_6, SF_4, S_2F_{10}
CH_3SCN	packed[6]/95	CF_3SF_5, SF_5CN, $SF_5CF_2NF_2$, $CF_2{=}NF$, CF_4, SF_6, S_2F_{10}

* With fluorine diluted with nitrogen or helium.
[1] So-called "jet fluorination reactor".
[2] Copper turnings or ribbon coated with silver difluoride.
[3] Copper gauze or shot
[4] Mole %.
[5] Gold-plated copper turnings.
[6] Fitted with a special concentric-tube injection port and packed with copper shot.

b) Use of high-valency metallic fluorides in the "metallic fluoride process" (Stacey and Tatlow 1960)

In general a saturated fluorocarbon is best prepared by passing the vapour of an aliphatic or aromatic hydrocarbon with the required carbon skeleton over a heated bed of cobaltic fluoride. In comparison with direct fluorination, much less heat is liberated in the substitution reaction

$$>CH— + 2\,CoF_3 \rightarrow >CF— + 2\,CoF_2 + HF \quad \Delta H \approx -56\ \text{kcal}$$

thus relatively less C—C bond fission occurs and good yields (50—75 %) of product can be obtained without much difficulty, *e.g.*,

$$\text{n-}C_7H_{16} \xrightarrow{CoF_3,\ 300^\circ} \text{n-}C_7F_{16} \quad (75\%)$$

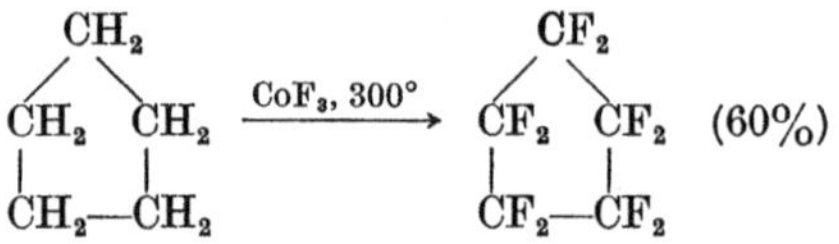

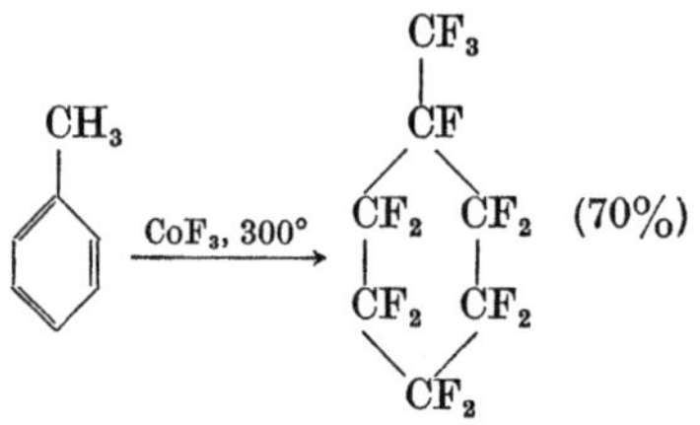

The apparatus need consist simply of a heated copper tube containing a layer of cobalt trifluoride, although the efficiency of the fluorination is increased if the latter is stirred. When reaction is complete, the hydrocarbon feed is discontinued and the cobalt trifluoride is regenerated by passing fluorine over the difluoride:

$$2\,CoF_2 + F_2 \xrightarrow{200^\circ} 2CoF_3$$

Unfortunately much decomposition occurs in the fluorination of organic compounds containing functional groups with cobalt trifluoride, and complex mixtures containing only small amounts, if any, of the corresponding fluorocarbon derivatives are obtained, *e.g.*,

$$CH_3COCH_3 \xrightarrow{CoF_3,\ 60^\circ} CHF_3,\ CH_2F_2,\ CH_3F,\ CH_2FCOF,\ CH_3COF,\ COF_2$$

$$CH_3SH \xrightarrow{CoF_3,\ 250^\circ} CF_3SF_5\,(20\%),\ CF_4,\ CHF_3,\ SF_6$$

$$(CH_3)_3N \xrightarrow{CoF_3,\ 250^\circ} (CF_3)_3N\,(6\%),\ (CF_3)_2NF\,(1\%),\ CF_3NF_2\ (0.8\%)$$

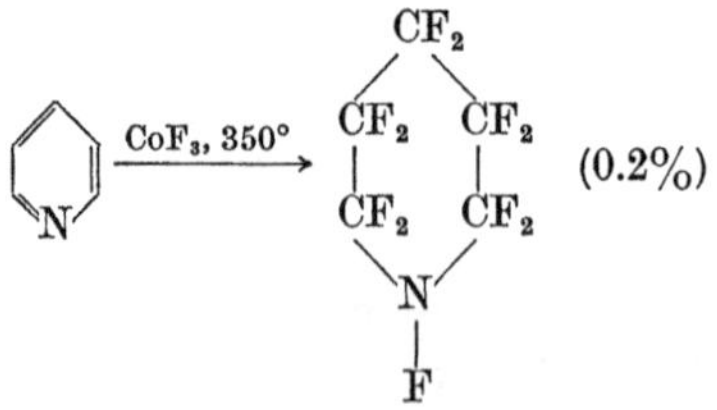

Hydrofluorocarbons can be prepared by fluorination of hydrocarbons with cobalt trifluoride under mild conditions, but the mixed products obtained are usually difficult to separate.

Silver difluoride, manganese trifluoride, cerium tetrafluoride, and lead tetrafluoride are also capable of use in the "metallic fluoride process" for the preparation of fluorocarbons, but they have received less attention than cobalt trifluoride.

c) Halogen fluorides

(MUSGRAVE 1960)

The halogen fluorides are highly reactive compounds, and like fluorine, from which they are prepared, must be used with caution. Relatively little use is made of the ability of these compounds to replace hydrogen in organic compounds by fluorine, since reactions are complicated by the tendency for the second halogen present to be introduced into the substrate molecule, particularly when the latter is unsaturated. Such complications are avoided if the organic substrate is a perhalogenated compound in which the halogen is the same as the second halogen in the halogen fluoride, *e.g.*,

$$CBr_4 \xrightarrow{BrF_3} CF_3Br \qquad (94\%)$$

$$CI_4 \xrightarrow{IF_5} CF_3I \qquad (95\%)$$

$$ICN \xrightarrow{IF_5} CF_3N{=}NCF_3 \qquad (60\%)$$

Saturated chlorofluorocarbon lubricants *(Florubes*[1]*)* which resist attack by halogens, oxygen, and strong acids are made by treating high-boiling aromatic chlorocarbons, *e.g.*, decachlorodiphenyl, octachloronaphthalene, with chlorine mono- and tri-fluoride.

Interest in halogen fluorides as reagents for the preparation of organic fluorides may be stimulated by the recent discovery that controlled fluorination of some hydrocarbon derivatives can be effected by bromine trifluoride or iodine pentafluoride under certain conditions (STEVENS 1961), *e.g.*,

$$CH_3COCH_3 \xrightarrow[-20^\circ]{BrF_3\text{ in HF}} CH_3CF_2CH_3 \qquad (90\%)$$

$$CH_3CN \xrightarrow[-20^\circ]{BrF_3\text{ in HF}} CH_3CF_3 \qquad (70\%)$$

d) Electrochemical fluorination

(BURDON and TATLOW 1960)

Many organic compounds, particularly those containing polar groups, dissolve in anhydrous hydrogen fluoride to give conducting solutions; when such a solution is electrolysed at a low voltage (usually 5—6 V) so that free fluorine is not generated, hydrogen is liberated at the cathode and the organic solute is fluorinated by some unknown anodic process. This electrochemical method of fluorination was discovered by SIMONS in 1941; it resembles fluorination with elementary fluorine or cobalt trifluoride since all hydrogen is replaced, double bonds are saturated, and fragmentation of molecules occurs, but in general functional groups are retained to a much greater extent. Thus, electrochemical fluorination is usually the method of choice for the preparation of fluorocarbon derivatives from hydrocarbon type precursors.

---

[1] Trade name, Imperial Chemical Industries Ltd., England.

Table 7. *Examples of the use of electrochemical fluorination*

Starting material	Product (yield %)	Starting material	Product (yield %)
CH_3COF	CF_3COF (85)	$(C_2H_5)_3N$	$(C_2F_5)_3N$ (27)
$C_7H_{15}CO_2H$	$C_7F_{15}COF$ (4)	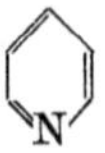	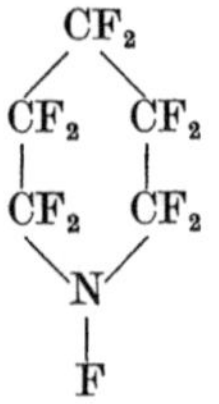 (10)
CH_3SO_2F	CF_3SO_2F (96)	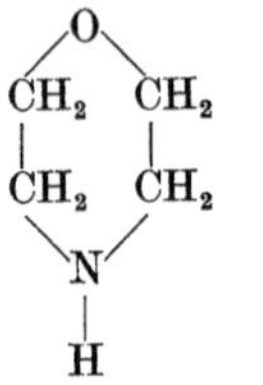	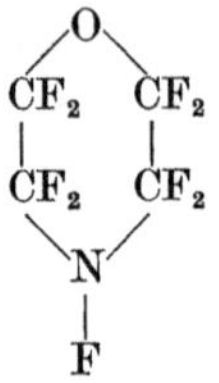 (13)
n-$C_3H_7SO_2Cl$	n-$C_3F_7SO_2F$ (68)	$(CH_3)_2NCOCl$	$(CF_3)_2NCOF$ (37)
n-$C_8H_{17}SO_2Cl$	n-$C_8F_{17}SO_2F$ (25)	$(CH_3)_2NCON(CH_3)_2$	$(CF_3)_2NCON(CF_3)_2$ (2) $(CF_3)_2NCOF$ (13)
CS_2	CF_3SF_5 (>90) $CF_2(SF_5)_2$ (0.5) $CF_2(SF_3)_2$ (0.5)	$C_2H_5OC_2H_5$	$C_2F_5OC_2F_5$ (*)
$(CH_3)_2S$	CF_3SF_5 (54) $(CF_3)_2SF_4$ (5)	$C_4H_9OCH_2CH_2OH$	$C_4F_9OC_2F_5$ (30)
(n-$C_3H_7)_2S$	n-$C_3F_7SF_5$ (18) (n-$C_3F_7)_2SF_4$ (16)	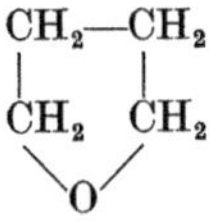	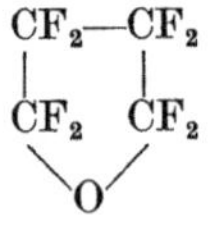 (42)
n-$C_8H_{17}SH$	n-$C_8F_{17}SF_5$ (21)		
$(CH_3)_2SO_2$	$(CF_3)_2SO_2$ (4) CF_3SO_2F (60)		
$HSCH_2CO_2H$	SF_5CF_2COF (2) $SF_3CF_2CO_2H$ (3) CF_3SF_5 (3)		
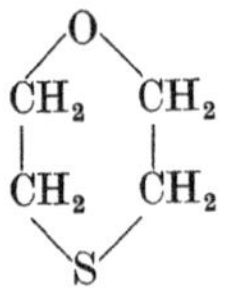	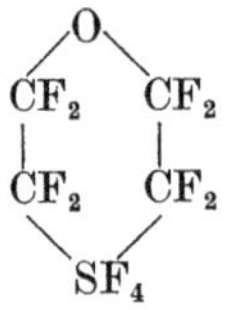 (20) $C_2F_5O(CF_2)_2SF_5$ (4) $C_2F_5SF_5$ (4)		

* No yield given.

Some examples of the preparation of fluorocarbon derivatives by electrochemical fluorination are listed in Table 7; the products are always accompanied by fully-fluorinated breakdown products, *e.g.*,

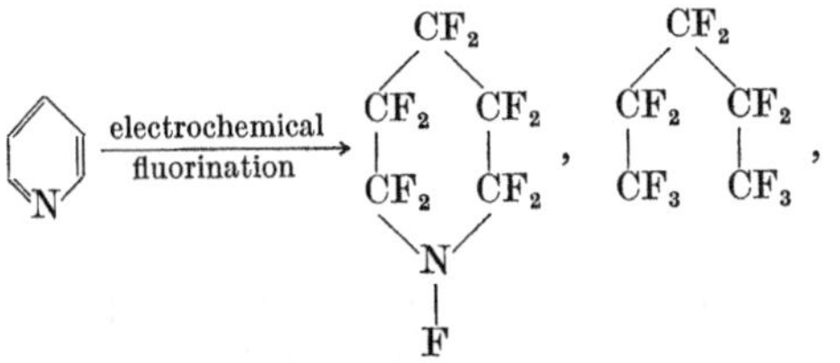

, NF_3, plus C_1—C_4 fluorocarbons

and this can lead to purification difficulties. Electrochemical fluorination is used commercially (RUDGE 1962) to prepare perfluoroalkanoyl fluorides, R_FCOF, and hence perfluoroalkanecarboxylic acids, R_FCO_2H ($R_F = CF_3$, C_2F_5, n-C_3F_7, n-C_7F_{15}), which are basic starting materials in the synthesis of a wide variety of fluorocarbon derivatives, and of long-chain perfluoroalkanesulphonyl fluorides, *e.g.*, n-$C_8F_{17}SO_2F$, for conversion to alkali-metal and chromium salts of the parent acids for use in the electroplating and textile industries, respectively (see Table 13, p. 46).

The apparatus used in electrochemical fluorination is relatively simple and inexpensive; it consists basically of an iron or, preferably, nickel cell containing a pack of alternate nickel anodes and cathodes and surmounted by a reflux condenser cooled to about —20° to prevent escape of hydrogen fluoride (b.p. 19.5°). The perfluorinated products are either swept out of the cell by the cathodic hydrogen or, being dense and insoluble in hydrogen fluoride, accumulate at the bottom of the cell and can be drained off periodically.

2. Fluorinating agents based on hydrogen fluoride

The most important reagents for the introduction of fluorine at specific sites in organic molecules are hydrogen fluoride, potassium fluoride, antimony fluorides, sulphur tetrafluoride, perchloryl fluoride, and tetrafluoroboric acid. The scope of each of these reagents will be defined and exemplified, and several other inorganic fluorides which find use as fluorinating agents will be mentioned briefly.

a) Hydrogen fluoride

(HUDLICKÝ 1961; STEPHENS and TATLOW 1962)

Apart from its use in electrochemical fluorination (see p. 21), anhydrous hydrogen fluoride is mainly employed (a) to effect exchange of chlorine or bromine in organic compounds for fluorine, (b) to add the elements HF across unsaturated bonds in olefins and acetylenes, and (c) to open epoxide rings to yield fluorohydrins. Diazotisation of aromatic amino-compounds in hydrofluoric acid or, preferably, anhydrous hydrogen fluoride can be used to prepare aromatic fluorides, but generally these compounds are best prepared *via* diazonium tetrafluoroborates as described below. Reaction of hydrogen fluoride with an alcohol gives only low yields, if any, of alkyl fluoride and has no value as a method of synthesis.

Anhydrous hydrogen fluoride (b.p. 19.5°) and aqueous hydrofluoric acid are hazardous chemicals and must be used with caution in metal or plastic equipment.

α) Halogen-exchange reactions. Anhydrous hydrogen fluoride substitutes fluorine for chlorine or bromine in organic compounds only with difficulty unless these halogens are activated, as, for example, in the case of compounds containing allylic or benzylic chlorine:

$$CCl_2{=}CClCCl_3 + 3\,HF \xrightarrow{155^\circ} CCl_2{=}CClCF_3\,(33\%) + 3\,HCl$$

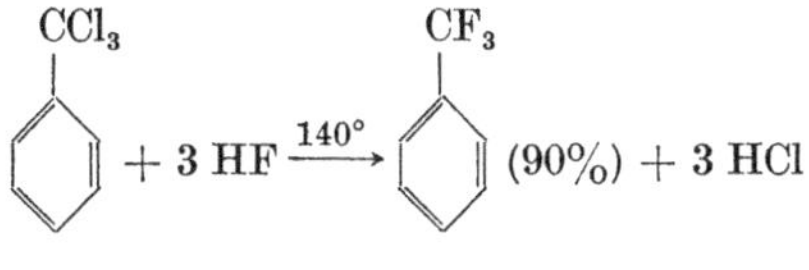

In the presence of a catalyst such as antimony pentachloride, chromic fluoride, or ferric fluoride, however, anhydrous hydrogen fluoride will substitute fluorine for chlorine or bromine in unreactive organic polyhalogeno-compounds with relative ease. Examples of the preparation of commercially-important organic chlorofluoro-compounds with the widely-used HF/$SbCl_5$ system are given below; presumably, the effective fluorinating agent is antimony trifluoridedichloride, SbF_3Cl_2, which is constantly regenerated. It is difficult, and often impossible, to replace all the chlorine in a chlorocarbon, *e.g.*, C_2Cl_6, by fluorine with HF/catalyst systems and thus obtain a fluorocarbon, *e.g.*, C_2F_6.

$$CCl_4 \xrightarrow[110^\circ,\ 30\ atm.]{HF,\ SbCl_5} CFCl_3\,(9\%),\ CF_2Cl_2\,(90\%),\ CF_3Cl\ (0.5\%)$$

$$CHCl_3 \xrightarrow[60^\circ]{HF,\ SbCl_5} CHF_2Cl\,(75\%) + CHFCl_2\,(20\%)$$

β) Reaction of anhydrous hydrogen fluoride with unsaturated compounds. Anhydrous hydrogen fluoride reacts readily with olefins and acetylenes in a manner analogous to the other hydrogen halides, *e.g.*,

$$CH_3CH{=}CH_2 + HF \xrightarrow{0^\circ} CH_3CHFCH_3 \quad (61\%)$$

$$CH_2{=}CHCl + HF \xrightarrow{150^\circ} CH_3CHFCl$$

$$CH{\equiv}CH + 2\,HF \xrightarrow{FSO_3H,\ 0^\circ} CH_3CHF_2 \quad (94\%)$$

It has been found that *trans*-addition of the elements of BrF or IF to an olefinic double bond can be effected with a mixture of *N*-bromoacetamide or *N*-iodosuccinimide (sources of the electrophilic species Br^+ and I^+, respectively) and anhydrous hydrogen fluoride in tetrahydrofuran (source of the nucleophilic F^-) (BOWERS 1959; ROBINSON et al. 1959; BOWERS et al. 1960a, b), *e.g.*,

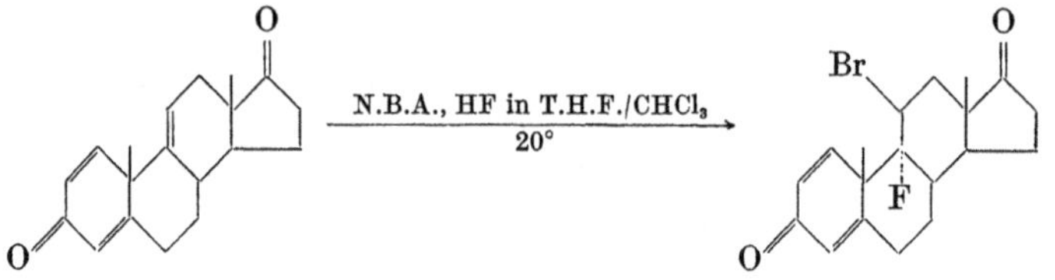

(41%)

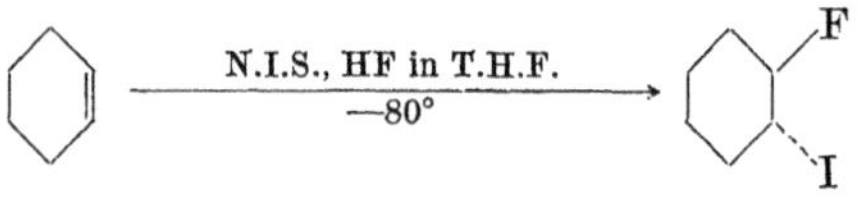

(73%)

The *cis*-addition of fluorine to a double bond in a steroidal olefin has recently been achieved in quantitative yield using a mixture of anhydrous hydrogen fluoride and lead tetra-acetate; it is presumed that lead tetrafluoride, generated *in situ*, is the active fluorinating agent (BOWERS et al. 1962):

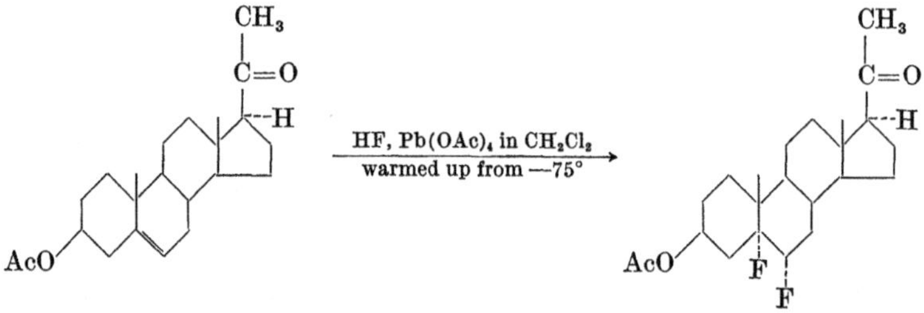

This work stems from the earlier discovery of HENNE and his co-workers that a mixture of anhydrous hydrogen fluoride and lead dioxide can be used to add fluorine indirectly across double bonds in halogeno-olefins, *e.g.*,

$$CCl_2{=}CCl_2 \xrightarrow[\text{warmed up from } -78^\circ]{HF,\ PbO_2} CFCl_2CFCl_2 \quad (59\%)$$

γ) Reaction with olefin oxides. In the presence of an organic proton acceptor, anhydrous hydrogen fluoride converts olefin oxides to fluorohydrins in good yield, *e.g.*,

$$\overbrace{CH_2{-}CH_2}^{O} + HF \xrightarrow{C_2H_5OC_2H_5,\ 100^\circ} CH_2FCH_2OH \quad (40\%)$$

This is an important reaction for the preparation of monofluorosteroids (FRIED and SABO 1957; HIRSCHMANN et al. 1956; see papers quoted by BOWERS et al. 1962), *e.g.*,

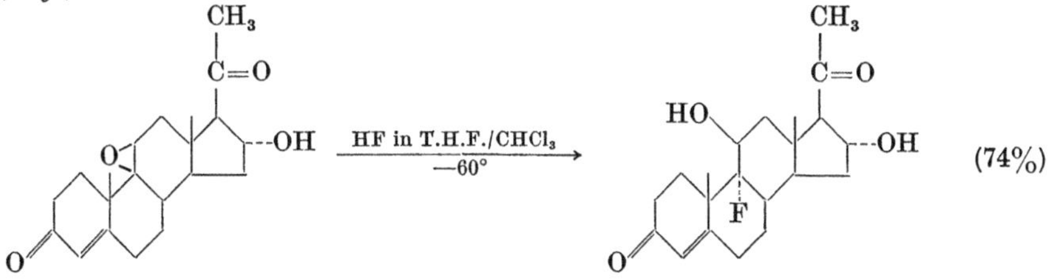

and is applied twice in the synthesis (MILLS et al. 1960) of 6α,9α-difluoro-16α-hydroxyprednisolone-16,17-acetonide *(Synalar*[1]*)*, an important new corticoid for topical therapy of the inflammatory dermatoses. Boron trifluoride etherate also cleaves epoxides to fluorohydrins (see papers quoted by BOWERS et al. 1962).

b) Potassium fluoride

(HUDLICKÝ 1961; STEPHENS and TATLOW 1962)

Common dry potassium fluoride is used extensively to convert alkyl and activated aryl monohalides, and alcohols in the form of sulphonate esters, usually tosyl esters, into the corresponding monofluorides; conventional glass apparatus can often be used, and reactions are normally facilitated by use of a solvent such as ethylene glycol, β, β′-dihydroxydiethyl ether, acetamide, dimethyl formamide, or dimethylsulphoxide, *e.g.*,

$$CH_3OTs + KF \xrightarrow{160\text{—}250^\circ} CH_3F\ (90\%) + TsOK$$

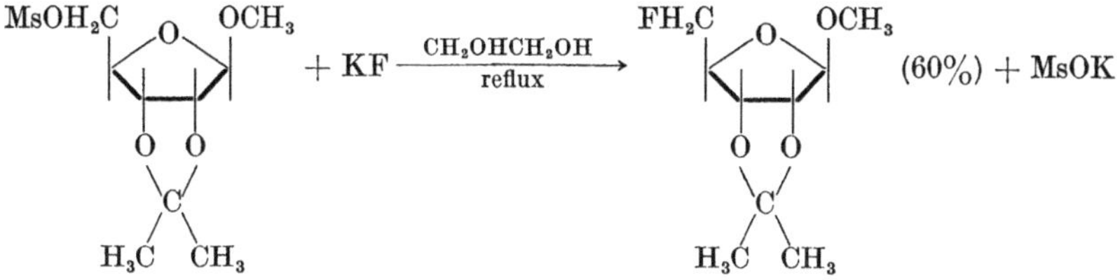

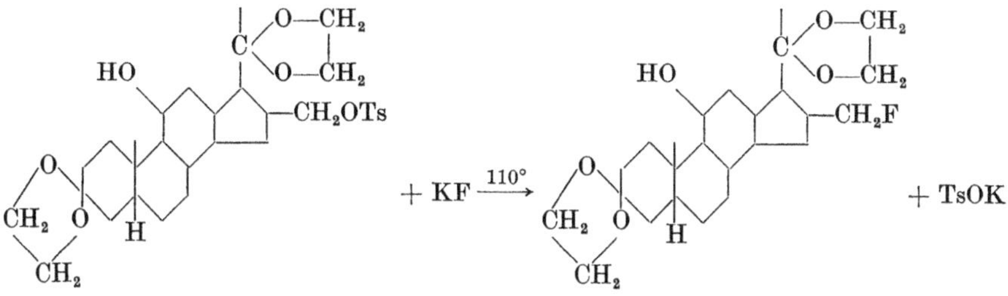

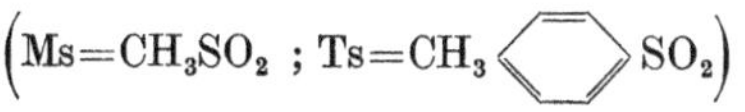

$$CH_2ClCO_2C_2H_5 + KF \xrightarrow[110\text{—}140^\circ]{CH_3CONH_2} CH_2FCO_2C_2H_5\ (63\%) + KCl$$

$$n\text{-}C_6H_{13}Cl + KF \xrightarrow[175\text{—}185^\circ]{HOCH_2CH_2OH} n\text{-}C_6H_{13}F\ (54\%) + KCl$$

[1] Trade name, Syntex Corporation, Mexico City.

$$CH_2BrCH_2Br + KF \xrightarrow{90^\circ} CH_2FCH_2Br\ (24\%) + KBr$$

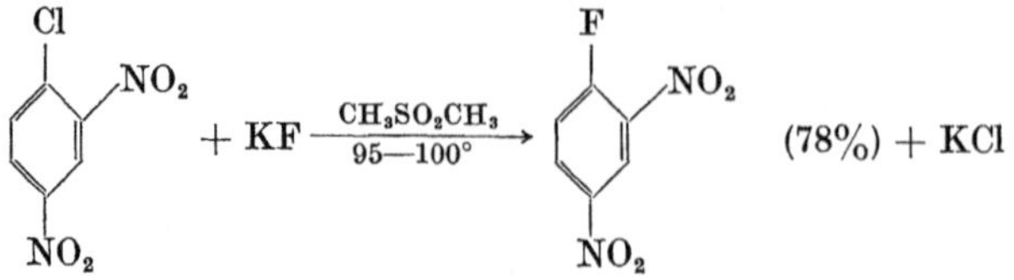

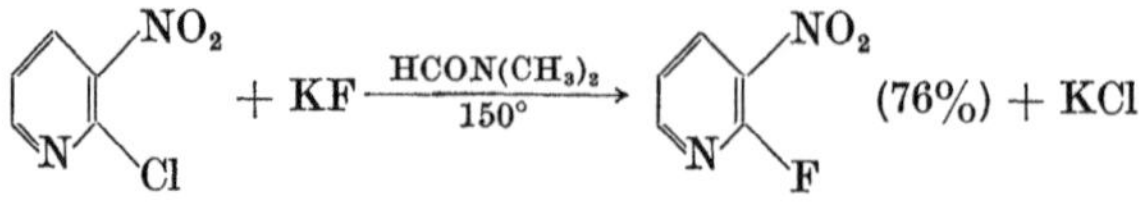

Several organic di- and poly-fluorides have been prepared with potassium fluoride, *e.g.*,

$$CH_2Cl(CH_2)_2CH_2Cl \xrightarrow[170^\circ]{KF,\ CH_2OHCH_2OH} CH_2F(CH_2)_2CH_2F\ (44\%) + CH_2F(CH_2)_2CH_2Cl\ (7\%)$$

$$CHCl_2CO_2CH_3 \xrightarrow[220-230^\circ]{KF} CHF_2CO_2CH_3\ (18\%)$$

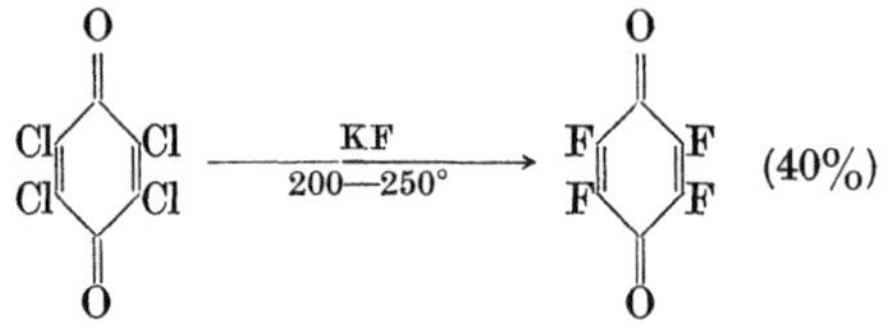

Acid potassium fluoride, KHF_2, is used to prepare acyl and sulphonyl fluorides, *e.g.*,

$$CH_3CO_2H \xrightarrow[100^\circ]{KHF_2,\ C_6H_5COCl} CH_3COF\ (82\%)$$

The other alkali-metal fluorides find little use as fluorinating agents; lithium and sodium fluoride are less efficient in their action than potassium fluoride, and while the fluorides of rubidium and caesium are more efficient, their cost is often prohibitive.

c) Antimony fluorides

(Hudlický 1961; Stephens and Tatlow 1962)

Reference was made earlier (p. 23) to the industrial use of anhydrous hydrogen fluoride in the presence of catalytic amounts of antimony(V) fluorides for the preparation of organic polyfluorides by the halogen-exchange technique. In the laboratory, antimony fluorides alone are used to replace halogen atoms of the groups $-CX_3$ and $>CX_2$ (X=Cl, Br, I) by fluorine; in general, they are not satisfactory for the preparation of monofluorides by exchange of halogen with the groups $-CH_2X$, $>CHX$, and $\geqslant CX$. Many fluorinations with antimony fluorides can be carried out in glass apparatus, but some require the use of metal autoclaves.

Antimony(V) fluorides are the most efficient fluorinating agents of their type. Thus, while antimony trifluoride is suitable mainly for the fluorination of compounds containing active chlorine or bromine atoms, antimony pentafluoride is a powerful halogen-exchange agent and will also add fluorine to double bonds, *e.g.*,

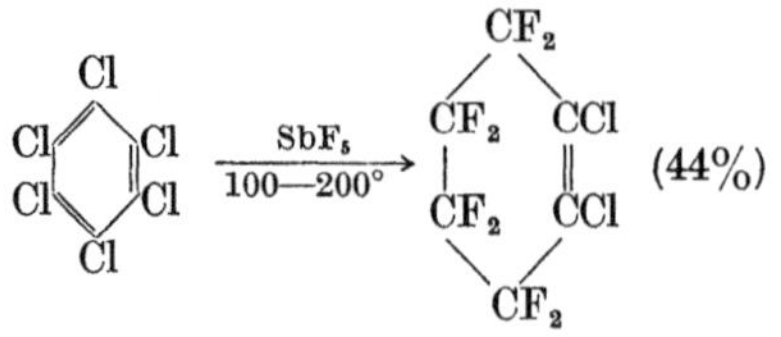

In practice, most polyhalogen-exchange reactions are carried out with commercial antimony trifluoride which has been activated by addition of antimony pentachloride or by part conversion (5—10%) into the pentavalent salts SbF_3Cl_2 or SbF_3Br_2 with chlorine or bromine, respectively. Difficult halogen-exchanges are effected with antimony trifluoridedichloride prepared by addition of the correct amount of chlorine to the trifluoride. Some examples are given below.

$$CHBr_3 \xrightarrow[160^\circ]{SbF_3,\ Br_2} CHF_2Br\ (80\%)$$

$$CCl_3CH_2Cl \xrightarrow[\Delta]{SbF_3,\ Cl_2} CF_2ClCH_2Cl + CFCl_2CH_2Cl$$

$$CCl_3CH_3 \xrightarrow[\Delta]{SbF_3,\ SbCl_5} CF_3CH_3$$

$$CCl_3CCl_3 \xrightarrow[\Delta]{SbF_3Cl_2} CF_3CF_2Cl,\ CF_2ClCF_2Cl,\ CF_2ClCFCl_2,\ CFCl_2CFCl_2,\ CFCl_2CCl_3$$

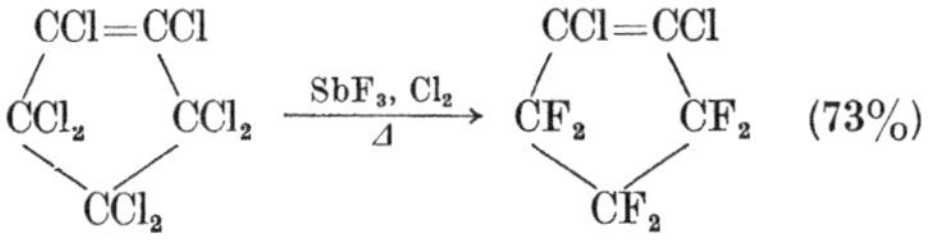

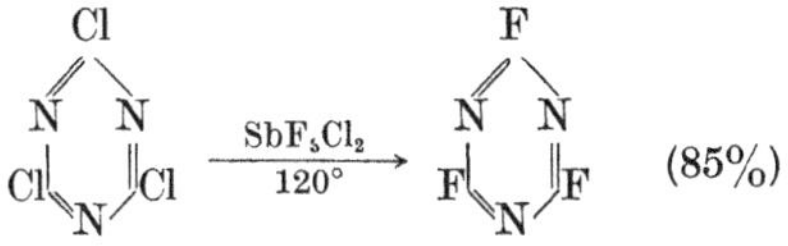

d) Sulphur tetrafluoride

(SMITH 1962)

Sulphur tetrafluoride, a toxic gas, b.p. —40°, is a unique reagent for the direct replacement of carbonyl oxygen by fluorine. Its main use lies in the preparation of *gem.*-difluorides from aldehydes and ketones, and in the conversion of carboxylic acids *via* acid fluorides into trifluoromethyl compounds:

$$R\overset{\overset{O}{\|}}{C}R' + SF_4 \xrightarrow{\Delta} RCF_2R' + SOF_2$$
$$(R' = R \text{ or } H)$$

$$RCO_2H + SF_4 \xrightarrow[\text{or below}]{\text{room temp.}} HF + SOF_2 + RCOF \xrightarrow{SF_4,\ \Delta} RCF_3 + SOF_2$$

Group R can be alkyl, alkenyl, alkynyl, cycloalkyl, cycloalkenyl, aryl, or heterocyclic and, under certain conditions, contain functional groups such as chloro, bromo, nitro, and methoxycarbonyl which remain unaltered. Sulphur tetrafluoride will also substitute fluorine for carbonyl oxygen in carboxylic acid anhydrides, amides, esters, quinones, amino acids, and fluoroformates, and for sulphur in thiocarbonyl compounds. In addition, it will effect certain halogen-exchange reactions, convert compounds containing multiple C—N bonds into organoiminosulphur difluorides, substitute fluorine for oxygen doubly bound to phosphorus or arsenic in organic derivatives, and replace hydroxyl groups, particularly those with an acidic nature, by fluorine. All these uses are illustrated by the examples given in Table 8; reactions are usually carried out under pressure in metal autoclaves, and in some cases it is necessary to add a Lewis-acid catalyst, *e.g.*, HF, BF_3, AsF_3, TiF_4, to facilitate fluorination.

The recently discovered phenylsulphur trifluoride, $C_6H_5SF_3$, will also convert carbonyl and carboxyl groups to difluoromethylene and trifluoromethyl groups, respectively, and is somewhat more convenient to use than sulphur tetrafluoride

Table 8. *Fluorinations with sulphur tetrafluoride*

Starting material	Reaction temp. (°C)	Product (yield %)	
CH_3CHO	50	CH_3CHF_2	(35)
C_6H_5CHO	150	$C_6H_5CHF_2$	(81)
CH_3COCH_3	110	$CH_3CF_2CH_3$	(60)
$C_6H_5COC_6H_5$	180 (HF catalyst)	$C_6H_5CF_2C_6H_5$	(97)
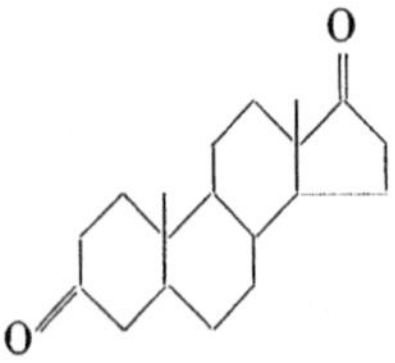	40 (HF catalyst, $CHCl_3$ soln.)	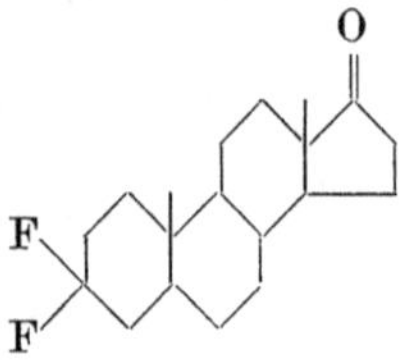	(37)
		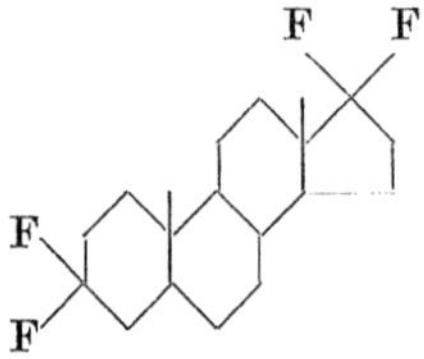	(11)
$CH_2(CO_2H)_2$	40	$CH_2(COF)_2$	(70)
$CH_2(CO_2H)_2$	150	$CF_3CH_2CF_3$	(57)
$HO_2CC{\equiv}CCO_2H$	170	$CF_3C{\equiv}CCF_3$	(80)
$C_6H_5CO_2H$	120	C_6H_5COF	(41)
		$C_6H_5CF_3$	(22)
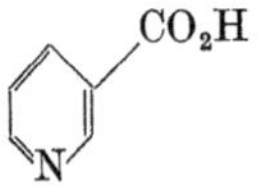	120 (HF as solvent)	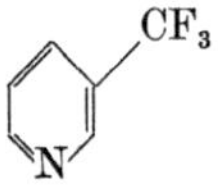	(25)
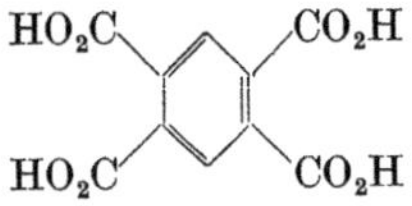	150	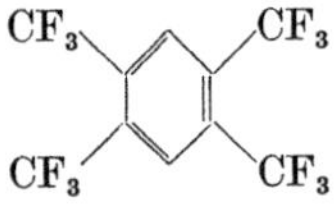	(77)
$HO_3S(CH_2)_{10}CO_2H$	130	$FO_2S(CH_2)_{10}CF_3$	(42)
$(CH_3CO)_2O$	300	CH_3CF_3	(50)
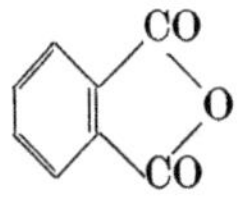	350	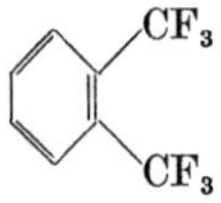	(45)
$C_6H_5CONH_2$	150	$C_6H_5CF_3$	(13)
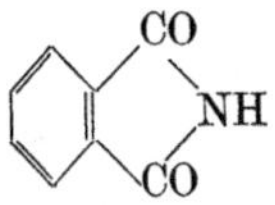	100	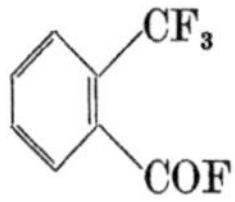	(58)
$H_2NCH_2CO_2H$	120 (HF as solvent)	$CF_3CH_2NH_2$	(24)
$C_6H_5CO_2CH_3$	300	$C_6H_5CF_3$	(55)
		CH_3F	
C_6H_5OCOF	150—175	$C_6H_5OCF_3$	(60—80)
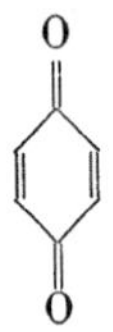	200 (HF catalyst)	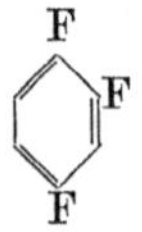	(30)

Table 8 (contd.)

Starting material	Reaction temp. (°C)	Product (yield %)	
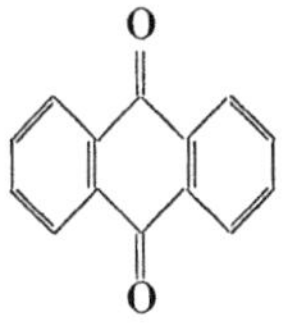	255 (HF cataylst)	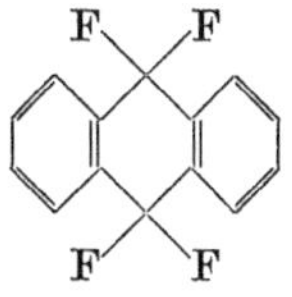	(78)
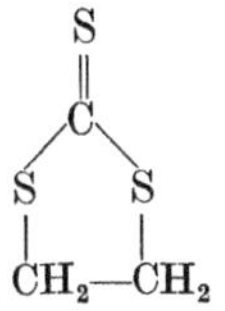	110	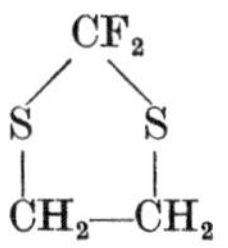	(82)
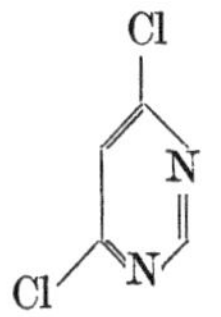	150	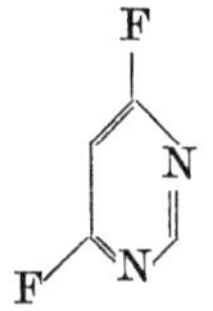	(70)
C_6H_5NCO	150	$C_6H_5N{=}SF_2$	(88)
C_6H_5CN	250	$C_6H_5CF_2N{=}SF_2$	(48)
$(C_6H_5)_3P{=}O$	150 (benzene as solvent)	$(C_6H_5)_3PF_2$	(67)
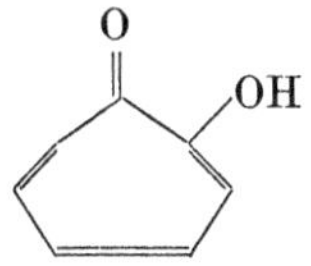	60	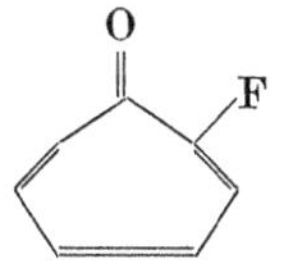	(28)

since it boils at 60°/5 mm and fluorinations can be run in glass apparatus at atmospheric pressure (Sheppard 1962). It is readily prepared in 60 % yield by fluorination of phenyl disulphide with silver difluoride in the inert solvent $CF_2ClCFCl_2$ at 40°.

e) Perchloryl fluoride

Depending on its type, a nucleophilic species N may attack perchloryl fluoride either at the chlorine to form a substituted chlorate and fluoride ion:

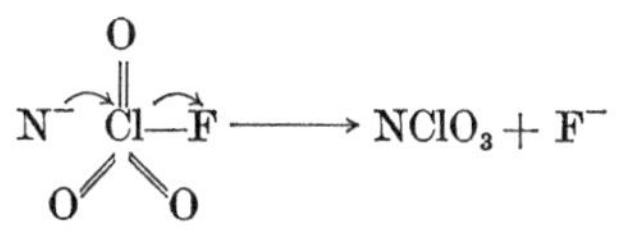

or at the fluorine to form a fluoride and chlorate ion:

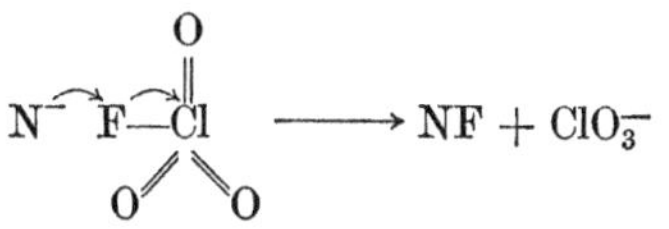

In general, nucleophiles with a localised charge or uncharged nucleophiles with localised non-bonding electrons, *i.e.*, *highly basic nucleophiles*, give products which are derived from initial attack on chlorine, *e.g.*,

$$C_2H_5O^-Na^+ + FClO_3 \longrightarrow NaF + C_2H_5OClO_3 \xrightarrow{C_2H_5O^-Na^+} NaClO_4 + C_2H_5OC_2H_5$$

$$2NH_3 + FClO_3 \longrightarrow NH_4F + H_2NClO_3 \xrightarrow{NH_3} NH_4^+(HNClO_3)^-$$

whereas resonance-stabilised carbanions or neutral organic molecules which have a canonical form with a free electron pair on carbon, *i.e.*, *highly polarisable nucleophiles*, apparently attack at fluorine, *e.g.*,

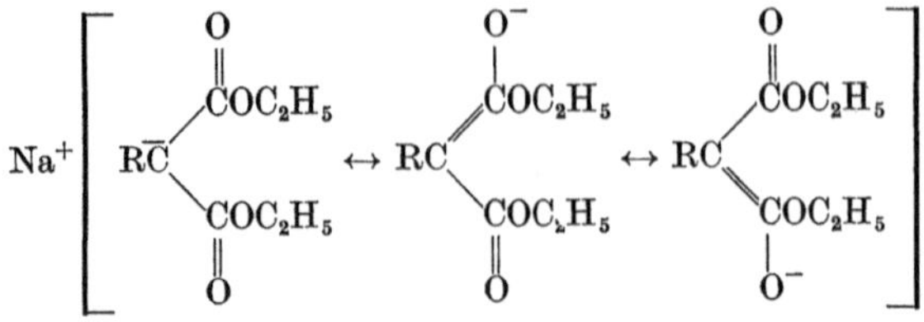

$$Na^+R\bar{C}(CO_2C_2H_5)_2 + FClO_3 \rightarrow RCF(CO_2C_2H_5)_2 + NaClO_3 \qquad (R = \text{alkyl})$$

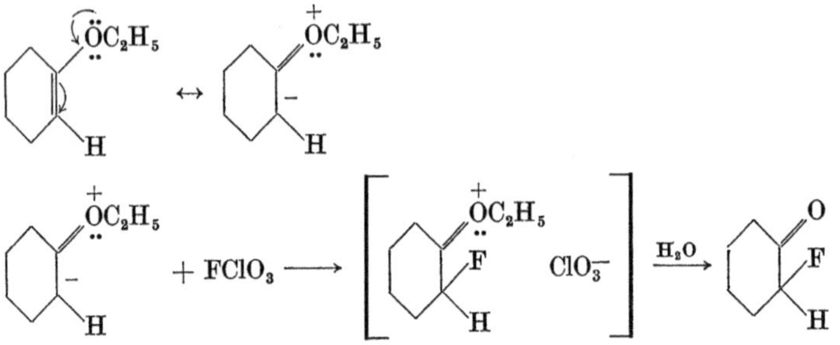

Thus, perchloryl fluoride is a novel reagent for the introduction, in good yield, of one fluorine atom at a known site in β-dicarbonyl compounds[1] (Inman et al. 1958; Kissman et al. 1960), α-hydroxymethylketones (Edwards and Ringold 1959; Robinson et al. 1960), secondary aliphatic nitro-compounds (Freeman 1960; Shechter and Roberson 1960), vinyl ethers (Nakanishi et al 1959, 1960), enol esters (Bloom et al. 1959; Allen and Austin 1961; Nakanishi and Jensen 1962), enamines (Gabbard and Jensen 1958; Nakanishi and Jensen 1962), enamides (Nakanishi and Jensen 1962), and certain phenols (Mills et al. 1960; Taub 1962; Taub et al. 1962). Most of the work so far has concerned the preparation of monofluorinated steroids, *e.g.*,

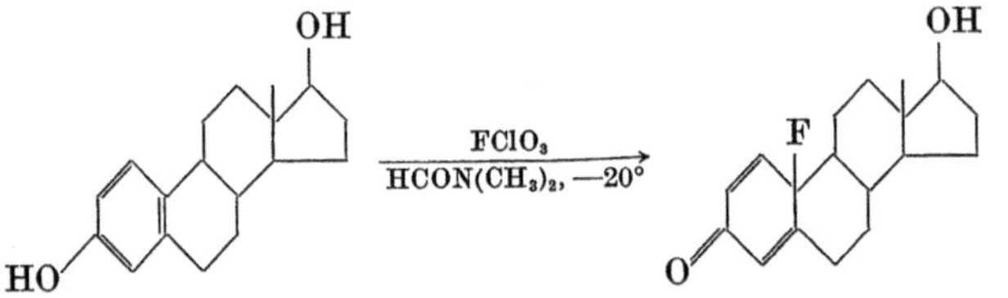

(68%)

Fluorinations with perchloryl fluoride, a commercially available gas[2], b.p. —46.8°, are carried out in the liquid phase at low temperatures, usually near 0°; organic substrates containing active methylene groups are usually dissolved in methanol or ethanol containing sodium in order to form sodium salts, while others are dissolved in suitable basic solvents, *e.g.*, pyridine, dimethylformamide, aqueous dioxan. Perchloryl fluoride is toxic and a powerful oxidising agent, therefore it is essential that potential users should acquaint themselves with safe handling procedures[2].

[1] β-dicarbonyl compounds containing two active hydrogens yield difluoro-derivatives, *e.g.*,

$$CH_3COCH_2CO_2C_2H_5 \xrightarrow[FClO_3,\ 0^\circ \text{ to} -10^\circ]{CH_3ONa/CH_3OH} CH_3COCF_2CO_2C_2H_5\ (59\%)$$

[2] Pennsalt Chemicals Corporation (U.S.A.) Booklet DC-1819, "Perchloryl Fluoride".

f) Tetrafluoroboric acid

(ROE 1949; HUDLICKÝ 1961)

In general, the best method of preparation of aromatic monofluorides involves the formation, isolation (in the majority of cases), and controlled thermal decomposition of solid diazonium tetrafluoroborates. This method, known as the Balz-Schiemann reaction, has been used to prepare fluoro-benzenes, -biphenyls, -naphthalenes, -fluorenes, -phenanthrenes, -pyridines, -quinolines, -isoquinolines, -benzothiazoles, and -carbazoles, *e.g.*,

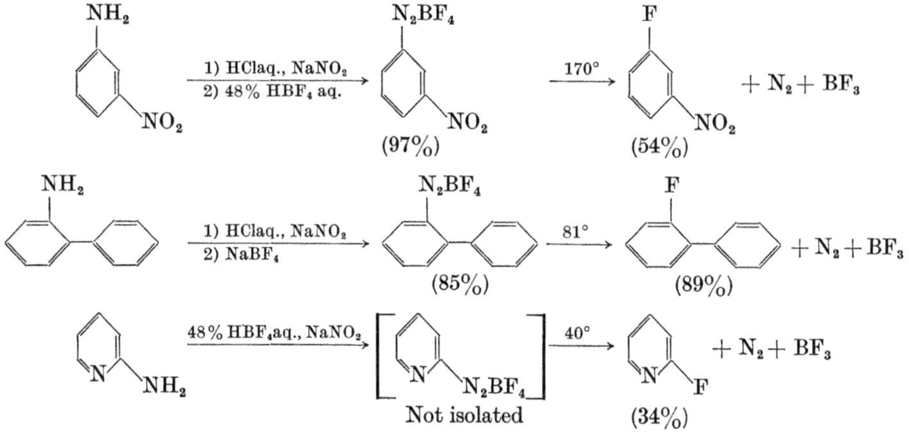

It is possible, in certain cases, to introduce more than one fluorine atom into an aromatic nucleus by the Balz-Schiemann technique (see p. 34).

Diazonium hexafluorophosphates and hexafluorosilicates also decompose to yield aromatic fluorides; the former are used when the analogous diazonium tetrafluoroborate is very soluble in aqueous solution and therefore difficult to isolate and purify (RUTHERFORD et al. 1961).

g) Other inorganic fluorides

The compounds AgF, CaF_2, COF_2, HgF, HgF_2, KSO_2F, Na_2SiF_6, NH_4F, NOF, TlF, and ZnF_2 have been used to introduce fluorine into organic compounds, but none of these has achieved much importance yet. With the exception of carbonyl fluoride (FAWCETT et al. 1962) and nitrosyl fluoride (ANELLO et al. 1961), their uses have been reviewed recently (HUDLICKÝ 1961; STEPHENS and TATLOW 1962).

B. Synthesis in organic fluorine chemistry

(HUDLICKÝ 1961)

1. Polyfluoro-compounds

Since very few fluorocarbons containing functional groups can be prepared satisfactorily by fluorination of hydrocarbon derivatives, and replacement of fluorine in fluorocarbons by other atoms or groups through chemical attack is impossible (see p. 35), a great effort has been spent on the development of methods for the synthesis of fluorocarbon derivatives from readily available fluorohalogeno-methanes and -ethanes, and from perfluoroalkanecarboxylic acids. As a result, fluorocarbon analogues of members of nearly all of the individual homologous series of organic chemistry are known (notable exceptions are amines

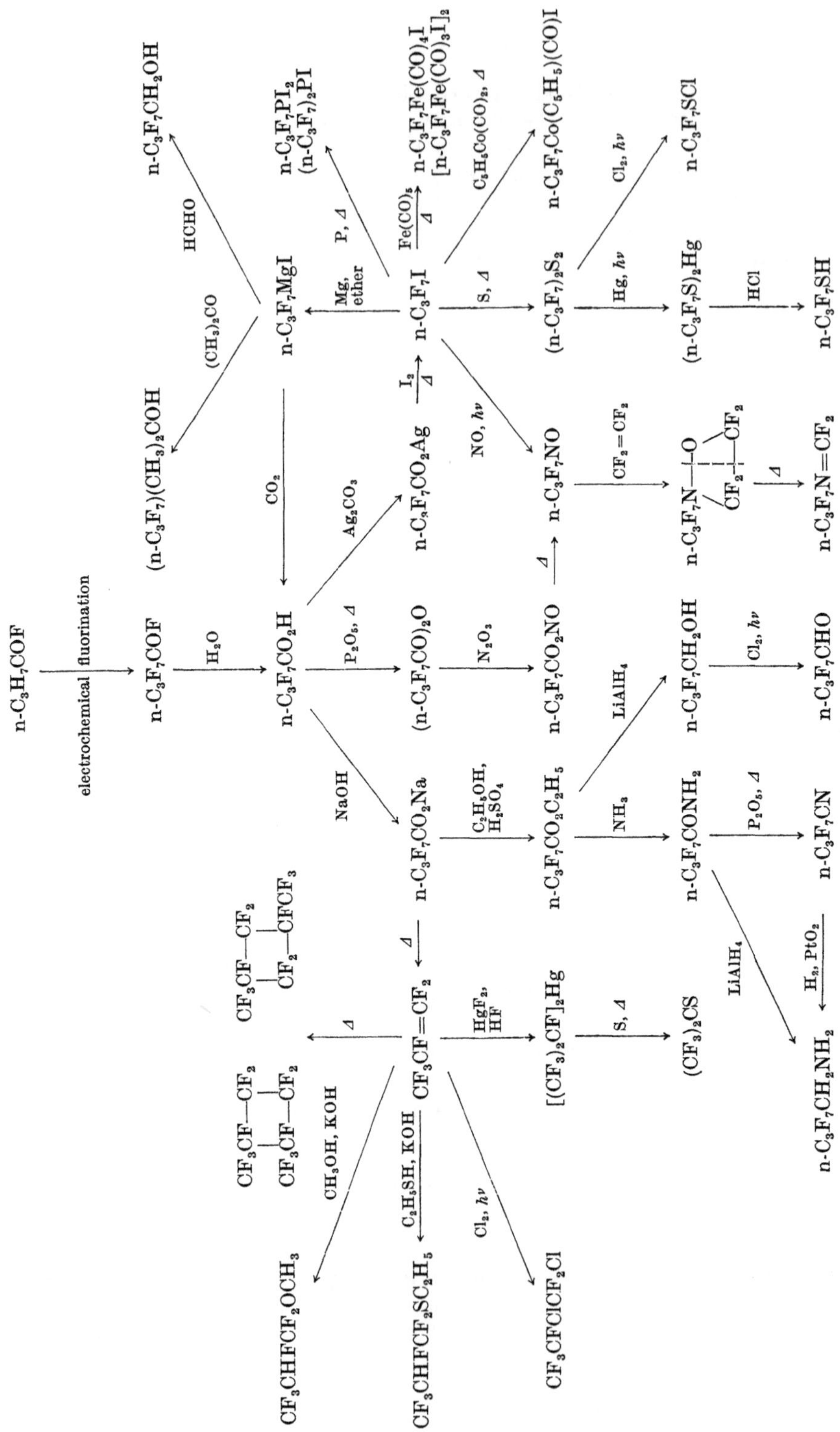

Fig. 1. Preparation of some derivatives of octafluoropropane

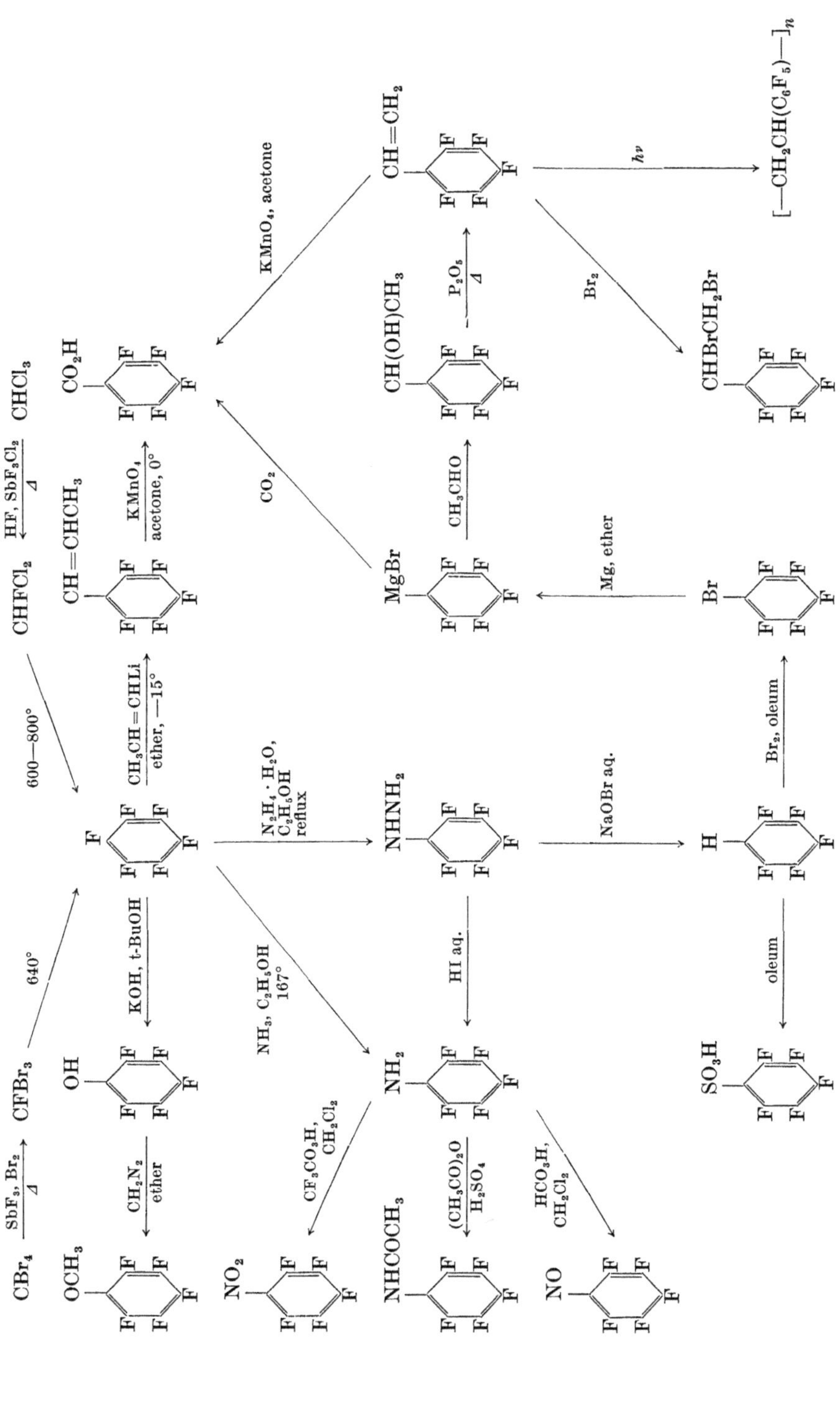

Fig. 2. Preparation of some derivatives of hexafluorobenzene

and alcohols of type $R_FCF_2NH_2$ and R_FCF_2OH, respectively, where $R_F = F$, CF_3, C_2F_5, *etc.*), and perfluoroalkyl derivatives of the following elements have been prepared: Li, Mg, Zn, Hg, B, Al, Si, Ge, Sn, Pb, N, P, As, Sb, Bi, O, S, Se, Fe, Co, Pd. In addition, many fluorohydrocarbon derivatives have been prepared.

The reactions shown in Figs. 1 and 2 illustrate some of the preparative methods used in fluorocarbon chemistry; many of these parallel familiar reactions used in hydrocarbon chemistry (*e.g.*, permanganate oxidation of olefins to acids), but some are peculiar to fluorocarbon chemistry in particular (*e.g.*, thermal dimerisation of olefins to cyclobutanes) or to halogenocarbon chemistry in general (*e.g.*, nucleophilic displacement of fluorine from hexafluorobenzene). Noteworthy is the fact that perfluoroalkyl Grignard reagents, *e.g.*, CF_3MgI, and perfluoroalkyl-lithium compounds, *e.g.*, n-C_3F_7Li, are usually troublesome to prepare and manipulate, with the result that their use tends to be avoided.

2. Compounds of low fluorine content

In general, the synthesis of a monofluorinated organic compound presents no special problems: one of the methods for the introduction of fluorine at a specific site must be applied at an appropriate stage, and care must then be taken to ensure that no reagents used in any subsequent stages will effect fluorine removal. *Gem.*-difluoro-compounds and trifluoromethyl compounds can be prepared by treatment of appropriate substrates with antimony fluorides or sulphur tetrafluoride (see p. 26), but the introduction of two, three, or, in some cases, four fluorine atoms at different sites must normally be effected by multiple use of monofluorination procedures. For example, 1,2,4,5-tetrafluorobenzene can be prepared as shown in the annexed scheme, but it is not possible to apply the reaction sequence once more and thus obtain pentafluorobenzene since the tetrafluorobenzene is converted into 2,5-difluorobenzoquinone on treatment with a nitrating mixture.

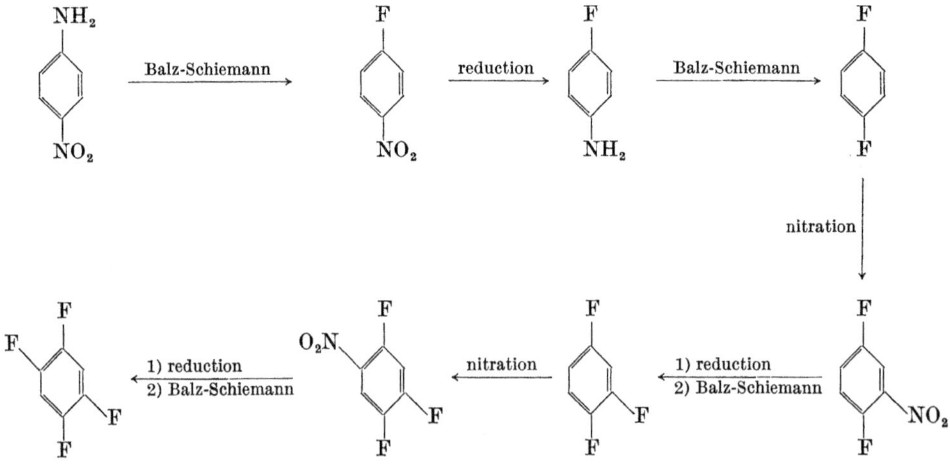

C. Properties and reactions of organic fluorine compounds

The factors responsible for the characteristic properties and reactions of organic fluorine compounds are: (i) the great strength of the C—F bond [for example, D(C—F) in $C_6H_5F = 115$ kcal/mole; *cf.* D(C—Cl) in $C_6H_5Cl = 86$ kcal/mole, D(C—Br) in $C_6H_5Br = 71$ kcal/mole], (ii) the relatively small size of the fluorine atom (van der Waals radius 1.35 Å; *cf.* hydrogen 1.2 Å, chlorine 1.8 Å), and (iii) the powerful electronic effects, inductive and resonance, associated with the presence of fluorine in a molecule. In the following discussion these factors will be used to explain some of the characteristic properties of fluorocarbons, a few fluorocarbon derivatives, and some organic compounds of low fluorine content.

1. Fluorocarbons and their derivatives

a) Alkanes

Saturated fluorocarbons, both acyclic and cyclic, are characterised by outstanding chemical and thermal stabilities. They are unaffected by boiling concentrated acids and alkalis, and by oxidising and reducing agents under normal conditions — properties which are due partly to steric shielding of the carbon backbone by the fluorine atoms, and partly to the inability of an attacking agent to coordinate on to the fluorine atoms because of the octet restriction. Fluorocarbons react with glass or silica at temperatures above 400° to give carbon dioxide and silicon tetrafluoride, and fusion with sodium or potassium at 550° converts them quantitatively into carbon and the appropriate alkali fluoride. Other active metals will also strip fluorine from fluorocarbons at elevated temperatures, and use is made of this for the controlled defluorination of alicyclic fluorocarbons to perfluoro-aromatic compounds, *e.g.*,

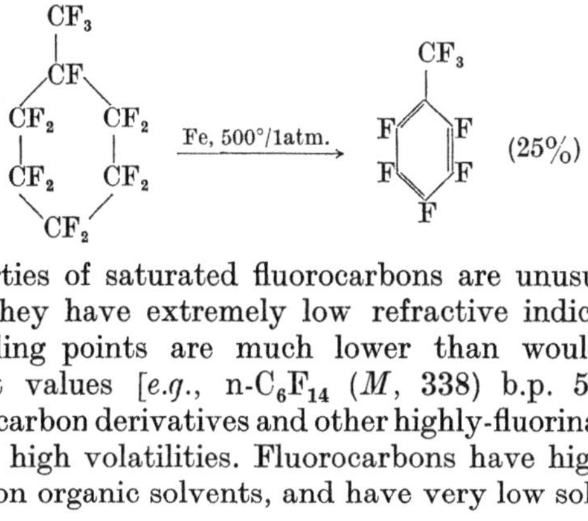

The physical properties of saturated fluorocarbons are unusual; due to low intermolecular forces, they have extremely low refractive indices and surface tensions, and their boiling points are much lower than would be expected from molecular weight values [*e.g.*, n-C_6F_{14} (*M*, 338) b.p. 57°; *cf.* n-C_6H_{14} (*M*, 86) b.p. 69°]. Fluorocarbon derivatives and other highly-fluorinated compounds also have unexpectedly high volatilities. Fluorocarbons have high densities, are poorly soluble in common organic solvents, and have very low solvent power.

b) Arenes

The only readily-prepared perfluoro-aromatic compound is hexafluorobenzene. It is a colourless liquid, b.p. 80.5° (*cf.* C_6H_6, b.p. 80°), which is readily attacked by nucleophilic reagents to yield pentafluorophenyl derivatives and fluoride ion (see Fig. 2):

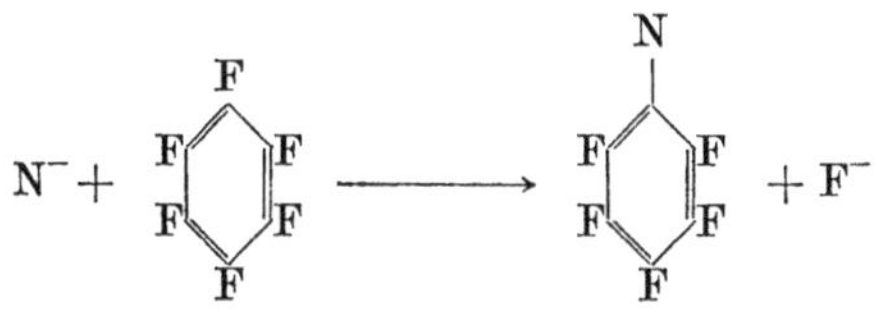

(N=H, NH_2, OH, SH, CH_3, *etc.*)

Neither hexafluorobenzene nor any other perfluoro-aromatic compound would be expected to undergo electrophilic substitution since this would require the elimination of fluorine as a cation, F^+ (see p. 4). This may be the reason why such reactions do not appear to have been studied, although electrophilic reagents have been used to hydrolyse perfluorotoluene to pentafluorobenzoic acid and to replace the hydrogen in pentafluorobenzene by bromine or iodine:

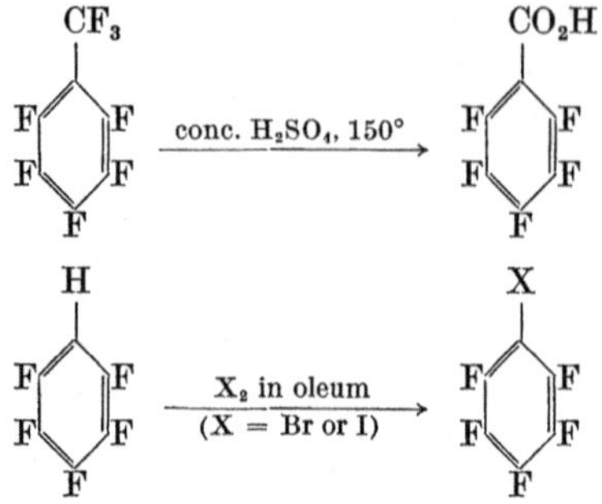

Information in the literature on free-radical attack on perfluoroarenes appears to be restricted to the photochemical chlorination of hexafluorobenzene to 1,2,3,4,5,6-hexachlorohexafluorocyclohexane.

At the present time, industrial interest in hexafluorobenzene derivatives runs high, mainly because polymers prepared from monomers belonging to this class of compound may meet some of the current demands for chemically inert materials with exceptionally high thermal stabilities.

c) Hydrides

Compounds of type R_FH (R_F = perfluoro-alkyl or -cycloalkyl) can be considered as fluorocarbon hydrides just as methyl fluoride, for example, is a hydrocarbon fluoride. The hydrogen in a fluorocarbon hydride is only weakly acidic and resists removal by basic reagents, but it can undergo homolytic substitution. Fluoroform, for example, exchanges $< 0.05\%$ of its hydrogen for deuterium when shaken with a 4% solution of sodium hydroxide in deuterium oxide for 1,121 hours; similar treatment converts chloroform completely into deutero-chloroform in < 2 hours. Undecafluorocyclohexane can be dehydrofluorinated to decafluorocyclohexene by prolonged heating with $10N$ potassium hydroxide solution. Chlorination and bromination of fluoroform at 500—700° yields the halides CF_3Cl and CF_3Br, respectively; the former product can also be obtained by photochemical chlorination of fluoroform.

d) Halides

A halogen atom (Cl, Br, or I) in a perfluoro-alkyl or -cycloalkyl halide shows unusual stability and cannot be displaced by nucleophilic reagents. The C—Cl and C—Br bonds in these compounds also resist homolytic cleavage, but the C—I bond in a perfluoroalkyl iodide breaks homolytically under the influence of heat or light. Trifluoroiodomethane, for example, is inert to moist silver oxide, silver cyanide, silver nitrite, aqueous potassium hydroxide, or potassium phthalimide at temperatures up to 150° (*cf.* CH_3I), and at higher temperatures complete destruction of the iodide occurs with the formation of fluoride ion. When heated or exposed to ultraviolet light, however, trifluoroiodomethane decomposes to yield trifluoromethyl radicals and iodine atoms:

$$CF_3I \xrightarrow{\Delta \text{ or } h\nu} CF_3\cdot + I\cdot$$

and this property has enabled it to be used in the synthesis of many fluorocarbon derivatives. In particular, use of trifluoroiodomethane has enabled many trifluoromethyl derivatives of metals, metalloids, and non-metals to be prepared (LAGOWSKI 1959; BANKS and HASZELDINE 1961; EMELÉUS 1962).

Fluoroform is formed when trifluoroiodomethane is heated with alcoholic potash — a result which demonstrates the positive nature of the iodine:

$$OH^- \; \overset{\delta+}{I}\text{—}\overset{\delta-}{C}F_3 \longrightarrow HOI + CF_3^- \xrightarrow[\text{solvent}]{H^+ \text{ from}} CHF_3$$

It might be expected that the powerful inductive effect of the fluorine atoms in trifluoroiodomethane, in addition to reversing the normal polarity of the C—I bond, would increase the positive nature of the carbon and thus encourage nucleophilic attack on this atom; such attack must be effectively prevented by the size of the fluorine atoms.

Perfluoroalkyl iodides react with magnesium under special conditions at low temperatures to yield Grignard reagents. These undergo the normal reactions associated with Grignard reagents, but must be used at temperatures below 0° to prevent their decomposition, which probably proceeds *via* fluorocarbanion formation (HASZELDINE 1956), *e.g.*,

$$CF_3CF_2CF_2MgI \longrightarrow CF_3CF_2\overset{-}{C}F_2 + \overset{+}{Mg}I$$

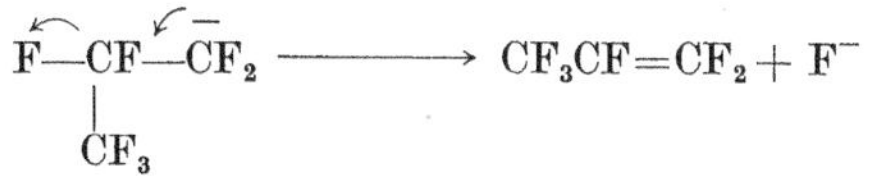

$$CF_3CF_2\overset{-}{C}F_2 \xrightarrow{\text{solvent}} CF_3CF_2CHF_2$$

Perfluoroalkyl-lithium compounds are also known but are only stable at low temperatures (LAGOWSKI 1959).

Fluorocarbon *vic.*-dihalides can be dehalogenated by metals, notably zinc, to fluoro-olefins:

$$\text{—CFXCFY— } + Zn \rightarrow \text{—CF=CF— } + ZnXY$$
$$(X, Y = Cl, Br, \text{ or } I)$$

Cases are known where X = F, Y = Cl, Br, or I, *e.g.*,

$$CF_3CF_2CHClF \xrightarrow[C_2H_5OH]{\text{Zn in refluxing}} CF_3CF{=}CHF$$

e) Olefins

In contrast to hydrocarbon olefins, highly-fluorinated olefins characteristically react with nucleophiles under mild conditions and resist electrophilic attack; this is a direct consequence of the electronegativity of fluorine, which renders the olefinic bond electron-deficient. Even fluoride ion, a relatively weak nucleophile, will attack a fluoro-olefin, and MILLER et al. (1960) have pointed out that for unsaturated fluorocarbons, fluoride ion occupies a position as a nucleophile which is analogous to that of a proton as an electrophile for unsaturated hydrocarbons:

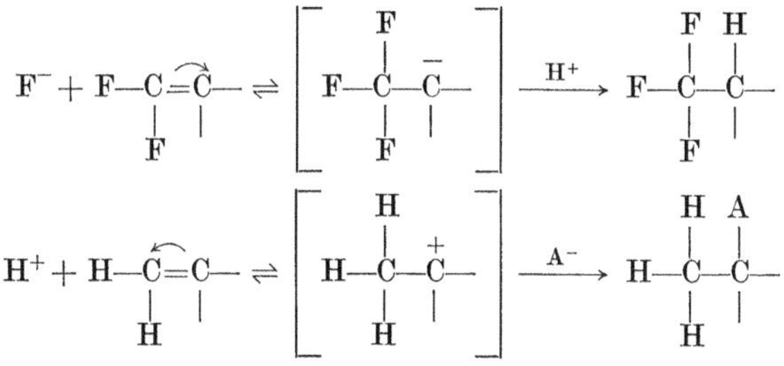

Some examples of additions to the double bonds of fluoro-olefins that are initiated by nucleophilic attack are annexed. It will be noted that the anionic part of the addendum becomes attached to the difluoromethylene group of a fluoro-olefin $CF_2{=}CXY$ ($X, Y = H$, Cl, Br, or fluoroalkyl), and it is concluded that the olefin must be polarised in the sense $\overset{\delta+}{CF_2}{=}\overset{\delta-}{C}XY$ due to mesomeric interaction of the lone pairs on fluorine with the double bond:

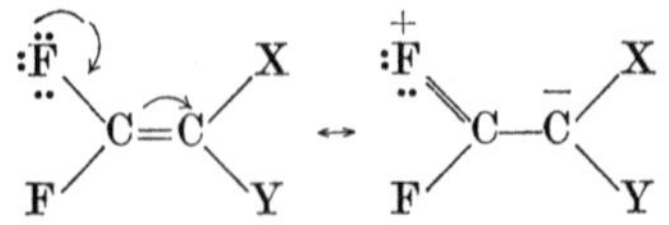

$$CH_3SH + CF_2{=}CF_2 \xrightarrow{\text{NaOH aq.}} CH_3SCF_2CHF_2$$

$$C_2H_5OH + CF_2{=}CFCl \xrightarrow{C_2H_5ONa} C_2H_5OCF_2CHFCl$$

$$C_6H_5OH + CF_2{=}CCl_2 \xrightarrow{\text{KOH aq.}} C_6H_5OCF_2CHCl_2$$

$$(C_2H_5)_2NH + CF_2{=}CFCl \longrightarrow (C_2H_5)_2NCF_2CHFCl$$

$$CF_2{=}CFCF_3 \xrightarrow{KF,\ HCONH_2} CF_3CHFCF_3$$

Fluoro-olefins are susceptible to attack by free radicals, and much use is made of this property in synthesis. Several industrially-important materials are made by free-radical addition polymerisation of fluoro-olefins (BANKS and HASZELDINE 1959; BANKS et al. 1961) (see Table 13, p. 47).

A remarkable property of fluoro-olefins of the type $CF_2{=}CFR$ ($R = H$, F, Cl, CN, CF_3, $CF{=}CF_2$, C_6H_5) is their ability to dimerise to cyclobutane derivatives under the influence of heat; apparently, in all cases except those of trifluoroethylene and hexafluoropropene, only the head-to-head adducts are formed (ROBERTS and SHARTS 1962):

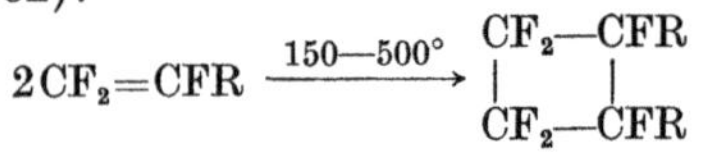

Tetrafluoroethylene and chlorotrifluoroethylene have been co-dimerised with a variety of olefinic compounds to yield cyclobutane derivatives, and a reaction of particular interest is that between tetrafluoroethylene and cyclopentadiene since this forms the first stage of a novel synthesis of tropolone in 20 % yield (DRYSDALE et al. 1958):

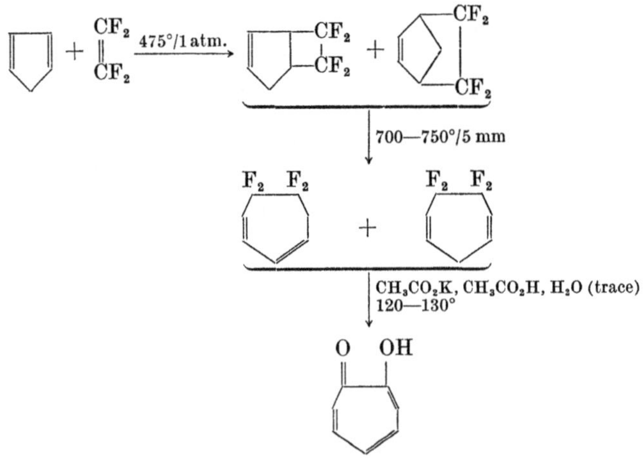

The facile hydrolysis of the two difluoromethylene groups in the final stage is noteworthy.

f) Carboxylic acids

The saturated perfluoro-carboxylic acids are very strong organic acids because of the powerful inductive effect of the perfluoroalkyl group (see Table 9). Chemically, they undergo many of the reactions associated with alkanoic acids (see Fig. 1 for examples); a reaction which has no direct hydrocarbon counterpart is the pyrolysis of an alkali-metal salt of a perfluoroalkanecarboxylic acid to yield a perfluoro-olefin, *e.g.*,

$$CF_3CF_2CF_2CO_2Na \xrightarrow{200^\circ} CF_3CF{=}CF_2 + NaF$$

This reaction probably proceeds *via* a fluorocarbanion produced by decarboxylation of the carboxylate ion, *e.g.*,

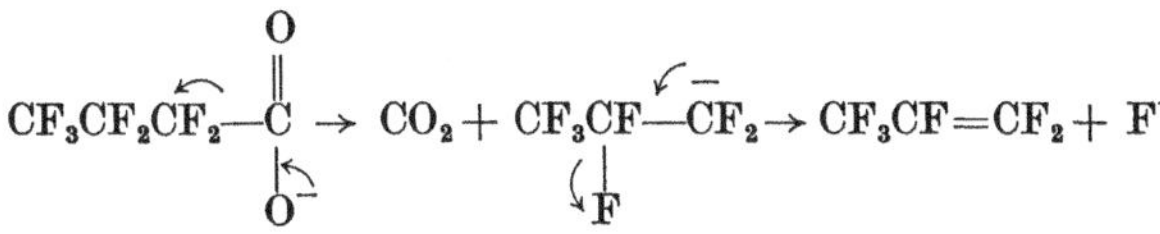

The hydrocarbon counterpart of this reaction is olefin formation by loss of a proton from a carbonium ion.

Trifluoroacetic acid, b.p. 72°, is the most important perfluoroalkanecarboxylic acid. In addition to being the starting point in the synthesis of many compounds containing a trifluoromethyl group, this acid, in the form of trifluoroacetic anhydride and of peroxytrifluoroacetic acid, finds use as a reagent in organic chemistry (MUSGRAVE 1954; HUDLICKÝ 1961). Trifluoroacetic anhydride is most frequently used in the esterification of hydroxy compounds: when it is added to an acid, a mixed anhydride is formed which, by virtue of the electron-attracting power of a trifluoromethyl group, ionises slightly to provide an acylium cation and is therefore a powerful acylating agent, *e.g.*,

Table 9. *Dissociation constants of some fluorinated acids*

Acid	Dissociation constant (K_a)
CH_3CO_2H	1.8×10^{-5}
CH_2FCO_2H	2.2×10^{-3}
CHF_2CO_2H	5.7×10^{-2}
CF_3CO_2H	5.5×10^{-1}
$CF_3CH_2CO_2H$ . . .	1.0×10^{-3}
$CF_3CH_2CH_2CO_2H$ . .	3.2×10^{-5}
$CF_3CH_2CH_2CH_2CO_2H$	1.56×10^{-5}
n-$C_3H_7CO_2H$	1.5×10^{-5}
n-$C_3F_7CO_2H$	6.8×10^{-1}

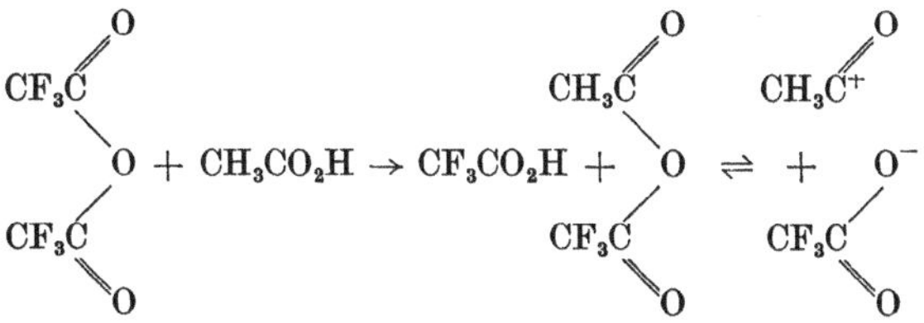

Acylation of alcohols and phenols often proceeds spontaneously at room temperature and is complete within a few minutes, so the method is particularly valuable for use with acid-labile hydroxy-compounds. Trifluoroacetic anhydride alone reacts readily with alcohols to yield trifluoroacetyl derivatives which, by virtue of the inductive effect of the trifluoromethyl group, can be hydrolysed back to the parent alcohol and trifluoroacetic acid merely by treatment with water or very weak alkali at room temperature; this leads to the use of the trifluoroacetyl group as a protecting group in carbohydrate and nucleic acid chemistry. Peroxytrifluoroacetic acid, made by adding 90% hydrogen peroxide to trifluoroacetic acid or its anhydride, is a powerful oxidising and hydroxylating agent.

2. Organic compounds of low fluorine content

a) Aliphatic fluorides

In 1936, HENNE and MIDGLEY wrote: "The first four members of the normal alkyl monofluoride series are stable and distil without decomposition. Members of the series higher than amyl fluoride show a tendency to decompose spontaneously to hydrogen fluoride and ethylenic hydrocarbons. This tendency increases with structural complexity and becomes so marked in secondary and tertiary fluorides that it is impossible to prepare them free from olefins. Similarly cyclohexyl fluoride decomposes spontaneously to cyclohexylene." Not unnaturally, this statement gave rise to a popular belief (even asserted by some authors to be a "general rule") that the presence of a single fluorine atom in an aliphatic compound causes instability. Since 1948, however, it has been amply demonstrated that *all* 1-fluoroalkanes are very stable compounds, and that secondary and tertiary alkyl fluorides can be prepared although they are often thermally unstable. PATTISON and his co-workers, for example, have prepared several hundred primary monofluorides during the course of their study of toxic aliphatic fluorine compounds, and found no evidence for instability that can be associated with the presence of a C—F bond.

The order of reactivity of a C-halogen bond in alkyl halides is $C—I > C—Br > C—Cl \gg C—F$, as would be expected from the values of the bond dissociation energies (49, 60, 78, and 105 kcal/mole). Thus, primary alkyl fluorides show remarkable resistance to attack by nucleophilic reagents, and even secondary and tertiary alkyl fluorides are relatively unreactive. The data presented in Table 10 are for the bimolecular substitution and elimination reactions which occur when alkyl monofluorides and their bromo-analogues are treated with alcoholic sodium ethoxide. These show that the fluorides react far more slowly than the bromides, and that the influence of alkyl-group structure on the rates of substitution and elimination is normal, *i.e.*, for substitution the rate sequence is primary > secondary > tertiary, and *vice versa* for elimination. Examination of the activation energies and Arrhenius parameters for these reactions has led to the important conclusion that solvation of incipient fluoride ion in the transition state allows a

Table 10. *Elimination and substitution in alkyl fluorides and bromides*
(From CHAPMAN and LEVY 1952)

k_s = velocity coefficient for bimolecular substitution in l. mole^{-1} sec^{-1}
k_E = velocity coefficient for bimolecular elimination in l. mole^{-1} sec^{-1}

Alkyl group	Bromides (at 55.0°)		Fluorides (at 120.0°)	
	$10^5 k_s$	$10^5 k_E$	$10^5 k_s$	$10^5 k_E$
$CH_3CH_2CH_2CH_2CH_2—$	35.7	3.5	1.41	0.02
$(CH_3)_2CHCH_2CH_2—$	—	—	0.49	0.05
$CH_3CH_2CH(CH_3)CH_2—$	—	—	0.30	0.04
$CH_3CH_2CH(CH_3)—$	2.3	10.3	0.027	0.067
$CH_3CH_2CH_2CH(CH_3)—$	2.0	8.3	0.014	0.060
$(CH_3)_3C—$	3	90	0.007	0.139
$(CH_3)_2(C_2H_5)C—$	6	177	0.006	0.121
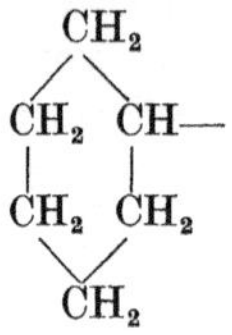	—	—	0.005	0.038

reaction to follow a course much more economical of activation energy than would otherwise be possible in view of the great strength of the C—F bond (CHAPMAN and LEVY 1952).

Grignard reagents will readily displace fluorine from primary alkyl fluorides as fluoride ion (HOFFMANN 1950; PATTISON and HOWELL 1956; MIROSEVIC-SORGO and SAUNDERS 1959).

Alkyl monofluorides resist solvolysis under neutral conditions; thus no detectable reaction occurs when molar ethanolic solutions of cyclohexyl fluoride or tertiary amyl fluoride are heated at 140° for 200 hours and 120° for 4 hours, respectively (CHAPMAN and LEVY 1952). Acid catalysis has been observed in solvolyses of benzyl fluoride, cyclohexyl fluoride, tertiary amyl fluoride, and tertiary butyl fluoride, however, and the rate-determining steps proposed for these reactions were (i) direct reaction of alkyl fluoride with hydronium ion to give a carbonium ion (CHAPMAN and LEVY 1952):

$$RF + H_3O^+ \rightarrow R^+ + HF + H_2O$$

and (ii) reaction of a hydrogen-bonded fluoride-hydronium ion complex with solvent (MILLER and BERNSTEIN 1948):

$$RF\cdots\cdots H_3O^+ + H_2O \rightarrow RO^+H_2 + HF + H_2O$$

More recently, SWAIN and SPALDING (1960) have investigated the solvolysis of benzyl fluoride in 90 % aqueous acetone solution containing perchloric or sulphuric acid and concluded that hydrolysis proceeds *via* a transition state structurally close to $C_6H_5CH_2FH^+$.

Strong Lewis acids promote heterolytic cleavage of the C—F bonds in alkyl monofluorides, which thus exhibit a high order of reactivity in Friedel-Crafts alkylations (CALLOWAY 1937), and in the presence of boron trifluoride will promote isomerisation, disproportionation, and self-alkylation of *iso*alkanes (MUSGRAVE 1954). An interesting reaction is the conversion of 3-fluoro-1-methyl-cyclohexa-1,4-diene into toluene by boron trifluoride (OLAH et al. 1958):

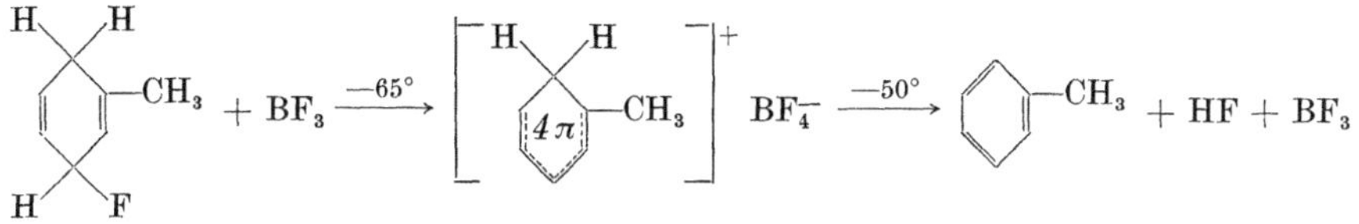

So far, all attempts to prepare a Grignard reagent from an alkyl monofluoride appear to have failed, although PATTISON and HOWELL (1956), using special reaction conditions, have found evidence for the formation of Grignard reagents of the type $X(CH_2)_nMgF$ ($X =$ Cl, Br, or I; $n = 6$—10) from the appropriate α-fluoro-ω-halogenoalkanes.

With the exception of the first two members of the series, α, ω-difluoroalkanes resemble 1-fluoroalkanes in reactivity. 1,2-Difluoroethane is reported to react with water to yield ethylene glycol and to decompose at 0° into butadiene and hydrogen fluoride (HENNE and MIDGLEY 1936). 1,3-Difluoropropane is much more stable, but does lose fluorine as fluoride ion fairly readily when refluxed with ethanolic sodium ethoxide; however, it is less reactive than the corresponding dichloro-compound (HOFFMANN 1949).

gem.-Difluoroalkanes are normally very stable compounds and resist dehydrofluorination to olefins and hydrolysis to carbonyl compounds. For instance, the compound $CH_3CF_2CH{=}CH_2$ cannot be dehydrofluorinated with solid potassium hydroxide at 200°; and 1,1-difluoro-2-bromoethane must be heated to 200° with water and mercuric oxide before the CF_2 group is attacked (note the resistance of the bromine towards replacement — see p. 43):

$$CH_2BrCHF_2 \xrightarrow[150^\circ]{H_2O,\ HgO} CH_2OHCHF_2$$

$$CH_2BrCHF_2 \xrightarrow[200^\circ]{H_2O,\ HgO} CH_2OHCHO$$

However, a difluoromethylene group lying in the β-position in a carboxylic acid, or adjacent to an olefinic bond or a nitrogen, oxygen, or sulphur atom is activated and can be readily hydrolysed, *e.g.*,

$$CHFClCF_2N(C_2H_5)_2 \xrightarrow{H_2O} CHFClCON(C_2H_5)_2$$

$$CH_2ClCF_2OC_2H_5 \xrightarrow{H_2O} CH_2ClCO_2C_2H$$

The presence of fluorine or perfluoroalkyl substituents on the β-carbon atom of the ether reduces the susceptibility of the α-CF_2 group to hydrolysis; thus the ether $CHF_2CF_2OC_2H_5$ requires treatment with concentrated sulphuric acid to hydrolyse it to ethyl difluoroacetate, and perfluoro-ethers, *e.g.*, $CF_3CF_2OCF_2CF_3$, show a hydrolytic stability comparable with that of fluorocarbons.

Aliphatic trifluoromethyl groups are normally very stable and unreactive, and it is interesting to note the difference in hydrolytic stability between the CF_3 and CCl_3 groups in 1,1,1-trichloro-4,4,4-trifluorobut-2-ene:

$$CF_3CH{=}CHCCl_3 \xrightarrow[80^\circ]{\text{conc. } H_2SO_4} CF_3CH{=}CHCO_2H$$

Due to the inductive effect of the fluorine atoms, a hydrogen atom adjacent to a CF_3 or CF_2 group is strongly acidic and readily eliminated as a proton; thus treatment of compounds such as $CF_3CH_2CH_2X$ and $CF_3CH{=}CHX$ ($X{=}Cl$, Br, or I) with a base enables fluoro-olefins and -acetylenes, respectively, to be synthesised, *e.g.*,

$$CF_3CH_2CH_2Br \xrightarrow[62^\circ]{\text{powdered KOH}} CF_3CH{=}CH_2$$

In such a dehydrohalogenation reaction, the ease of elimination of halogen hydracid usually decreases in the order $HI > HBr > HCl > HF$. A halogen atom on the carbon atom adjacent to the polyfluoro-group, *e.g.*, CF_3CHXCH_3, $CF_3CX{=}CH_2$, is stabilised, making its removal as halogen hydracid HX difficult. Furthermore, elimination of halogen hydracid does not occur readily when either the hydrogen atom or the halogen atom taking part is attached to a CF_2 group (LOVELACE et al. 1958).

A hydrogen atom adjacent to a polyfluoro-group is substantially protected from attack by atomic reagents. For example, in the photochemical chlorination of 1,1,1-trifluoropropane, $CF_3CH_2CH_3$, attack occurs mainly on the terminal CH_3 group, and at low temperatures the halogenation proceeds step-wise to yield the trichloro-compound $CF_3CH_2CCl_3$ before attack on the central carbon atom begins (HUDLICKÝ 1961). That even a single fluorine substituent can exert a directive influence in free-radical halogenation reactions is illustrated by the values quoted for the relative selectivities shown by the different halogen atoms when abstracting hydrogen from 1-fluorobutane (TEDDER 1960):

	CH_2F—	—CH_2—	—CH_2—	—CH_3
Fluorination at 20°	<0.3	0.8	1.0	1
Chlorination at 78°	0.9	1.7	3.7	1
Bromination at 146°	10	9	88	1

Halogen atoms on carbon atoms adjacent to polyfluoro groups are stable and difficult to replace or eliminate (see the above discussion on dehydrohalogenation), but this stabilising effect does not extend beyond the adjacent carbon atom. Thus it is difficult to effect nucleophilic displacement of chlorine, bromine, or iodine from halides of the type CF_3CH_2X and CHF_2CH_2X (X = Cl, Br, or I), but the C—X bonds in halides of the type $CF_3CH_2CH_2X$ and $CHF_2CH_2CH_2X$ show normal reactivity.

Grignard reagents cannot be prepared from the halogeno-ethanes CF_3CH_2Cl and CF_3CH_2Br, but at low temperatures the corresponding iodo-compound will combine with magnesium to yield 1,1,1-trifluoroethyl magnesium iodide, which is unstable and decomposes into vinylidene fluoride, $CH_2{=}CF_2$, presumably *via* loss of fluoride ion from the carbanion $CF_3\overline{C}H_2$ (see p. 37). Halides of the type $R_F(CH_2)_nCH_2X$ ($R_F = CHF_2$ or perfluoroalkyl; n = 1,2,3, *etc.*; X = Cl, Br, or I) form normal Grignard reagents.

b) Aromatic fluorides

Although the halogens are capable of withdrawing electron density from saturated carbon chains by induction, they are also capable of supplying π-electron density to conjugated systems by a mechanism called the mesomeric effect and their ability to do this decreases in the order F > Cl > Br > I. In the case of an aromatic system, mesomeric release of electrons from a halogen substituent in the nucleus causes an increase in electron density at the ortho and para positions (resonance forms of type I, II, and III may be drawn)

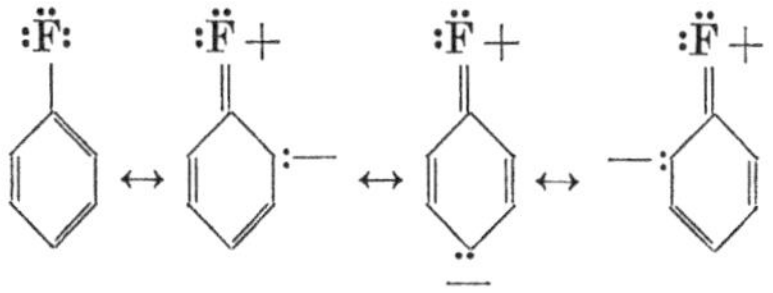

(I) (II) (III)

and offsets the strong inductive effect. Evidence for this is provided by the acidity and basicity constants quoted in Table 11. It will be seen that a para-fluorine substituent only slightly strengthens benzoic acid, weakens phenol as an acid, and barely succeeds in weakening aniline as a base. Fluorine, like the other halogens, brings about ortho-para substitution in, accompanied by deactivation of, the aromatic nucleus in which it is located.

Table 11. *Dissociation constants* (From Ingold 1953)

X =	F	Cl	Br	I	H	
p-$XC_6H_4CO_2H$ . .	7.22	10.5	10.7	11.8	6.27	$K_a \times 10^5$ in H_2O/25°
p-XC_6H_4OH . . .	0.26	1.32	1.55	2.19	0.32	$K_a \times 10^{10}$ in 30% aq. ethanol/25°
p-$XC_6H_4NH_2$ . . .	120	28.8	21.9	15.1	126	$K_b \times 10^{12}$ in 30% aq. ethanol/25°

The many studies of the comparative ease of displacement of the halogens in various nucleophilic substitution reactions show that the four halogens do not stand in any constant order of replaceability (Bunnett and Zahler 1951). In reactions of unsubstituted monohalogenobenzenes with nucleophilic reagents such as sodium ethoxide, potassium amide, and piperidine, the ease of halogen displacement increases in the order F < Cl < Br < I. On the other hand, fluorine is by far the most easily displaced halogen when it lies ortho or para to an electron attracting group; for example, the reactivities of the *p*-nitrohalogenobenzenes toward sodium ethoxide are in the ratio F:Cl:Br:I= 3,100:13.6:11.8:1 at 90.8°. The reason for this appears to be that the controlling factor in these substitutions is the positiveness of the carbon atom adjacent to the halogen and not the ease of fission of the carbon-halogen bond. The lability of the fluorine in 2,4-dinitrofluorobenzene is responsible for the use of this compound for identification of the amino terminal units in proteins and polypeptides.

IV. Analysis of fluorine compounds

This topic is so wide that only the barest outline can be given here. It can be divided into two main sections — the determination of fluorine in its compounds, and the application of physical methods to analysis of fluorine compounds.

A. Determination of fluorine

(Horton 1960; Macdonald 1962)

This can be considered under two headings:

1. Conversion of fluorine into a determinable form

Fluorine is generally determined as fluoride ion, and the conversion of the fluorine in fluorinated compounds into fluoride ion is often difficult. For organic fluorine compounds, methods include fusion with sodium or potassium, combustion with silica to give volatile silicon tetrafluoride, and decomposition by a sodium/diphenyl complex.

2. Determination of fluoride ion

The classical gravimetric procedure, applicable to relatively large amounts, is precipitation as calcium fluoride. Lead chlorofluoride is another convenient form for gravimetric or titrimetric determination.

For smaller amounts of fluoride, titration with thorium nitrate has been widely used, but other methods, including ion-exchange techniques and colorimetric methods, are probably more reliable.

B. Physical methods

1. Infrared spectroscopy

No recent attempt to correlate infrared spectra with structure in compounds containing fluorine has been made. The subject is a difficult one since the stretching frequencies for, say, carbon-fluorine bonds, occur in a region where many other absorption bands are found. However a number of empirical correlations are available (Bellamy 1958; Weiblen 1954).

2. Nuclear magnetic resonance spectroscopy

(Pople et al. 1959; Muetterties and Phillips 1962)

^{19}F has a nuclear spin quantum number of $^1/_2$, like ^1H, and is one of the most easily examined nuclei. A considerable amount of work on fluorine resonance has already appeared, and this method is a very powerful one for examining the structures of fluorine compounds. The technique is also potentially a method of quantitive analysis for fluorine, but few examples of this particular use have been reported.

3. Mass spectroscopy

(MAJER 1961)

This technique has been applied with some success to a limited number of highly-fluorinated organic compounds, but more information on a wider range of compounds is needed.

V. Industrial aspects of fluorine chemistry

(LEECH 1960; BARBOUR 1961; FINGER 1961; RUDGE 1962)

In the foregoing discussion frequent mention has been made of industrially important fluorine compounds. The vital intermediate in the manufacture of these is anhydrous hydrogen fluoride, obtained from fluorspar, and the fact that 160,000 tons of this were produced in America during 1961 (1955 output: 66,600 tons; 1960 output: 115,000 tons) gives some idea of the healthy size of the fluorine-chemical industry. The main outlets for anhydrous hydrogen fluoride are shown in Table 12; some important commercially available fluorides and their uses are listed in Table 13. The intensity of current research in the area of fluorine chemistry must surely result in the development of many more useful products, new applications for established materials, and the continued growth of the fluorine-chemical industry.

Table 12. *Uses of anhydrous hydrogen fluoride in the U.S.A.* (Consumption during 1961)

Use	Short tons	% of total
Preparation of organic fluorides	64,000	40.0
Production of aluminium	53,000	33.1
Uranium production	18,000	11.3
Petroleum alkylation	7,000	4.4
Preparation of inorganic fluorides	5,000	3.1
Production of special metals	3,000	1.9
Etching and frosting of glass	2,000	1.3
Other uses	3,000	1.9

Table 13. *Some commercially available fluorine compounds and their uses.*

Compound	Uses
Inorganic fluorides	
Aluminium fluoride, AlF_3	Aluminium production. Flux and opacifier in ceramics production. Coatings for arc welding rods.
Antimony trifluoride, SbF_3	Preparation of organic fluorides.
Barium fluoride, BaF_2	Light metal industry. Ingredient of some ceramic enamels.
Boron trifluoride, BF_3	Catalyst in alkylation, esterification, and polymerisation reactions (*e.g.*, preparation of coumarone-indene resins). Gaseous flux in the internal brazing of hollow steel propellers.
Calcium fluoride, CaF_2 (fluorspar)	Hydrogen fluoride production. Flux in steel industry. Flux and opacifier in glass and ceramics production.
Chlorine trifluoride, ClF_3	Uranium production. Potential rocket fuel. Chemical cutter for drilling oil wells. Preparation of chlorofluorocarbon lubricants.

(Continued Table 13)

Compound	Uses
Chromium trifluoride, CrF_3	Mordant for treatment of wool before dyeing.
Fluorine, F_2	Uranium production. Potential rocket fuel. Preparation of high-valency metal fluorides.
Hydrogen fluoride, HF	See Table 12.
Lead fluoride, PbF_2	Flame colorant in pyrotechnics.
Magnesium fluoride, MgF_2	Production of "bloomed" optical components.
Perchloryl fluoride, $FClO_3$	Preparation of monofluoro steroids. Potential rocket fuel. Gaseous dielectric.
Potassium fluoride, KF	Preparation of organic fluorides.
Sodium fluoride, NaF	Wood preservative, fungicide, and insecticide. Fluoridation of water. Production of ceramics. As an electrolyte modifier in light metal production.
Stannous fluoride, SnF_2	Toothpaste additive — prevents dental caries.
Sulphur hexafluoride, SF_6	Gaseous dielectric in high-voltage equipment.
Ammonium bifluoride, $NH_4F \cdot HF$	Frosting of glass. Brewery sanitation. Electrodeposition of special alloys. As an ingredient of proprietary cleaning and polishing solutions for aluminium and its alloys.
Fluoroboric acid, HBF_4 and its salts (Na^+, K^+, NH_4^+)	Cleaning and pickling of metals—fused KBF_4 is a good solvent for many metallic oxides. Electroplating, especially of lead and tin.
Fluosilicic acid, H_2SiF_6 and its salts (Na^+, K^+, NH_4^+, Ba^{++}, Mg^{++}, Pb^{++}, Zn^{++})	Water fluoridation. Electroplating. Concrete hardeners. Wood preservatives. Textile sours. Flux in casting of light metals. Production of synthetic mica. Extraction of zirconium. Ingredients of acid-resisting cements.
Potassium fluotitanate, K_2TiF_6	Additive to light metals to produce alloys containing definite amounts of titanium. Production of Al-Ti master alloys.
Sodium hexafluoroaluminate, Na_3AlF_6, (cryolite)	Electrolyte in the production of aluminium. Flux in steel making and production of light metals. Opacifier and flux in production of enamels, ceramic glazes, and glasses.
Organic fluorides	
Chlorofluoro-methanes and -ethanes, *e.g.*, CF_2Cl_2, CHF_2Cl, CF_2ClCF_2Cl.	Refrigerants. Aerosol propellents. Blowing agents for polyurethane foams. Intermediates in production of fluoropolymers.
Bromofluoromethanes, CF_3Br and CF_2Br_2	Fire extinguishing agents.
Bromochlorodifluoromethane, CF_2BrCl	Fire extinguishing agent.
1-Bromo-1-chloro-2,2,2-trifluoroethane, $CF_3CHBrCl$	Inhalation anaesthetic.
Octafluorocyclobutane, $\overline{CF_2CF_2CF_2CF_2}$	Aerosol propellent for foodstuffs.
Alkali-metal salts of long-chain perfluoroalkanesulphonic acids, *e.g.*, $C_8F_{17}SO_3K$	Inert surface-active agent for use in chromium plating industry.
Chromium salts of perfluoroalkanesulphonic acids $(R_FSO_3)_3Cr$	Used for imparting combined oil and water repellency to paper and textiles.
Perfluoroalkanecarboxylic acids, mainly CF_3CO_2H and n-$C_3F_7CO_2H$	Intermediates in chemical synthesis.
Sodium monofluoroacetate, CH_2FCO_2Na	Rodenticide.

(Continued Table 13)

Compound	Uses
Fluorinated steroids	Pharmaceuticals.
Dyes containing trifluoromethyl groups	Dyestuffs of increased light fastness.
Polychlorotrifluoroethylene $[-CF_2CFCl-]_n$	Inert oils, greases, waxes, and thermoplastic resins.
Polytetrafluoroethylene $[-CF_2CF_2-]_n$	Resin with outstanding chemical and thermal stability and excellent electrical characteristics. Very low coefficient of friction leads to non-stick applications.
Poly(vinylidene fluoride), $[-CH_2CF_2-]_n$	Thermoplastic resin.
Poly(vinyl fluoride), $[-CH_2CHF-]_n$	Thermoplastic resin.
Copolymer of tetrafluoroethylene with hexafluoropropene, $[-CF_2CF_2CF_2CF(CF_3)-]_n$	Thermoplastic resin similar to polytetrafluoroethylene but with lower softening point.
Copolymer of vinylidene fluoride with hexafluoropropene, $[-CH_2CF_2CF_2CF(CF_3)-]_n$	Chemically and thermally stable elastomer.
Copolymer of vinylidene fluoride with chlorotrifluoroethylene, $[-CH_2CF_2CF_2CFCl-]_n$	Chemically and thermally stable elastomer.
Methyl-3,3,3-trifluoropropyl silicone rubber, $[-(CF_3CH_2CH_2)(CH_3)SiO-]_n$	Chemically and thermally stable elastomer.

Text books on fluorine chemistry

BANKS, R. E.: Fluorocarbons and their Derivatives. London: Oldbourne Press 1965.

A small (161 pages) and inexpensive monograph containing a fully comprehensive account of the preparation and reactions of fluorocarbons and their derivatives (408 references).

FORCHE, E.: Herstellung, Reaktivität und Umwandlung von Fluorverbindungen. In: E. MÜLLER, Ed., Methoden der organischen Chemie (HOUBEN-WEYL), Halogenverbindungen, Band V/3, 1—502. Stuttgart: Georg Thieme Verlag 1962.

An excellent, fully comprehensive, account of the preparation and reactions of organic fluorine compounds.

HASZELDINE, R. N.: Fluorocarbon Derivatives. Royal Institute of Chemistry Monograph. No. 1, 1956.

A small (49 pages) monograph containing an account of some of the novel chemistry associated with fluorocarbons and their derivatives.

HASZELDINE, R. N., and A. G. SHARPE: Fluorine and Its Compounds. London: Methuen 1951.

A small (153 pages) inexpensive book containing a concise account of inorganic and organic fluorine chemistry. A good starting point for beginners.

HUDLICKÝ, M.: Chemistry of Organic Fluorine Compounds. Oxford, New York, Paris: Pergamon 1961 (Note: CZECH and GERMAN editions are also available).

A full account, with 1105 references, of organic fluorine chemistry; some actual experimental procedures are quoted, together with details of the preparation and methods of manipulation of inorganic fluorinating agents. This standard text should be consulted by all workers in the field. Mechanistic aspects of reactions involving fluorine compounds are seldom mentioned.

LOVELACE, A. M., D. A. RAUSCH, and W. POSTELNEK: Aliphatic Fluorine Compounds. American Chemical Society Monograph No. 138. New York: Reinhold 1958.

A reference book containing a collection of facts, mainly methods of preparation and physical constants, relating to aliphatic fluorides.

MELLOR, J. W.: Comprehensive Treatise on Inorganic and Theoretical Chemistry. Supplement II, Part I, 1—261. London: Longmans 1956.

A full account of inorganic fluorine chemistry, with a brief mention of fluorocarbons and analytical, biological, and spectroscopic aspects of fluorine chemistry.

PATTISON, F. L. M.: Toxic Aliphatic Fluorine Compounds. Amsterdam, London, New York, Princeton: Elsevier 1959.

This monograph provides the most complete survey yet published of the toxic effects of monofluorinated organic compounds.

PAVLATH, A. E., and A. J. LEFFLER: Aromatic Fluorine Compounds. New York: Reinhold 1962.

A comprehensive (820 pages) treatment of all aspects of the chemistry of aromatic compounds containing fluorine.

RUDGE, A. J.: The Manufacture and Use of Fluorine and Its Compounds. London: Oxford University Press 1962.

This small (87 pages) inexpensive book deals with industrial preparations and uses of inorganic and organic fluorides.

SAUNDERS, B. C.: Some Aspects of the Chemistry and Toxic Action of Organic Compounds containing Phosphorus and Fluorine. London: Cambridge University Press 1957.

SIMONS, J. H. (Ed.): Fluorine Chemistry. New York: Academic Press 1950 (vol. I), 1954 (vol. II), 1963 (vol. III), 1964 (vol. V).

Vol. I contains the following chapters:

Nonvolatile Inorganic Fluorides by H. J. EMELÉUS.
Volatile Inorganic Fluorides by A. B. BURG.
The Chemistry of the Fluoro Acids of Fourth, Fifth, and Sixth Group Elements by W. LANGE.
The Halogen Fluorides by H. S. BOOTH and J. T. PINKSTON.
Boron Trifluoride by H. S. BOOTH and D. R. MARTIN.
Hydrogen Fluoride by J. H. SIMONS.
Hydrogen Fluoride Catalysis by J. H. SIMONS.
Preparation of Fluorine by G. H. CADY.
Physical Properties of Fluorine by G. H. CADY.
The Theoretical Aspects of Fluorine Chemistry by G. GLOCKLER.
The Action of Elementary Fluorine upon Organic Compounds by L. A. BIGELOW.
Fluorocarbons and Their Production by J. H. SIMONS.
Fluorocarbons — Their Properties and Wartime Development by T. J. BRICE.
Fluorocarbon Derivatives by W. H. PEARLSON.
Aliphatic Chlorofluoro Compounds by J. D. PARK.
Fluorine Compounds in Glass Technology and Ceramics by W. A. WEYL.

Vol. II contains the following chapters:

Fluorine-containing Complex Salts and Acids by A. G. SHARPE.
Halogen Fluorides — Recent Advances by H. J. EMELÉUS.
Analytical Chemistry of Fluorine and Fluorine-containing Compounds by P. J. ELVING. C. A. HORTON and H. H. WILLARD
Organic Compounds Containing Fluorine by P. Tarrant.
Metallic Compounds Containing Fluorocarbon Radicals and Organometallic Compounds Containing Fluorine by H. J. EMELÉUS.
Fluorocarbon Chemistry by J. H. SIMONS.
The Infrared Spectra of Fluorocarbons and Related Compounds by D. G. WEIBLEN.

Vol. III:

Biological Effects of Organic Fluorides by H. C. HODGE, F. A. SMITH, and P. S. CHEN.

Vol. V contains the following chapters:

General Chemistry of Fluorine-Containing Compounds by J. H. SIMONS.
Physical Chemistry of Fluorocarbons by T. M. REED III.
Radiochemistry and Radiation Chemistry of Fluorine by JOHN A. WETHNGTON JR.
Industrial and Utilitarian Aspects of Fluorine Chemistry by A. G. BRYCE.

SLESSER, C., and S. R. SCHRAM (Eds.): The Preparation, Properties, and Technology of Fluorine and Organic Fluoro Compounds. National Nuclear Energy Series, Division VII, vol. I. New York, Toronto, London: McGraw-Hill 1951.
An account of the work carried out in America during the Second World War in connection with the Atomic Bomb (Manhattan) Project.

STACEY, M., J. C. TATLOW, and A. G. SHARPE (Eds.): Advances in Fluorine Chemistry. London: Butterworths 1960 (vol. 1), 1961 (vol. 2), 1963 (vol. 3).

Vol. 1 contains the following chapters:

The Halogen Fluorides — Their Preparation and Uses in Organic Chemistry by W. K. R. MUSGRAVE.
Transition Metal Fluorides and Their Complexes by A. G. SHARPE.
Fluoroboric Acids and Their Derivatives by D. W. A. SHARP.
The Electrochemical Process for the Synthesis of Fluoro-organic Compounds by J. BURDON and J. C. TATLOW.
Exhaustive Fluorinations of Organic Compounds with High-valency Metallic Fluorides by M. STACEY and J. C. TATLOW.

Vol. 2 contains the following chapters:

The Thermochemistry of Organic Fluorine Compounds by C. R. PATRICK.
Fluorine Resources and Fluorine Utilization by G. C. FINGER.
Mass Spectrometry of Fluorine Compounds by J. R. MAJER.
The Fluorination of Organic Compounds using Elementary Fluorine by J. M. TEDDER.
The Fluorides of the Actinide Elements by N. HODGE.
The Physiological Action of Organic Compounds Containing Fluorine by B. C. SAUNDERS.

Vol. 3 contains the following chapters:

Effects of Adjacent Perfluoroalkyl Groups on Carbonyl Reactivity by H. P. BRAENDLIN and E. T. MCBEE.
Perfluoroalkyl Derivatives of the Elements by H. C. CLARK.
Mechanisms of Fluorine Displacement by R. E. PARKER.
Nitrogen Fluorides and their Inorganic Derivatives by C. B. COLBURN.
The Organic Fluorochemicals Industry by J. M. HAMILTON.
The Preparation of Organic Fluorine Compounds by Halogen Exchange by A. K. BARBOUR, L. J. BELF and M. W. BUXTON.

TOPCHIEV, A. V., S. V. ZAVGORODNII, and YA. M. PAUSHKIN: Boron Fluoride and Its Compounds as Catalysts in Organic Chemistry. London, New York, Paris, Los Angeles: Pergamon 1959.

Pharmacologically-active Fluorine Compounds have been fully reviewed by N. P. BUU-HOÏ: Les Derivés Organiques du Fluor d'Intérêt Pharmacologique. In: E. JUCKER (Ed.), Drug Research, vol. 3, 9—74. Basel und Stuttgart: Birkhäuser Verlag 1961.

References

Many of the references quoted here are review articles or textbooks where the locations of original publications can be found.

ALLEN, G. R., and N. A. AUSTIN: Halogenated progesterones. A preferential reaction of perchloryl fluoride. J. Org. Chem. **26**, 5245—5247 (1961).

ANELLO, L. G., J. GORDON, H. R. NYCHKA, and C. WOOLF: Nitrosyl fluoride-HF complexes and the fluorination of organic compounds. Abstracts of the 140th. Amer. Chem. Soc. Meeting, Chicago, Illinois, Sept. 1961, p. 18 M.

BANKS, R. E., and R. N. HASZELDINE: Polymers containing fluorine. J. Oil Col. Chem. Assoc. **42**, 591—611 (1959).

— J. M. BIRCHALL, and R. N. HASZELDINE: Polymers containing fluorine. Chem. & Ind. (London) Monograph No. **13**, 270—294 (1961).

—, and R. N. HASZELDINE: Polyfluoroalkyl derivatives of metalloids and nonmetals. In: H. J. EMELÉUS and A. G. SHARPE (Eds.), Advances in Inorg. Chem. Radiochem. **3**, 337 — 433 (1961).

BARBOUR, A. K.: Industrial aspects of fluorine chemistry. Chem. & Ind. (London) **1961**, 958—972.

BARTLETT, N.: Xenon hexafluoroplatinate(V). Proc. chem. Soc. 218 (1962).

BELLAMY, L. J.: The Infrared Spectra of Complex Molecules. London: Methuen 1958.

BLOOM, B. M., V. V. BOGERT, and R. PINSON: A new synthesis of 6-fluoro steroids. Chem. & Ind. (London) **1959**, 1317.

BOWERS, A.: Steroids. CXXIX. A new general route to fluorinated steroids. J. Amer. Chem. Soc. **81**, 4107—4108 (1959).

— L. C. IBÁÑEZ, E. DENOT, and R. BECERRA: Steroids. CXXXIX. New fluorination procedures. Part I. The addition of Br—F and I—F to cyclohexene and a variety of unsaturated steroids. J. Amer. Chem. Soc. **82**, 4001—4007 (1960a).

— E. DENOT, and R. BECERRA: Steroids. CXLII. New fluorination procedures. Part 2. The abnormal addition of I—F to Δ^5-steroids. J. Amer. Chem. Soc. **82**, 4007—4012 (1960b).

— P. G. HOLTON, E. DENOT, M. C. LOZA, and R. URQUIZA: Steroids. CLXXXVIII. New fluorination procedures. Part 3. *cis*-Addition of fluorine to a steroid olefin. A new route to 6α-fluoro-Δ^4-3-ketones. J. Amer. Chem. Soc. **84**, 1050—1053 (1962).

BUNNETT, J. F., and R. E. ZAHLER: Nucleophilic substitution reactions. Chem. Rev. **49**, 273—412 (1951).

BURDON, J., and J. C. TATLOW: The electrochemical process for the synthesis of fluoro-organic compounds. In: M. STACEY, J. C. TATLOW, and A. G. SHARPE (Eds.), Advanc. Fluorine Chem. **1**, 129—165 (1960).

CADY, G. H.: Fluorine-containing compounds of sulfur. In: H. J. EMELÉUS and A. G. SHARPE (Eds.), Advanc. Inorg. Chem. Radiochem. **2**, 105—157 (1960).

CALLOWAY, N. O.: Reactions in the presence of metallic halides. II. The behavior of fluorides and the reactivity of the halogens. J. Amer. Chem. Soc. **59**, 1474—1479 (1937).

CHAPMAN, N. B., and J. L. LEVY: Nucleophilic displacement of fluorine from organic compounds. Part II. Kinetics of the reactions of alkyl fluorides with ethanolic sodium ethoxide. Part III. Acid-catalysed solvolysis of alkyl fluorides in aqueous ethanol. J. Chem. Soc. **1952**, 1673—1677, 1677—1682.

CLAASSEN, H. H., H. SELIG, and J. G. MALM: Xenon tetrafluoride. J. Amer. Chem. Soc. **84**, 3593 (1962).

DRYSDALE, J. J., W. W. GILBERT, H. K. SINCLAIR, and W. H. SHARKEY: A new synthesis of tropolone. J. Amer. Chem. Soc. **80**, 3672—3675 (1958).

EDWARDS, J., and H. J. RINGOLD: Steroids. CXXXII. 2-Fluoro and 21,21-difluoro steroids. J. Amer. Chem. Soc. **81**, 5262 (1959).

EMELÉUS, H. J.: Recent studies on fluoroalkyls and related compounds. Angew. Chemie (International Edition) **1**, 129—133 (1962).

FAWCETT, F. S., C. W. TULLOCK, R. D. SMITH, and D. D. COFFMAN: Chemistry of carbonyl fluoride. Preprints of the Second International Fuorine Symposium. Estes Park, Colorado, U.S.A., July 1962. Pp. 124—137. J. Amer. Chem. Soc. **84**, 4275—4288 (1962).

FINGER, G. C.: Fluorine resources and fluorine utilization. In: M. STACEY, J. C. TATLOW, and A. C. SHARPE (Eds.), Advanc. Fluorine Chem. **2**, 35—54 (1961).

FREEMAN, J. P.: The reactions of certain oxidized nitrogen compounds with perchloryl fluoride. J. Amer. Chem. Soc. **82**, 3869—3873 (1960).

FRIED, J., and E. F. SABO: Halogenated corticoids. I. 9α-Halogen derivatives of cortisone and hydrocortisone. J. Amer. Chem. Soc. **79**, 1130—1141 (1957).

GABBARD, R. B., and E. V. JENSEN: 2α-fluorocholestanone. J. Org. Chem. **23**, 1406 (1958).

GEORGE, J. W.: Halides and oxyhalides of the elements of groups Vb and VIb. In: F. A. COTTON (Ed.), Progr. in Inorg. Chem. **2**, 33—107 (1960).

HASZELDINE, R. N.: Fluorocarbon derivatives. Royal Institute of Chemistry Monograph. No. 1, 1956.

HENNE, A. L., and T. MIDGLEY: Reactivity and influence of fluorine in aliphatic compounds. J. Amer. Chem. Soc. **58**, 882—884 (1936).

HIRSCHMANN, R. F., R. MILLER, J. WOOD, and R. E. JONES: The reactions of epoxides with anhydrous hydrogen fluoride in the presence of organic bases. The preparation of 9α-fluoro-4-pregnene-11β, 17α, 21-triol-3,20-dione 21-acetate and its 1-dehydro analog. J. Amer. Chem. Soc. **78**, 4956—4959 (1956).

HOFFMANN, F. W.: Aliphatic fluorides. I. ω,ω'-Difluoroalkanes. II. 1-Halogeno-ω-fluoroalkanes. J. Org. Chem. **14**, 105—110 (1949); **15**, 425—434 (1950).

HOFFMAN, C. J., and R. G. NEVILLE: Nitrogen fluorides and their organic derivatives. Chem. Rev. **62**, 1—18 (1962).

HOLLOWAY, J. H., and R. D. PEACOCK: A simple preparation of xenon tetrafluoride. Proc. Chem. Soc. 389—390 (1962).

HORTON, C. A.: Trends in the Determination of Fluorine. In: CHAS. REILLEY (Ed.). Advances in Analytical Chemistry and Instrumentation, vol. 1, 151—183. New York: Interscience 1960.

HUDLICKÝ, M.: Chemistry of Organic Fluorine Compounds. Oxford, London, New York, Paris: Pergamon 1961.

INGOLD, C.: Structure and Mechanism in Organic Chemistry. New York: Cornell Univ. Press 1953.

INMAN, C. E., E. A. TYCZKOWSKI, R. E. OESTERLING, and F. L. SCOTT: A novel fluorination reaction: The interaction of perchloryl fluoride with active methylene compounds. Experientia **14**, 355 (1958).

— R. E. OESTERLING, and E. A. TYCZKOWSKI: Reactions of perchloryl fluoride with organic compounds. II. Fluorination of certain active methylene compounds. J. Amer. Chem. Soc. **80**, 6533—6535 (1958).

KATZ, J. J., and I. SHEFT: Halides of the actinide elements. In: H. J. EMELÉUS, and A. G. SHARPE (Eds.), Advances in Inorg. Chem. Radiochem. **2**, 195—236 (1960).

KISSMAN, H. M., A. M. SMALL, and M. J. WEISS: Fluorinated steroids. II. The reaction of perchloryl fluoride with alkoxalylated steroids. Synthesis of certain 2α-fluro and 21,21-difluoro steroids. J. Amer. Chem. Soc. **82**, 2312—2317 (1960).

LAGOWSKI, J. J.: Perfluoroalkyl derivatives of metals and non-metals. Quart. Rev. **13**, 233—264 (1959).

LEECH, H. R.: The physical and chemical properties of fluorine, and the physical, and chemical properties and uses of hydrogen fluoride and its aqueous solutions. In: H. V. A. BRISCOE, A. A. ELDRIDGE, and G. M. DYSON (Editorial Board), Mellor's Comprehensive Treatise on Inorganic and Theoretical Chemistry, Suppl. II, Part I, 46—71 and 85—146. London: Longmans, Green 1956.

LEECH, H. R.: Some aspects of inorganic fluorine compounds in chemical industry. Chem. & Ind. (London) **1960**, 242—250.
LOVELACE, A. M., D. A. RAUSCH, and W. POSTELNEK: Aliphatic Fluorine Compounds. American Chemical Society Monograph No. 138. New York: Reinhold 1958.
MACDONALD, A. M. G.: Seventh main group. 7a. Fluorine. In: C. L. WILSON and D. W. WILSON (Eds.), Comprehensive Analytical Chemistry, vol. 1C, 319—340. Amsterdam: Elsevier 1962.
MAJER, J. R.: Mass spectrometry of fluorine compounds. In: M. STACEY, J. C. TATLOW, and A. G. SHARPE. Advances in Fluorine Chem. **2**, 55—103 (1961).
MILLER, W. T., and J. BERNSTEIN: The relative reactivities of some substituted benzyl fluorides. J. Amer. Chem. Soc. **70**, 3600—3604 (1948).
— J. H. FRIED, and H. GOLDWHITE: Substitution and addition reactions of the fluoroölefins. IV. Reactions of fluoride ion with fluoroölefins. J. Amer. Chem. Soc. **82**, 3091—3099 (1960).
MILLS, J. S., A. BOWERS, C. DJERASSI, and H. J. RINGOLD: Steroids. CXXXVII. Synthesis of a new class of potent cortical hormones. 6α, 9α-Difluoro-16α-hydroxyprednisolone and its acetonide. J. Amer. Chem. Soc. **82**, 3399—3404 (1960).
— J. BARRERA, E. OLIVARES, and H. GARCÍA: Steroids. CL. 10β-Halo steroids. J. Amer. Chem. Soc. **82**, 5882—5889 (1960).
MIROSEVIC-SORGO, P., and B. C. SAUNDERS: Toxic fluorine compounds containing the C—F link. X. Rupture of the C—F link by alkali and other reagents. Tetrahedron **5**, 38—43 (1959).
MUERTTERTIES, E. L., and W. D. PHILLIPS: The use of nuclear magnetic resonance in inorganic chemistry. In: H. J. EMELÉUS and A. G. SHARPE (Eds.). Advances in Inorg. Chem. Radiochem. **4**, 231—292 (1962).
MUSGRAVE, W. K. R.: The reactions of organic fluorine compounds. Quart. Rev. **8**, 331—354 (1954).
— The halogen fluorides — Their preparation and uses in organic chemistry. In: M. STACEY, J. C. TATLOW, and A. G. SHARPE (Eds.). Advances in Fluorine Chem. **1**, 1—28 (1960).
NAKANISHI, S., K. MORITA, and E. V. JENSEN: The reaction of perchloryl fluoride with enol ethers. J. Amer. Chem. Soc. **81**, 5259—5260 (1959).
— R. L. MORGAN, and E. V. JENSEN: 4-Fluorinated steroids from the reaction of perchloryl fluoride with steroidal enamines. Chem. & Ind. (London) **1960**, 1136—1137.
—, and E. V. JENSEN: 16α-Fluorinated steroids from the reaction of perchloryl fluoride with an enamide. J. Org. Chem. **27**, 702—703 (1962).
OLAH, G. A., A. E. PAVLATH, and J. A. OLAH: Aromatic substitution. V. The synthesis of a protonated toluene tetrafluoroborate complex. J. Amer. Chem. Soc. **80**, 6540—6545 (1958).
PATTISON, F. L. M., and W. C. HOWELL: Organometallic reactions of ω-Fluoroalkyl halides. I. Preparation of ω-Fluoroalkylmagnesium halides. J. Org. Chem. **21**, 879—882 (1956).
PAYNE, D. S.: Halides of the phosphorus group elements. Quart. Rev. **15**, 173—189 (1961).
PEACOCK, R. D.: Some fluorine compounds of the transition metals. In: F. A. COTTON (Ed.). Progress in Inorganic Chem. **2**, 193—249 (1960).
POPLE, J. A., W. G. SCHNEIDER, and H. J. BERNSTEIN: High-resolution nuclear magnetic resonance. New York: McGraw-Hill 1959.
ROBERTS, H. L.: The chemistry of compounds containing sulphur-fluorine bonds. Quart. Rev. **15**, 30—55 (1961).
ROBERTS, J. D., and C. M. SHARTS: Cyclobutane derivatives from thermal cycloaddition reactions. In: R. ADAMS, A. H. BLATT, V. BOEKELHEIDE, T. L. CAIRNS, A. C. COPE, D. Y. CURTIN, and C. NIEMANN (Eds.). Org. Reactions **12**, 1—56 (1962).
ROBINSON, C. H., L. FINCKENOR, E. P. OLIVETO, and D. GOULD: A new class of potent anti-inflammatory agents; synthesis of 9α, 11β-dihalocorticosteroids. J. Amer. Chem. Soc. **81**, 2191—2195 (1959).
— N. F. BRUCE, E. P. OLIVETO, S. TOLKSDORF, M. STEINBERG, and P. L. PERLMAN: 16,16-Difluoroestrone derivatives. A new series of cholesterol lowering agents. J. Amer. Chem. Soc. **82**, 5256—5257 (1960).
ROE, A.: Preparation of aromatic fluorine compounds from diazonium fluoborates. The Schiemann reaction. In: R. ADAMS, W. E. BACHMANN, A. H. BLATT, L. F. FIESER, J. R. JOHNSON, and H. R. SNYDER (Eds.). Org. Reactions **5**, 193—228 (1949).
RUDGE, A. J.: The Manufacture and Use of Fluorine and Its Compounds. London: Oxford University Press 1962.
RUTHERFORD, K. G., W. REDMOND, and J. RIGAMONTI: The use of hexafluorophosphoric acid in the Schiemann reaction. J. Org. Chem. **26**, 5149—5152 (1961).
SAUNDERS, B. C.: The physiological action of organic compounds containing fluorine. In: M. STACEY, J. C. TATLOW, and A. G. SHARPE (Eds.). Advances in Fluorine Chem. **2**, 183—210 (1961).

SCOTT, F. L., R. E. OESTERLING, E. A. TYCZKOWSKI, and C. E. INMAN: Reaction of perchloryl fluoride with nitrogenous bases. Chem. & Ind. (London) **1960**, 528—529.

SHARP, D. W. A.: Fluoroboric acids and their derivatives. In: M. STACEY, J. C. TATLOW, and A. G. SHARPE (Eds.). Advances in Fluorine Chem. **1**, 68—128 (1960).

SHARPE, A. G.: Some general aspects of the inorganic chemistry of fluorine. Quart. Rev. **11**, 49—60 (1957).

— Transition metal fluorides and their complexes. In: M. STACEY, J. C. TATLOW, and A. G. SHARPE (Eds.). Advances in Fluorine Chem. **1**, 29—67 (1960).

SHECHTER, H., and E. B. ROBERSON: Reactions of perchloryl fluoride and salts of mononitro compounds. J. Org. Chem. **25**, 175—177 (1960).

SHEPPARD, W. A.: Alkyl- and arylsulfur trifluorides. J. Amer. Chem. Soc. **84**, 3058—3063 (1962).

SMITH, W. C.: The chemistry of sulfur tetrafluoride. Angew. Chemie (International Edition) **1**, 467—475 (1962).

STACEY, M., and J. C. TATLOW: Exhaustive fluorinations of organic compounds with high-valency metallic fluorides. In: M. STACEY, J. C. TATLOW, and A. G. SHARPE (Eds.). Advances in Fluorine Chem. **1**, 166—198 (1960).

STEPHENS, R., and J. C. TATLOW: Fluorocarbon chemistry. Part I. The fluorination of organic compounds. Quart. Rev. **16**, 44—70 (1962).

STEVENS, T. E.: Fluorination of some nitriles and ketones with bromine trifluoride. J. Org. Chem. **26**, 1627—1630 (1961).

SWAIN, C. G., and R. E. T. SPALDING: Mechanism of acid catalysis of the hydrolysis of benzyl fluoride. J. Amer. Chem. Soc. **82**, 6104—6107 (1960).

TAUB, D.: Fluorination of phenols. Chem. & Ind. (London) **1962**, 558—559.

— C. H. KUO, and L. WENDLER: Synthesis in the griseofulvin series: 7-fluoro-7-dechloro-griseofulvin, an active analogue. Chem. & Ind. (London) **1962**, 557—558.

TEDDER, J. M.: The interaction of free radicals with saturated aliphatic compounds. Quart. Rev. **14**, 336—356 (1960).

— The fluorination of organic compounds using elementary fluorine. In: M. STACEY, J. C. TATLOW, and A. G. SHARPE (Eds.). Advances in Fluorine Chem. **2**, 104—137 (1961).

WEEKS, J. L., C. L. CHERNICK, and M. S. MATHESON: Photochemical preparation of xenon difluoride. J. Amer. Chem. Soc. **84**, 4612—4613 (1962).

WEIBLEN, D. G.: The infrared spectra of fluorocarbons and related compounds. In: J. H. SIMONS (Ed.). Fluorine Chem. **II**, 449—503 (1954).

WIEBENGA, E. H., E. E. HAVINGA, and K. H. BOSWIJK: Structures of interhalogen compounds and polyhalides. In: H. J. EMELÉUS, and A. G. SHARPE (Eds.). Advances in Inorg. Chem. Radiochem. **3**, 133—169 (1961).

Chapter 2

Metabolism of Inorganic Fluoride[1]

By

FRANK A. SMITH

With 17 Figures

I. Introduction

The presence of fluoride has been recognized in biological materials since 1803 when MORICHINI demonstrated the presence of fluorine in fossilized elephant teeth. Its presence has been reported in biological samples of every type submitted to analysis, though admittedly, some of the early analytical methods employed left something to be desired when applied to such materials.

Early biological interest in fluorides centered around the effects of acutely and subacutely toxic doses, which perhaps is only logical. Interest in the metabolism of doses low enough to be considered of no more than chronic toxicity, or better yet, low enough to be in the range of normal intake, did not come until much later. Several reasons have contributed to this. One of these assuredly was the lack of anything other than passing academic interest in compounds of an element of little or no industrial significance, and so difficult to prepare. A second important reason is the difficulty inherent in quantitatively measuring microgram amounts of fluoride in the presence of many grams of extraneous matter, frequently organic in nature. With the publication of Willard and Winter's method (1933) based on separation of the fluoride by steam distillation and subsequent titration of F in the distillate with alizarin and thorium nitrate, the stage was set for a fresh surge of interest in the biological behavior of fluorides.

The impetus was not long in coming. In 1932 MØLLER and GUDJONSSON had reported unusual roentgenological observations in certain cryolite workers, which in turn led to the now classical report by KAJ ROHOLM on the effects of fluoride in Danish cryolite workers and in experimental animals (1937). About this same period fluorine in drinking water was established first as the causative agent of mottled enamel, and later of a reduced incidence of dental caries in persons using fluorine-containing water supplies. Finally, the steadily increasing demand for phosphate and superphosphate fertilizers, and for phosphoric acid, led to the evolution into the atmosphere of increasing amounts of fluorine and fluorides during the roasting of rock phosphate, which in turn led to deleterious effects in livestock pastured down wind from such operations.

[1] The author is most appreciative of the kindness of Dr. HAROLD C. HODGE in reading and commenting upon the manuscript of this chapter. He also expresses his thanks to Dr. DONALD A. MORKEN for stimulating and helpful discussions of certain aspects of the dynamics of fluoride metabolism.

Part of the work reported herein was done under contract with the U.S. Atomic Energy Commission at the University of Rochester Atomic Energy Project.

Interest in each of these areas, spurred on and expanded by the enormously increased industrial use of both inorganic and organic fluorides in the past twenty-five years, has led to numerous studies employing a variety of experimental approaches. From these there is emerging an ever more comprehensive picture of the absorption, distribution and excretion of fluoride. Unfortunately, the state of knowledge in this area has not benefited to any extensive degree from the spate of post World War II work with isotopes. This situation stems from the fact that the only practically useable isotope of fluorine, F^{18}, has a half-life of only 109 min; moreover, there are few facilities where the isotope can be prepared. The few studies which have been done have proven invaluable in confirming and extending the picture developed from the voluminous work with stable fluoride.

The literature dealing with biological effects of fluoride is extensive; currently, bibliographies may contain more than 3000 entries in this field. Much of this has been reviewed recently by HODGE and SMITH (in press) in a somewhat selective fashion. Therefore, using chiefly the more recent literature and certain of the especially appropriate earlier references, the presentation here will attempt to build upon and possibly extend the general picture developed earlier.

II. Absorption

A. Absorption from the gastrointestinal tract

An apparently never-ending stream of papers in the literature continues to offer indirect proof that fluorides are absorbed from the gastrointestinal tract following ingestion, as evidenced by increased urinary excretion of fluoride and increased storage of fluoride in the bone. However, there are very few instances in which gastrointestinal absorption has been measured directly. Determination of blood fluoride concentrations does indicate that absorption has occurred. However, such data do not permit estimation of the magnitude or rate at which fluoride is absorbed, since these concentrations are the resultant of several simultaneous processes, viz. passage of fluoride into the blood from the gut, removal from blood to the urine, and removal of F to and from bone. Consequently, only those experiments in which fluoride remaining in the digestive tract is measured at various time intervals after ingestion are of value in quantitating the rate and magnitude of alimentary absorption. Only rarely has this been the primary objective of the experimental design.

Absorption at early intervals was investigated by ZIPKIN and LIKINS (1957), who showed in rats that absorption was 50 % complete after 30 min. HEIN et al. (1956) obtained reasonably good agreement at 30 min (43 %), but STOOKEY et al. (1962a) found only 30 % absorption in the first half hour. In a study of the organ distribution of F^{18} at different time intervals after ingestion, WALLACE (1953) determined the percentage of the dose remaining in the alimentary canal at 1, 4 and 9 hours and showed that the fractions absorbed were 72.5, 84.8 and 84.2 %, respectively. Comparable figures were obtained by ZIPKIN and LIKINS (1957) at 1 and 1.5 hours (72 and 86 %, respectively). ERICSSON (1958a) measured absorption at 4, 8 and 10 hours, and confirmed the observations of WALLACE at similar time intervals.

The results of these various studies are summarized in Table 1, where both the percentage of dose absorbed and percentage of dose remaining are tabulated.

The cumulative absorption is plotted in Figure 1. It is evident that absorption is rapid during the first hour and a half, and furthermore, that maximal absorption, about 85 %, is attained in this time; very little absorption occurs thereafter in the succeeding 8.5 hours. It is unlikely that the 10—15 % of dose remaining in the gastrointestinal tract up to 10 hours after administration represents unabsorbed fluoride. The rats had been fasted prior to dosing, and the presence of intestinal contents which might interfere with absorption would be expected to be minimal. Maintenance of a constant fraction of the dose in the intestinal tract for a prolonged period more likely reflects a state of equilibrium between fluoride leaving and fluoride entering the intestinal canal. The rate of turnover evidently is such that

Table 1. *Absorption of ingested fluoride from the gastrointestinal tract of the rat* (fluoride as NaF)

Time interval	Percentage of dose		Isotope used	Reference
	absorbed	remaining		
0 min	12	88	stable	Zipkin and Likins (1957)
5	22	78	stable	Zipkin and Likins (1957)
15	36	64	stable	Zipkin and Likins (1957)
30	50	50	stable	Zipkin and Likins (1957)
30	43.3	56.7	F^{18}	Hein et al. (1956)
30	29.9	70.1	stable	Stookey et al. (1962a)
1 hr	72	28	stable	Zipkin and Likins (1957)
1	72.5	27.5	F^{18}	Wallace (1953)
1.5	86	14	stable	Zipkin and Likins (1957)
2	45.2	54.8	stable	Stookey et al. (1962a)
2	52.8	47.2	stable	Stookey et al. (1963)
4	64.3	35.7	stable	Stookey et al. (1963)
4	63.9	36.1	stable	Stookey et al. (1963)
4	84.8	15.2	F^{18}	Wallace (1953)
4	83.6	16.4	F^{18}	Ericsson (1958a)
8	88.8	11.2	F^{18}	Ericsson (1958a)
	89.6	10.4	F^{18}	Ericsson (1958a)
9	84.2	15.8	F^{18}	Wallace (1953)
10	88.7	11.3	F^{18}	Ericsson (1958a)

approximately 10—15 % of the dose is being recycled. Support for this concept comes from several sources. Wallace (1953) and Hein et al. (1956) have demonstrated the presence of fluoride within the intestinal tract of the rat after intravenous injection of fluoride as F^{18}. There are several routes by which fluoride could have been brought to the lumen of the intestinal canal, viz. from swallowed saliva containing fluoride, from secretion through the mucosa of the stomach and passage into the intestine, by way of the bile, pancreatic juices or intestinal juices, and by diffusion from the blood into the intestine. In a series of carefully designed experiments Wallace (1953) demonstrated that of these various pathways, the most significant was passage from the blood by a process or processes resembling diffusion. She considered

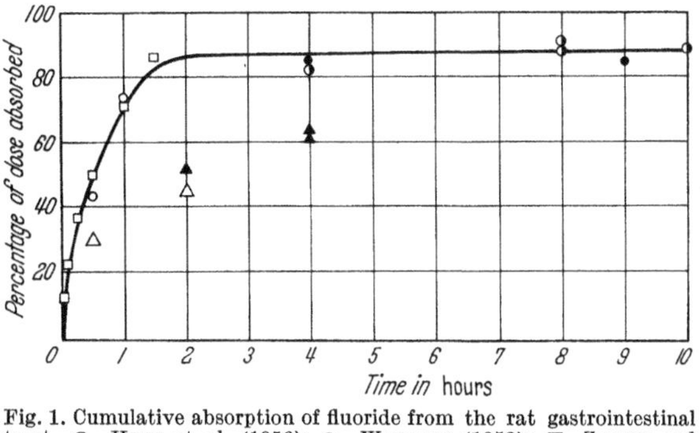

Fig. 1. Cumulative absorption of fluoride from the rat gastrointestinal tract. ○, Hein et al. (1956); ●, Wallace (1953); □, Zipkin and Likins (1957); △, Stookey et al. (1962a); ◐, Ericsson (1958a); ▲, Stookey et al. (1963)

the extent of passage in this manner to be dependent upon the level of fluoride in the blood and the rate of blood flow in the vessels supplying the intestine. The appearance of a nearly constant percentage of the dose after 1.5 hour sis consistent with the suggested influence of the blood level; by this time post ingestion, the concentration of fluoride in blood would be expected to have returned to more nearly normal and constant levels. ERICSSON and ULLBERG (1958) also demonstrated autoradiographically that F^{18} was not excreted via the bile or by the intestinal wall, but PERKINSON et al. (1955) and BELL et al. (1961) showed that in ruminants, the rumen wall plays an important role in the passage of fluoride into and out of the gastrointestinal tract.

1. Absorption in different portions of the gastrointestinal tract

Absorption of fluoride from various segments of the gastrointestinal tract has been the subject of several investigations. WAGNER (1962a) isolated the stomach *in situ* in a series of rats, injected fluoride directly into the stomach, and determined the amount remaining at various time intervals up to five hours. After a 15-minute delay, absorption proceeded rapidly for the next 15—20 min, and then declined in rate; 51 % had left the stomach after the first hour and 58 % after the second hour under these unphysiological conditions. FOSTER and RUSH (1961) found 44 and 58 % of fluoride to be absorbed in one and two hours, respectively, from the rat stomach *in vitro*. CARLSON et al. (1960a) showed that fluoride ingested by normal human subjects disappeared from the stomach after approximately 150 min; in these instances the fluoride was cleared both by absorption and normal mechanical emptying into the intestine.

STOOKEY et al. (1962a) reported 25—30 % to be absorbed in 30 min from the rat stomach isolated *in situ* and 31—49 % was absorbed in 30 min when fluoride was introduced into the first, second or third 5 cm length of intestine.

ARMSTRONG et al. (1961) and DELLINGER (1961) investigated the passage of fluoride across the intestinal wall. Using isotopic tracers, the former authors found the order of transport to be $H_2^3O > Cl^{36} > F^{18}$ in the small intestine of the rat *in vivo*. The rate of transport of F^{18} was the same in the upper, middle and lower segments, and was not affected by equivalent concentrations of iron, calcium and magnesium; 10-fold greater concentrations of Fe^{+++} and magnesium did reduce the transport. DELLINGER, on the other hand, reported that passage from isolated intestinal segments *in vitro* to the surrounding medium varied from segment to segment along the gastrointestinal tract, and was much less when the stomach was used; he also found the presence of calcium and magnesium to affect the passage.

In ruminant species, PERKINSON et al. (1955) showed that F^{18} crossed the wall of the rumen of lambs and BELL et al. (1961) demonstrated this transfer in cattle.

2. Rate of absorption

Ingested fluoride is rapidly absorbed and distributed throughout the body. Using data from Table 1, the percentage of dose remaining in the gastrointestinal tract has been plotted on a logarithmic scale against time on an arithmetic scale for the period of active absorption (Fig. 2). During the first 90 min post-administration, a straight line fits the data reasonably well. The data thus are typical of a first order reaction: the amount of fluoride leaving the gastrointestinal tract at any given time is proportional to the amount present at that time. The first order reaction kinetics indicate that 30 min are required to reduce by half the amount remaining at any instant after ingestion. The velocity constant for the processes involved is 0.0231 min^{-1}, indicating that during the first 90 min 2.31 % of that remaining is removed per minute.

ZIPKIN and LIKINS (1957) investigated the absorption of a number of inorganic compounds of fluoride by the rat, and found the absorptions of Na_2SiF_6, Na_2PO_3F and SnF_2 to be very similar to that of NaF, while absorption of KPF_6, $(C_2H_5)_4NPF_6$ and KBF_4 is appreciably more rapid. If it is assumed that the absorption of these latter three compounds also obey first order reaction kinetics, it can be shown that the rates of absorption are approximately 4.8, 3.6 and 4.6 % of the dose per minute, respectively. Thus, these compounds, which are physiologically inert are absorbed at rates approximately twice as fast as is the F of NaF. ZIPKIN and LIKINS attribute this difference at least in part to differences in electronic structure; fluoride in the rapidly absorbed compounds is held covalently and does not behave as the fluoride ion, whereas in the more slowly absorbed compounds exemplified by NaF, it is held electrovalently and is present in the ionic form.

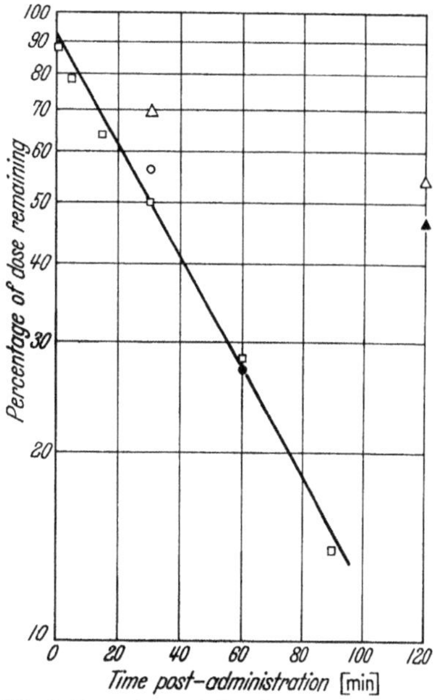

Fig. 2. Percentage of the dose remaining in the gastrointestinal tract of the rat at various times after dosing. ○, HEIN et al. (1956); ●, WALLACE (1953); □, ZIPKIN and LIKINS (1957); △, STOOKEY et al. (1962a); ▲, STOOKEY et al. (1963)

Additional, indirect evidence of the rapidity of absorption is found in studies where F was determined in blood or urine after oral administration of fluoride. For example, PERKINSON et al. (1955) found F^{18} in the blood 5 min after ingestion of an oral dose of NaF^{18} by the lamb; peak concentrations were obtained at approximately three hours. Fluoride also appeared promptly in the blood of a cow given F^{18}, though the maximal level was not seen until 5 hours post-administration. CARLSON (1959) showed the presence of F^{18} in plasma 22 min after ingestion by man; this was the earliest blood sample collected. Peak concentrations were noted after one hour.

Table 2. *Mean urinary excretion of ingested soluble fluoride by man*

Time post-ingestion	Percentage of dose		Reference[2]
	excreted	remaining[1]	
0.5 hr	1.7	98.3	SMITH et al. (1963a)
1	10.1	89.9	ERICSSON (1958a)
	6.2	93.8	SMITH et al. (1963a)
1.5	4.1	95.9	WAGNER and MUHLER (1959a)
	10.5	89.5	SMITH et al. (1963a)
2	14.4	85.6	SMITH et al. (1963a)
	15.7	84.3	ERICSSON et al. (1958a)
2.5	16.3	83.7	SMITH et al. (1963a)
3	17.8	82.2	SMITH et al. (1963a)
	19.8	80.2	ZIPKIN et al. (1957)
	9.5	90.5	WAGNER and MUHLER (1959a)
4	28, 33	72, 67	CARLSON (1959)
	21.7	78.3	ERICSSON (1958a)

[1] This fraction includes F remaining in the gastrointestinal tract as well as F absorbed and remaining elsewhere, *e.g.* bone, tissue, fluids.

[2] SMITH et al., 6 subjects; ERICSSON, 7; ZIPKIN et al., 8; CARLSON, 2; WAGNER and MUHLER, 5.

Appearance of fluoride in the urine is also indicative of absorption following ingestion, and in Table 2 are summarized results reported by a number of workers.

The data are plotted in Fig. 3. Agreement among four of the studies is remarkably good, and indicates that in general, approximately 20 % of the dose is excreted in four hours. CARLSON finds nearer 30 % excreted in this time. WAGNER and MUHLER, however, found less than 10 % excreted after three hours.

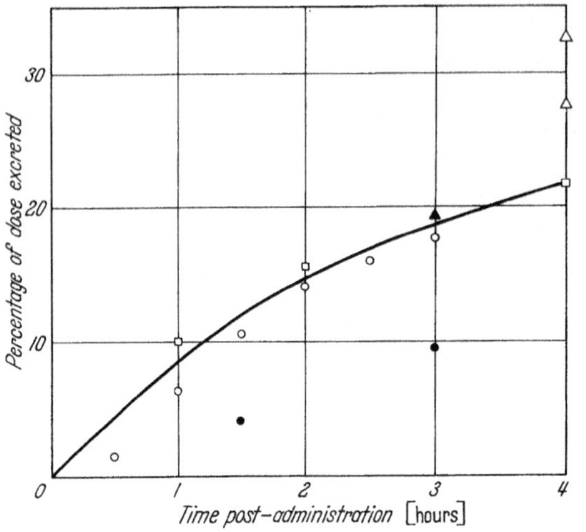

Fig. 3. Percentage of dose of ingested fluoride excreted by man at various times after ingestion. ○, SMITH et al. (1963a); □, ERICSSON (1958a); △, CARLSON (1959); ▲, ZIPKIN et al. (1957); ●, WAGNER and MUHLER (1959a)

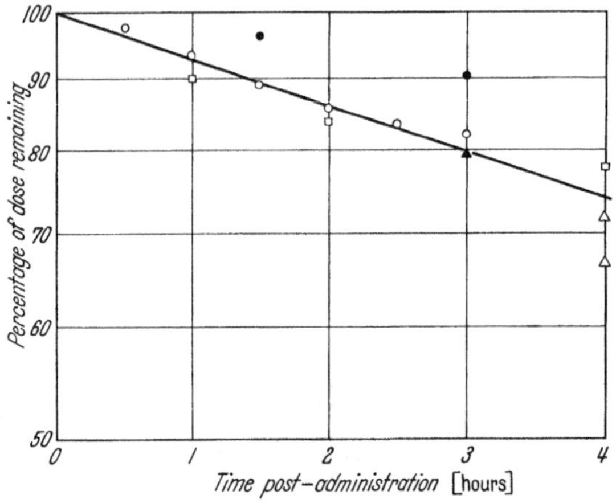

Fig. 4. Percentage of dose remaining after ingestion of fluoride by man. ○, SMITH et al. (1963a); □, ERICSSON (1958a); △, CARLSON (1959); ▲, ZIPKIN et al. (1957); ●, WAGNER and MUHLER (1959a)

The percentage of the dose remaining in the gastrointestinal tract, bone, and elsewhere (from Table 2) is plotted on a semilogarithmic scale against time on a linear scale in Fig. 4.

The straight line obtained indicates that the passage of fluoride from the gastrointestinal tract to the urine can be described by first order kinetics. It will be appreciated of course, that the removal of a portion of ingested F to the urine involves a number of processes. It is the net result of these processes, over the four hours for which data are available, which is characterized by the stright line. The net process is characterized by a half time of 9.6 hours and a rate constant corresponding to 7.2 % per hour.

3. Extent of absorption

a) Normal dietary fluoride

The ubiquitous distribution of fluoride in nature makes it virtually impossible to prepare a diet or find a ration for man or animal which does not contain at least trace amounts of fluoride. The occurrence of fluoride in foods and waters has been reviewed by CHOLAK (1959), who states that the average general diet in the United States supplies 0.2—0.3 mg fluoride daily. To this must be added fluoride ingested with the drinking water if the water supply contains fluoride; in areas where drinking water contains 1 ppm F (1 mg F/liter) this can be expected to contribute an additional 1.0—1.5 mg (McCLURE, 1949). In our experience, commercially available pellet rations for laboratory animals have been found to contain 15—40 ppm F. A recent survey of the literature suggests that the usual diet of livestock ranges from a few ppm to 50 ppm F (HODGE and SMITH, in press).

In view of the fact that practically all fluoride absorbed from the alimentary canal eventually is deposited in the skeleton or passes through the kidneys and into the urine, it becomes of interest to have some estimate of the extent to which naturally occurring dietary fluoride is absorbed. Data pertaining to this point are summarized in Table 3.

Table 3. *Absorption of fluoride occurring naturally in the normal daily ration of various species*

Species	mg F ingested daily range or mean	Percentage absorbed	Reference
Man . . . . . (6—14 wks. age)	0.100—0.171 (milk formula)	45—71	HAM and SMITH (1954a)
Man, adult . .	0.429—0.792	65—88	HAM and SMITH (1954b)
Man, adult . .	0.390—0.480	38—93	LARGENT (1961)
Man, adult . .	1.5	70	MC CLURE et al. (1945)
Lamb	3.6	61	HOBBS et al. (1954)
Rabbit	3.42—4.20	48—58	GARDNER et al. (1957)
Rabbit	5.85	56	SMITH et al. (1955)
Rat	0.010—0.038	41—74	TAYLOR et al. (1961)
Rat	0.007	64	WEDDLE and MUHLER (1955)

It is evident that man usually absorbs at least 45 % of fluoride normally present in his diet, and may absorb nearly all of it. In one instance LARGENT reported only 38 % absorbed, but this value is not in agreement with other data reported by him. Age in man seems to have little effect on the efficiency of absorption. Absorption by the guinea pig appears to be comparable to that in man in the one instance reported, while in the rat and rabbit appreciably less dietary fluoride is absorbed.

The form(s) in which fluoride is normally present in foods is not known, though it is reasonable to expect that a large proportion of the total is present in inorganic combinations; availability of this fluoride may be expected to differ, depending upon the form present. TAYLOR et al. (1961) found 10—15 % of fluoride present in a commercial rat diet to be stored in the skeleton, while GARDNER et al. (1957) found 26—48 % of fluoride in a commercial rabbit ration to be so retained.

Absorption of ingested fluoride is a function of a number of factors. Physical chemical properties of the compound are important, in that these govern its solubility and the extent and manner of its dissociation. Whether it is ingested in food or in water is important, inasmuch as more water often is drunk than food is eaten, and also because either medium may contain elements with a particularly high affinity for fluoride, thus decreasing the amount of fluoride ion available. The availability of fluoride added to milk also is of interest.

In Table 4 is listed the absorption of fluoride from a variety of sources incorporated in food or water; in each instance listed here absorption was measured directly in balance studies.

The salient features of Table 4 may be commented upon briefly. Bone meal and rock phosphate are seen to be poor sources of fluoride, though in some instances bone meal may furnish appreciable amounts. When equal amounts of cryolite were fed rats in food and in water, the percentages absorbed were slightly greater for water borne F (LAWRENZ et al., 1939b). Moreover, man was shown also to absorb cryolite from food or water to approximately the same extent as did the rat (LARGENT, 1961). In the experiments listed, F from CaF_2 was poorly absorbed from food, but was taken up efficiently from solution. In general, NaF is well absorbed from

Table 4. *Absorption of fluoride administered as different compounds and in food or water*

Compound	Species	Mg F ingested daily		Per cent absorbed	Reference
		food	water		
Bone meal[1]	man	0.946—1.435		19—76	HAM and SMITH (1954b)
Bone meal	man	6.31		37	LARGENT (1961)
Cryolite	rat	0.054—0.084		63—87	LAWRENZ et al. (1939b)
			0.054—0.084	72—90	
Cryolite	man	6.41—36.40		62—77	LARGENT (1961)
			25.4	93	
Rock phosph.	rat	19.7—21.4		39—41	KICK et al. (1935)
Tea	man		1.200—1.368	79—88	HAM and SMITH (1954b)
CaF_2	man	6.43		62	LARGENT (1961)
			6.25	96	
CaF_2	rat	20.8		1.9	KICK et al. (1935)
NaF	man		6.47—19.4	96—97	LARGENT (1961)
NaF	calf		491	68—72	MARIAKULANDAI and VENKATARAMAIAH (1955)
NaF	lamb	3.6, 6.1		61—62	HOBBS et al. (1954)
		27.4, 40.6		86—87	
		74.9—107.4		90—92	
NaF	rat	11.7		45	KICK et al. (1935)
NaF	rat		0.066—12.1	47—89	TAYLOR et al. (1961)
NaF	rat	0.0315		90	WEDDLE and MUHLER (1957)
$NaBF_4$	man	6.40		98	LARGENT (1961)
Na_2SiF_6	rat	11.2—11.7		65	KICK et al. (1935)
Na_2SiF_6	rat		0.032	89	WEDDLE and MUHLER (1957)
SnF_2	rat		0.0318	91	WEDDLE and MUHLER (1957)

[1] As Pablum, a bone meal-containing baby food.

solutions or from diets; the results of HOBBS et al. (1954) in the lamb are of interest in that they suggest that the percentage absorbed is a function of the intake. Fluoride as NaF is not necessarily readily absorbed, as is brought out by the data of KICK et al. (1935) and of TAYLOR et al. (1961). Na_2SiF_6 is absorbed from either food or water, and F from SnF_2 appears to be well absorbed in the one instance in which absorption was measured directly. $NaBF_4$ appears to be absorbed almost completely though in this instance the fluoride does not appear as F ion.

b) Fluoride in food vs. fluoride in water

Comparison of the availability of fluorine added to food and to water has been the subject of several studies. In a carefully controlled experiment LAWRENZ et al. (1939b) fed the same amount of F as cryolite to rats in the food and in the water, and compared the two routes in terms of F stored in soft and hard tissues, F excretion, effects on incisor enamel, and growth. Fluoride ingested in the food was retained to a lesser extent in the bones and teeth and soft tissues than was the same amount of F taken in the drinking water; assimilability of the food borne F was approximately 20% less than that of F in the water. The authors have suggested that this difference is due to a difference in the absorbability of the food borne F from the alimentary canal. They also point out however, this may be the result of interference with absorption by the food residues present and not necessarily due to differences in the extent of dissolution of the cryolite. In this experiment the F was fed in amounts equivalent to 10 ppm in the solid food. In a later paper LAWRENZ and MITCHELL (1941b) compared equal amounts of F as NaF fed in the diet and in the water supply; concentrations were of the order of 8 to 10 ppm. Again, assimilation was depressed approximately 21% by admixture with food.

WEDDLE and MUHLER (1954) essentially repeated the experiment of LAWRENZ and MITCHELL referred to above, when they fed identical amounts of F as NaF in food and in water at a concentration of 5 ppm. Again, total carcass storage of F from food fed fluoride was approximately 20 % less than that from water borne fluoride.

In contrast to these reports, several studies have shown no differences in availability when fluoride is given in food or in water. MCCLURE (1939) fed rats equal amounts of fluoride as NaF in the two media, at concentrations corresponding to 90.4, 45.2 and 22.6 ppm F in the water, and concluded that F in food was no more detrimental than F in water as regards daily gain in body weight, ash and fluorine content of bones and teeth, total F retained and appearance of the teeth.

More recently WUTHIER and PHILLIPS (1959, 1961) found no appreciable differences in the concentrations of F stored in hard tissues (femurs and teeth) when F was given in food or water at concentrations ranging up to 90 ppm F. Deposition of F appeared to be related only to the daily intake in terms of μg F/g of body weight. However, in these studies with rats a given concentration of F in water caused approximately the same F deposition as twice this concentration in food due to the fact that the intake of water was almost exactly twice that of food.

LAWRENZ and MITCHELL (1941b) noted and commented upon the difference between their results and those of MCCLURE (1939). In their opinion, MCCLURE did not see a clear-cut difference in the two routes because he did not separate in time the ingestion of F-containing water and food, with the result that the presence of food residues in the gastrointestinal tract possibly interfered with the absorption of water borne F. WEDDLE and MUHLER (1954) somewhat fortuitously obtained some degree of separation in time, which contributed to the success of their experiment. In justice to MCCLURE, it should be pointed out that he recognized that a maximal effect would have been demonstrated by widely separating the periods of eating and drinking; as he remarked however "... conditions in practice were more nearly duplicated by allowing ad libitum eating and drinking so far as time was concerned."

WUTHIER and PHILLIPS (1959) also recognized that the practical conditions of ad libitum feeding, where considerable mixing of food and water in the digestive tract was expected, resulted in little difference in availability being evident.

c) Fluoride in milk vs. fluoride in water

Comparisons of the availability of F in milk and in water have been made by several investigators. MUHLER and WEDDLE (1955a) fed rats nearly identical amounts of F in milk and in water, thereby eliminating effects due to differences in the amounts of milk and water ingested, and reported that when the concentration of F in the two vehicles was 10 ppm, no differences in skeletal or carcass storage of F were evident; however, at 2 ppm the F of milk was much less available than that of water. They suggest that at the lower concentration Ca and Mg interfere with the availability of F, but that this effect is not apparent at 10 ppm F. Using F^{18}, ERICSSON (1958a) demonstrated that the absorption of milk borne F is slower than that of water-born F, as evidenced by lower blood and femur levels of F^{18} in rats given F in milk, and by the more rapid urinary excretion in man of F^{18} given in water. ERICSSON suggests however, that these differences are not such that fluoridation of milk cannot be considered as a means of administering fluoride to reduce dental caries. Indeed, at concentrations of 1 ppm F, only 17—19 % and 10—11 % of fluoride is unabsorbed by the rat after 8—10 hours when F is given in milk and water, respectively. KONIG (1960) has also shown that the skeletal storage of fluoride is greater when F is given in water than when it is given in milk.

d) Nature of the compound

LAWRENZ and MITCHELL (1941 b) have remarked that the relative toxicities of different compounds are not constant but vary with the amounts fed, and that at lower dietary concentrations marked variations would not be expected. The data of Table 4 bear this out; under appropriate conditions NaF, CaF_2, Na_2SiF_6, SnF_2 and cryolite are all absorbed equally well (89—97 %), or equally poorly (61—65 %).

Using visible changes in the enamel of the rat's incisor as a criterion, DEEDS and THOMAS (1933—1934) demonstrated that F was equally effective when supplied as NaF, Na_2SiF_6, or Na_3AlF_6. SMITH and LEVERTON (1934) showed this to be true for NH_4F, KF, $BaSiF_6$, K_2SiF_6 and Na_2SiF_6, using the same criterion.

In a thorough and careful series of studies LAWRENZ et al. have investigated the availability of F present in NaF, CaF_2 and natural and synthetic cryolite (LAWRENZ, MITCHELL and RUTH, 1939a; LAWRENZ and MITCHELL, 1941a, b). Using dose levels low enough to be of significance in human nutrition, *i.e.* 7—13 ppm F, these authors showed that F was equally available from NaF, CaF_2 and cryolite. However, the F of synthetic cryolite was more available than was that of natural cryolite; the difference was attributed to a greater solubility of the cryolite present in the former product. Criteria employed included F retention, storage in bone and tooth, and effects on the incisor enamel.

MCCLURE (1950) and ZIPKIN and MCCLURE (1951, 1954) have measured the effects of various compounds of fluorine on caries reduction, skeletal and tooth storage, and incisor enamel in rats, using NaF, Na_2SiF_6, $(NH_4)_2SiF_6$, Na_2PO_3F, KPF_6 and CF_3COONa. The F of the two latter compounds was considered to be unavailable when measured by these standard fluoride effects. All other compounds were adjudged to be equally effective, *i.e.* the fluoride was equally available.

ZIPKIN and LIKINS (1957) compared the gastrointestinal absorption of a series of fluorine compounds in the rat, by measuring the amount of F still present in the alimentary canal 30 min after administering a standard dose by stomach tube. By this criterion, the compounds examined fell into two classes, viz. those in which the fluoride was releasable as the F^- and which were absorbed to the extent of about 48% in 30 min, and those in which the F was held covalently, which were absorbed to the extent of about 74%. In other words, the physiologically inactive compounds were absorbed at a faster rate than was the F ion. The results raise interesting questions as to the mechanism(s) by which the ion and the compounds are transported across the intestinal wall. Perhaps the slower passage of the F ion is a clue to the involvement of this active ion in a greater variety of vital reactions not directly concerned with its transport. The data obtained by these authors are reproduced in the following table, taken from their paper.

Table 5. *Absorption of various fluorine compounds from the gastrointestinal tract of the rat* (ZIPKIN and LIKINS, 1957)

Compound	% of fluorine intake absorbed[1]	Compound	% of fluorine intake absorbed[1]
1. NaF	49.6 ± 4.3	5. KPF_6	77.2 ± 3.2
2. Na_2SiF_6	50.9 ± 3.1	6. Et_4NPF_6	67.7 ± 3.7
3. Na_2PO_6F	43.2 ± 2.8	7. KBF_4	75.8 ± 2.7
4. SnF_2	50.0 ± 1.7		
Mean	48.4 ± 1.6	Mean	73.6 ± 2.0

[1] Mean $\pm$ std. error based on 10 rats/compound.

The picture with respect to the absorption of F from Na_2PO_3F is not yet clear. SHOURIE et al. (1950) found NaF to be three times more toxic than Na_2PO_3F, yet the two compounds were comparable in reducing dental decay in the hamster. The authors interpreted these findings to mean that there was little release of F^- from the Na_2PO_3F and that F need not exist as the free ion to reduce dental caries.

Zipkin and McClure (1951) also found NaF and Na_2PO_3F to be equivalent with regard to skeletal and tooth storage of F, and reduction in caries, and Ericsson et al. (1961) showed that the F^{18} of $Na_2PO_3F^{18}$ and of NaF^{18} was taken up equally well by bone. These latter authors suggest that if F is transported via blood to the bone as PO_3F ion, bone must either take it up as $PO_3F^{=}$ or split the complex ion to release F^-. This experiment also demonstrated that the two compounds were absorbed equally well from the intestine (*cf.* also Table 5). Evidence for splitting of the $PO_3F^{=}$ was obtained by Ericsson et al. (loc. cit.) by using the doubly labeled compound, $Na_2P^{32}O_3F^{18}$. When this material was administered to rats, significant differences in F^{18} and P^{32} levels in blood, femur, urine, and the digestive tract were obtained. The *in vivo* splitting of Na_2PO_3F was thus demonstrated, through the mechanism and rate of the process were not investigated. Ericsson et al. suggest that despite the fact that both NaF and Na_2PO_3F are absorbed equally well, F is released slowly enough from the $PO_3F^{=}$ that it can be reasonably well excreted or deposited in the skeleton, thus accounting for the lower toxicity of the latter compound.

Indirect methods, *i.e.* determination of effects on teeth and/or storage in bone, have been employed to investigate the availability of F in a variety of other compounds. Fluoride was shown to be readily available from Na_3AlF_6 and $AlFSO_4 \cdot 2\,H_2O$ (Flural) (Hein et al., 1951), $CaSiF_6$ and CuF_2 (Kempf and Nelson, 1936; Kempf et al., 1937), but not from KPF_6 (Hein et al., 1951; Zipkin and McClure, 1951), AlF_3 and ZnF_2 (Kempf and Nelson, 1936). Likins et al. (1957) also demonstrated the lack of *in vivo* hydrolysis of KPF_6, using P^{32}-labeled compound. Anbar et al. (1960) showed that the F^{18} of NaF^{18} was not taken up by the rat thyroid, whereas F^{18} of BF_4^-, as KBF_4^{18}, was accumulated in this gland; similar though lesser differences were noted in the fraction of the dose going to the liver and brain. A difference was thus shown in the ease with which these two forms of F cross cell membranes.

4. Alleviators

The toxic effects of fluorine have led to a number of attempts to alleviate or mitigate these effects by the concurrent ingestion of salts which might be expected to complex or combine with F, thereby reducing its availability.

Hobbs et al. (1954) appear to have made the most extensive study of this feature, from the points of view of long-term efficacy and of the variety of compounds considered. The effectiveness of aluminum sulfate hydrate, $Al_2(SO_4)_3 \cdot 18\,H_2O$, in reducing the absorption of ingested fluoride by sheep and cattle was shown by the increased fecal excretion of F, the decreased urinary excretion of F, and indirectly by the lesser skeletal storage of F and decreased incisor effects. Aluminium trichloride also led to good alleviation. These authors investigated the effectiveness of aluminium salts in removing F already deposited in bone, but were not able to demonstrate such an effect in rats.

A number of compounds tested for their effectiveness in decreasing the retention of ingested fluoride are listed in Table 6.

Practically without exception, the effective compounds are seen to be salts of calcium and aluminium. It is interesting to note that Weddle and Muhler (1954) found Mg to be effective only at concentrations of 1000 ppm or 10,000 ppm, and not at 100 ppm; Wagner and Muhler found Mg to be ineffective at 160 ppm or less. Hobbs et al. (1954) found $Al_2(SO_4)_3 \cdot 18\,H_2O$ to be appreciably effective only at concentrations of 1000 ppm Al or more. Dietary concentration of the alleviator clearly plays a role in its effectiveness.

Table 6. *Compounds tested for their effectiveness in reducing the availability of ingested fluoride*

Effective		Little or no effect	
Compound	Reference	Compound	Reference
$AlCl_3$	Hobbs et al. (1954)	Al salt	Ranganathan (1944)
	Sharpless (1936a)		
	Weddle and Muhler (1954)	Al_2O_3	Weddle and Muhler (1954)
$Al_2(SO_4)_3$	Hobbs et al. (1954), Majumdar and Ray (1946a, b)	$Al_2O_3 \cdot H_2O$	Hobbs et al. (1954)
	Venkataramanan and Krishnaswamy (1949)	Amberlite	Hobbs et al. (1954)
$Al(OH)(C_2H_3O_2)_2$	Hobbs et al. (1954)	B salt	Sharpless (1936b)
$CaCO_3$	Boddie (1957)	Ba salt	Ranganathan (1944)
	Ranganathan (1944)		
	Sharpless (1936a)	boric acid	Hobbs et al. (1954)
	Suttie et al. (1957)		
$CaCO_3 + Al_2O_3$	Boddie (1957)	$CaCO_3$	Harkins et al. (1963)
$CaCl_2$	Ranganathan (1944)	$CaCl_2$	Sharpless (1936a)
	Wagner and Muhler (1958)	$Ca_2P_2O_7$	Weddle and Muhler (1954)
Ca lactate	Ranganatgan (1944)	Ce salt	Sharpless (1936b)
Ca gluconate	Ranganathan (1944)	$FeSO_4$	Wagner and Muhler (1958)
CaO	Ranganathan (1944)	iodinated casein	Hobbs et al. (1954)
$Ca_3(PO_4)_2$	Ranganathan (1944)	La salt	Sharpless (1936b)
$MgCl_2$	Weddle and Muhler (1954)	$MgCO_3$	Ranganathan (1944)
		$MgCl_2$	Hobbs et al. (1954)
			Wagner and Muhler (1958)
		Th salt	Sharpless (1936b)

5. Increased retention of fluoride

Several different circumstances have been described as leading to an increase in the retention of fluoride.

Muhler (1958) has described experiments interpreted as showing that on vitamin C-deficient diets fluoride storage is minimal and is improved by supplements of vitamin C; when vitamin C intake is increased, fluoride retention also increases. This view is diametrically opposed to those put forward by Pandit and Rao (1940), Pandit et al. (1940), and Wadhwani (1952, 1954). These latter authors have interpreted their investigations as demonstrating that vitamin C-deficient diets lead to increased absorption of dietary F and to enhanced severity of skeletal fluorosis; moreover, they consider these conditions to be alleviated by supplemental ascorbic acid. The data for either view of the role of vitamin C are not particularly impressive, however. Indeed, Venkateswarlu and Narayana Rao (1954, 1957a) could find no evidence for an effect of ascorbic acid on fluoride metabolism and retention. They suggest (1957) that the beneficial effects reported for this vitamin may have been due in part to improvement of a scorbutic state concurrently present or imposed upon the fluorotic state. Several of the difficulties reported improved, viz. osteophytic outgrowths, periosteal thickening, stiffness of limbs and restricted movements, are similar in both fluorosis and chronic vitamin C deficiency.

Stookey and Muhler (1959, 1962) have suggested that molybdenum in drinking water increases the availability of the fluoride ion which may explain the decrease in dental caries seen in a population whose drinking water was low in F but which did contain appreciable amounts of Mo. Büttner (1963) however, demonstrated that molybdenum administered in the drinking water alone or with F was without effect on utilization and absorption of F, since no significant changes in F retention were noted. Similar conclusions were reached with regard to the effects of vanadium, manganese, and selenium on fluoride metabolism.

WAGNER and MUHLER (1958, 1960) are of the opinion that phosphate increases fluoride retention.

High dietary fat has been shown to increase the retention of ingested fluoride (MILLER and PHILLIPS, 1955; BUTTNER and MUHLER, 1958a; BIXLER and MUHLER, 1960).

B. Other routes of entry

There is no reason to expect that once fluoride has gained access to the extracellular water, it will be distributed in different fashions depending upon its original route of entry. The metabolic fate of this ion is governed by the interrelationships between its physical chemical properties and the biological properties of the host organism. ZIPKIN and McCLURE (1951), for example, administered F as NaF to rats in the drinking water, and gave the same total ingested dose to other rats by intraperitoneal injection; differences in skeletal deposition of F were not statistically significant.

Inhalation as a route of entry for fluorides assumes special importance where these materials are handled in industry, and absorption from the lung has been repeatedly demonstrated. COLLINGS et al. (1951) were able to show increased urinary excretion of F within the first two hours of an eight-hour industrial exposure. Moreover, they found absorption of gaseous HF and SiF_4 to be closely similar in extent and rapidity to that of F in rock phosphate dust. RYE (1960) also found rapid absorption of gaseous HF and SiF_4 in phosphate workers, but in this instance the maximal urinary excretion appeared earlier than after inhalation of the phosphate dust. DERRYBERRY et al. (1963) have reported an extensive study of elevated urinary F excretion in phosphate fertilizer workers inhaling dusts and gases containing fluoride.

LYON (1962) analyzed urine specimens of 61 individuals employed up to seven years in the handling of gaseous compounds of fluorine, and found the average excretion of F to be 1.1 ppm; atmospheric concentrations of F ranged up to 24.7 ppm.

LARGENT (1961) found both urinary and fecal excretion of F to be increased as the result of inhaling HF.

The effects of inhaled hydrogen fluoride have been reported by MACHLE et al. (1934), MACHLE and KITZMILLER (1935), and MACHLE and SCOTT (1935), by STOKINGER (1949), by LYON (1962), and by ROSENHOLTZ et al. (1963).

C. Species differences

Despite the vast literature on the biological effects of fluorides, there are distressingly few data which permit a direct comparison of F metabolism in different species. One might expect certain differences between ruminants and non-ruminants in the extent to which F is absorbed with respect to time, but this possibility appears not have been explored. PERKINSON et al. (1955) have shown that orally administered fluoride is absorbed more rapidly by sheep than by cattle, but both species are ruminants. Differences in metabolic patterns or rates among non-ruminants are suggested by the observation that the LD_{50} of NaF in the mouse, hamster, rabbit and rat ranges from 46—250 mg/kg, a variation of approximately 5-fold. These species are nonruminant herbivores.

III. Transport

The manner in which fluoride is transported in the blood has received attention from surprisingly few investigators, despite its fundamental importance to the questions of how fluoride is made available to the bone crystals for deposition and to the renal tubules for excretion.

Chen et al. (1956) prepared ultrafiltrates of normal dog plasma, using seamless visking tubing, and compared F concentrations in the ultrafiltrates and in the original plasma. These were found to be identical, indicating that the fluoride in these plasmas was completely diffusible and not protein-bound. Results were the same when concentrations of F in the plasma were increased to 1.4, 6.6 or 10.5μg/ml.

Seppili et al. (1957) reported that at "low" concentrations of fluoride in serum, a greater portion is free than is "anchored," and that the "anchored" fraction is bound to serum albumin; at higher concentrations of total F the bound fraction exceeded the free or "directly titratable" F. However, these *in vitro* studies used unrealistically high concentrations of added fluoride (6.45 and 21.0 mg %, resp.), nor has it been convincingly demonstrated that the free F is directly titratable in serum.

Bell et al. (1961) found the protein-free filtrate of blood to contain more F^{18} than did the plasma or cells, when F^{18} was given intravenously to cattle. Tosteson (1959) found F about equally divided between cells and a cell-free medium.

The most careful and thorough study currently available of the state of fluoride in blood is that of Carlson et al. (1960c). *In vivo* experiments with tracer levels of F^{18} in dogs demonstrated that 74 % of the total F^{18} in either venous or arterial blood was contained in the plasma. Similar *in vitro* experiments gave a corresponding value of 79 %.

Effects of variations in CO_2 tension of dog plasma were investigated, to determine if a plasma fluoride shift exists similar to the well-known plasma chloride shift. In these experiments the ionic distribution was first measured *in vitro* at pH 7.4, after which varying amounts of CO_2 were bubbled through the blood to produce changes in blood pH. Pertinent data are set forth in Table 7. At pH 7.7 the percentage increase in plasma chloride content was three times the percentage increase in plasma F^{18}; at lower pH's the percentage decrease of Cl was about half that of F^{18}. Fluoride does thus undergo a halide shift qualitatively similar, but quantitatively different from that of Cl. The concentration of F^{18} in the red cells at physiological pH, expressed as cpm per ml of water, was 56 % and increased as pH decreased.

The fraction of F^{18} in dog plasma which was nondiffusible across a collodion membrane was found to be 4.8 % at pH 7.4, after correction for the Donnan membrane effect.

Table 7. *Changes in plasma contents of chloride and fluoride induced by changes in whole blood* CO_2 *tension in vitro* (Carlson et al., 1960c)

Parameter	Blood pH			
	7.7	7.4	7.1	6.8
Plasma Cl, mEq/l	120.2	109.0	105.3	104.3
Δ in plasma Cl from initial value at pH 7.4[1]	+10%	—	—3.4%	—4.3%
Plasma F^{18} cpm/ml	37,480	36,414	33,723	33,210
Δ in plasma F^{18} from initial value at pH 7.4[1]	+2.9%	—	—7.4%	—8.8%
Ratio, mEq Cl/ml RBC H_2O to mEq Cl/ml plasma H_2O	0.31	0.62	0.72	0.72
Ratio, cpm F^{18}/ml RBC H_2O to cpm F^{18}/ml plasma H_2O	0.56	0.66	0.90	0.93

[1] A plus value indicates a migration from erythrocytes to plasma, and a negative value indicates migration in the other direction.

Addition of bovine albumin at the iso-electric point of this protein increased the nondiffusible fraction of F^{18} to approximately 11%. Addition of Mg to a synthetic plasma containing bovine albumin and the major ions except Ca and Mg increased the nondiffusible fraction of F^{18} but when Ca was added the nondiffusible fraction increased markedly. CARLSON (1959) suggests that perhaps the molecular species which binds F in plasma may be a positively charged Ca-protein, or that possibly F is bound as CaF^+.

IV. Distribution

A. Volume of distribution

The lack of a convenient radioisotope of fluoride surely has contributed to the singular lack of data on the volume of distribution of F. The most pertinent data appear to be those of CARLSON et al. (1960b), who were geographically and technically able to avail themselves of this shortlived isotope (half-life, 109.7 min). These authors administered F^{18} intraperitoneally to rats, and measured the concentrations of F^{18} and of Cl in the tissue and plasma water 80 min later. Their data for normal rats are summarized in Table 8. Equilibration of F^{18} between the extracellular and intracellular compartments is believed to have been achieved within the 80 min post injection. Hence, the F^{18} tissue water: plasma water ratios of less than 1.00 noted for all tissues except tendon indicate that fluoride is somewhat restricted in its entry into the intracellular compartment. The accumulation of F in the tendon is thought perhaps to be related to its Ca content. This has also been suggested by WALLACE (1953), by ANBAR et al. (1960), and by ERICSSON and ULLBERG (1958) with respect to calcification in cartilage. The ratios in the last column of Table 8 compare the distribution of the F^{18} with that of the predominantly extracellular Cl. Ratios greater than one indicate entry of F into a volume greater than the volume of distribution of Cl, and this is seen to be the case in each tissue examined except the brain. Thus, the volumes of distribution in the soft tissue fluid compartments are not the same for these two halogens. For brain, perhaps the volume of distribution really is less than that of Cl, or perhaps equilibrium had not yet been attained.

The data listed in Table 8 indicate that F crosses cell membranes with ease, and in fact, CARLSON et al. (1960c) showed that when F^{18} was added to whole dog blood, equilibrium between the erythrocyte and plasma F^{18} contents was attained within two minutes (the earliest time interval studied).

TOSTESON (1959) has investigated this process in an elegant experiment, wherein red blood cells labeled with radioisotopes of each of the halogens were

Table 8. Ratio of *F^{18} in tissue water to F^{18} in plasma water, and of F^{18} per μeq Cl in tissue to F^{18} per μeq Cl in plasma* (Data of CARLSON et al., 1960b)

Tissue	Ratio $\frac{F^{18}\text{ per ml tissue }H_2O}{F^{18}\text{ per ml plasma }H_2O}$	Ratio $\frac{F^{18}\text{ per }\mu\text{eq tissue Cl}}{F^{18}\text{ per }\mu\text{eq plasma Cl}}$
Plasma	1.00	1.0
Tendon	1.86	2.1
Skin	0.90	1.1
Testes	0.79	1.3
Liver	0.68	2.1
Muscle	0.51	2.9
Heart	0.49	1.4
Brain	0.17	0.4

Average of three rats.

suspended in a chloride-phosphate medium containing no tracer, and the rate constant for outflux of the isotope measured. In addition, the ratio of isotope concentrations in cells and medium, and the isotope flux were determined; pertinent data are summarized in Table 9. The equilibrium ratio of F^{18} is seen to be 0.5, indicating that at equilibrium this halogen is distributed equally between the cells and medium. The relative rates of transport of the four halide ions in beef red cells are Cl > Br > F > I; the rate for F is only about one-tenth that of Cl. TOSTESON's analysis of his data led him to the conclusion that some F^{18} was bound in the cells, and F and the other halides are transported across the red cell membrane by passive diffusion, though the possibility of some exchange diffusion could not be ruled out. LINDEMANN and PASSOW (1960) have also suggested that the human red cell membrane binds F.

Table 9. *Distribution and transport of tracer halides in red blood cells* (Data of TOSTESON, 1959)

Characteristic	Cl^{38}		Br^{82}		F^{18}		I^{131}	
	beef	man	beef	man	beef	man	beef	man
Equilibrium ratio, cell to medium isotope concentration	0.58	0.54	0.63	0.63	0.50	—	1.06	1.21
Rate constant for outflux, sec^{-1}	3.1	3.1	0.6	0.6	0.3	—	0.06	0.07
Flux, $\mu\mu$moles cm^{-2} sec^{-1}	13,100		3100		2300		—	

The magnitude of this binding has not been determined, and it is not clear how great an effect this would have on the relative volumes of distribution suggested by CARLSON's data (Table 7).

The rapidity with which fluoride is distributed *in vivo* has been repeatedly demonstrated in a manner much more gross and less refined than that employed by TOSTESON in his *in vitro* experiments. For example, ERICSSON and ULLBERG (1958) were able to show autoradiographically that F^{18} administered intravenously to rats was heavily concentrated in the skeleton only two minutes later. BELL et al. (1961) found 46.5 % of intravenously administered F^{18} to have left the circulating blood of cattle in two minutes. PERKINSON et al. (1955) estimated the rate of disappearance of intravenously administered F^{18} to be about 32 % per minute for cattle and 41 % per minute for lambs, and WALLACE (1953) found only 8 % of an intravenous dose of F^{18} still in the circulating blood of rats after 15 min (the earliest interval which she investigated). Orally administered fluoride also is rapidly disseminated throughout the body. ZIPKIN and LIKINS (1957) found 22 % of a dose of fluoride introduced into the stomach to be absorbed in 5 min, and PERKINSON et al. (1955) detected F^{18} in the blood of sheep 5 min after ingestion. CARLSON (1959) working with the human, found F^{18} in the urine 5 min after ingestion.

B. Organ distribution of absorbed fluoride

Values reported for the "normal" content or concentration of fluoride in tissues and organs are fraught with qualifications all too frequently ignored or glossed over (and sometimes unrecognized, one suspects). The absorption of fluoride ingested in the normal diet is influenced by a number of factors, including chemical form, whether it is ingested in food or in water, and the presence or absence of fluoride complexers. Effects of these factors on absorption have already been discussed. In addition, normal animal diets are known to vary considerably in natural fluoride content; analyses of stock laboratory animal rations have shown concentrations of 15—30 ppm, occasionally as much as 50 ppm, of fluoride;

moreover, the chemical form of this fluoride is seldom known. Normal human diets are estimated to contain approximately 1 ppm F. These factors must have some influence upon the amounts of fluoride in various organs; these, as well as others such as age, sex, previous encounters with fluoride, and time all have a clear-cut and appreciable effect on the storage of fluoride in bone, as will be discussed later. Their effect on soft tissue fluoride however, while real enough, is very much smaller in magnitude and far more difficult to demonstrate convincingly.

The problem stems chiefly from the fact that under any conditions fluoride concentrations in soft tissue are low — at most only a very few parts per million, frequently less than one ppm — and many analytical methods for these small amounts of fluoride leave much to be desired when applied to biological samples. All too frequently reagent and distillation blanks constitute a sizeable fraction of the total fluoride being determined. Attempts are sometimes made to improve matters by pooling organs, especially the smaller organs of laboratory animals, but in so doing one loses valuable information regarding the spread of values about the mean and also eliminates (or makes difficult) the possibility of statistical analysis of the data.

Analysis of total carcass ash is sometimes resorted to with small laboratory animals, to show changes in soft tissue fluoride content. This approach has limitations however, because usually 75 % or more of the carcass ash is derived from the relatively fluoride-rich skeleton and only a small proportion of the total fluoride present has come from the soft tissue. Because bone concentrations may increase to several thousands of micrograms per gram whereas soft tissue concentrations under any circumstances have been reported to increase only slightly (still of the order of 10 ppm or less), the ratio may be as great as milligrams to micrograms.

VENKATESWARLU and NARAYANARAO (1957b) have aptly stated "It need, however, be emphasized that the values reported for fluorine content of the soft tissues are only approximate ... Undoubtedly, there is still a large scope for improvement in fluoride analytical methods applicable to soft tissues."

1. Studies with radioactive fluoride

Turning now to specific studies, the distribution of F^{18} among the organs and tissues of a number of different species has been described (VOLKER et al., 1941; WALLACE, 1953; PERKINSON et al., 1955; HEIN et al., 1956; BELL et al., 1961; and ERICSSON and MALMNÄS, 1962). The data are summarized in Table 10; in order to facilitate comparison among the several studies, the results have all been listed here as per cent of dose per gram, though in several of the original publications the data are also presented as per cent of dose per organ. It is apparent (Table 10) that no organ has a particular and lasting affinity for fluoride; in general, tissue concentrations reflect the blood levels. The data of Table 10, and the work of APPELGREN et al. (1961), ERICSSON and ULLBERG (1958) and of ERICSSON (1958a) all point to the rapid disappearance of fluoride from the blood. As WALLACE (1953) has pointed out, this probably is the resultant of several processes such as equilibration in the extracellular and intracellular fluids, deposition in bone, and excretion through the kidneys. WALLACE suggests that the time necessary to attain equilibrium between the F^{18} in the blood and in the tissues depends upon the vascularity of the tissues and organs; thus, the percentage of dose per gram of liver, spleen, or small intestine is nearly the same as that in blood after only 15 min, whereas less vascular tissues such as skin and muscle required perhaps an hour to reach equilibrium. BELL et al. (1961) however, found in cattle the highly vascular liver

Table 10. *Distribution of F^{18} in tissues of various species as per cent of dose per gram of tissue*

Species, route	Rat, intravenous									Rat, oral			
weight	147 g	185 g		250 g	171 g	185 g	250 g	185 g	250 g	170 g	185 g	185 g	185 g
reference	HEIN et al. (1956)	WALLACE (1953)			HEIN et al. (1956)	WALLACE (1953)				HEIN et al. (1956)		WALLACE (1953)	
time	10 min	0.25 hr	1 hr	1 hr	1.5 hr	4 hr	4 hr	9 hr		0.5 hr	1 hr	4 hrs	9 hrs
Skeleton	1.26	2.98—1.76	3.79	2.32	1.92	5.17—4.33	2.74	3.31 —3.17	2.46	—	3.20	4.53	3.00
Muscle	0.25	0.28—0.19	0.08	0.06	0.04	0.01	0.008	0.006—0.004	0.004	0.16	0.07	0.01	0.006
Skin	—	0.39—0.29	0.07	0.08	—	0.01—0.008	0.01	0.005—0.003	0.01	—	0.06	0.008	0.01
Blood	2.98	0.65—0.50	0.08	0.08	0.11	0.015—0.008	0.008	0.005—0.003	0.004	0.93	0.10	0.01	0.005
Spleen	0.48	0.52—0.39	0.06	—	0.10	0.009	—	0.003—0.01	—	0.14	0.08	0.01	0.004
Lung	0.48	0.58—0.48	0.11	—	0.07	0.04	—	0.03 —0.01	—	0.18	0.10	0.04	0.02
Liver	0.67	0.49—0.43	0.06	0.06	0.06	0.03—0.01	0.008	0.005—0.006	0.005	0.19	0.10	0.01	0.006
Kidney	2.29	2.45—0.84	0.18	0.15	1.20	0.04—0.03	0.02	0.02 —0.01	0.01	0.45	0.19	0.04	0.04
Stomach	0.27	0.32—0.30	0.07	0.06	0.02	0.009	0.01	0.003—0.005	0.008	9.16	1.48	0.76	0.56
sm. Intest.	0.28	0.37—0.28	0.07	0.06	0.16	0.009	0.008	0.004—0.002	0.004	1.61	0.72	0.02	0.01
lg. Intest.	0.02	0.37—0.35	0.07	0.04	0.06	0.04	0.01	0.006—0.004	0.01	0.08	0.07	0.03	0.02
Bile										—	—	—	—
Brain	0.05	—	0.02	—	0.03	0.009	—	0.004	—	0.03	0.02	0.008	—
Thyroid	2.17	—	—	—	0.09	—	—	—	—	1.17	—	—	—
Adrenal	0.69	—	—	—	0.14	—	—	—	—	0.23	—	—	—
Parotid gl.	0.16	1.23—0.69	0.08	0.08	0.14	0.01	0.009	0.005—0.01	0.003	0.21	0.10	0.01	
Submax.,sublingl.gl.	0.64				0.06					0.15			
Uterus	0.15	—	—	—	0.07	—	—	—	—	0.22	—	—	—
Heart	0.37	—	—	—	0.03	—	—	—	—	0.13	—	—	—
Pancreas	—	0.41	0.04	—	—	0.009	—	0.002	—	—	0.07	0.008	0.004
Lymph node	—	—	—	—	—	—	—	—	—	—	—	—	—
Pituitary													
Mammary gl.													
Molar teeth													
Incisors													
Salivary gl.													
Teeth													

Table 10 (Continend)

Species, route	Rat, I.P.	Cat, I.V.	Cattle, I.V.		Lamb, oral	Rabbit, I.V.					Man, I.V.
weight	250 g	2.6—4.0 kg	yearling	mature	36 kg						adult females
reference	VOLKER et al. (1941)	VOLKER et al. (1941)	BELL et al. (1961)		PERKINSON et al. (1955)	ERICSSON and MALMNAS (1962)					ERICSSON and MALMNÄS (1962)
time	0.5 hr	—	4 hrs		2 hrs	15 min	19 min	35 min	25.5.min	38 min	0.25 hr.
Skeleton	0.371—1.327	0.020—0.101	0.0002—0.0006	—	0.0008–0.0048						
Muscle			0.0001	—	0.00015						
Skin			0.0001	—							
Blood	0.128—0.370	0.015—0.060	0.0001	—	0.00061	0.066	0.058	0.048	0.037	0.040	0.004—0.01
Spleen			—	—	0.00016						
Lung			0.0005	0.0009							
Liver			0.00009	0.00005	0.00033						
Kidney			0.0003	0.0002							
Stomach			0.00008–0.0003	0.00003–0.0007							
sm. Intest.			0.00006	0.00003							
lg. Intest.			0.00006	0.00005							
Bile			—	—	0.00050						
Brain			—	—							
Thyroid			0.0001	0.0001				0.051	0.013	0.023	
Adrenal			0.00005	0.00005							
Parotid gl.			0.00007								
Submax.,sublingl. gl.			—	—							
Uterus			—	—							
Heart			0.00004	0.00002							
Pancreas			0.00006		0.00033						
Lymph mode			—	—	0.00028						
Pituitary								0.076	0.046	0.023	
Mammary gl.						0.027	0.024				
Molar teeth	0.229—0.435										
Incisors	0.786—1.197										
Salivary gl.	0.098										
Teeth		0.014—0.032									

to contain only two-thirds the blood level of F^{18}. BELL et al. also found appreciable amounts of F^{18} in mucus from the cows' nostrils; perhaps this might account in part for the high concentrations found in the lungs.

The survey autoradiograms of ERICSSON and ULLBERG (1958) are in essential agreement with the data of Table 10, in that they failed to show any notable uptake of F^{18} in the parenchymatous organs, nor was there evidence of secretion via the bile or intestinal wall. Concentrations were low in muscle and depot fat, and especially so in the central nervous system.

There is no clear-cut evidence that the kidney is especially rich in fluoride content (see also Tables 11 and 12). As the data in Table 10 indicate, appreciable fractions of a single dose appear promptly in the kidney, reflecting the prompt removal of absorbed fluoride to the urine; but it is also evident that each influx of fluoride into the kidney is soon cleared from that organ. ERICSSON and ULLBERG (1958) showed autoradiographically that the concentration of F^{18} appeared to follow the anatomical localization of the collecting tubules; they also demonstrated that the whole kidney may contain up to three times as much F^{18} as a corresponding weight of blood during the first 30 min following an intravenous injection.

Throughout the years, special concern has been given to the question of whether or not F is stored preferentially in the thyroid gland. Obviously, this interest stems from the fact that this gland does have a special affinity for iodine—does this also apply to the fellow halogen, fluorine? Data in Table 10 indicate that thyroid concentrations of F^{18} in every instance but one were equal to or less than that in blood, *i.e.* the gland does not concentrate fluoride. GALLETTI and JOYET's study (1958) with F^{18} also failed to demonstrate any thyroidal uptake of F. The reasons for this distinction in behavior of the thyroid toward I^- and F^- are not known at present. ULLBERG et al. (1964) have demonstrated failure of the thyroid to accumulate radiochloride and radiobromide. They do not consider the thyroid to be "halide blind." The work of ANBAR et al. (1959, 1960), LEWITUS et al. (1962) and of WOLFF and MAUREY (1963) all suggest that ionic size, valency and shape are important in determining those anions which are capable of entering the iodide transport system and thus being accumulated by the thyroid. If these are governing factors, then fluoride evidently fails to qualify in some respect, perhaps in size.

The effects of Na ethylenediamine tetraacetate, zirconium, scandium and yttrium on the distribution of F^{18} in the rat was studied by ANBAR and ERNST (1962), who injected mixtures of each of the complexers with NaF^{18}. EDTA caused a decrease in the concentration of F^{18} in the liver, kidney, and brain and especially in bone; the authors interpret the results as a retarded uptake of F^{18} in bone owing to the induced decalcification caused by EDTA. In the presence of Zr, an extremely stable complex with F is formed, and apparently a major portion of the F is bound to Zr and shares the metabolic fate of the latter element. Clearance of F from the circulation is augmented, as evidenced both by decreased specific activity in the tissues, and by increased relative specific activities in liver, spleen, kidney and bone. When Sc was added to the injected F^{18}, clearance of the fluoride was enhanced, and storage in bone was reduced. Yttrium decreased the rate of clearance of F from the blood and its skeletal uptake. ANBAR and ERNST (loc. cot.) suggest that alterations in F^{18} distribution in different regions of bone formation, achievable with complexers, may be useful for medical diagnostic purposes.

Distribution of KBF_4 labeled with F^{18} has been reported by ANBAR et al. (1960, 1961), ANBAR and ERNST (1962) and by ASKENASY et al. (1962); in each instance, relative specific activities were reported. KBF_4 is distributed reasonably uniformly throughout the liver, spleen, muscle and bone; concentrations are somewhat higher in kidney and lung, very much higher in the thyroid, and very much lower in the brain. These findings have led ANBAR et al. (1961) and ASKENASY et al. (1962) to propose the use of KBF_4^{18} for the localization of brain tumors. Blood/brain ratios for KBF_4^{18} were compared with those for several other isotopes considered for the localization of intracranial lesions (As^{74}, as Na arsenate, Cu^{64} as Cu versenate, I^{131} as NaI, and F^{18}-labeled fluorescein) and found to be appreciably higher, whereas muscle/brain were comparable to those for Na arsenate and Cu versenate. This combination of factors, *i.e.* low concentration in brain as compared to blood, no affinity for bone, and ready penetration of muscle (assumed comparable to that of brain lesions) recommend KBF_4^{18} to these authors as superior to other tracers for the detection and localization of disturbances in the blood-brain barrier. Fluorofluorescein, with a very limited permeability into muscle was considered useful in detecting changes in brain vascularization rather than in tissue permeability. In this connection, it is interesting to note that KETY (1963) has described the use of I^{131}-labeled trifluoroiodomethane in blood-flow studies in the brain.

In a beautiful series of experiments APPELGREN et al. (1961) have visually demonstrated the distribution of F^{18} in mice and rats and compared this with distribution of calcium. In these experiments, autoradiographs of sections of the entire animal were prepared after the successive injection of F^{18} and Ca^{45}. Both isotopes were rapidly removed from the blood, while F^{18} accumulated more rapidly in hard tissues; Ca^{45} appeared in appreciable amounts in some soft tissues. The principal excretory organ for F^{18} was the kidney, while high concentrations of Ca^{45} were seen in the mucosa and contents of the small intestine. Very low concentrations of F^{18} were evident in the central nervous system of the mouse after 30 min (see also ERICSSON and ULLBERG, 1958). This is interesting, in view of the report by BIXLER and MUHLER (1960) of high concentrations of F in chick brain following administration of fluoride for several weeks. CARLSON (1959) found concentrations of F^{18} in the tissue water of rat brain to be significantly lower than in any other tissue, suggesting an effective blood-brain barrier against F in nervous tissue.

Both autoradiographic and tracer experiments with F^{18} have been helpful in demonstrating the role of calcification in fluoride uptake in non-skeletal tissue. WALLACE (1953) found cartilage to be a significant site of deposition of F^{18}, tracheal cartilage containing about twice as much as xiphoid cartilage. The latter apparently does not calcify; hence, WALLACE was led to comment that cartilage takes up F^{18} to an extent related to its potentialities for calcification. ERICSSON and ULLBERG (1958), and APPELGREN et al. (1961) found no uptake of F^{18} in non-calcified cartilage. ANBAR et al. (1960) did report that tracheal cartilage accumulated F^{18}, and pointed out that this must be considered when attempting to follow the behavior of F^{18} by external counting in the vicinity of the thyroid. ERICSSON and ULLBERG (1958) also showed conclusively that areas of localized calcification, as in the placenta for instance, take up F^{18} leading to localized fluoride deposits. The significance of this in selecting portions of organs for analysis is obvious; this may well explain in part the widely divergent values frequently seen in soft tissue concentrations of F regardless of whether portions or total organs are analyzed.

2. Studies with nonradioactive fluoride

a) Normal fluoride intake

Fluoride concentrations in various organs as determined not by F^{18} measurements but by chemical analyses of the tissues for the stable isotope, are listed in Tables 11 and 12. The former table represents a summary of earlier data reported in detail in HODGE and SMITH (in press), whereas data published since then or not included in the earlier compilation are shown in Table 12. A considerable variation

Table 11. *Summary of fluoride concentrations in soft tissues of different species*[1]. *Data as parts per million of fluoride*[2]

Organ or tissue	Cat	Chicken	Cow	Dog	Guinea pig	Man	Pig	Rabbit	Rat	Sheep	Turkey
Blood . . .		12	0.69—37	0—0.61	0.13— 3.3	0—40	0.7—0.97	0—7.5	0—0.4		
Brain . . .			4.4 —16.6	0.31 0.97	6.6 — 7.2 0.52	1.8 —43 0.40—0.68		2.0 — 3.2	3.0—3.4 4.3—4.4	5.0 —19.2	
Duodenum .						2.8				3.4[3]	
Fat		0.9				3—4		0.5—0.7			
Gall bladder						3.9					
Hair			6.1 —7.0[3]			14—30 2.4 2.1					
Heart . . .			1.8 — 2.5 2.3 — 2.7[3]	0.44 0.46	7.9 —11.5 0.24	1.3 — 6.6 0.44—0.60		1.1—2.7 0.9	5.9—6.8 2.6	4.0 —12.7 2.2 — 3.1[3] 3.0[3] 0.34—0.36	
Kidney. . .	1.1	6.0—6.5	2.5 — 2.8 6.8 —10.1[3]	0.42 0.52	4.4 — 5.8 0.06	2.1 —94 0.56—0.78		0.8—10.6 1.7	3.2—3.5 28.7 0.62	2.2 —11.4 2.3 — 4.5[3] 4.2[3] 1.0 — 1.3	2.6—6.5
Liver . . .	0.5	6.0—6.5	0.19 0.66[3] 0.6 — 2.0 5.2 — 5.8[3]	0.1 — 0.3 0.26—0.48 0.63 0.1 — 0.3	1.4 — 1.7 0.4	2.5 —19 0.36—0.70	13.3	0.8—1.7 0—1.8 0.2	1.2 21.3 0.21	3.7 —18.6 0.6 — 1.0[3] 3.5[3] 0.23—0.30	1.6—2.7
Lungs . . .	0.9		1.9 — 5.6 2.67[3]	0.40 0.56	3.9 — 9.6 0.4	4.5 —23 0.16—0.42		0.7—3.4 4.8—6.5	14.1 1.5	3.1 — 7.1 0.54—0.59	
Marrow . .						44					
Muscle . . .		4.6	0.7 —0.75	0.8 — 2.0 0.30 0.13 0.6 — 1.1	2.5 — 4.0	2—3.7		1.1—5.9 0.6—1.0	3.1—8.1 0.53	2.0[3]	1.2—2.2[3]
Nails. . . .						3.6					
Nerve . . .						16					

Table 11. (Continued)

Pancreas . .		6.9 —10.3[3]	0.27		2.8 —38		0.5		2.8[3]	
Skin				0.3	5					
Spleen . . .			0.41 0.37	22.5—36.5	2.6 —18 0.25—0.30		19.5—26.2	3.4	2.2 0.43—0.62	
Stomach . .			0.43	0.2	2.9 —6.7					
Thyroid . .		6.8[3]			1.5 —95		9		3.0[3]	
Tendon . .		5.4 — 7.5[3]			24					

[1] Summary of data from the literature described in detail in HODGE and SMITH (in press).
[2] Assumed to be fresh weight unless stated otherwise.
[3] Dry weight basis.

is evident from organ to organ, and also from species to species. Nevertheless, it is apparent that all organs are usually found to contain less than 10 ppm F, regardless of species.

b) Chronic ingestion of fluoride

Table 13 lists values reported for F in soft tissues following the chronic ingestion of fluoride. Data reported here are limited to representative, recent experiments, and include the control data in each instance. The data of BELL et al. (1961), of SUTTIE et al. (1958) and of HARVEY (1952) represent experimental periods of 2—8 years, while those of BIXLER and MUHLER (1960) and HOBBS et al. (1954) represent periods of 1—4 months. In general, the kidney is seen to be relatively high in fluoride concentration; as has been indicated previously, this probably reflects the role of this organ in excreting fluoride rather than a special affinity for F. The high values reported for brain (BIXLER and MUHLER, 1960) are unusual, in view of the failure of autoradiographic technics to demonstrate any localization of F^{18} in this organ. The experiments reported with cattle and sheep comprise studies by four different laboratories, continued for periods of one month to eight years, and include dietary levels of 5—200 ppm F, yet they are remarkably uniform in demonstrating that in nearly every instance (and even at 200 ppm in the diet) the organs and tissues analyzed did not increase in fluoride content by more than about three-fold. In the two studies wherein blood concentrations were measured, the increases were 1.6—2.8-fold. Moreover, the individually reported data of SUTTIE et al. (1958) show that F concentrations in the same organ from animal to animal on the same level of dietary supplement may vary by factors of 1.0 to 4.8 or more. Indeed, the latter authors (loc. cit.) state that fluorine concentration of soft tissues is a very poor index of fluorosis because of the narrow margin between fluorotic and non-fluorotic animals. HOBBS et al. (1954) noted that differences were found in F concentrations in the organs analyzed, but that these could not be attributed to differences in dietary fluoride even though these ranged up to 200 ppm. WAGNER (1962b) suggests

Table 12. *Normal concentrations of fluoride in the organs of various animal species*

Species	Organ	ppm F	Comment	Reference
Chicken	femur	404	Basis for concn. not stated. Age, 8 wks.	BIXLER and MUHLER (1960)
	carcass	378	As above	
	heart	0.2	As above	
	liver	0.2	As above	
	kidney	0.2	As above	
	brain	2.5	As above	
	muscle	0.5	As above	
Cow	reticular wall	2.03	Wet basis. Stock ration contained 7 ppm F	BELL et al. (1961)
	rumen wall	1.29		
	abomasal wall	0.44		
	lg. intest. wall	5.33		
	aorta	0.74		
	heart	0.14		
	lung	0.38		
	liver	0.18		
	kidney	0.38		
	pancreas	0.11		
	thyroid	0.45		
	placenta	0.41		
	fetal placenta	0.32		
	blood	0.05		
Cow	blood	17.9	Whole blood. On expt. 10 mo. Ingested 288 mg F daily from normal stock ration.	MARIAKULANDAI and VENKATARAMAIAH (1955)
	brain	72	Ash basis; as above	
	lungs	349		
	heart	307		
	stomach	404		
	sm. intestines	310		
	lg. intestines	330		
	liver	102		
	kidneys	265		
	spleen	220		
	gall bladder	355		
	muscle	218		
	skin + hair	260		
	bone	1683–2150		
	incisors	514		
	molars	667		
	hoofs	924		
	horn	1351		
Cow	heart	2.3	Basal ration contained 3—5 ppm F for 5.5 yrs. Dry wt. of organ; av. of 3 animals	SUTTIE et al. (1958)
	liver	2.3	As above	
	kidney	3.5	As above	
	pancreas	2.8	As above; dry, fat-free	
	thyroid	2.1	As above; dry, fat-free	
	adrenal	5.3	As above; dry, fat-free	
	blood	0.34	Whole blood	
Dog	lung	7.5	Basis for concn. not stated; assumed to be ash wt.	MINOGUCHI and IWAMOTO (1957)
	blood	0.1		
	heart	3.5		
	liver	7.3		
	pancreas	5.1		

Table 12. (Continued)

Species	Organ	ppm F	Comment	Reference
Dog	spleen	5.6		
	kidney	4.8		
	stomach	2.0		
	intestine	5.7		
	muscle	4.5		
	bone	531—821		
	teeth	660		
Dog	blood	0—0.25	95% of 84 samples from 35 dogs within this range	SMITH and GARDNER (1951)
Guinea pig	carcass	317—319	Basis for concn. not stated. Stock diet contained 3 ppm F, water was F-free	MUHLER (1958)
Sheep	liver	0.6—1.0	Dry wt. basis. Age 6 wks.	HARVEY (1952)
	kidney	2.3—4.5	As above	
	heart	2.2—3.1	As above	
	spleen	2.2	As above	
	bone	57—76	Ash basis. Age 6 wks.	
	teeth	40—70	As above	
Sheep	liver	3.5	Dry wt. basis. Age 2 yrs. 8 mo.	HARVEY (1952)
	kidney	4.2	As above	
	pancreas	2.8	As above	
	thyroid	3.0	As above	
	heart	3.0	As above	
	gastrocnemius muscle	2.0	As above	
	duodenum	3.4	As above	
	bone	150—225	Ash basis	
	teeth	84—120	As above	
	dentine	210	As above	
	enamel	60	As above	
Sheep	liver	0.23	Wet wt. basis. Initial age 8—12 mo., 1 mo. on stock ration containing 6 ppm F	HOBBS et al. (1954)
		0.30	As above after 4 mo.	
	heart	0.36	As above after 1 mo.	
		0.34	As above after 4 mo.	
	kidney	1.04	As above after 1 mo.	
		1.32	As above after 4 mo.	
	lung	0.54	As above after 1 mo.	
		0.59	As above after 4 mo.	
	spleen	0.43	As above after 1 mo.	
		0.62	As above after 4 mo.	
Rabbit	bone	312	Wet wt. basis. 46 ppm F in stock diet. Fetal carcass from these mothers contained 3 ppm F	MAPLESDEN et al. (1960)
Rat	femur	280—300 Av. 297	Ash. 0.2 ppm F in food; dist'd. H_2O; non-pregnant females	BRZEZINSKI et al. (1962)
	blood	0.09; 0.12		
	femur	270—300 Av. 289	As above, but pregnant	
	blood	0.10	As above	
Rat	carcass	53	Ash basis. Mothers' diet contained 1 ppm F. Age 1 day	BUTTNER and MUHLER (1958b)
		48	As above; age, 10 days	

Table 12. (Continued)

Species	Organ	ppm F	Comment	Reference
Rat	femur	168	Basis of concn. not stated. Stock corn diet, redist'd. water. Weanling males 4 wks. on expt.	BUTTNER and MUHLER (1957)
	carcass	123	As above	
Rat	carcass	0.2	Food contained 0.2 ppm F. Initial age 1 mo.; on expt. 1 mo. Concn. on wet wt. basis	JACKSON (1955)
		0.7	As above; on expt. 2 mo.	
		1.0	As above; on expt. 3 mo.	
		0.7	As above; on expt. 4 mo.	
		1.0	As above; on expt. 5 mo.	
		1.5	As above; on expt. 6 mo.	
Rat	carcass	9—11	Wet wt. basis. 3 ppm F in stock diet. F not detectable in fetal carcasses from these mothers	MAPLESDEN et al. (1960)
	carcass	9.2	Wet wt. basis; 3 ppm F in stock diet. Fetal carcasses contained 0.2—1 ppm F	
Rat	carcass	19—95	Basis for concn. not stated; probably ash. Food, 0.05 ppm F; water F-free	MUHLER et al. (1959)
	femur	21—145	As above	
Rat	femur	42	Ash basis; drinking water pH 2	MUHLER and WEDDLE (1955b)
		43	As above; water, pH 4	
		109	As above; water, pH 6	
Rat	carcass	60	Basis for concn. not stated. Diet contained 0.08 ppm F; drinking water F-free	STOOKEY and MUHLER (1962)
	femur	63	As above	
Rat	carcass	26.4	Basis for concn. not stated. Diet contained 0.5 ppm F	STOOKEY and MUHLER (1959)
	femur	35.5	As above	
Rat	femur	218	Basis for concn. not stated; probably ash. Water supply F-free	STOOKEY et al. (1962b)
	incisor	52	As above	
	carcass	144	As above	
Rat	femur	111	Basis for concn. not stated; probably dry wt. Old males; age 1.5—2.5 yrs. Diet and water low in F	WAGNER (1962b)
	carcass	88	As above; basis not stated	
	heart	6.1	As above	
	liver	2.3	As above	
	kidney	3.1	As above	
Rat	femur	133	Basis for concn. not stated; probably dry wt. Young males aged 91 days. Diet and water low in F	WAGNER (1962b)
	carcass	100	As above; basis not stated	
	heart	1.6	As above	
	liver	0.3	As above	
	kidney	0.7	As above	

Table 12 (Continued)

Species	Organ	ppm F	Comment	Reference
Rat	carcass	214	Basis for concn. not stated. Weanling males	WAGNER and MUHLER (1960)
Rat	carcass	74—178	Basis for concn. not stated; probably ash. Food, 0.5 ppm F; water 1.2 ppm F	WAGNER and MUHLER (1959b)
Rat	carcass	29	Basis for concn. not stated. Diet contained 0.5 ppm F. Age, ca. 2 mo.	WAGNER and MUHLER (1958)
		116	As above. Water supply contained 1 ppm F	
Rat	liver	0.21	Fresh wt. Av. of 6 young rats	VENKATESWARLU and NARAYANARAO (1957b)
	muscle	0.53		
	kidney	0.62		
	lung	1.50		
	heart	2.60		
	spleen	3.40		
	bone	775		

that soft tissue deposition of retained F increases in older rats due to the well-known slower rate of skeletal storage in older animals (see, for example, WALLACE-DURBIN, 1954). However, a more extensive ectopic tissue calcification could account for this increase (ERICSSON and ULLBERG, 1958).

The mean concentrations reported in Table 13 indicate a trend toward higher levels as the dietary intake is increased. It would be expected that fluoride treatment would increase the soft tissue level when the level of absorbed fluoride became sufficient to increase the amount of fluoride in the extracellular fluid. Data of SINGER and ARMSTRONG (1960) pertain to this point, and show that "fluoride homeostasis" as indicated by relatively constant concentrations (0.1—0.2 ppm) of F in plasma, *i.e.*, extracellular fluid is maintained despite variations in concentration of water borne fluoride in the range of 0.15—2.5 ppm. At 5.4 ppm F in drinking water, the capacity of these mechanisms is somewhat exceeded and a new state of equilibrium characterized by a slightly greater plasma concentration (0.24 ppm of F) is achieved. SINGER and ARMSTRONG (1960), and ARMSTRONG (1961) suggest that fluoride homeostasis is achieved by regulation of the intestinal absorption of F, renal excretion, and skeletal uptake of F. More recently, STOOKEY et al. (1963) purport to have shown a renal effect in regulating intestinal absorption.

The data in Table 13 clearly indicate that accurate and precise analytical methods are essential to demonstrate the relatively slight changes in tissue fluoride concentrations to be expected from even drastic treatment with fluoride. Analysis of any single organ (other than bone), or indeed of all organs of a single animal, is not sufficient to prove whether or not the animal in question was receiving supplemental fluoride in addition to the "normal" dietary intake. SMITH et al. (1950) have called attention to this uncertainty with regard to blood fluoride concentrations.

Table 13. *Concentrations of fluoride in organs of different*

Experimental conditions	Heart	Liver	Kidney	Pancreas	Lung
					Chicken, BIXLER
Controls	0.2	0.2	0.2	—	—
2 mg F orally, daily; 8 wks.	0.8	1.6	3.7	—	—
20% cottonseed oil in diet; 8 wks.	1.6	0.7	2.9	—	—
2 mg F orally, daily; 20% cottonseed oil, 8 wks.	1.2	0.8	1.7	—	—
20% oleic acid in diet 8 wks.	2.6	0.2	2.0	—	—
2 mg F orally, daily; 20% oleic acid; 8 wks.	1.4	0.5	1.3	—	—
20% stearic acid in diet 8 wks.	0.5	2.3	4.4	—	—
2 mg F orally, daily; 20% stearic acid; 8 wks.	1.8	2.3	7.6	—	—
20% lard in diet; 8 wks.	0.6	0.4	2.9	—	—
2 mg F orally, daily; 20% lard; 8 wks.	0.7	0.6	2.1	—	—
					Cow, BELL
7 ppm F in stock ration 8 yrs.	0.14 ± 0.01	0.18 ± 0.04	0.38 ± 0.06	0.11 ± 0.04	0.38 ± 0.05
40 ppm F added to above ration 8 yrs.	0.23 ± 0.04	0.34 ± 0.07	1.10 ± 0.42	0.16 ± 0.09	0.83 ± 0.17
50 ppm F added to above ration 8 yrs.	0.23 ± 0.03	0.25 ± 0.02	0.96 ± 0.16	0.17 ± 0.03	0.62 ± 0.11
					Cow, SUTTIE
Stock diet containing 3—5 ppm F	1.7—3.3 2.3[5]	1.9—3.1 2.3[5]	2.9—4.4 3.5[5]	1.7—4.0 2.8[6]	—
20 ppm F added to stock diet 5.5 yrs.	2.5—4.4 3.4[5]	2.1—3.9 2.7[5]	6.0—12.8 8.6[5]	1.7—3.2 2.2[6]	—
30 ppm F added to stock diet 5.5 yrs.	2.7—4.7 3.5[5]	2.5—5.1 4.1[5]	9.1—12.5 10.7[5]	2.0—5.0 3.5[6]	—
40 ppm F added to stock diet 5.5 yrs.	2.9—5.5 4.0[5]	3.0—5.6 3.8[5]	7.8—20.4 16.0[5]	3.0—5.1 3.8[6]	—
50 ppm F added to stock diet 5.5 yrs.	3.2—6.3 4.6[5]	2.1—4.8 3.6[5]	13.7-28.9 19.3[5]	4.0—4.5 4.2[6]	—
					Dog, MINOGUCHI
Control dog	3.5	7.3	4.8	5.1	7.5
Fed 13.6 mg F daily for 26 months[8]	37.7	29.5	95.3	62.9	15[8]
					Lamb,
Control lambs[10]	2.2—3.1	0.6—1.0	2.3—4.5	—	—
One lamb; drinking water of mother contained 2 ppm F[10]	2.7	0.7	2.2	—	—
Drinking water of mothers contained 10 ppm F[10]	1.8—4.0 2.9	1.0—1.3 1.2	6.0—7.3 6.7	—	—
Controls 2 yrs. old[11]	3.0	3.5	4.2	2.8	—
Drinking water contained 5 ppm F 2 yrs. Oaten chaff diet[11]	2.4	2.8	14.8	1.0	—

animal species after ingestion of fluoride; values in ppm F

Spleen	Thyroid	Muscle	Intest.	Adrenal	Aorta	Brain	Stomach	Blood
and MUHLER (1960)[1]								
—	—	0.5	—	—	—	2.5	—	—
—	—	2.5	—	—	—	17.5	—	—
—	—	3.7	—	—	—	5.8	—	—
—	—	12.7	—	—	—	13.0	—	—
—	—	1.8	—	—	—	8.0	—	—
—	—	0.5	—	—	—	4.6	—	—
—	—	0.6	—	—	—	3.6	—	—
—	—	3.8	—	—	—	5.2	—	—
—	—	0.7	—	—	—	6.3	—	—
—	—	0.7	—	—	—	1.7	—	—
et al. (1961)[2]								
—	0.45 ± 0.03	—	533[3] ± 1.66	—	0.74 ± 0.08	—	—	0.05 ± 0.01
—	0.86 ± 0.31	—	5.50[3] ± 0.49	—	4.09 ± 3.22	—	—	0.09 ± 0.04
—	0.62 ± 0.06	—	9.00[3] ± 2.00	—	4.99 ± 2.63	—	—	0.14 ± 0.06
et al. (1958)[4]								
—	0.6—2.9 2.1[6]	—	—	2.0—11.9 5.3[6]	—	—	—	0.22–0.49 0.34
—	2.9—11.2 6.9[6]	—	—	3.3—3.8 3.5[6]	—	—	—	0.34–0.84 0.54
—	2.4—4.1 3.5[6]	—	—	3.3—3.3 3.3[6]	—	—	—	0.30–0.89 0.55
—	4.9—7.6 5.8[6]	—	—	2.5—8.8 4.7[6]	—	—	—	0.31–0.94 0.66
—	4.4—12.2 7.3[6]	—	—	4.1—8.7 6.4[6]	—	—	—	0.38–0.84 0.67
and IWAMOTO (1957)[7]								
5.6	—	4.5	5.7	—	—	—	2.0	—
95.6	—	51.0	89.3	—	—	—	52.6	—
HARVEY (1952)[9]								
2.2—2.2	—	—	—	—	—	—	—	—
1.7	—	—	—	—	—	—	—	—
0.8—1.7 1.3	—	—	—	—	—	—	—	—
—	3.0	2.0	3.4	—	—	—	—	—
—	4.6	1.2	2.0	—	—	—	—	—

Table 13.

Experimental conditions	Heart	Liver	Kidney	Pancreas	Lung
					Lamb,
Drinking water contained 10 ppm F 2 yrs. Oaten chaff[11]	3.0	2.2	22.6	5.2	—
Drinking water contained 5 ppm F 2 yrs. Lucerne chaff[11]	2.0	1.0	6.2	1.0	—
Drinking water contained 10 ppm F 2 yrs. Lucerne chaff[11]	1.5	2.0	5.4	2.0	—
					Lamb, HOBBS
Controls; stock diet contained 6 ppm F; 1 month	0.36	0.23	1.04	—	0.54
As above; 4 months	0.34	0.30	1.32	—	0.59
25 ppm F added to stock ration containing 6 ppm F; 1 month	0.92	0.63	1.11	—	0.48
As above; 4 months	0.54	1.64	1.16	—	0.48
50 ppm F added to stock ration containing 6 ppm F; 1 month	0.14	0.33	1.27	—	0.40
As above; 4 months	0.49	0.21	1.22	—	1.53
75 ppm F added to ration containing 6 ppm F; 1 month	0.21	0.34	0.86	—	0.28
As above; 4 months	0.40	0.34	1.68	—	0.38
100 ppm F added to ration containing 6 ppm F; 1 month	0.11	0.16	0.43	—	0.27
As above; 4 months	0.66	0.62	1.29	—	0.80
200 ppm F added to ration containing 6 ppm F; 1 month	0.47	0.47	1.42	—	0.05
As above; 4 months	0.48	0.42	2.73	—	0.81
					Rat, VENKATESWARLU
Controls	2.60	0.21	0.62	—	1.50
2 mg F daily in milk 76 days; sac. on 77th day	5.40	0.28	1.50	—	2.30
					Rat,
Old controls (1.5—2.5 yrs.) On low-F water and diet throughout life	6.1	2.3	3.1	—	—
Young controls (45 days old). Low-F water and diet throughout life	1.6	0.3	0.7	—	—
Old rats ingesting total of 66.5 mg F in water	21.4	4.5	8.9	—	—
Young rats ingesting total of 66.5 mg F in	9.0	1.7	3.8	—	—

[1] Concn. basis not stated; pooled 3 or 6 organs for each analysis.
[2] Concn. basis not stated; presumed to be fresh wt. Mean and std. error of mean, 4 animals.
[3] Large intestine, wall.
[4] Mean of 3 or 4 cows, and range.
[5] Concn. basis dry wt.
[6] Concn. basis dry, fat-free wt.
[7] Concn. basis not stated; presumed to be ash wt.
[8] Pregnant during last two months.

(Continued)

Spleen	Thyroid	Muscle	Intest.	Adrenal	Aorta	Brain	Stomach	Blood
HARVEY (1952)[9]								
—	13.0	5.5	2.5	—	—	—	—	—
—	7.5	2.4	1.2	—	—	—	—	—
—	10.0	2.0	4.0	—	—	—	—	—
et al. (1954)[12, 13]								
0.43	—	—	—	—	—	—	—	—
0.62	—	—	—	—	—	—	—	—
0.71	—	—	—	—	—	—	—	—
0.44	—	—	—	—	—	—	—	—
0.65	—	—	—	—	—	—	—	—
0.76	—	—	—	—	—	—	—	—
0.58	—	—	—	—	—	—	—	—
0.53	—	—	—	—	—	—	—	—
0.05	—	—	—	—	—	—	—	—
1.08	—	—	—	—	—	—	—	—
0.50	—	—	—	—	—	—	—	—
0.44	—	—	—	—	—	—	—	—
and NARAYANARAO (1957b)[14]								
3.40	—	0.53	—	—	—	—	—	—
7.27	—	1.60	—	—	—	—	—	—
WAGNER (1962b)[15]								
—	—	—	—	—	—	—	—	—
—	—	—	—	—	—	—	—	—
—	—	—	—	—	—	—	—	—
—	—	—	—	—	—	—	—	—

[9] Concn. basis dry wt.; range and/or mean, 2 animals.
[10] Six weeks of age.
[11] Initial age, 4 months.
[12] Concn. basis fresh wt.; each value, average of 2 lambs.
[13] Age range, 8—12 months.
[14] Concn. basis fresh wt.; average of six rats.
[15] Concn. basis dry wt. Means of 9 or 10 male rats.

C. Distribution of total body fluoride

1. Distribution in animals

The determination of total body fluoride and its distribution among body compartments has seldom been attempted.

In one instance, WADHWANI (1953) administered 0.9 mg F as NaF daily to 12 young rats for 20 weeks, then sacrificed three of the animals and determined the total F content. This proved to be, on the average, 68.80 mg, in excellent agreement with the average total of 73.34 mg calculated from fluoride balance data on these same animals. A second group of 3 rats was also sacrificed at the same time, and the F content determined for different structures and organs. Finally, when the daily administration of fluoride was terminated after 20 weeks, the remaining six animals were returned to normal F intake for 12 weeks. They were then sacrificed, total fluoride determined in three of them (47.52 mg, contrasted with 51.97 mg calculated from balance data) and the F content of organs and bones measured in the other three. WADHWANI's data, expressed as percentages of the total F, are listed in Table 14.

Table 14. *Distribution of total body fluoride in the rat as percentage of the total*
Data of WADHWANI (1953)[1]

Total F: 68.80 mg				Total F: 47.52 mg[2]			
Soft tissue	Per cent	Bone	Per cent	Soft tissue	Per cent	Bone	Per cent
Stomach	0.06	fibula	0.17	Stomach	0.02	fibula	0.21
Small intest.	0.27	radius	0.67	Small intest.	0.11	radius	0.74
Duodenum	0.04	ulna	0.95	Duodenum	0.02	ulna	1.04
Kidney	0.25	humerus	2.34	Kidney	0.23	humerus	2.56
Liver	0.25	scapula	1.12	Liver	0.15	scapula	0.84
Heart	0.27	femur	2.62	Heart	0.12	femur	2.85
Spleen	0.10	tibia	2.32	Spleen	0.07	tibia	2.35
Aorta	0.02			Aorta	0.01		
Lungs	0.10	total	10.19	Lungs	0.02	total	10.59
Brain	0.37			Brain	0.21		
Pelt	1.45			Pelt	0.90		
Thyroid	0.02			Thyroid	0.01		
Pancreas	0.14			Pancreas	0.01		
Adrenals	0.17			Adrenals	0.12		
Total	3.51			Total	2.00		
Grand total	13.70			Grand total	12.59		

[1] Expressed in terms of fresh, whole organs.
[2] These rats had been fed F, then returned to a normal diet prior to sacrifice (see text).

It is apparent that the fluoride content of the vital organs constitutes only a small percentage of the total F in the body. Unfortunately, data are not available for the entire skeleton and teeth, nor for the remainder of the bone-free carcass. These fractions, *i.e.* those not analyzed, together contain 86.30 % of the total of 68.80 mg in one instance and 87.41 % of the 47.52 mg in the other. Rough assumptions as to weight of carcass remainder and average fluoride in the remaining soft tissue will readily demonstrate that F in the remaining soft tissue is likewise a small fraction of the total, *e.g.* less than 6 % if one assumes 200 g of soft tissue containing as much as 20 ppm F (an unusually high concentration). In other words, 90 % or more of the total F in WADHWANI's rats was localized in the skeleton.

It should be evident from these figures that attempts to assess changes in soft tissue fluoride from analyses of whole carcass ash, which consists primarily of skeletal ash, are very likely to prove meaningless. Ninety per cent or more of the F retained will be localized in the bony tissue, whereas not more than ten per cent will appear in the soft tissues. Of the total carcass F being measured then, 90 % or more is of no significance with regard to the soft tissue changes being sought; these changes are to be found in only one-tenth of the total being measured. The situation is analogous to that of an analytical method in which the value of the reagent and procedure blank is nine times greater than the experimental value being determined.

In a somewhat similar experiment MARIAKULANDAI and VENKATARAMAIAH (1955) investigated the compartmentation of F in three calves. One animal served as a control, a second received sodium fluoride solution per os, and the third was given fluoride together with bone meal; the initial daily dose was one gram of NaF daily, which was varied from time to time depending upon the condition of the animals, and the respective regimens were continued 37—46 weeks. At sacrifice "individual analyses of every part" of the animals were done. This experiment is as remarkable for the enormity of the undertaking as for its scientific merit.

The data resulting are listed in Table 15.

Table 15. *Distribution of total body fluoride in calves.* Data of MARIAKULANDAI and VENKATARAMAIAH (1955)[1]

Tissue	Per cent of total body fluoride		
	Control	Fluoride	Fluoride + bone meal
	total F, 13.369 g	total F, 43.780 g	total F, 22.290 g
Skull and teeth	25.2	21.5	25.3
Skeleton . . .	73.1	78.0	74.0
Hoofs and horns	0.05	0.03	0.04
Pelt	0.37	0.08	0.17
Muscle	1.32	0.08	0.21
Organs	0.27	0.26	0.35
Total	100.31	99.95	100.07

[1] In fresh tissue.

Again it is apparent that the vital organs contain only a small fraction of the total fluoride, less than one per cent in these animals. In fact, 98 % of the total is localized in the calcified structures. Of this, about one-fourth is present in the skull and teeth. Muscle, the major bulk of the animal carcass, contains only one per cent of the F or less.

2. Distribution in man

Ultimately, concern regarding the *in vivo* distribution of fluoride centers about the question of its distribution in the organs and tissues of man. Compared to the data cited from animal studies, however, there is a great paucity of data relating to this question.

In Table 16 are listed concentrations found in a few investigations in which a number of organs were analyzed. The difficulties referred to previously in making rigorous comparisons are again evident; concentrations among the three studies differ by an order of magnitude or more. Nevertheless, it is also apparent that in man as well as in lower species no single organ is unusually rich in fluoride.

In a number of other studies miscellaneous individual organs have been analyzed, with the following results (expressed as ppm F in fresh tissue): placenta, 0.07—0.27 (GEDALIA et al., 1961a) and 0—6 (GARDNER et al., 1952); hair 2.4, nails, 3.6 (VON FELLENBERG, 1948); cornea, lens, usually not detected but as high as 383 in the cornea in one instance (SCASSELLATI-SFORZOLINI and SCASSELLATI-SFORZOLINI, 1956); thyroid, 1.5—95 (EVANS and PHILLIPS, 1938); urinary tract calculi, less than 1 to 1790 but concentration basis not stated (HERMAN, 1956; HERMAN et al.,

Table 16. *Normal concentrations of fluoride in the organs of man.* ppm F in *fresh tissue*

Organ or tissue	MATUURA et al. (1955)	GETTLER and ELLERBROOK (1939)	HERMAN et al. (1958)[1]
Bladder . . .	—	0.40—0.68	15—185
Brain	1.8—4.3		
Fat	3—4		<5—145
Gall bladder .	3.9		
Hair	14—30		13—171
Heart	1.3—6.6	0.44—0.60	
Intestine . . .	2—8		
Kidney	2.1—94	0.56—0.78	<5—181
Liver	2.5—19	0.36—0.70	
Lung	4.5—23	0.16—0.42	
Marrow . . .	44		
Muscle	2—3.7		
Nails			10—186
Nerve	16		
Pancreas . . .	2.8—38		
Prostate gland	—		<5— 86
Skin	5		10—290
Spleen	2.6—18	0.25—0.30	
Stomach . . .	2.9—6.7		
Tendon	24		

[1] Concentration basis not stated; assumed to be fresh weight.

Table 17. *Normal concentrations of fluoride in human blood*

ppm F	Comment	Reference
2.55—3.12	Adults	AGATE et al. (1949)
2.17—3.48	Children	
2.77	Water supplies contained 0.07 and 0.18 ppm F	BOWLER et al. (1947)
0.04—0.36; av. 0.18	Non-pregnant women; 0.55 ppm F in drinking water	GEDALIA et al. (1961 a)
0.02—0.21; av. 0.09	Pregnant women; 0.55 ppm F in water	
0.03—0.25; av. 0.11	Cord blood of above pregnant women	
0.40—0.68	—	GETTLER and ELLERBROOK (1939)
0.17—0.39	Pregnant women; cord (fetal) blood contained 0.24—0.32 ppm F	HELD (1952)
0.23—0.36	Normal hospital diet; 0.092—0.098 ppm F in water. Milk of these mothers contained 0.08—0.147 ppm F	
0.19—0.24	Pregnant women	HELD (1954)
10—18	—	MATUURA et al. (1955)
0.14 plasma	0.15 ppm F in water supply	SINGER and ARMSTRONG (1960)
0.15 plasma	1.1 ppm F in water supply	
0.19 plasma	As above	
0.16 plasma	2.5 ppm F in water supply	
0.26 plasma	5.4 ppm F in water supply	
0—0.09; av. 0.014	Water supply contained 0.06 ppm F	SMITH et al. (1950)
0—0.09; av. 0.04	Water supply contained 1 ppm F	
1.36	Water supply contained 1 ppm F. Urine of these persons contained 1.02 ppm F	YUDKIN et al. (1954)
0.78	Drinking water and urine contained 0.1 and 0.30 ppm F, resp.	
1.70	Water supply contained 1 ppm F. Nephritic patients whose urine contained 0.64 ppm F	
0.77	Water supply contained 0.1 ppm F. Nephritics whose urine contained 0.32 ppm F	

1958), 200—11,100 on a dry basis (ZIPKIN et al., 1958a); biliary tract calculi none—60 (ZIPKIN et al., 1958a).

Values reported in the literature for fluoride in human blood are summarized in Table 17. With the exception of the data of MATUURA et al. (1955), AGATE et al. (1949) and BOWLER et al. (1947), there is general agreement that blood contains only small concentrations of fluoride, *i.e.*, generally less than 0.5 ppm. As has been discussed in a preceding section, fluoride absorbed into the blood is rapidly removed.

More recently, data have become available describing concentrations of fluoride found in organs and bones obtained in several extended series of autopsies. CALL and GREENWOOD (1958) have analyzed the brain, thyroid, heart, aorta, lung, liver, spleen, pancreas, kidney, calvarium, sternum, rib, iliac crest and vertebra from 59 human subjects who were residents of Utah (see Tables 18 and 19). In addition, SMITH et al. (1963a) have analyzed rib and vertebral samples taken at autopsies of long-term residents of Rochester, N. Y. (see SMITH et al., 1953 for a preliminary report) and SMITH and GARDNER (1963) have measured fluoride content in the total ash of 20 cadavers (Tables 20 and 21).

The subjects of CALL and GREENWOOD all received approximately the same daily dose of fluoride, *i.e.* the dose corresponding to that ingested daily by the populations of Utah, Weber and Salt Lake counties of Utah, plus that inhaled from the atmospheres of these three industrial counties. According to GREENWOOD (personal communication) the water supplies used by these individuals contained < 0.5 ppm F. This study furnishes data on a much more meaningful number of individual organs than has been available heretofore; consequently, a better insight is afforded into the range of F concentrations to be expected in the tissues of a population exposed to fluorides in the normal course of their lives.

The data of Table 18 give no indication of a regular increase in fluoride concentration with increasing age in the organs analyzed, nor is any tissue other than aorta unusually high in fluoride concentration. Average concentrations range from 2.0 ppm for liver to 5.9 for thyroid; average concentration in the aorta is 18.5. Variations among concentrations in a given organ, or from organ to organ are somewhat greater than that seen for comparable data from animal studies (see Table 13), but this is to be expected since appreciably greater numbers of human samples were available for analysis. The greater concentrations of F found in aorta are not surprising, in view of the known propensity for calcification in this tissue and the accumulation of F at local sites of calcification (ERICSSON and ULLBERG, 1958). Similar accumulation in the aorta in a more limited series of autopsy samples was encountered by SMITH et al. (1960).

Fluoride concentrations in dry, fat-free bone as found by CALL and GREENWOOD (loc. cit.) are summarized in Table 19. In general concentrations in all bones of both sexes tend to increase with increasing age. No other patterns are apparent in these data; no one bone consistently contains more fluoride than another, nor are there consistent sex differences. Estimates of the daily fluoride intakes of these subjects are not available except as described above.

SMITH et al. (1963a) analyzed rib and vertebral samples from long-term residents of Rochester, N. Y. These samples were obtained during 1950—1952, prior to the addition of supplemental fluoride to the water supply. During the period of residence of these subjects (life span, in most instances) the drinking water contained less than 0.1 ppm of F. The data are set forth in Table 20. Fluoride concentrations in both rib and vertebra proved to correlate well with the age of

Table 18. *Normal concentrations of fluoride in human dry, fat-free organs from 59 autopsies. Parts per million of fluoride, range and mean*[1] (CALL and GREENWOOD, 1958)

Age, yrs.	Brain	Thyroid	Heart	Aorta	Lung	Liver	Spleen	Pancreas	Kidney
0—9	— —	— —	0.4 0.4 (1)	0.8 0.8 (1)	1.2 1.2 (1)	0.2 0.2 (1)	1.3 1.3 (1)	— —	— —
10—19	— —	5.0 5.0 (1)	0.6 0.6 (1)	0.7 0.7 (1)	0.6 0.6 (1)	0.4 0.4 (1)	1.5 1.5 (1)	— —	0.6 0.6 (1)
20—29	— —	1.6—8.1 4.85 (2)	1.7—5.7 3.35 (4)	3.5—15.1 10.15 (4)	1.0—6.7 4.22 (4)	0.8—5.6 2.25 (4)	0.9—5.5 3.47 (3)	1.1—4.1 2.30 (4)	1.6—7.2 3.97 (4)
30—39	— —	5.0—11.8 8.40 (2)	0.8—21.3 11.05 (2)	10.9—21.2 16.1 (2)	6.0 6.0 (1)	0.9—23.0 12.0 (2)	1.4—10.2 5.80 (2)	3.4 3.4 (1)	9.0—38.0 23.5 (2)
40—49	0.4—3.0 2.0 (3)	0.6—12.0 5.78 (6)	0.5—3.4 1.87 (6)	2.1—21.1 7.92 (6)	1.3—8.5 3.47 (6)	0.1—1.3 0.77 (6)	0.3—2.1 1.20 (6)	1.0 1.0 (1)	1.1—10.0 3.43 (7)
50—59	0.4—2.7 1.57 (9)	1.8—11.0 4.01 (8)	0.4—2.8 1.44 (9)	1.0—15.6 6.42 (9)	1.1—4.2 2.73 (10)	0.3—7.7 2.09 (10)	0.5—4.0 1.89 (10)	1.0—2.9 1.97 (3)	0.7—6.6 2.91 (9)
60—69	0.2—3.0 1.52 (5)	0.5—13.0 4.60 (8)	0.5—12.0 2.29 (10)	0.3—17.0 6.76 (9)	0.8—7.9 4.42 (11)	0.4—4.0 1.43 (10)	0.5—5.1 1.84 (10)	0.2—4.0 1.52 (5)	0.6—7.0 3.02 (10)
70—79	0.7—3.0 3.17 (6)	2.0—30.0 8.47 (9)	0.5—4.0 1.61 (13)	0.6—125.5 50.3 (9)	1.2—17.0 4.24 (14)	0.4—8.6 1.78 (14)	0.5—5.0 1.82 (13)	0.9—8.2 2.33 (7)	1.1—9.5 2.89 (14)
80—89	0.9—12.0 3.98 (5)	0.7—15.0 6.01 (8)	0.8—13.0 3.15 (8)	11.5—57.0 24.8 (5)	0.8—11.0 4.19 (8)	0.2—3.1 1.10 (8)	0.4—8.6 2.64 (5)	3.5 3.5 (1)	1.5—8.8 3.30 (7)

[1] Numbers in parentheses refer to number of samples analyzed.

Table 19. *Normal concentrations of fluoride in human dry, fat-free bone from 59 autopsies. Parts per million of fluoride, range and mean*[1] (CALL and GREENWOOD, 1958)

Age, yrs.	Calvarium		Sternum		Rib		Iliac crest		Vertebra	
	male	female	male	female	male	female	male	female	male	female
0—9	— —	190 190 (1)				230 230 (1)				230 230 (1)
10—19	— —	— —	90 90 (1)		90 90 (1)		60 60 (1)		90 90 (1)	
20—29	200 200 (1)	— —	200—360 263 (3)	340 340 (1)	170—300 235 (2)	120 120 (1)	200 200 (1)	270 270 (1)	320—360 340	150 150 (1)
30—39	— —	— —	280 280	490 490 (1)	140—240 190 (2)	450 450 (1)		460 460 (1)	250—260 255	340 340 (1)
40—49	420 420 (1)	360—960 575 (4)	220—690 460 (4)	350—500 403 (3)	220—600 400 (4)	260—770 445 (4)	200—630 440 (4)	300—480 327 (3)	300—740 497	300—650 450 (4)
50—59	550—800 643 (4)	220—420 296 (5)	250—850 584 (5)	240—390 312 (5)	320—900 538 (5)	180—320 256 (5)	550—600 575 (2)	200—340 258 (5)	370—740 550	220—480 333 (5)
60—69	340—500 420 (2)	500—640 570 (2)	240—1370 519 (7)	330—730 523 (4)	200—1190 466 (7)	330—610 430 (4)	250—470 316 (5)	350—570 470 (4)	250—1550 600	350—700 525 (4)
70—79	270—600 407 (3)	240—720 458 (4)	250—730 414 (5)	360—1680 846 (7)	260—730 405 (6)	300—1440 696 (8)	260—560 374 (5)	350—1160 624 (5)	260—790 392	350—940 674 (8)
80—89	530—840 615 (4)	440—600 507 (3)	520—880 635 (4)	320—690 513 (3)	400—580 508 (4)	460—610 537 (3)	420—700 570 (4)	560—590 575 (2)	470—620 535	300—760 523 (3)

[1] Numbers in parentheses refer to number of samples analyzed.

Table 20. *Concentrations of fluoride in human rib and vertebral samples taken from 158 autopsies in Rochester, N. Y. during 1950—1952.* Parts per million of fluoride in ash (SMITH et al., 1963a)[1]

Age	Rib	Vertebra	Age	Rib	Vertebra	Age	Rib	Vertebra	Age	Rib	Vertebra
Males											
Stillborn	0	58	24 yrs.	287	411	52 yrs.	1058	904	74 yrs.	1269	970
Newborn	134	175	25	270	254	52	698	782	76	1139	1015
Newborn	67	50	26	267	300	53	892	753	76	1146	1127
Newborn	162	111	28	189	267	54	542	498	76	1336	1393
2 days	0	29	31	655	890	55	712	777	77	1358	1308
3 days	77	60	31	1043	1217	55	739	830	79	1501	1409
4 weeks	89	65	32	388	431	56	452	507	80	1533	1383
8 months	38	46	34	800	933	57	1207	948	80	1637	1458
9 months	95	123	36	453	632	57	773	788	80	778	1065
1.5 yrs.	96	148	36	870	932	60	533	775	81	487	612
2	194	268	42	1058	946	61	580	651	82	1570	2020
3	161	193	44	1098	1017	62	1748	1472	82	1239	1512
4.5	381	627	44	2200	1977	63	1188	1790	84	1790	2140
6	94	119	44	1151	1275	63	492	706	85	929	1084
10	139	203	45	1259	1296	64	710	571	86	2520	3310
11	109	210	46	1452	1822	65	628	552	86	1080	789
14	69	91	47	842	750	67	1146	1209	87	2150	2120
15	128	180	47	1030	986	68	1262	1334	91	1536	809
15	118	181	47	1332	1298	71	931	983	91	708	1062
17	112	151	48	891	990	72	1323	828			
22	877	640	49	476	510	72	1197	1344			
23	1823	1540	51	1336	1485	73	386	949			
Females											
Stillborn	105	93	39	532	531	59	1223	1287	76	597	620
Newborn	63	82	40	1121	1520	60	716	740	77	839	978
Newborn	102	85	41	635	441	62	528	460	80	765	860
8 hrs.	306	110	41	1633	1432	63	1110	980	81	608	635
1 month	0	321	43	481	456	65	1727	1890	82	381	668
9 months	366	216	44	875	981	65	1104	1040	84	1651	1920
2 yrs.	106	152	44	824	789	67	580	702	84	562	573
2.5 yrs.	56	79	45	680	688	68	974	1112	85	990	1240
4	158	179	49	371	306	68	1018	922	86	671	828
7	70	128	49	1093	1238	69	548	650	88	1134	1360
7	96	94	50	418	429	69	492	576	88	2250	2750
8	67	150	52	911	988	70	656	548	89	1050	972
17	250	173	52	644	726	72	1845	2060	90	960	1000
19	248	305	53	948	1040	72	1228	919	92	1374	1200
20	232	184	54	836	956	74	796	706	93	1107	945
26	261	361	54	560	631	74	1010	1063	93	1310	1310
28	253	345	56	975	1112	75	1800	1260			
31	764	742	58	622	575	75	996	1196			
33	286	301	58	668	701	76	1096	1326			

[1] A preliminary report of this study has been published in SMITH et al. (1953).

the subject, the correlation coefficient being 0.70 for both bones[1]. The equations of the lines fitting the data were calculated to be

$$\text{for males:}\quad R = 144.5 + 14.6\ A$$

$$\text{for females:}\quad R = 123.9 + 11.9\ A$$

[1] We are much indebted to Dr. S. LEE CRUMP, now deceased, of the Statistics Section of the University of Rochester Atomic Energy Project for the statistical analysis of the data.

where R is ppm F in the rib ash and A is the age in years. The range in individual samples about the fitted line is about ± 50% of the value on the line. Concentrations in the rib and vertebra were highly correlated, the coefficient of correlation being 0.95. The two are related by the equation

$$V = 100 + 0.97\,R$$

where V and R are the ppm F in vertebral and rib ash, respectively. The equation is the same for each sex.

In summary then, the data of Table 20 indicate: a) fluoride concentrations in human bones are related to age, *i.e.* to the total dose of fluoride received; b) concentrations differ in the rib and vertebra; c) concentrations in either bone differ between males and females; d) there is considerable variation in skeletal F concentration among individuals of the same age and sex in either bone analyzed here; e) fluoride is found in the bones of stillborn and newborn infants, indicating that F can be and is transmitted from the mother to the fetus.

In these subjects, skeletal deposition of F apparently increased steadily throughout the life span, whereas other investigators have reported that bone concentrations reach a constant value after a period of time and do not increase further despite continuing intake, *i.e.* a steady state is attained, wherein only sufficient fluoride is deposited to replace that which is lost from the bone. JACKSON and WEIDMANN (1958) for example, found F concentrations in human bone to reach a plateau after approximately 50—60 years of age. The magnitude of the bone concentration at the steady state increased as the concentration of F in the drinking water increased, *i.e.* as the total F intake or dosage was increased. But, subjects of SMITH et al. (1963a) used water containing less than 0.1 ppm F (approximately 0.06 ppm) during their life time; whereas JACKSON and WEIDMANN's subjects used waters containing, respectively, less than 0.5 ppm, 0.8 or 1.9 ppm F. Evidently then, the daily intake of F determines not only the magnitude of the concentration at the steady state, but also the time required for its attainment. At very low levels of intake, it may not become apparent in the normal life span.

Table 21. *Fluoride content of ash of human Cadavers*[1] (SMITH and GARDNER, 1963)

Age, yrs.	Sex	Total Ash wt., kg	ppm F in Ash	Total F g
fetal	—	—	140	—
fetal	—	—	29	—
36	M	2.48	918	2.27
48	M	4.41	744	3.28
54	M	2.50	659	1.65
55	M	2.50	1480	3.70
57	M	2.10	2270	4.76
60	M	2.50	550	1.37
65	M	3.35	828	2.78
66	M	1.97	1006	1.98
68	M	2.50	1020	2.55
74	M	2.26	1485	3.36
74	M	2.31	717	1.66
75	M	2.00	1187	2.39
76	M	2.00	1144	2.29
77	M	1.70	2145	3.65
77	F	0.79	933	0.74
81	M	1.57	988	1.55
82	M	2.58	1494	3.86
83	M	2.20	1506	3.31
85	F	1.50	567	0.85
85	M	2.57	1288	3.31

[1] The bodies had been used for instruction purposes; samples of the ash were made available through the kindness of Dr. C. E. TOBIN, Dept. of Anatomy, University of Rochester School of Medicine and Dentistry, Rochester, N. Y.

The role of the skeleton in sequestering fluoride, the manner in which this is done, and various factors influencing skeletal uptake are described in detail by Dr. WEATHERALL in a later chapter.

SMITH and GARDNER (1963) have measured F in the total ash of a series of exsanguinated human cadavers; though residential histories of these subjects are not on record, but it is probable that at least a large portion of their lives were spent in western New York, where the water supplies generally contain not more than about 0.1 ppm F. Concentrations of F found in these cadavers are listed in Table 21.

In this limited series of samples, there appears to be no relation between F content and total ash weight. The age span in this series is quite limited for the most part, and no relation is evident between F concentration and age. The data do indicate however, that total F in the human body is appreciable, ranging from 0.74 to 4.76 g with an average of 2.57 g in this series. This is comparable to the total body stores of iron or of zinc, and appreciably more than the totals of manganese, copper or iodine.

Using the available data presented in this Section for fluoride concentration in different human tissues, and by making certain reasonable assumptions, one may calculate the distribution of total body fluoride in man.

a) Vital organs

The data of CALL and GREENWOOD (1958) for concentrations of F in the kidney, lung, spleen, thyroid, heart, brain, pancreas and liver indicate an average concentration of 3 ppm in these organs on a dry, fat-free basis. Using values reported in the *Handbook of Biological Data* (SPECTOR, 1956) for water and lipid content, it can be calculated that the average concentration of 3 ppm corresponds to approximately 0.5 ppm F in the fresh organs. Data for the standard 70 kg man listed in the recommendations of the International Commission on Radiological Protection (ICRP, 1959) indicate that these eight organs constitute a total of 5040 g. Total fluoride in these combined organs then, is 2.5 mg.

b) Muscle and skin

Muscle and skin of standard man comprise 30 kg and 2 kg, respectively, or 32 kg total. Applicable F concentration data are lacking for man, but because of the reasonable uniformity in concentrations among the organs analyzed by CALL and GREENWOOD (1958) it seems reasonable to assume that muscle and skin also contain approximately 0.5 ppm F in the fresh tissue. Accordingly, the total F in this combined pool is about 16 mg.

c) Blood

In the standard man, the weight of the blood volume is taken to be 5.4 kg. According to SINGER and ARMSTRONG (1960), an average plasma F concentration may be taken as 0.16 ppm, while CARLSON et al. (1960a) have shown that plasma contains 72 % of the whole blood fluoride. Using a hematocrit value of 45, it may be calculated that whole blood F concentration is about 0.11 ppm. The total blood volume then, contains approximately 0.59 mg F.

Plasma constitutes about 4.3 % of body weight (HERNANDEZ-PEON, 1960) or about 3.01 kg in standard man. Using SINGER and ARMSTRONG's value of 0.16 ppm in plasma, this pool is seen to contain 0.48 mg of F. If whole blood contains 0.59 mg F, then the cellular components must contain 0.11 mg F, by difference.

d) Extracellular fluid

According to HERNANDEZ-PEON (loc. cit.) extracellular fluid comprises 17.5 % of the body weight. In the standard 70 kg man this corresponds to 12.25 kg, and if the concentration of F in extracellular fluid is considered to be the same as that in plasma, the extracellular fluid is seen to contain about 1.96 mg F.

e) Bone

The exsanguinated cadavers analyzed by SMITH and GARDNER (1963) contained on the average, 2.566 g of F. These cadavers represented bones and teeth, skin, muscle, and vital organs. Since skin, muscle and vital organs contain a total of 0.019 g F, the bones and teeth must therefore contain 2.547 g of fluoride.

Table 22 summarizes the above data on the distribution of F as calculated for man. Certain basic assumptions made should be reiterated at this point, *viz.* a) the soft tissue concentrations used are for individuals whose water supplies contained < 0.5 ppm F; however, SINGER and ARMSTRONG's data (1960) for blood suggest that tissue concentrations would not be affected appreciably until the water levels reached 5 ppm F or more. b) Data for F in bones and teeth are based on individuals using water containing less than 0.1 ppm F. For individuals using drinking water containing more F, the total skeletal F will be increased and the percentages of total body F found in the various non-calcified compartments will decrease accordingly.

Table 22. *Calculated distribution of total body fluoride in man*

Compartment	Grams F	Per cent of total F	Percentage distribution of non-skeletal F[1]
Bones and teeth	2.547	99.3	—
Skin and muscle	0.016	0.62	81.7
Vital organs	0.003	0.12	15.3
Whole blood	0.0006	0.02	3.0
cells	0.0001	0.003	0.5
plasma	0.0005	0.017	2.5
Extracellular fluid	0.002	0.08	10.0
Total[2]	2.5666	100.06	100.0

[1] Extra-skeletal F = 2.5666 — 2.547 = 0.0196 g or 20 mg.

[2] For purposes of summation, cells and plasma are included in whole blood, and extracellular fluid is included in whole blood and in fresh skin, muscle and organs.

As was noted previously for the rat and the calf, almost the entire body fluoride of man is localized in the calcified structures. Circulating whole blood is calculated to contain approximately 0.02 % of the total F. The calculated distribution agrees well with that of MARIAKULANDAI and VENKATARAMAIAH (1955) for the calf, whereas WADHWANI (1953) found a slightly higher proportion of F in the soft tissues of the rat (*cf.* Tables 14 and 15).

When the distribution of the non-skeletal fluoride is considered, it is seen that four-fifths of this F is to be found in the skin and muscle, while the organs and extracellular fluid contain 15.3 and 10.0 %, respectively of the extra-skeletal F. Whole blood contains 3 % of this F.

D. Maternal-fetal exchange of fluoride

Interest in the maternal-fetal exchange of fluoride arises, naturally enough, from concern over the question of whether or not fluoride ingested during pregnancy would be likely to have any effects in the developing fetus. Mineralization of bone and teeth commences *in utero*, and F has long been known to affect this process. At present there seems to be little or no question that fluoride does indeed appear in the fetus, but the part played by the placenta in this transfer is not fully resolved. Some authors describe the role of the placenta as that of a barrier insuring that excessive amounts of F do not reach the developing fetus, while others appear convinced the placenta functions in a manner intended to insure that the fetus does indeed receive its due share of F. The proper interpretation of the placental role would be immensely aided by resolution of the question of whether or not fluorine is an essential trace element.

Table 23. *Normal concentrations of fluoride in fetal organs*

Species	Age of Fetus	Organ	ppm F	Comment	Reference
Man	3 mo. 4 mo. 5 mo. 6 mo. 7 mo. 8 mo. 9 mo.	femur femur femur femur femur femur femur	2.5 4—6; av. 5 20—40; av. 32 50—60; av. 56.2 70—90; av. 77.5 95—105; av. 100 110—140; av. 130	Ash basis. Mothers' water supply contained 0.55 ppm F	Brzezinski et al. (1960)
Rat	term	bone	0.300—0.330; av. 0.317	Ash basis. Mothers' food contained 0.2 ppm F; distilled water	Brzezinski et al. (1962)
Dog	newborn	lung heart liver spleen kidney stomach intestine muscle meconium bone teeth	5.5 2.1 4.5 3.1 2.5 4.2 4.8 7.3 1.6 256—549 130	Dry wt. basis	Minoguchi and Iwamoto (1957)
Rat	term	carcass	0—1.0	Wet basis. Diet of mothers contained 3 ppm F	Maplesden et al. (1960)
Rabbit	term	carcass	3.1	Wet basis. Diet of mothers contained 46 ppm F	Maplesden et al. (1960)
Man	term	blood	0.24—0.32	Maternal blood contained 0.17—0.39 ppm F	Held (1952)
Cow	term fetal	placenta placenta	0.41 0.32	Stock ration of mother contained 7 ppm F	Bell et al. (1961)
Rabbit	term	carcass	0.127 10.4	Mother in "fluorine-less" region. Mother fed 0.6 ml of 2% NaF soln. daily for 37 days	Soejima et al. (1957)
Cattle	7 mos.	rib metacarpus	330—620 230—400	Ash basis. Cows may have been exposed to F-containing industrial effluents; age 5—8 yrs.	Hobbs et al. (1954)
		rib metacarpus	250—550 190—470	As above; age 9—12 yrs.	
		rib metacarpus	260—390 220—300	As above; age 13–16 yrs.	
		rib metacarpus	440—750 460—970	Beef heifers	
		rib metacarpus	320—810 270—430	Cows and heifers	
		metacarpus	500	Ash basis. Cow on stock ration containing 7 ppm F	
Rat	newborn	whole body	1.1	Fresh wt. basis	Murray (1936)
Cattle	newborn	metacarpus	11	Dry, fat-free basis. Stock ration of mothers contained 3—5 ppm F	Suttie et al. (1957)

Table 23. (Continued)

Species	Age of Fetus	Organ	ppm F	Comment	Reference
Rat	newborn	whole body	53±9	Ash basis	BÜTTNER and MUHLER (1958b)
Man	term	femur mandible, maxilla tooth buds	10.6—29.0 9.3—27.0 8.0—17.0	Dry, fat-free basis; 8 fetuses. Water supply of mothers contained <0.05 ppm F	MARTIN (1948)
Man	newborn	rib	160	Dry, fat-free basis. Mother's drinking water contained 1.9 ppm F	JACKSON and WEIDMANN (1958)
Man	term	total ash	29 and 140	Ash basis. Mothers' water supply contained <0.06 ppm F	SMITH et al. (1963a)
		rib vertebra	not det'd.—162 50—175	As above; 4 male fetuses	
		rib vertebra	63—105 82— 93	As above; 3 female fetuses	
Man	term	placenta	0.07—0.27, av. 0.15	Water supply contained 0.55 ppm F	GEDALIA et al. (1961a)
		cord blood	0.03—0.25, av. 0.11	As above. Maternal blood contained 0.02—0.21, 0.09 ppm F. Blood of non-pregnant women contained 0.04—0.36, av. 0.18 ppm F	
Dog	term	entire fetus	not detected	Assumed to be ash basis. Mother rec'd. 4 ppm F in water for 8 wks. of gestation	KNOUFF et al. (1935—1936)
		entire fetus	730	Assumed ash basis. Mother rec'd. 25 ppm F in water throughout gestation	

In 1936 the question of whether or not there was placental passage of F was not at all clear. The very rare occurrence of mottled deciduous enamel was offered in support of the view that the placenta was impervious to F, while the appearance of mottling in breast-fed infants whose mothers' drinking water contained high F concentrations suggested that F either entered the fetal circulation or the milk of the mother (MURRAY, 1936). Direct evidence for or against the placental passage of fluoride thus was lacking.

In 1936 Murray initiated a series of experiments designed to measure directly placental transference, or lack thereof, of fluoride. In these experiments the diet fed pregnant female rats was moistened with 0.05 % NaF solution, and at delivery the litters were sacrificed and analyzed *in toto* for F content. Control data were obtained on the litters of mothers not given the NaF-moistened diet. On the average, the litters of the fluoride-fed mothers contained five times as much F as did control litters.

In the same year KNOUFF et al. (1936) administered different levels of F in drinking water to pregnant dogs, and determined the F content of the newborn pups. Fluoride was not detected in the fetus of the mother receiving 5 ppm NaF

(2.3 ppm F) during the last eight weeks of gestation, but was measurable in the fetus of the mother whose drinking water contained 25 ppm NaF (11.3 ppm F) throughout pregnancy. The authors concluded that the absence of F in the first instance was due to fixation of all of the NaF in the maternal tissues, rather than to any impermeability of the placenta and that when this capacity for fixation was exceeded, F did pass the placenta into the fetus.

The placental passage of fluorine was thus proven in direct fashion, and the concept introduced of the placenta acting in a barrier role to retard the passage of F.

Since these reports, an appreciable amount of data pertaining to the maternal-fetal exchange of F has accumulated, much of which is summarized in Tables 23 and 24.

The barrier-threshold concept is still extant in current thinking. HARVEY (1952) reported that 2 ppm F in the drinking water of ewes did not increase concentrations of F in the offspring above those seen in control lambs, but at 10 ppm, fluoride concentrations in the offspring definitely were increased. At 15 ppm transmission to the fetus was considered to be deleterious to the unborn lamb. HOBBS et al. (1954) determined concentrations of F in fetal calf bones; the mothers had pastured 5—16 years on high phosphatic soil, and where some F may have been ingested from industrial sources. No correlation between fetal bone concentrations of F and duration of the mother's exposure was apparent, and the authors concluded that elevated maternal ingestion of F had little effect on increasing the placental transfer. In a number of other studies these authors fed cows rations containing up to 300 ppm F and upon analysis of bones of the calves produced by these mothers, concluded that there was little transfer of F to the young via the placenta or the milk. At levels of 600—1200 ppm F in the diet however, they did find an appreciable transfer from the dam to the fetus. On the other hand, SUTTIE et al. (1957) found increasing amounts of F in the metacarpal bone at birth of calves whose mothers had received 20—50 ppm F in their ration, and SHUPE et al. (1963a) found F in the ribs of calves to be correlated with the maternal intake over the range 12—93 ppm F. BELL et al. (1961) administered F^{18} to pregnant cows, and determined the uptake of the isotope in fetal bone and in fetal and maternal placentae. A higher percentage of the dose appeared in the fetal metatarsus than in the maternal metatarsus, but the reverse was true for mandible and rib. Maternal placentae contained $0.60 \times 10^{-4}\%$ of the dose per gram at 4 hours, while the fetal placenta contained only $0.25 \times 10^{-4}\%$ per gram. They concluded "... that part of the F^{18} passes to the fetus but there appears to be a barrier to the free passage of F^{18}..."

MINOGUCHI and IWAMOTO (1957), in an investigation of placental transfer of F in the dog, showed that some of the fluoride stored in the female prior to pregnancy was transferred to the developing fetus. Within the fetus itself, not all of the F was stored in the bone and tissue, as was evidenced by the finding of F in the meconium.

Mention has already been made of MURRAY's experiments (loc. cit.) which demonstrated placental passage of F in the rat. WALLACE (1953), using F^{18}, also found F to pass the placenta in this species; concentrations of F^{18} in the placenta and fetuses proved to be less than half that in the maternal blood. In 1958 ERICSSON and ULLBERG showed autoradiographically that F^{18} passes the mouse placenta. They state "... the placenta constitutes a partial barrier to the fluorine, and that the fetus is protected to a considerable degree against overdosage."

BUTTNER and MUHLER (1958b) found water-borne fluoride concentrations of 1, 3 or 5 ppm did not increase the amount of F in the carcass of 1-day-old pups

Table 24. *Fluoride concentrations in organs of offspring whose parents received fluoride*

Species	Age	Organ	ppm F	Comment	Reference
Cattle	fetus	metacarpus rib	2200 2400	Ash basis; 8—9 mos. in utero; 907 ppm F in ration for 71 da.	HOBBS et al. (1954)
	fetus	metacarpus rib	960 960	Ash basis; 8 mos. in utero; 1207 ppm F in ration for 40 days	
Cattle (calf)	133 da.	metacarpus	330	Ash basis. Mother rec'd. stock ration contg. 7 ppm F 422 da.	HOBBS et al. (1954)
	126–182 da.	metacarpus	190—250	Ash basis. Mother rec'd. ration 107 ppm F 422 da.	
	166–170 da.	metacarpus	270—330	Ash basis. Mother rec'd. ration contg. 207 ppm F 423 da.	
	171–172 da.	metacarpus	290—320	Ash basis. Mother rec'd. 307 ppm F 422 da.	
	45 da.	metacarpus mandible	1200 770	Ash basis. Mother rec'd. 607 ppm F 130 da.	
	6 da.	metacarpus mandible rib	650 460 640	Ash basis. Mother rec'd. 907 ppm F 88 da.	
Cattle	adult fetus	placenta placenta	0.50—0.59 0.23—0.24	Fresh basis. Ration contained 47 or 57 ppm F	BELL et al. (1961)
Rat	22 da.	humeri	30—39	Dry, fat-free basis. With mother until sac.; mothers' diet contained 6.7 ppm F	KONIG (1960)
			76	Mothers given water containing 25 ppm F	
			83	Mothers given milk containing 15 ppm F	
			73	Mothers given diet contg. 50 ppm F	
Dog	newborn	lung heart liver spleen pancreas kidney stomach intestine muscle meconium bone teeth	9 8 8.6 5.8 6.5 2.4 7.4 10.4 17.9 85 1425—2560 1186	Dry wt. basis. Mother rec'd. 13.6 mg F/kg daily for preceding 2 yrs. (before and during pregnancy)	MINOGUCHI and IWAMOTO (1957)
Dog	newborn	lung heart liver spleen kidney stomach intestine muscle meconium bone teeth	8.2 5.2 4.3 2.1 4.4 5.8 10.8 8.7 72 349—644 425	Dry wt. basis. Mother rec'd. 13.6 mg F/kg daily during pregnancy only	MINOGUCHI and IWAMOTO (1957)

Table 24. (Continued)

Species	Age	Organ	ppm F	Comment	Reference
Lamb	6 wks.	bone	45—76	Ash basis. Rec'd. F via mothers' milk and by placental transfer	HARVEY (1952)
		teeth	40—47	Mothers on stock diet, F-free water	
		liver	0.6—1.0	Dry wt. basis. As above	
		kidney	2.3—4.5		
		heart	2.2—31		
		spleen	2.2		
		bone	33—67	As above; mothers rec'd.	
		teeth	55—69	2 ppm F in water	
		liver	0.7	Dry wt. basis	
		kidney	2.2		
		heart	2.7		
		spleen	1.7		
		bone	128—163	As above; mothers rec'd.	
		teeth	86—141	10 ppm F in water	
		liver	1.0—1.3	Dry wt. basis	
		kidney	6.0—7.3		
		heart	1.8—4.0		
		spleen	0.8—1.7		
Rat	newborn	whole body	5.1	Fresh wt. basis. Mothers' daily ration moistened with 15 ml of 0.05% NaF soln.	MURRAY (1936)
Cattle	newborn	metacarpus	86	Dry, fat-free basis. Ration of mother contained 20 ppm added F	SUTTIE et al. (1957)
			136	30 ppm F added to mothers ration	
			104	40 ppm F added to ration	
			140	50 ppm F added to ration	
			130	50 ppm F + 200 g $CaCO_3$ added to ration	
Rat	newborn	whole body	50± 8	Ash basis. Mothers rec'd. 1 ppm F in water	BUTTNER and MUHLER (1958b)
			51± 5	Mothers water supply cont'd. 3 ppm F	
			45± 9	Mothers water cont'd. 5 ppm F	
			77± 6	Mothers water cont'd. 10 ppm F	
			81± 7	Mothers water cont'd. 25 ppm F	
			115±14	Mothers water cont'd. 50 ppm F	
Man	term	fetal blood	0.21—0.29	Mothers' blood cont'd. 0.20–0.46 ppm F; mothers rec'd. 36.5–92.5 mg F during last 19–55 days of pregnancy	HELD (1954)
Rat	term	carcass	1.0	Wet basis. Mothers rec'd. 50 ppm F in ration	MAPLESDEN et al al. (1960)
			1.8	Mothers rec'd. 100 ppm F F in ration	
			4.1	Mothers rec'd. 200 ppm F in ration	

Table 24. (Continued)

Species	Age	Organ	ppm F	Comment	Reference
Rabbit	term	carcass	5.8	Wet basis. Mothers rec'd. 50 ppm F in ration	MAPLESDEN et al. (1960)
			0.3	Mothers rec'd. 100 ppm F in ration	
			14.8	Mothers rec'd. 200 ppm F in ration	
			21.5	Mothers rec'd. 300 ppm F in ration	
Cattle	2 days	rib	50—130	Dry fat-free basis. Five successive calvings. Mothers' ration cont'd. 12 ppm F (dry basis)	SHUPE et al. (1963a)
			70—160	As above; 27 ppm F in mothers' ration	
			100—160	As above; 49 ppm F in mothers' ration	
			165—270	As above; 93 ppm F in mothers' ration	

over that found in control pups, but increases were noted when the water contained 10, 25 or 50 ppm. An increase from 1 to 50 ppm in the drinking water resulted in only a two-fold increase in F concentration in the pups at birth; they considered that at least 10 ppm F must be present in water before fluoride in the newborn pups will show a detectable increase. BRZEZINSKI et al. (1962) also believe that a daily intake of at least 10—15 ppm F is required in order to appreciably increase fetal concentrations of F in the rat, and KONIG (1960) attributes a "partial barrier" action to the placenta of rats.

MAPLESDEN et al. (1960) concluded that "... the placenta maintained its function as an effective barrier even under extreme conditions." In their experiments they "saturated" female rats with fluoride by maintaining them on high dietary levels of F while at the same time continuing them through repeated whelpings. However, the increasing amounts of fluoride thus made available in the mothers, *i.e.* F which could not be accommodated in the increasingly "saturated" skeleton, were not passed to the fetuses, since fetal F did not increase in the successive litters. One should not lose sight of the fact however, that the maternal skeletal system and the kidneys have extraordinary capacities to sequester and to excrete fluoride, respectively; moreover, no data are reported in this paper permitting an evaluation of the degree of skeletal "saturation".

The contribution of these maternal factors to the maintenance of low fetal levels of F must be kept in mind in stress situations of this nature. SHUPE et al. (1963a) also did not find F passing the placenta to increase in successive gestations in cattle.

In other experiments MAPLESDEN et al. (loc. cit.) fed rats 50—300 ppm F for 196—208 days, the last 21 of which the rats were pregnant; rabbits also were fed these dietary levels for 128—157 days, being pregnant the final 30 days. At term the fetuses were removed and analyzed for F. Fluoride in the fetus was found to increase with increasing dietary F, in both species. Their data are presented graphically in Fig. 5.

The figure indicates a greater placental passage of F in the rabbit than in the rat. MAPLESDEN et al. state that this difference is difficult to explain on the basis of morphological structure of the two placentae; they suggest it may be due to differences in permeability of the placentae, to the molecular size of compounds to which F may have become fixed, or to other factors affecting placental transfer. However, there may be a more simple explanation for the greater concentrations of F in the fetal rabbit. The rabbit ingests approximately ten times more food than does the rat, the average gestation period for the rabbit is ten days longer than for the rat, and the extent of calcification of the skeleton of the newborn rabbit is greater than for the rat; all of these factors may be expected to contribute to the differences in fluoride concentration in the newborn rabbit and rat.

HELD (1954) noted the similarity between the concentrations of F in human fetal and maternal blood, and interpreted this to mean that the placenta behaves with regard to F as an organ of transport, rather than as a gland with a specific regulatory function. GEDALIA et al. (1961a) however, felt because the average concentration of F in placental tissue exceeded that in cord blood, and because the two were correlated (there was no correlation between placental and maternal blood F concentrations in their series of patients) that the placenta must play an active role in accumulating fluoride and transferring it to the fetus.

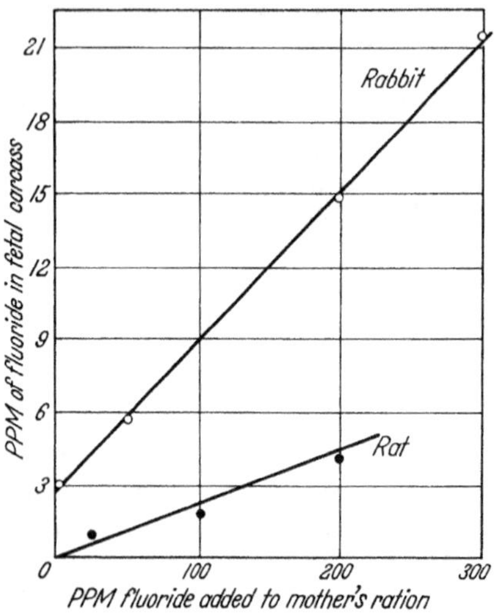

Fig. 5. Relation between dietary fluoride and fluoride in the fetal rat and rabbit. Data of MAPLESDEN et al. (1960)

Some of the extensive investigations of the group at Hebrew University Hadassah Medical School in Jerusalem have been reported by GEDALIA et al. (1959), BERCOVICI et al. (1960), and by BRZEZINSKI et al. (1960). Fluoride concentrations have been determined in human fetuses aged 3–9 months, in maternal urine from the fourth month of pregnancy on, and in milk for several weeks after delivery. Urinary excretion of F decreased steadily during the course of pregnancy, beginning at the fifth month, and concurrently, fetal concentrations of F were found to increase. GEDALIA et al. (1959) point out that mineralization of the deciduous teeth also begins at about the fifth month of gestation. Shortly before delivery urinary excretion of F begins to increase again, but approximately four months are required to restore the levels to pre-pregnancy concentrations. It is suggested (BERCOVICI et al., 1960; BRZEZINSKI et al., 1960) that there appears to be little fetal need of F during the first months of gestation, but that this need increases during the latter half of pregnancy. These fetal demands are met by drawing on the mother's fluoride intake and stores, as evidenced by the decline in urinary excretion during the later months; the placenta is not a barrier to fluoride transfer. After delivery, the mother's depleted stores are gradually replenished and her urinary excretion reflects this by returning gradually to pre-pregnancy levels. The lag in normalization of the post-delivery excretion is considered not to be due to loss of F via the milk, since concentrations here are low and constant.

The finding of MINOGUCHI and IWAMOTO (1957) that maternal F in the dog is transferred to the fetus is in agreement with the above suggestion. The possibility might be tested further by determining whether or not there is a more avid uptake of F^{18} by the skeleton in women during the first several months after delivery. The technic proposed by BLAU et al. (1962) for bone scanning with F^{18}

might prove appropriate here. The essentiality of F for both the developing fetus and the mother implied by BERCOVICI et al. (loc. cit.) is interesting to note. BRZEZINSKI et al. (1962) point out that the human tends to retain F during pregnancy, whereas the pregnant rat does not. WUTHIER and PHILLIPS (1961) however, have reported increased concentrations of fluoride in the femur of rats during pregnancy and lactation, which they attribute to increased consumption of food and water.

The data of BRZEZINSKI et al. (1960) relating to concentrations of F in the fetus and in the maternal urine are shown in Fig. 6. A surprisingly good correlation between these two parameters is apparent, from which one might expect to predict the amount of fluoride in the fetus from analysis of the mother's urine. One should hasten to point out that the relationship depicted applies only to mothers whose drinking water contains an average of 0.55 ppm F. Also, GEDALIA et al. (1959) have drawn attention to the wide individual variation in urinary F concentrations at each month of pregnancy and thereafter.

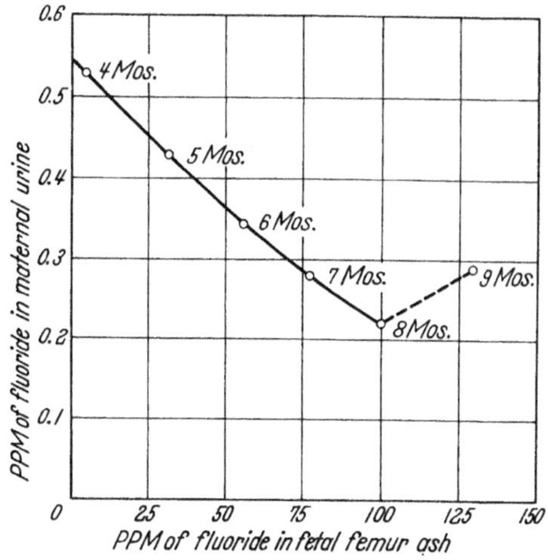

Fig. 6. Concentrations of fluoride in human maternal urine and fetal ashduring the course of pregnancy. Months of pregnancy indicated at each point. Data of BRZEZINSKI et al. (1960)

Salivary concentrations of F were also noted by BERCOVICI et al. (1960) to decrease progressively during pregnancy, beginning at about the fourth to fifth month and continuing through eight months.

ERICSSON and MALMNÄS (1962) have made a very important, and so far, unique contribution to our knowledge of placental transfer of fluoride, by demonstrating the extent and rapidity with which F^{18} crosses the placenta in the human. In their experiment F^{18} was administered intravenously to women immediately prior to undergoing a therapeutic abortion; during the course of the operation successive samples of maternal blood, single samples of fetal blood, and several samples of placental tissue were taken for F^{18} analysis. The per cent of dose of F^{18} per gram of fetal blood varied between one-fourth and one-tenth of that in the maternal blood, while concentrations in the placenta in each instance were intermediate between the maternal and feta concentrations.

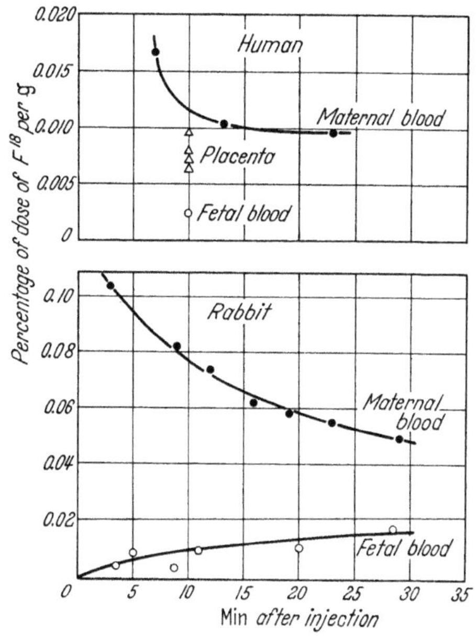

Fig. 7. Concentrations of F^{18} in maternal and fetal blood of the human and of the rabbit. From ERICSSON and MALMNÄS (1962)

In experiments with rabbits, F^{18} was administered intravenously two days short of delivery, and the fetuses removed sequentially during the next 30–35 min. Transfer of F^{18} to the fetal blood was slow and maximal concentrations never reached one-third of those determined simultaneously in the maternal blood. Representative figures from the paper of ERICSSON and MALMNÄS (1962) are shown in Fig. 7.

These authors consider the placenta to form a partial barrier to F, effective to such an extent that even sudden increases in maternal F concentration, such as those achieved by intravenous injection, do not result in any great rise in fetal blood F. They failed to find an accumulation of F in the human placentae in their four cases, in which the fetuses were only 12–15 cm in length; they consider it probable that placental concentrations do increase toward the end of pregnancy, as evidenced by their autoradiographic studies with mice (ERICSSON and ULLBERG, 1958), and the work of GARDNER et al. (1952) with human placentae sampled at parturition.

ERICSSON and MALMNÄS (1962) have pointed out that the ease with which the halogens cross the placenta seems to be inversely related to their atomic weights, the order of transfer being I > Br > Cl > F.

E. Fluoride in milk

Closely related to the preceding discussion are the questions of how and to what extent fluoride enters the maternal milk, and how effectively this may be transmitted to the young.

WALLACE (1953) administered F^{18} orally to female rats who were still nursing 16-day-old litters, and determined the distribution of the isotope in the organs of the mothers. Concentrations in the mammary glands were found to be nearly equal to those in the maternal blood. BELL et al. (1961) confirmed this similarity several years later with F^{18} given to cattle. WALLACE (loc. cit.) was led to suggest that the similarity in concentrations in the blood and in the mammary gland indicated that the passage of F^{18} into the milk more closely resembles a diffusion process than it does true secretion. PERKINSON et al. (1955) also demonstrated the appearance of F^{18} in milk of cows following oral or intravenous administration, but considered that there was not free passage of the isotope into milk.

ERICSSON (1958a) investigated the state of fluoride in milk, using F^{18} added to cows' milk. He found that there was no appreciable sedimentation of the added F over a five-hour period, nor was the added F completely diffusible in ultrafiltration experiments, suggesting that the fluoride is present in both ionic and bound forms. Separation of the milk fats and proteins showed that only traces were bound to the fat and to the albumin plus globulin, whereas the casein contained about one-fifth of the total activity.

Milk from a variety of species has now been analyzed for fluorine content. Some of the values reported in the literature are summarized in Table 25 below. In most instances the concentrations are below 0.5 ppm F; only rarely do the reported concentrations exceed this level. As would be expected, cows' milk has been analyzed with the greatest frequency; in those few instances where the milk of the dog, goat and sheep have been examined, the concentrations have been found not to differ from those reported for cows' milk.

Higher levels of fluorine intake may be associated with increases in the amount of F in the milk, though this is not always evident as the data of Table 25 demonstrate. Whether or not appreciable increases are produced probably depends in part upon availability of the ingested F. MINOGUCHI and IWAMOTO (1957) for

Table 25. *Concentrations of fluoride found in milk of different species*

Species	Concn., ppm F	Comment	Reference
Cow	0.031	hay contained 1 ppm F	LINDBERG (1956)
	0.046	hay contained 3 ppm F	
	0.05—0.44; av. 0.138	—	PHILLIPS et al. (1934)
	0.08—0.33	88 dairies throughout Sweden	NOMMIK (1953)
	0.09—0.19	diet contained 25 ppm F 40 months	STODDARD et al. (1956)
	0.10—0.19	diet contained 12 ppm F	
	0.1	water contained 0.1 ppm F	MINOGUCHI and IWAMOTO (1957)
	0.11—0.14	water contained 0.2 ppm F 5 days	NOMMIK (1953)
	0.11—0.15	water contained 3.2 ppm F 5 days	
	0.11—0.15	diet contained 440 ppm F 5 years	PHILLIPS et al. (1934)
	0.11—0.18	—	AGATE et al. (1949)
	0.11—0.44	pastured near aluminium plant	
	0.12	water supply contained 0.17 ppm F	NOMMIK (1953)
	0.13—0.21	diet contained 50 ppm F 40 months	STODDARD et al. (1956)
	0.13—0.35	diet contained 100 ppm F 40 months	
	0.14—0.26; av. 0.192	diet contained 880 ppm F 5 years	PHILLIPS et al. (1934)
	0.15—0.16	water supply contained 0.53 ppm F	NOMMIK (1953)
	0.16	water supply contained 0.27 ppm F	
	0.16	water supply contained 0.38	
	0.16	diet contained 3—5 ppm F	SUTTIE et al. (1957)
	0.17	water supply contained 0.19 or 1.12 ppm F	NOMMIK (1953)
	0.18	water supply contained 0.99 ppm F	
	0.19	water supply contained 0.18 ppm F	
	0.2 —0.4	water contained 0.2—500 ppm F	SMITH, M. C. et al. (1941)
	0.21—0.35	pastured 4—9 yrs. near rock phosphate plant	LARGENT (1951)
	0.21	water supply cont'd. 0.24 or 0.85 ppm F	NOMMIK (1953)
	0.22	water supply contained 0.98 ppm F	
	0.24	water supply contained 0.17 ppm F	
	0.27—0.44	diet contained 50 ppm F 5 years	SUTTIE et al. (1957)
	0.29—0.31	diet contained 20 ppm F 5 years	
	0.30—0.38	diet contained 30 ppm F 5 years	
	0.31—0.51	removed from vicinity of phosphate plant	LARGENT (1951)
	0.32—0.51	diet contained 50 ppm F plus $CaCO_3$	
	0.37	hay contained 24 ppm F	LINDBERG (1956)
	0.46	water contained 0.82 ppm F	MINOGUCHI and IWAMOTO (1957)
	0.54	water contained 0.7 ppm F	
	0.55—1.02	—	VON FELLENBERG (1951)
	<1	severe industrial fluorosis	BLAKEMORE et al. (1948)
Dog	0.1	—	MINOGUCHI and IWAMOTO (1957)
Goat	0.11—0.15	—	MINOGUCHI and IWAMOTO (1957)
Sheep	0.2	water supplies cont'd. up to 10 ppm F	HARVEY (1952)
	0.28—0.62	pastured near aluminium plant	AGATE et al. (1949)
	0—0.79	—	

example, found F in cows' milk to be increased 4- to 5-fold when F in the water supply was increased 7- to 8-fold, and SUTTIE et al. (1957) found the concentration to be roughly doubled when the amount of NaF added to the diet was increased by a factor of 4 to 10. On the other hand PHILLIPS et al. (1934) found little or no increase when the cows were fed 220—880 ppm F as rock phosphate.

The investigations of WALLACE (1953) with F^{18} demonstrated that in her rats about one per cent of the F^{18} absorbed by the mothers appeared in the nursing young and STOOKEY et al. (1962c) showed increased F in the femurs of nursing rats whose mothers were ingesting fluoride. HOBBS et al. (1954) concluded there was little transfer of F to the young calf by way of maternal milk. In their experiments F in the skeletal ash of control calves sacrificed at weaning, and whose mothers had received the control ration containing 7 ppm F, was only slightly less than that of calves whose mothers had ingested rations containing 10–100 ppm of F added as sodium fluoride.

Fluoride concentrations in human milk have been investigated with far less frequency than is the case for cows' milk. Available data are listed in Table 26, below.

Table 26. *Concentrations of fluoride found in human milk*

Concn., ppm F	Comment	Reference
0—0.35; av. 0.131	4—5 days post-delivery; 0.55 ppm F in drinking water	BERCOVICI et al. (1960)
0—0.24; av. 0.107	4—32 wks. post-delivery; 0.55 ppm F in drinking water	
0.08—0.147	maternal blood contained 0.23 to 0.36 ppm F	HELD (1952)
0.115–0.168	mothers given 5 mg F daily 2—6 days	
0.10—0.18	drinking water contained 0.055 ppm F	ZIEGLER, quoted by BERCOVICI et al. (loc. cit.)
0.25	drinking water contained 1.13 ppm F	
0.13—0.25	control subjects	LINDBERG (1956)
0.45—0.60	non-workers living near superphosphate factory	
1.05—1.88	workers in superphosphate factory	
0—12	dry basis	WALDO and ZIPF (1952)
not detected –0.12	3—8 days post-delivery; 0.06 ppm F in water supply	SMITH et al. (1963a)

A constancy in F concentrations is again evident, though the magnitude of this plateau may vary with the level of fluoride ingested. HELD (1952) found milk to contain 0.08–0.147 ppm F in mothers consuming a normal hospital diet and drinking water containing 0.09–0.10 ppm F. When these mothers were given 5 mg F daily in tea for 2 days, F increased about 15% in both blood and milk, but there was no further increase in milk concentrations when the 5 mg was continued for five days despite an increase of 55% in blood F levels. HELD (loc. cit). considered the mammary gland to function in a selective fashion with regard to secretion of F.

BERCOVICI et al. (1960) also were impressed with the constancy of the levels of F in milk during a 32-week post-delivery period, and SMITH et al. (1963a) demonstrated stable F levels in milk both within a given day and from day to day. The data of SMITH et al. are listed in Table 27. In the former study the mothers used water containing 0.55 ppm F, while in the latter investigation the mothers' water supply contained only 0.06 ppm F.

Limited data suggest that ingested F appears promptly in the milk. PERKINSON et al. (1955) found F^{18} to appear in the milk of a cow within minutes (30 min and less) after either ingestion or intravenous injection of the isotope. MINOGUCHI and IWAMOTO (1957) fed fluoride to a lactating goat and found increased concentrations of F in the milk as early as three hours thereafter, with maximal concentrations at 6 hours. Values were normal again after three days.

Table 27. *Concentrations of fluoride in human milk during succeeding days post-partum.* Water supply contained approximately 0.06 ppm F (data of SMITH et al., 1963a)

Subject	Comment		Concn., ppm F
D	3rd day post-partum		not detected
J	3rd day post-partum,	2:00 PM	0.06
		10:00 PM	0.05
	4th day post-partum	6:00 AM	0.03
		4:00 PM	not detected
		10:00 PM	0.02
	5th day post-partum	6:00 AM	0.02
	7th day post-partum	time unknown	0.02
		time unknown	0.02
		time unknown	0.02
K	day post-partum unknown		0.12
	next day	6:00 AM	0.02
		2:00 PM	0.04
		10:00 PM	0.06
	next day	6:00 AM	0.03
		2:00 PM	0.05
		10:00 PM	0.02
	next day	6:00 AM	0.03
A	5th day post-partum		not detected
B	5th day post-partum		not detected
C	5th day post-partum		0.05
G	8th day post-partum		0.09
E	post-partum interval unknown		not detected
F	post-partum interval unknown		0.04
H	post-partum interval unknown		0.02
I	post-partum interval unknown		0.003

F. Fluoride in saliva, plaque and calculus

The secretion of F in saliva was first investigated with the aid of isotopes by WILLS (1940), who compared the secretion of F^{18} and radiochloride in saliva of the cat. An appreciable portion of F^{18} given intravenously appeared in the saliva within the first minute, with lesser amounts being secreted during the succeeding twenty minutes. A total of 0.082% of the dose was recovered in the submaxillary saliva during a period of 21 min. In contrast, little or no radiochloride appeared in the first minute, peak concentrations were achieved in the ensuing ten minutes, and a total of 0.365 % was secreted in the 23 min post-administration. The average ratio of salivary to plasma F in successive ten-minute intervals was 0.098, while the corresponding ratio for Cl was 0.387. Thus, F appears to cross from blood to saliva to a lesser extent than does Cl, despite the more prompt appearance of the former in the saliva.

There was insufficient F^{18} in the salivery glands of Wills' cats to permit its quantitation (VOLKER et al., 1941). In other experiments however, concentrations of F in the salivary glands have been measured and found to be quite low. Using rats, VOLKER et al. (1941) found the salivary glands to contain 0.098% of the dose per gram (the blood contained 0.370 % per gram) 35 min after intraperitoneal injection. WALLACE-DURBIN (1954) found parotid glands of rats to contain twice as much F^{18} as blood, 15 min after intravenous injection. HEIN et al. (1956) found F^{18} in the salivary glands of rats to be present in concentrations equal to or less than that in blood, and BELL et al. (1961) found F^{18} in the parotid and mandibular glands of cattle at concentrations below those prevailing in blood. The autoradiograms of ERICSSON and ULLBERG (1958) show no appreciable concentration of F^{18} in salivary glands of mice and rats.

Table 28. *Concentrations of fluoride in human saliva*

ppm F in		Comment	Reference
saliva	water		
None	—	mottled enamel area	BOISSEVAIN and DREA (1933)
0.07	—	4 hrs. after ingesting 8 mg F as NaF	BUTTNER and MUHLER (1962)
Not detected	—	0.5 hrs. after ingesting 8 mg F	
Not detected	—	prior to ingesting 8 mg F	
0.04—0.46; av 0.18	—	males, 18—30 yrs.	GEDALIA et al. (1961b)
0.06—0.41; av. 0.16	up to 1	calculus-free adults 20—38 yrs. old	GEDALIA et al. (1963)
0.04—0.14	—	adults	McCLURE (1941)
0.06	—	14—21 yrs.	
0.06—0.1	—	children, 12—14 yrs.	
0.10	—	children, 8—13 yrs.	
0.111	—	carious non-gypsies	HATTYASY et al. (1956)
0.15	—	caries-resistant gypsies	
0.15	—	12—22 yr. old persons with mottled enamel	
0.248	—	gypsies with arrested caries	
0.08	0.2	carious subjects	HATTYASY (1954)
0.74	0.2	caries-free gypsies	
0.12	0.2	av. of 3 children, 8 yrs. of age	COX (1940)
0.07—0.37	0.5—0.6	children, 12—14 yrs.	DVIR et al. (1962)
0.11—0.13	0.7	children, 9—14 yrs.	McCLURE (1941)
0.11—0.29	1	children, 12—14 yrs.	MARTIN and HILL (1950)
0.1	1.2—1.3	children, 12—14 yrs.	
0.095	1.8	av. of 3 children, 8 yrs. of age	COX (1940)
0.16	1.8	children, 12—14 yrs.	McCLURE (1941)
0.13—0.24	3.8—4.0	children	McCLURE (1941)

The evidence suggests then, that levels of F in saliva would be expected to be low, and indeed they are. Salivary F levels reported by a number of investigators are summarized in Table 28. The rather limited data do not indicate a very strong correlation between concentrations of F in the saliva and in the drinking water. The data listed are comparable to those reported by SINGER and ARMSTRONG (1960) for plasma fluorides in persons using water supplies containing up to about 5 ppm F. CARLSON et al. (1960a) found levels of F^{18} in saliva to be less than those in plasma in humans ingesting a small quantity of the isotope. Peak concentrations in both fluids were achieved within an hour of taking the fluoride and the course of its appearance and disappearance in saliva paralleled that in plasma. BELL et al. (1961) also found F^{18} levels in saliva to be less than those in plasma when F^{18} was given intravenously to cattle; the peak concentration in saliva was reached in five minutes. Evidently, the mechanisms acting to keep plasma fluoride concentrations low also indirectly succeed in keeping the concentrations of F low in the salivary glands and thus in the saliva.

Present thinking concerning the mechanism(s) whereby fluoride succeeds in reducing the incidence of dental caries attributes a role to F at the enamel surface, perhaps to inhibit bacterial production of acid and/or to produce an apatite more resistant to the attack of acids. Investigations intended to furnish data relevant to these possibilities have now afforded data describing the concentrations of F in dental plaque and calculus.

HARDWICK (1961) found concentrations up to 30 ppm in fresh plaque, with half of the 30 samples analyzed containing 6 ppm or more. Later HARDWICK and LEACH (1963) reported plaque from 51 individuals living in a low fluoride area to contain 6—180 ppm F (fresh wt. basis). KUDAHL (1963) found that more than half of a series of 24 samples from persons using water containing 0.05 ppm F contained little or no F. The significance of F in plaque with respect to caries has been discussed by JENKINS (1963) and by HARDWICK (1963).

SPEIRS (1959) has reported that dental calculus from persons residing in a non-fluoride area contained 1070—1200 ppm F (dry wt. basis), whereas calculus of persons in a fluoride area contained 2000—2020 ppm F. Speirs considers F in calculus to be related to that in the drinking water, and that there is a continuing deposition and adsorption from fluoride in the mouth, *e.g.* from tea and water. GEDALIA et al. (1963) found calculus from persons using water supplies containing up to 1 ppm F to contain 220—775 ppm F (average 465 ppm; ash basis). They point out that concentrations of this order are comparable to those reported for dentin, enamel, intact deciduous teeth, and bone, and consider this to be in accordance with the similarity in composition of these various calcified structures. Fluoride in calculus is considered by these authors to be derived from saliva and from drinking water, perhaps as the result of a slow incorporation during precipitation of the calculus. Subgingival calculus has been reported to contain less F (113—350 ppm) than supragingival calculus (160—733 ppm), probably because of its lesser contact with saliva and drinking water (YARDENI et al., 1963).

G. Skeletal storage of fluoride

The two mechanisms whereby the body disposes of absorbed fluoride are i) deposition in the calcified structures, and ii) excretion through the kidneys into the urine. The importance of these processes will be evident when it is recalled that 99 % or more of fluoride retained in the body is localized in the skeleton, and that fluoride appears promptly in the urine after ingestion, as much as 20 % being found there in the next 3—4 hours. Excretion of fluoride is discussed in the next Section, and a detailed discussion of skeletal uptake of F is given by Dr. JOHN WEATHERALL in a later chapter. Because of the importance of the subject however, it is necessary to present a general description of the principal aspects at this time. Fluoride in teeth is considered by Brudevold elsewhere in this volume.

1. Rapidity of skeletal deposition

Fluoride appears promptly in the bone, as has been shown by a number of investigators. ERICSSON and ULLBERG (1958) demonstrated the presence of F^{18} autoradiographically in the skeleton 2 min after intravenous injection in mice. HEIN et al. (1956), and WALLACE (1953) found F^{18} in the rat skeleton 10 and 15 min, respectively, after intravenous injection, and VOLKER et al. (1941) found the isotope in the bones of rats 30 min after intraperitoneal injection.

To date, the data of WALLACE (1953) are the most appropriate for demonstrating the time course of skeletal uptake of F^{18}, though one could wish for more frequent time intervals in her experiment. Her data, obtained in rats following ingestion or intraperitoneal injection of the isotope are shown in Fig. 8. It is evident from the figure that the initial rate of uptake by the skeleton is quite rapid regardless of the route of administration, and also that in young rats the skeletal concentrations achieved after ingestion are only slightly less than those obtained when the F is given intravenously. Wallace's data indicate that the fraction of the dose appearing in the skeleton is 1.5—4.5 times greater than that appearing in the urine. Skeletal deposition then, is the more rapid process and thus regulates the size of the fractions deposited and excreted.

Carlson et al. (1960a) demonstrated that rapid skeletal uptake of F obtains in man, also. In their experiments subjects ingested F^{18} in a small volume of water, following which a portable crystal scintillation counter was positioned over the right femur and tibia. F^{18} was detected in the tibia 25–46 min later, and in the femur (region of the greater trochanter) after 31–34 min. Counts in the femur had decreased only 15% from the maximal value after 250 min, indicating that the calcified tissues retained their F, even though the plasma activity had decreased approximately 85%.

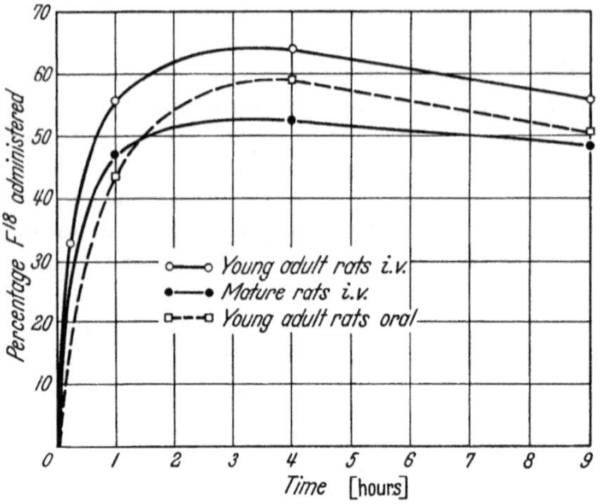

Fig. 8. Uptake of F^{18} by the rat skeleton. Data of Wallace (1953)

2. Skeletal concentrations of fluoride

A number of factors have been shown to affect bone fluoride concentrations. Consequently, quotations of "normal" levels must be qualified by the inclusion of additional information such as F content of the stock diet, the interval during which this diet was ingested, the age of the subject or animal when the dietary regimen was started, and sex. Other factors as well may also be influential.

Bone F concentrations have been reported in literally hundreds of experiments in the literature, in most of which control groups were included. These control data have served their intended purpose of furnishing a base line against which to measure changes produced in the experimental groups, but all too frequently pertinent data such as concentration of F in the stock diet and animal age and sex have been omitted, since these were comparable in both groups. Consequently, there are surprisingly few data available which describe skeletal fluoride concentrations produced by the daily ingestion of known amounts of fluoride naturally present in the normal diet of different species.

In Table 29 are listed bone fluoride concentrations from the literature which are adequately related to normal dietary F. It is immediately evident that there are all too few such data; approximately 15 such reports are available in the literature of the past 15 years. Two-thirds of these deal with the rat, and only two other species, viz. the cow and the rabbit are included. Comparisons are further complicated by the fact that concentrations may be reported for bone ash, for dry fat-free bone, for dry bone, or the basis may not be stated at all. Nevertheless, certain aspects of skeletal uptake of fluoride are apparent.

The effect in cattle of prolonged ingestion of low levels of F is seen in the experiments of Miller and Shupe (1962) and of Suttie et al. (1957). The former investigators found a regular increase in F in the rib of cattle with increasing time, whereas Suttie et al. (1957) found the increase to be somewhat less regular but nevertheless clearly evident. In the latter experiment the animals were started as 18–24 month old heifers; the fact that rib concentrations first declined after the animals were placed on Suttie's stock ration and did not exceed the initial values until after 24 months, suggests that the prior ration contained more than the

Table 29. *Skeletal fluoride concentrations in several species*

Species	Tissue[1]	ppm F	Comment	Reference
Cow	rib	1300	started as 12—15 mo. old heifers; 54 mos. on stock diet cont'g. 7 ppm F	HOBBS et al. (1954)
Cow	rib[2]	425	started as 18—24 mo. old heifers; 9 mos. on stock diet cont'g. 3—5 ppm F	SUTTIE et al. (1957)
		360	as above; 19 mos.	
		400	as above; 24 mos.	
		498	as above; 30 mos.	
		512	as above; 37 mos.	
		495	as above; 49 mos.	
		590	as above; 63 mos.	
Cow	rib[3]	305	started as 6 mo. old heifers; 1 mo. on stock ration cont'g. 12 ppm F	MILLER and SHUPE (1962)
		425	as above; 13 mos.	
		515	as above; 25 mos.	
		614	as above; 37 mos.	
		681	as above; 49 mos.	
		819	as above; 61 mos.	
		895	as above; 73 mos.	
Rabbit	femur[3]	600	initial age, 8 wks., maintained 3 mos. on stock diet cont'g. 3ppm F	HOBBS et al. (1954)
Rabbit	tibia and femur[2]	275	initial wt. 750 g.; 4 mos. on diet cont'g. at least 8 ppm F. Both sexes	BRIGGS and PHILLIPS (1952)
Rat	humerus, femur[4]	25—41	started as weanlings, both sexes; 11 mos. on stock diet cont'g. 1 to 1.4 ppm F	AUSKAPS and SHAW (1955)
Rat	femur	74	started as weanling males; 140 days on stock diet cont'g. 0.3 ppm F	BIXLER et al. (1954)
		101	females, as above	
		133	started as weanling males; 140 da. on stock diet cont'g. 0.6 ppm F	
		149	females, as above	
Rat	tibia, mandible, incisors	150 to 160	started as weanlings; 30 days on stock diet cont'g. 1.5 pm F	HOBBS et al. (1954)
		180 to 380	started as weanlings; 6 wks. on stock diet cont'g. 10—20 ppm F	
Rat	jaw alveolar bone	1700	started as weanling males; 2 yrs. on stock diet cont'g. 18–19 ppm F	MAYNARD et al. (1949)
		1550	females as above	
	femoral epiphysis	1700	males as above	
		1800	females as above	
	femoral diaphysis	1850	males as above	
		1400	females as above	
Rat	femur	3.2	started as weanling males; 105 da. on stock diet cont'g. ca 0.007 ppm	MAURER and DAY (1957)
		4.5	as above; 165 days	
		1.9	as above; 325 days	
		0	females as above; 105—190 days	
		8.8	females as above; 195 days	
		4.7	females as above; 300 days	
		2.4	females as above; 325 days	

Table 29. (Continued)

Species	Tissue[1]	ppm F	Comment	Reference
Rat	femur	200	started as weanlings, both sexes; 100 da. on stock diet cont'g. 1 ppm F	McCann and Bullock (1957)
	humerus	200	as above	
	mandible	200	as above	
Rat	femur[2]	225	started as weanling females; 6 wks. on stock diet cont'g. 3—5 ppm F	Miller and Phillips (1953)
		250	as above; 10 wks.	
		240	as above; 14 wks.	
		270	as above; 18 wks.	
		305	as above; 22 wks.	
		305	as above; 26 wks.	
		350	as above; 38 wks.	
Rat	femur	31	started as weanling males; 3 mos. on stock diet cont'g. 0.2–0.3 ppm F	Smith et al. (1963b)
		59	as above; 6 mos.	
		72	as above; 12 mos.	
		130	as above; 24 mos.	
		38	started as weanling females; 3 mos. on stock diet cont'g. 0.2–0.3 ppm F	
		80	as above; 6 mos.	
		73	as above; 12 mos.	
		137	as above; 24 mos.	
Rat	femur[3]	23	started as weanling females; 94 da. on stock diet cont'g. 0.5 ppm F	Wuthier and Phillips (1961)
		22	males, as above	
		47	females as above; 184 days on expt.	
		34	males as above	
		84	females as above; 365 days on diet	
		57	males as above	
		66	females as above; 554 days	
		40	males as above	
		60	females as above; 622 days	
Rat	femur	1500	started as weanling females; 6 wks. on stock diet cont'g. 3 ppm F	Zipkin et al. (1959)
	mandible	1310		

[1] Ash basis unless otherwise indicated.
[2] Dry, fat-free bone.
[3] Dry basis.
[4] Not stated.

3–5 ppm F fed by Suttie and that F was being mobilized from the bone. The slightly higher concentrations reported by Miller and Shupe (1962) may be attributed to the slightly higher concentrations of F in their ration. The much younger age of these heifers when the experiment was started means that their prior use of a ration of unknown F content was considerably shortened, and this may have contributed to the more regular increase seen in this experiment.

The effects of prolonged feeding are also apparent in the data of Smith et al. (1963b) (Table 29), where rats were fed a low-F diet for two years, or nearly their life span. These data are represented graphically in Fig. 9. Increased bone concentrations with increasing time on diet are again apparent, as is also the fact that concentrations are slightly greater in the female rat than in the male. This may be accounted for by the observation that the femurs of the males usually were larger than those of the females; however, total micrograms of F per femur were greater in the males.

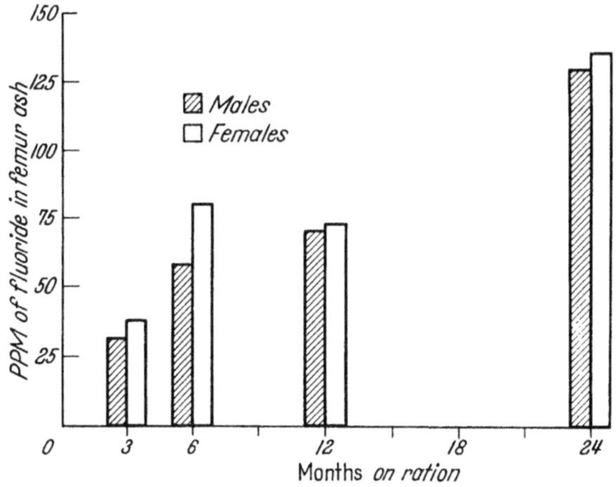

Fig. 9. Effect of prolonged ingestion of a ration low in fluoride (0.3 ppm) on storage of F in the rat femur. Data of SMITH et al. (1963b)

It is interesting to note that fluoride is present in bone even when the diet contains as little as 0.007 ppm F. MAURER and DAY (1957) found femoral ash to contain approximately 2–5 ppm F in rats fed such a diet for nearly one year.

3. Skeletal content vs. intake and duration of exposure

ZIPKIN et al. (1958b) and McCLURE et al. (1958) found increasing concentrations of fluoride in human bone with increasing concentrations of F in the drinking

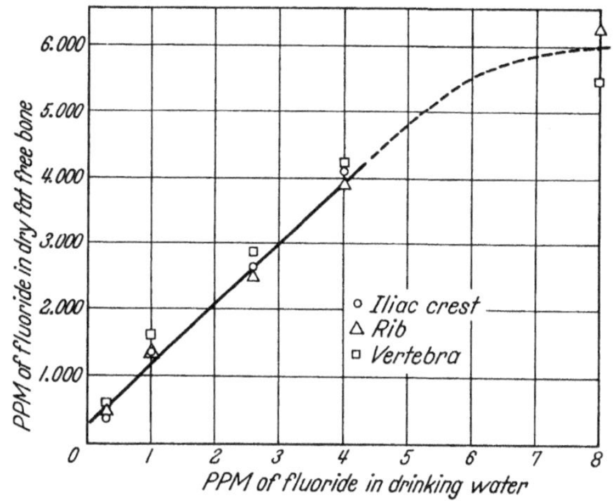

Fig. 10. Relation between fluoride in drinking water and fluoride in human bone. Data of ZIPKIN et al. (1958); McCLURE et al. (1958)

water. Their data have been compiled in one graph in Fig. 10. These were persons whose ages ranged from 26 to 90 years and whose use of their respective water supplies varied from 10 to 87 years.

There have been numerous studies in experimental animals which have demonstrated that concentrations of F in bones and teeth are increased with increasing levels of fluoride ingested. Recent reports include those of SUTTIE et al. (1957, 1958), WUTHIER and PHILLIPS (1959, 1961), MILLER and SHUPE (1962), HARRIS et al. (1963), SHUPE et al. (1963a) and SMITH et al. (1963b).

Data of the latter investigators are shown in Figs. 11 and 12 where concentrations of F in rat femurs are plotted arithmetically on the ordinate against months of F ingestion on a logarithmic abscissa. In these experiments groups of rats were maintained on a low-F diet (0.2–0.3 ppm F) and given access *ad libitum* to drinking water containing 1–10 ppm F for 24 months; other rats fed the same diet received 25–100 ppm F for 12–18 months. At successive time intervals rats were sacrificed and F determined in the femur ash. The data illustrate several points of importance in the skeletal uptake of fluoride.

It is clearly evident from the figures that as the daily level of fluoride ingested is increased,

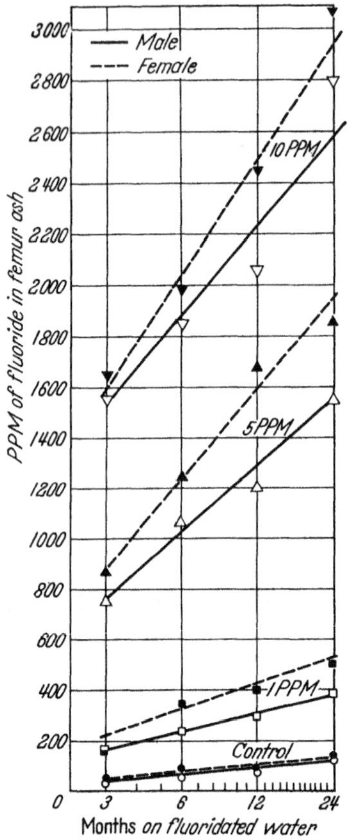

Fig. 11

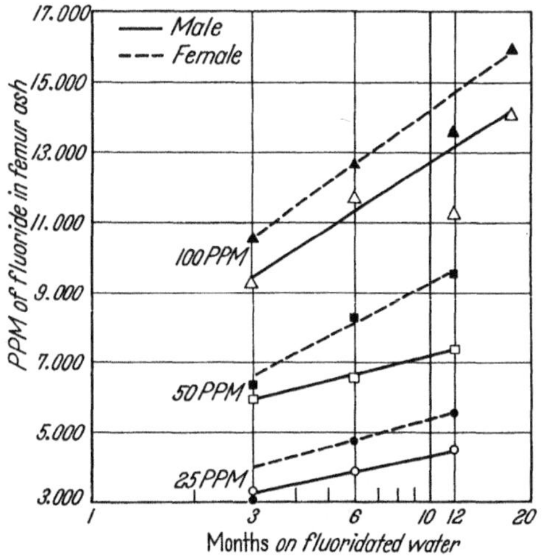

Fig. 12

Fig. 11. Skeletal deposition of fluoride in rats ingesting 1—10 ppm of fluoride in drinking water. Data of SMITH et al. (1963b)

Fig. 12. Skeletal deposition of fluoride in rats ingesting 25—100 ppm of fluoride in drinking water. Data of SMITH et al. (1963b)

the skeletal concentrations obtaining at any given time also increase, though this latter change is not strictly proportional to the increase in concentration of F in the water supply.

It is apparent also that the length of time during which fluoride is ingested has an effect on the skeletal concentrations achieved. Fluoride continued to be laid down in the bones of these rats throughout a 24-month period, virtually the life span of these animals, though the rate of uptake lessened as the experiments progressed.

Inasmuch as time can be considered a measure of the total dose of fluoride when the level of F in the water supply is kept constant, Figs. 11 and 12 indicate that in the rat the response (skeletal storage of F) to the ingestion of F is proportional to the logarithm of the dose (time), a not uncommon pharmacological response. While not as clear-cut, the data of CALL and GREENWOOD (1958) and of SMITH et al. (1963a) for F in the bones of man (*cf.* Tables 19 and 20) also demonstrate a reasonably good relationship between bone F and the logarithm of age. A similar relationship is to be found in the data of MILLER and SHUPE (1962) for cattle; in this instance however, it does not become apparent until the fluoride had been fed for 13 months or more.

4. Skeletal fluoride and age

With low doses of fluoride the skeleton continues to increase in fluoride content with age throughout life. The data of Table 20 illustrate this for man, while the control data shown in Fig. 11 show this for the rat.

Young rats deposit and retain greater amonts of dietary fluoride than do adult rats (SUTTIE and PHILLIPS, 1959; MILLER and PHILLIPS, 1956; ZIPKIN and MCCLURE, 1952; SAVCHUCK and ARMSTRONG, 1951). Typical data from MILLER and PHILLIPS (1956) are shown in Table 30. In this experiment, weanlings three weeks old, young adults 9 weeks old and adults 5 months old were fed a stock ration containing 450 ppm F as added NaF for a total of 18 weeks. At various time intervals during this period groups of rats were sacrificed and the total F in the femurs determined with the results shown in Table 30. It is apparent that in every instance but one the femurs of the weanling rats acquired more total F than did those of the young or old adults.

Table 30. *Effect of age upon deposition of fluorine in the femur of rats.* (Data of MILLER and PHILLIPS, 1956)

Weeks of fluoride feeding	Initial age of rats		
	3 wks.	9 wks.	5 mos.
	milligrams F per femur		
6	1.60	1.55	1.30
9	2.40	2.20	1.50
12	2.80	2.60	1.70
18	3.35	3.50	2.30

Fluoride in enamel and dentin may also increase with age (BRUDEVOLD et al., 1960; JACKSON and WEIDMANN, 1959).

5. Mechanism of skeletal deposition

From dilute solutions fluoride deposits in bone mineral by exchanging with hydroxyl ions of the hydroxyapatite lattice. This has been shown to be a simple exchange phenomenon described by the Mass Law (NEUMAN et al., 1950). Hydroxyl ions in solution and fluoride ions in solution compete for the OH^- loci in the lattice. The physical resemblance (ionic charge, ionic radius) between F^- and OH^- is so similar that F^- can then penetrate into the internal crystal structure.

6. Enamel deposition

Fluoride concentrations in enamel and cementum have been shown to increase with increasing levels of F in the food or water (SUTTIE and PHILLIPS, 1960; BRUDEVOLD et al., 1960). After calcification and eruption the enamel possesses little metabolic activity. Increasing the dietary F of cattle increased F in the enamel only if the teeth had not erupted prior to exposure to F, whereas F in the dentin increased with levels of dietary F and throughout the duration of ingestion (SUTTIE and PHILLIPS, 1960).

Uptake of F by intact enamel *in vitro* has been demonstrated using F^{18} (ERICSSON 1961, 1958b; HARDWICK et al., 1958; BRUDEVOLD et al., 1957; MUHLEMANN et al., 1955), and also by direct chemical analysis (SUNDVALL-HAGLAND et al., 1959).

7. Mobilization

The study of LARGENT (1952) offers an illustration of the mobilization of fluoride deposited in the human skeleton. At the end of a series of metabolic studies performed with himself as the subject, and extending over a period of more than two years, Largent knew that approximately 1.7 g of the total F ingested during this interval was retained in his skeletal system. Upon ceasing the intake of additional F, Largent then measured his daily fluoride intake and urinary excretion at intervals throughout the succeeding 100 weeks. During this time urinary excretion always exceeded the intake, thus demonstrating mobilization of a portion of the previously deposited F. Largent calculated that 4.7 years would be required to reach the point at which the excess of urinary fluoride would have decreased to the point where it could not be distinguished from the normal output. In other words, mobilization of previously stored fluoride in this individual would continue for at least 4.7 years after returning to a normal intake of F.

Mobilization to a limited degree has also been demonstrated in rats, as exemplified in the data of SAVCHUCK and ARMSTRONG (1951), and by MILLER and PHILLIPS (1953, 1956).

8. Steady state

The establishment of a steady state in the deposition of fluoride in the skeleton is described by ZIPKIN and MCCLURE (1952) in rats given 10 ppm F in the drinking water starting at 30 days of age and continuing for 420 days. Total femur F increased rapidly for about 200 days and more slowly for the next 100 days; little change occurred thereafter through the 420th day. The authors considered that a stabilized or saturation level of femur F had been reached.

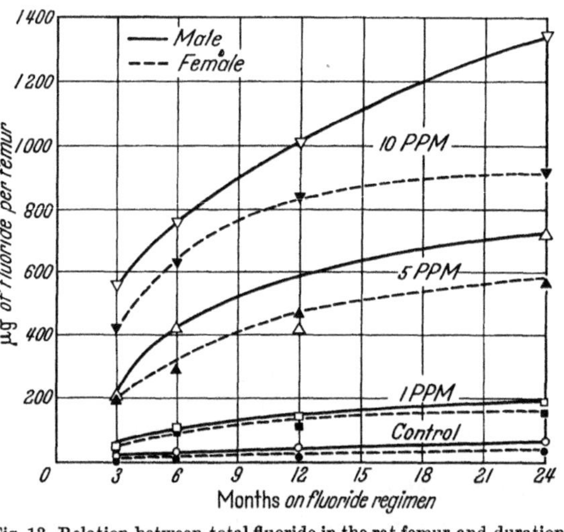

Fig. 13. Relation between total fluoride in the rat femur and duration of fluoride ingestion. Data of SMITH et al. 1963b)

SMITH et al. (1963b) found a somewhat similar pattern; their data for rats drinking water containing 1–10 ppm F are shown in Fig. 13 where total micrograms of fluoride per femur are plotted against time. The curves suggest, however, that in this experiment the steady state had not yet been achieved to the same degree as was found by ZIPKIN and MCCLURE (loc. cit.). In each instance, and especially in the males receiving 10 ppm F, the curves suggest that femur F was still increasing after 24 months, though at a greatly diminished rate.

JACKSON and WEIDMANN (1958) have demonstrated the achievement of a steady state in the human skeleton. Subjects in their study had used water supplies containing < 0.5, 0.8 or 1.9 ppm F, and at each level concentrations of F in rib samples taken at autopsy attained reasonably constant levels after 50–60 years.

9. Cartilage

The uptake of fluoride in the ossification centers of cartilage has been demonstrated by several investigators. WALLACE (1953) reported that F^{18} was taken up by rat cartilage, to an extent commensurate with its potentialities for calcification, and this has been verified by ERICSSON and ULLBERG (1958), ERICSSON et al. (1960), and APPELGREN et al. (1961).

ZIPKIN et al. (1958b) and MCCLURE et al. (1958) measured fluoride concentration in the intervertebral cartilage of persons who had ingested drinking water containing up to 8 ppm F for prolonged periods. Their results, shown in the text table below, indicate that concentrations of F in dry fat-free intervertebral cartilage increases somewhat with elevated levels of F in the water, but that these concentrations are much less than those of bone (*cf.* Fig. 10). According to ERICSSON and ULLBERG (1958) the fluoride found here probably is due to the presence of Ca salts in the samples analyzed.

ppm F in drinking water	ppm F in dry fat-free intervertebral cartilage
1.0	30 ± 0
1.0	40 ± 10
2.6	40 ± 10
4.0	70 ± 30
8.0	110

ENGLE et al. (1961) investigated the binding of various anions by rabbit rib cartilage, and showed that fluoride decreased the negative colloidal charge from a normal value of about 0.15–0.17 equiv./kg water to about 0.08 equiv./kg at pH 7.4. The effect was much more pronounced near the isoelectric point of pH 2–2.2.

10. Prediction of skeletal fluoride

It is readily apparent that some means other than preparation of the entire skeleton would be advantageous for estimating total skeletal F. The question has intrigued several investigators, but as yet their suggestions have not been widely tested.

SAVCHUCK and ARMSTRONG (1951) determined total fluoride in the skeletons of four rats varying widely in age, weight and past fluoride ingestion, as well as the fraction of the total skeletal F located in each of 10 component bones of the edentulous skeletons. Despite differences in age and past intake of F, the humerus (left or right) was found to contain an acceptably constant fraction of the total skeletal F, viz. 2.3 %, with a standard deviation of 0.12. Much larger variations were seen in the vertebra, thoracic skeleton and bones of the paw. These authors therefore recommend the humerus as a representative bone in studies of fluoride turnover, and as a basis for estimating total F in the skeletal system in the rat.

More recently, SINGER and ARMSTRONG (1962) compared fluoride concentrations in the ash of enamel, dentin, cementum, mandible, femur and iliac crest of 11 human cadavers ranging in age from 49 to 78 years. In all cases except one the cementum had the highest fluoride content of all the calcified tissues examined. A comparison of the ratios and standard deviations of fluoride contents of enamel, dentin and cementum to bones indicated the relative value of the dental tissues in estimating fluoride contents of the skeleton to be cementum > dentin = enamel. For example, knowledge of the F content of cementum would allow calculation of that of the iliac crest within 7.6 % of the determined concentration, in two-thirds of the cases. The authors emphasize that their results probably apply only to a population of relatively advanced age, whose fluoride intakes during life were not exceptionally large (probably less than 1 ppm in the drinking water).

RILEY et al. (1963) cite the work of BURNS and ALLCROFT (1962) in suggesting that analysis of vertebrae from the tails of cattle may be useful in estimating skeletal F in such animals. In a series of 57 animals values for F in the tail bone were within 30 % of that for the rib in 81 % of the cases.

H. Extraskeletal calcification

1. Soft tissues

The most conclusive evidence yet available for the deposition of fluoride in sites of calcification other than the bones or teeth, is that of ERICSSON and ULLBERG (1958). These authors demonstrated autoradiographically the presence of F^{18} localized in numerous discrete sites throughout the placentae of pregnant mice; upon staining some of these sections for Ca deposits, small calcified granules were found to coincide exactly with the locations of F^{18} appearing on the autoradiograms.

SMITH et al. (1960) have suggested that the increase seen in fluoride in the samples of human aorta analyzed by them could be associated with the increased calcification frequently seen in this tissue with advancing age. Calcium determinations were not made on these samples unfortunately, but the F concentrations did correlate with age as does Ca, increasing as the age increased.

Recently STOOKEY and MUHLER (1963) investigated the extraskeletal deposition of fluoride in rats and guinea pigs maintained on a "calcification-inducing" diet, and interpreted their results to indicate that increases in tissue Ca in heart, liver and kidney were associated with increases in tissue F. Careful examination of the data however, indicates that fluoride did not always increase when tissue Ca increased, and indeed, that tissue Ca did not always increase under the influence of the "calcification-inducing" diet. Several factors may have contributed to the partial lack of the expected results. Ca and F determinations were not made on the same portion of the organs, but on separate halves; if the ectopic Ca were not uniformly distributed throughout the organ, and it probably is not, then erroneously low Ca values would be obtained. Secondly, the "calcification-inducing" diet apparently contained severely toxic amounts of calciferol (186,000 units per gram) as evidenced by the fact that body weights of the animals on this diet were only about half those of the controls, after 30 days. Such a severe weight loss would be expected to be accompanied by some decrease in organ weights, so that expression of Ca and F data in terms of $\mu g/g$ could prove misleading.

2. Renal and biliary calculi

In 1956 Herman reported kidney stones from 10 human cases of urolithiasis to contain fluoride in concentrations ranging from 4 to 1560 ppm. It was noted that stones high in Ca were also high in F, and in two instances where Ca was not detected, the concentrations of F were 4–5 ppm. In a later paper HERMAN et al. (1958) examined stones from 100 cases of urolithiasis, and found < 5–1800 ppm F in these instances; there was no relation between F concentration and the portion of the tract (renal, ureteral or vesicle) from which the stone came. Fluoride concentrations were low in the uric acid calculi, which contained little or no Ca; in general, those stones containing 5 % or less of Ca contained less than 100 ppm F, whereas F concentrations exceeded 100 ppm where Ca contents were more than 5 %. Those calculi containing 241 ppm or more of F were shown by x-ray diffraction analysis to contain apatite in the stone; the apatite contained less than 0.3 % F, indicating only slight conversion to fluoroapatite.

In a more extensive study ZIPKIN et al. (1958a) measured F in urinary tract calculi of individuals whose water supplies contained a) 0.6 ppm F or less, or b)

2.6 ppm F. Stones from the former population contained 200–6700 ppm, average 2500 ppm (dry basis); in the latter population, corresponding values were 300–11,100, average 3700 ppm. These were considered not to be significantly different. In both groups the average concentration of F in the calculi exceeded that in bone from individuals residing in the same area. The apatite structure was identified in 9 of 11 stones submitted to x-ray diffraction analysis, but there appeared to be no relation between F and Ca concentrations.

A lesser number of biliary tract calculi from persons using water containing 2.6 ppm F contained 0–60 ppm F, averaging 20 ppm (dry basis). Calcium generally was present in very low concentrations in these stones. A sample of bile pooled from four individuals whose drinking water contained 1 ppm F, contained only 0.1 ppm F.

Herman and Papadakis (1960) found concentrations of 0.1–500 ppm F in drinking water to have no effect on experimental urolithogenesis in the rat.

V. Excretion

A. Urinary excretion

As has been indicated, the ultimate fate of absorbed fluoride is either excretion in the urine or deposition in bone and retention in the skeletion. Much lesser proportions are excreted in the feces or retained in the soft tissues. As with bone, there are difficulties inherent in establishing "normal" urinary concentrations of F. This parameter will reflect the total intake of available fluoride and in addition will be influenced by the extent and rate at which this is taken up by the skeleton.

1. Rapidity of excretion

Fluoride is rapidly excreted in the urine, as a number of studies have shown. Following intravenous administration of F^{18} to cats, Volker et al. (1941) found the greater share of urinary excretion to take place in the first 30 min or less. According to Wallace (1953) the rat excretes 31 % of an intravenously administered dose of F^{18} in 15 min, and 55 % in one hour; 13 % was present in urine one hour after an oral dose of F^{18}. After nine hours the total fraction of the dose appearing in the urine was very nearly the same by either route, being 31.4 and 25.6 % after intravenous and oral administration, respectively.

Man also appears to be capable of rapid excretion of F via urine. Carlson (1959) collected samples as early as 11 min after ingestion of NaF labeled with F^{18}, and found measureable amounts of the isotope at this time. A number of other studies have quantitated the amount excreted in the first few hours after ingesting F; these have been summarized in Table 2 and Fig. 3, from which it is evident that one-fifth of an ingested dose of soluble fluoride is excreted in the urine in the ensuing 3–4 hours.

McClure and Kinser (1944) noted during the course of field studies in which McClure briefly visited areas of the country where the local water supplies contained 0–4.5 ppm F, that concentrations of F in his urine rapidly approximated those in the local source of water. For example, 18 hours after arriving in Lubbock, Texas where the water contained 3.8 ppm F, urine concentrations had increased to 3.9 ppm.

Supposedly "unavailable" fluoride also appears surprisingly promptly in urine, *e.g.* Largent (1961) found increased concentrations two hours after ingesting 15.8 mg F as rock phosphate, the concentrations becoming maximal after an additional two hours. Collings et al. (1951) also found elevated urinary fluoride as early as two hours after inhalation exposure to either particulate or gaseous fluoride. It should be pointed out that inasmuch as neither LARGENT nor COLLINGS et al. collected samples earlier than two hours post ingestion or post exposure, at which times concentrations were increased, it is reasonable to suppose that F first appeared in the urine earlier than this, as indeed was shown by CARLSON (loc. cit.).

Several studies have shown the presence of fluoride in urine after using a fluoride-containing dentifrice or mouthwash (SCHWEINSBERGER and MUHLER, 1956; SCHWEINSBERGER and MUHLER, 1957; ERICSSON, 1961; BUTTNER et al., 1961; HELLSTROM, 1960; DUCKWORTH, 1963).

The data of ZIPKIN et al. (1957) afford an estimate of the rate at which man excretes fluoride in the urine. In this study frequent samples were collected from a group of volunteers over a 24-hour period, during which the principal source of F

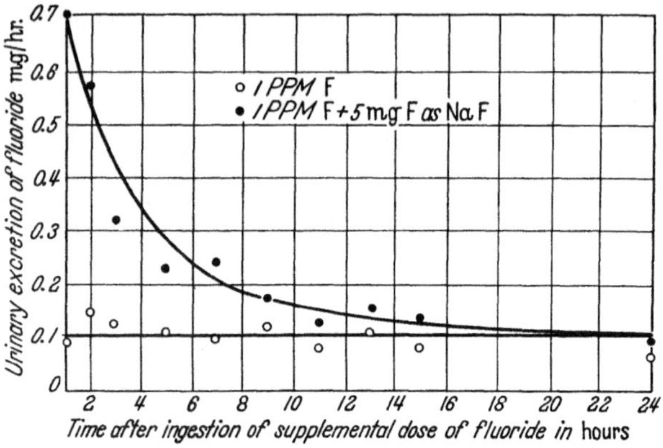

Fig. 14. Urinary excretion of fluoride in mg/hr in adults drinking water containing 1 ppm F and receiving a supplement of 5 mg F as NaF. From ZIPKIN et al. (1957)

intake was drinking water containing 1 ppm F. The average total intake was 3.2 mg. Of this, 65.1 % was excreted in the 24 hours and the average rate of excretion was 0.1 mg/hr. During a second 24-hour period, the subjects ingested 5 mg of F as NaF in 200 ml of water. Average total F intake was 8.1 mg of which 54.1 % was excreted in the 24 hours. During this interval the hourly excretion rate was greatest during the first hour after ingestion of the "challenge" dose, being 0.7 mg/hr. The rate dropped rapidly thereafter, and closely approached the control rate of 0.1 mg/hr approximately 11 hours after imbibing the test dose. Fig. 14, taken from the paper of ZIPKIN et al. (1957) illustrates the changing rate of excretion.

2. Urinary excretion as a function of intake

Concentrations of fluoride in the urine are reasonable reflections of the daily intake of fluoride, especially when the entering fluoride is in "available" forms. In fact, the analysis of spot urine samples of industrial workers exposed to fluorides is routinely used as a bioassay technic to ensure that engineering controls are operating effectively.

The relation between fluoride ingested and fluoride excreted in the urine is shown in Fig. 15 where data are plotted for cattle, sheep and the rat; the latter species received F in the drinking water, while the F was incorporated in the diet of the cattle and sheep. It is clearly evident that as the quantities of fluoride ingested are increased, the amounts of F excreted in the urine also increase. The data of SUTTIE et al. (1957) and of SHUPE et al. (1963) plotted here are from experiments in which fluoride as NaF was added to the ration of cattle. The graph suggests that the fluoride was less available to the cattle in the latter experiment, or that a greater proportion was stored in the skeleton, or both. The relationship indicated in Fig. 15 suggests that urinary concentrations of F should prove useful in estimating the amount of fluoride ingested. Indeed, many workers have considered urinary excretion as such an indicator. However, the use of such data for this purpose is subject to several limitations, as has been pointed out by SHUPE et al. (1963b), SUTTIE et al. (1957) and HOBBS et al. (1954). Several other factors in addition to current intake influence urinary excretion of F, *e.g.* past exposures, length of time on a given ration, present age and age when started on the ration in question. Some of these factors are to be commented upon shortly.

A close correspondence between the concentrations of F in drinking water and in urine has been noted for man by a number of investigators. MCCLURE and KINSER (1944) found a nearly 1:1 ratio over the range 1–4 ppm F in the water supply. This relationship has been confirmed by others, for example by SMITH et al. (1950), YUDKIN et al. (1954) and LARGENT (1961). However, the less soluble forms of fluoride are excreted via the urine to a lesser extent than are soluble fluorides. MCCLURE et al. (1945) found smaller percentages of fluoride in the urine of human subjects when F was ingested in the form of bone meal or as solid CaF_2, than when NaF or F-containing drinking water was ingested.

WEDDLE and MUHLER (1957) found the percentage of fluoride appearing in urine of rats to be quite similar regardless of whether NaF, Na_2SiF_6 or SnF_2 was administered in the drinking water.

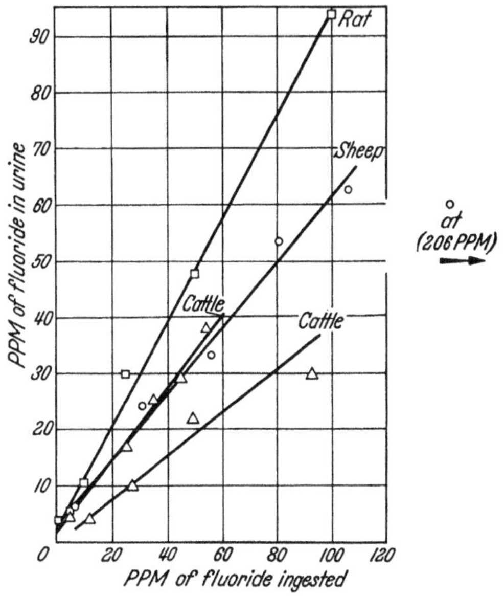

Fig. 15. Relation between fluoride ingested and fluoride excreted in the urine by different species. Rats received fluoride in drinking water; the other species ingested fluoride in the food

3. Physiological factors

Factors such as pregnancy and growth are recognized as influencing the urinary excretion of F.

GEDALIA et al. (1959) and BERCOVICI et al. (1960) have demonstrated that urinary F is decreased in pregnant women from the fifth to the eighth month, and that normal levels are not achieved again until several months post delivery. However in the rat, pregnancy did not affect urinary excretion of F (BRZEZINSKI et al., 1962).

According to GDALIA (1958), adults using a water supply containing 0.5 to 0.6 ppm F excreted 0.52 ppm F in their urine whereas children 4–6 years old and using the same water excreted 0.27 ppm F and young children 1–3 years of age excreted 0.14 ppm F. ZIPKIN et al. (1956) have also reported data showing the effect of skeletal age on the urinary excretion of F. In their study urines were collected periodically from adults and children during the approximately 3.5 years immediately following fluoridation of the water supply to a level of 1 ppm F. Urines of the adults reached a concentration of 1 ppm six weeks after fluoridation was started, whereas children 5—14 years of age required nearly three years to reach this concentration. Prior to fluoridation the water supply contained 0.2 to 0.3 ppm F. Growing rats maintained on diets containing a constant concentration of added fluoride excreted less fluoride initially than was the case after 30 weeks (LAWRENZ et al., 1940). Evidently, the younger individual, be he man or rat, has more skeletal sites available for fluoride deposition; consequently more is deposited in the bone and less is available for urinary excretion.

4. Extent of skeletal saturation

When the fluoride intake remains reasonably constant over a prolonged period of time, concentrations of fluoride in the skeleton of adult individuals or animals tends to approach a maximal or "plateau" concentration for the given level of intake. Thereafter skeletal concentrations tend to remain constant and urinary excretion accounts for all or nearly all of the daily intake of fluoride. When intake is increased above the previously established level, a portion of this increased intake is taken up by the bone, and only the remainder is left for removal in the urine, *i.e.* something less than 100 % of the increment is excreted in the urine. With time, the skeleton approaches a new level of "saturation" and again urinary excretion accounts for practically all of the ingested fluoride. In the case of children or young animals the situation is similar except that a longer time is required for the skeleton to reach a new level of relative saturation because of the greater capacity of the young skeleton to store fluoride.

Data are available from several sources to support this concept. For example, LARGENT (1961) has presented information relating to fluoride balance in a group of adult individuals who were long-term residents of communities whose water

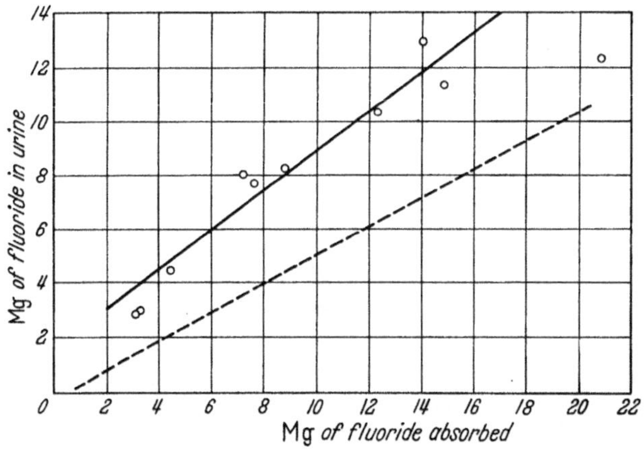

Fig. 16. Relation between fluoride absorbed and fluoride excreted in the urine by man. Fluoride ingested in the food. Data of LARGENT (1961) and MACHLE and LARGENT (1943)

supplies contained 2—20 ppm F. From the data pertaining to fluoride intake and excretion one may calculate the F absorbed, and in Fig. 16 the absorbed fluoride has been plotted against the corresponding urinary excretion of F. It is evident from the upper line shown in the figure, which represents data from the long-term residents in a steady state with respect to fluoride intake and excretion, that the ratio of fluoride excreted to that absorbed is approximately 0.98. The lower line of Fig. 16 is from data of MACHLE and LARGENT (1943). Here, an individual previously in fluoride balance increased his daily intake of F to a new level for a period of several weeks, several different levels of increased intake being employed. The amount excreted is seen to increase as the F absorbed is increased, but it is evident that the fraction excreted is not as great as the skeletal system attempts to achieve a new and higher steady state. The ratio of excreted to absorbed F is approximately 0.5.

The data of ZIPKIN et al. (1956) referred to just previously also illustrate the decrease in urinary excretion of F while the skeleton is adjusting to a new steady state.

SMITH et al. (1963b) have demonstrated the change in urinary excretion with approaching steady state, in rats. In this experiment rats were given drinking water containing 1–100 ppm F from weaning to age 12 months, or for approximately half the life span of this species. Fluoride balance data were obtained at three, six and twelve months, from which Fig. 17 was constructed. The ratio of fluoride excreted to fluoride absorbed is 0.36, 0.45 and 0.59 at 3,6 and 12 months, respectively. With increasing time then, the skeletons approached more nearly to the steady state commensurate with fluoride intake, and the fraction of absorbed fluoride excreted in the urine increased correspondingly.

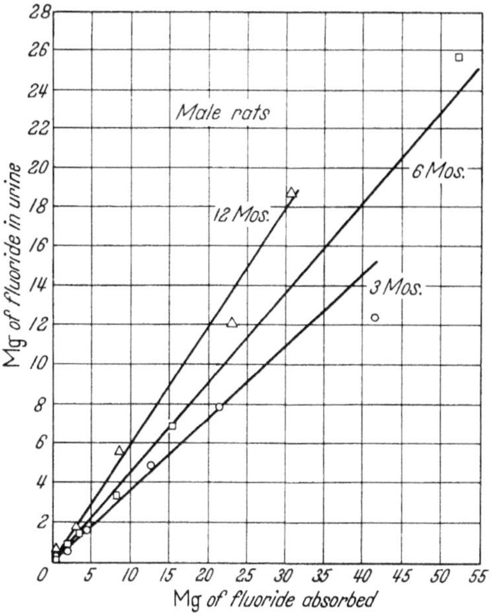

Fig. 17. Relation between fluoride absorbed and fluoride excreted in the urine of rats. Fluoride ingested in the drinking water. Data of SMITH et al. (1963b)

5. Renal clearance of fluoride

The promptness with which ingested fluoride appears in the urine suggests that perhaps a special mechanism may be present in the kidney to deal with fluoride. Measurements of the renal clearance of F in man and in the dog indicate that such an assumption is unnecessary. Such studies have been reported for the dog by CHEN et al. (1956) using stable fluoride and chemical analyses, and for the dog and man by CARLSON et al. (1960a, d) using F^{18}. In every instance the clearance of F never exceeded that of creatinine, and always exceeded that of Cl. CARLSON et al. (1960a) found that in man 51–63 % of the F appearing in the glomerular filtrate was resorbed in the tubules, and in the dog 23–78 % was resorbed. Using the less sensitive chemical analysis, CHEN et al. (1956) reported that tubular resorption was approximately 91–98 % (mean, 92 %) of that filtered. Mannitol diuresis and diuresis induced with hypertonic sodium chloride solution or chlorothiazide all increased the clearance of fluoride in the dog (CHEN et al., 1956; CARLSON et al., 1960d). The clearance of F^{18} in man under normal conditions was found to be approximately half that of creatinine and at least 45 times, often several hundred times, greater than that of chloride. Renal concentration ratios for F^{18} in man and in the dog were 7.8–118 and 3.4–14.5, respectively (CARLSON et al., 1960a, d). The kidney is evidently an efficient organ for the rapid removal of F from the blood.

The available evidence thus indicates that the kidney handles fluoride by means of glomerular filtration, with a variable amount of tubular resorption (Carlson et al., 1960d). Resorption is less efficient than that for chloride, and is inversely related to the urine flow, suggesting that possibly the fluoride ion is handled as is water, because of its extensive hydration (Carlson et al., 1960d). The kidney appears to discriminate between F and Cl, as evidenced by the fact that the clearance of F exceeds that of Cl, and that the former is concentrated in urine far more effectively than is Cl.

Data of Carlson et al. (1960a) describing the renal clearance of F^{18} in man are reproduced in Table 31.

Table 31. *Renal clearance of F^{18} in man* (Data of Carlson et al., 1960a)

Subject and wt.	ratio $\frac{F^{18}\text{ urine}}{F^{18}\text{ plasma}}$	urine flow, ml/min	$C_{F^{18}}$, ml/min	ratio $\frac{C_{F^{18}}}{C_{Cl}}$	ratio $\frac{C_{F^{18}}}{C_{creat.}}$	Tubular resorption of F^{18}, %
W.D.A., 80 kg	43.8	1.2	51	104	0.40	60
	46.2	1.4	65	112	0.39	61
	25.8	1.8	46	65	0.52	48
	35.8	1.9	68	106	0.40	60
	31.2	2.4	76	109	0.49	51
	37.5	3.3	125	93	0.47	53
	23.0	3.4	77	56	0.41	59
	14.7	4.9	71	45	0.41	59
	16.5	6.0	99	51	0.50	50
	19.4	6.9	133	61	0.40	60
	12.0	8.8	106	57	0.70	30
	11.8	11.0	129	69	0.68	32
	12.8	11.0	140	45	0.59	41
C.H.C., 74 kg	118.3	0.42	50	276	0.43	57
	111.0	0.57	63	176	0.43	57
	28.5	1.4	40	111	0.21	79
	29.4	1.5	44	102	0.31	69
	18.6	2.7	50	98	0.35	65
	14.4	2.7	38	98	0.33	67
	20.2	2.8	56	88	0.39	61
	15.8	3.1	49	126	0.29	71
	18.7	3.4	64	85	0.42	58
	15.0	3.8	57	58	0.42	58
	13.0	4.0	52	108	0.29	71
	16.0	4.2	67	97	0.36	64
	13.3	6.2	82	82	0.41	59
	11.1	6.9	77	171	0.28	72
	8.6	7.9	67	749	0.35	65
	7.3	8.2	60	142	0.35	65
	10.2	10.2	104	868	0.43	57
	8.2	10.4	85	947	0.53	47
	7.8	10.5	82	748	0.44	56
	8.6	11.7	101	1119	0.45	55

Clearance periods are arranged in order of increasing urine flow rates.

B. Fecal excretion

Fluoride excreted in the feces represents almost entirely that portion of ingested fluoride not absorbed from the gastrointestinal tract. Since nearly all soluble, or "available" fluoride does enter the systemic circulation, F appearing in feces must therefore represent that which was initially unavailable, or rendered so by virtue of combination with other components of the ingesta, *e.g.* calcium.

1. Man

Machle et al. (1942) and Largent and Heyroth (1949), in studies on the same human subject, estimated the fecal excretion of fluoride to range from 5 to 30 % of that ingested with an average value of 10.3 %. In one instance (not included in calculating the average) fecal excretion was 62.5 % of that ingested. Balance periods in these studies were 1–20 weeks in duration, and the F intake was that present in a normal, unselected diet. Ham and Smith (1954b) found three young women ingesting normal diets to excrete 12–35 % of the F in the feces, and when intake was approximately doubled by the inclusion of tea in the diet, fecal excretion was 12–21 % and the percentage excreted in the urine was increased. McClure et al. (1945) also found approximately 33 % of normally ingested F to be excreted in the feces by man.

Table 32. *Metabolic fluoride balance of subject E.L. during periods of elevated intake* (modified from Largent, 1961)

Source of added F	Av. F ingested mg/day	Per cent excreted		Per cent retained
		feces	urine	
NaF soln.	6.47	2.9	37	60
	12.40	3.6	51	45
	19.40	3.7	50	46
CaF_2 soln.	6.25	4.3	35	61
CaF_2 solid	6.43	38	28	34
Bone meal	6.31	63	17	20
Cryolite soln.	25.40	6.9	59	34
Cryolite solid	6.61	23	40	37
	18.40	30	38	32
	36.40	34	36	30
	12.40	32	44	24
	6.41	38	41	21
$NaBF_4$ solid	6.40	1.6	100	0

Physiological availability of fluoride in the ingesta must necessarily affect the proportion excreted in feces. The numerous metabolic studies of Largent and his colleagues have included a number of instances where fluoride was fed as CaF_2, cyrolite, bone meal or sodium fluoborate as a part of diets normally containing 0.39–0.48 mg/day. Certain of their balance data are summarized in Table 32. It is apparent from these data that when fluoride is ingested in solution, whether as NaF, CaF_2 or cryolite, very little appears in the feces. However, when added to the diet in solid form, fecal excretion of F is increased approximately ten-fold, viz. from 2.9–6.9 % to 23–63 % and the percentage retained in the body decreases correspondingly. The quantity of F ingested seems to have little or no effect on the percentage excreted in the feces, regardless of whether it is given in solid or solution form. In these instances it is interesting to note that the entire dose of sodium fluoborate was recovered unchanged in the urine; this compound does not yield the F ion *in vivo*.

McClure et al. (1945) have also investigated the fluoride balance in persons ingesting CaF_2, cryolite and bone meal. They found CaF_2 administered in water to be excreted via the feces to the extent of 15.8–19.6 %, whereas in food the corresponding range was 26.7–36.2. Fecal excretion of F from cryolite and bone meal fed in solid form was 32–56 %. The supplemental fluoride in these studies was generally 3 mg per day, considerably less than was employed by Largent.

In a later series Largent (1961) estimated the fluoride balance in ten subjects whose water supplies contained 2–20 ppm F; these data are summarized in Table 33. Under these conditions of long established residency (8–48 years) fecal excretion accounted for 5–12 % of the fluoride ingested. Eight of the ten subjects were in positive fluoride balance, and again the level of fluoride ingested does not appear to be related to the percentage excreted in feces. For these subjects, most of the total daily fluoride was in solution in the water supply, thereby ensuring its availability; this is reflected in the fact that urinary excretion ranged from 55 to 94 %.

Table 33. *Metabolic fluoride balance in ten human subjects using water supplies containing 2—20 ppm fluoride* (modified from LARGENT, 1961)

Subject	ppm F in water	Fluoride intake, mg/day			Per cent excreted			Per cent retained
		fluid	food	total	feces	urine	total	
L. L.	2.0	2.42	1.17	3.59	10.0	80.0	90.0	10.0
E. Lo.	2.0	2.55	0.94	3.49	5.4	82.5	87.9	12.1
McM.	5.5	8.14	1.35	9.49	7.0	88.0	95.0	5.0
M. W.	5.5	3.81	1.32	5.13	12.3	87.5	99.8	0.2
B. Le.	6.1	6.74	1.02	7.76	5.7	104	109.7	—9.7
T. B.	6.1	6.34	1.98	8.32	7.1	93.5	100.6	—0.6
A. G.	8.0	12.4	3.13	15.5	8.8	83.0	91.8	8.2
R. G.	8.0	11.3	2.47	13.8	10.3	75.2	85.5	14.5
L. H.	20.0	20.8	1.48	22.3	6.2	55.0	61.2	38.8
W.H.	20.0	15.6	1.16	16.8	11.2	67.6	78.8	21.2

2. Animal studies

Fluoride balance data in experimental animals, as reported in or derived from selected published papers, are listed in Table 34. It is apparent from these data that generally when fluoride is ingested in solution form, the proportion excreted in the urine exceeds that in the feces by factors of two to four, though occasionally urinary excretion may be 10—20 times greater. When F is ingested in food, fecal excretion may be the greater by a factor of 2—10, but at times the proportion may be nearly equal or even slightly in favor of urine. While several species are represented in Table 34, there are not sufficient examples available to demonstrate conclusively whether or not there are species differences in the excretory pattern. Adding Ca to the diet did not significantly alter the proportions excreted in feces and urine by sheep (HARVEY, 1952), but WEDDLE and MUHLER (1957) increased fecal excretion 7-fold by adding Ca to the fluoride-containing solution ingested by rats. SUTTIE et al. (1957) found fecal excretion of F to be increased by the concurrent addition of calcium to the ration, and HOBBS et al. (1954) described the increase in fecal F brought about in cattle and in sheep by the addition of aluminum salts to the diet. SHUPE et al. (1962) compared fluoride retention in cattle given NaF and CaF_2 in the diet and found retention of the former compound to be appreciably greater than that of the latter (184 vs. 21 mg per day).

C. Perspiration

The role of sweat in affecting fluoride balance has received some attention. MACHLE et al. (1942) reported that at normal levels of fluoride intake, sweat contained too little F to permit its determination whereas at levels of "high fluoride intake" sweat contained 0.066—0.514 ppm F. Shortly thereafter, MCCLURE et al. (1945) carried out a series of balance studies in young men maintained for eight hours out of the 24 in "comfortable" or in "hot-moist" conditions, and included analyses of the perspiration collected during the 8-hour intervals. The subjects ingested 3 mg F daily in the food. During the "hot-moist" periods appreciable quantities of a dilute sweat were obtained, which contained 0.28—0.34 ppm F. In "comfortable" periods up to 1 kg of insensible perspiration containing 0.85

Table 34. *Metabolic fate of fluoride in different species*

Species	Source	Ingested F mg/day	Per cent F excreted in feces	Per cent F excreted in urine	Per cent F excreted in total	Fluoride balance‘ %	Duration of experiment	Reference
Calf	normal food	288	68.0	7.9	75.9	+24.1	300 da.; initial wts., 110—190 lbs.	MARIAKULANDAI and VENKATARAMAIAH (1955)
	NaF, soln.	491	27.6—32.5	12.4—13.2	40.8—44.9	+55.1—59.2		
	NaF, soln.	528—540	41.4—45.2	6.1—8.9	50.3—51.3	48.7—49.7	as above; diet cont'd. added bone meal	
Guinea pig	NaF, oral	152[1]	12.3	18.9	31.2	+68.8	5 wks.; initial wts. 200—300 g	VENKATESWARLUa nd NARAYANARAO (1957a)
Hamster	NaF, soln.	0.086—0.122[1]	9.0—19.8	11.5—16.3	20.5—36.1	+63.9—79.5	old females; 10 day balance trial	LOVELACE et al. (1959)
		0.084—0.085[1]	9.4—14.3	7.1—8.3	16.5—22.6	+77.4—83.5	old males; as above	
		0.784—0.823[1]	2.4—3.1	3.6—4.6	6.0—7.7	+92.3—94.0	old females; as above	
		0.676—0.679[1]	3.5—3.8	4.3—5.2	8.1—8.7	+91.3—91.9	old males; as above	
Rabbit	NaF, soln.	65—80[1]	51—42	10—22	53—73	+27—47	19 days; males, initial wt., 2.9—3.8 kg	GARDNER et al. (1957)
		110—180[1]	34—44	12—18	53—56	+44—47		
		335—350[1]	28—32	10—17	44—49	+51—56	as above	
		455—565[1]	29—32	12—17	44—47	+53—56	as above	
		580—810[1]	32—27	7—16	34—48	+52—66	as above	
Rabbit	normal food	0.6	44.0	28.5	72.5	+27.5	40 days; young adults	SMITH et al. (1955)
Rat	rock phosphate food	217.2[1]	59.6	14.5	74.1	+25.9	11 da.; males, initial wt. 125 g	KICK et al. (1935)
		213.6[1]	62.2	9.6	71.8	+28.2	10 da.; as above	
	Na_2SiF_6, food	269.9[1]	34.9	34.6	69.5	+30.5	23 da.; as above	
	Na_2SiF_6, food	269.9[1]	34.9	33.3	68.2	+31.8	22 da.; as above	
	NaF, food	211.2[1]	55.0	12.2	67.2	+32.8	18 da.; as above	
	CaF_2, food	229.6[1]	98.0	1.8	99.8	+0.2	11 da.; as above	
Rat	cryolite, food	0.879[1]	27.0	37.5	64.5	+35.5	19—20 wks.; females, initial wt. 80—90 g	LAWRENZ et al. (1939b)
		1.170[1]	29.8	35.8	65.6	+34.4	as above; males	
	cryolite soln.	0.900[1]	19.1	34.7	53.8	+46.2	as above; females	
		1.170[1]	18.4	40.0	58.4	+41.6	as above; males	

Table 34. (Continued)

Species	Source	Ingested F mg/day	Per cent F excreted in feces	urine	total	Fluoride balance, %	Duration of experiment	Reference
Rat	NaF, soln.	0.29[2]	38	76	114	−14	12 mos.; males initially weanlings	SMITH et al. (1963b)
		0.74[2]	22	64	86	+14		
		3.09[2]	25	41	66	+34		
		8.88[2]	25	47	72	+28		
		23.17[2]	19	42	61	+39		
		30.73[2]	31	43	74	+26		
Rat	NaF, soln.	0.5	2.2	23.5	25.7	+74.3	4 days; weanlings	STOOKEY and MUHLER (1962)
		0.5	12.4	58.3	70.7	+29.3	100 days; initially weanlings	
		0.5	1.2—2.3	23.8—27.8	25.7—29.0	71.0—74.3	4 da.; weanlings. Mo. added to diet	
		0.5	7.2—11.4	51.8—59.1	59.4—69.7	30.3—40.6	100 da.; initially weanlings; Mo added to diet	
Rat	NaF, soln.	0.13[3]	54	15.4	69.4	+30.6	3 mos, males, initially weanlings	TAYLOR et al. (1961)
		0.64[3]	33	29.7	62.7	+37.3		
		2.45[3]	24	25.7	49.7	+50.3	as above	
		5.36[3]	18	30.3	48.3	+51.7	as above	
		14.50[3]	13	33.7	46.7	+53.3	as above	
		23.92[3]	11	33.8	44.8	+55.2	as above	
		47.36[3]	12	26.2	38.2	+61.8	as above	
Rat	NaF, soln.	0.9	2.0	42.3	44.3	+55.7	20 wks.; initial age 5—6 wks.	WADHWANI (1953)
		0.9	1.8	51.8	53.6	+46.4	3 wks.; initial age 5—6 wks.	
Rat	NaF, soln.	1.26[1]	10.3	47.8	58.1	+41.9	40 da.; initial age 30 da.	WEDDLE and MUHLER (1957)
	Na_2SiF_6, soln.	1.28[1]	10.9	43.6	54.5	+45.5	as above	
	SnF_2, soln.	1.27[1]	9.5	37.8	47.3	+52.7	as above	
	NaF, soln.	—	10.5	26.6	37.1	+62.9	14 da.; no Ca present in soln.	
	NaF, soln.	—	75.2	6.4	81.6	+18.4	as above; $CaCl_2$ included in soln.	
Rat	NaF, food	0.597[1]	36.2	31.2	67.4	+32.6	80 da.; initial age, 28 days Male	WEDDLE and MUHLER (1955)

Table 34. (Continued)

Species	Source	Ingested mg/day	Per cent F excreted in feces	urine	total	Fluoride balance, %	Duration of experiment	Reference
	NaF, soln.	0.443[1]	36.3	26.6	62.9	+37.1	as above; female	
		11.927[1]	8.9	27.4	36.3	+63.7	as above; male	
		8.756[1]	14.9	29.3	44.2	+55.8	as above; female	
Sheep	NaF, soln.	4.7—9.1	3.8—23.0	18.7—34.0	22.5—57.0	43.0—77.5	1 yr.; initial age 4 mo. Oat or lucerne ration	Harvey (1952)
		4.3—12.0	3.6—10.2	15.4—25.8	19.2—35.4	64.6—80.8	as above; Ca included in ration	
Sheep	NaF, food	3.6	39.0	16.6	55.6	+44.4	140 da.; lambs, initial age 8—12 mo.	Hobbs et al. (1954)
		6.1	37.6	62.2	99.8	+ 0.2	as above	
		27.4	13.1	33.0	46.1	+53.9	as above	
		40.6	14.5	25.7	40.2	+59.8	as above	
		74.9	7.8	15.8	23.6	+76.4	as above	
		86.1	8.8	25.7	34.5	+65.5	as above	
		107.4	10.6	17.3	27.9	+72.1	as above	

[1] Total intake of F during period of the balance trial.
[2] Total ingested by 3 rats in 5—7 days.
[3] Total ingested by 3 rats in 7 days.

to 1.38 ppm was produced each 8 hours. The proportions of absorbed F excreted via sweat and urine were found to vary according to environmental conditions. During "comfortable" periods perspiration accounted for 24 %, but during "hotmoist" periods sweat accounted for 44 %. Corresponding figures for the excretion in urine were 77 and 49 %, respectively.

Crosby and Shepherd (1957) investigated the role of perspiration in the excretion of F in two subjects taking 3 mg F orally in solution. Their male subject showed an increase in total F excreted (urine plus sweat) when sweating was induced, but in the female subject sweating was without effect on the total F excreted. Sweat of the male subject ingesting F contained 0.93–1.14 ppm F, while the concentration was not significantly increased in the female's perspiration. Also, renal excretion of F was decreased in the female during sweating but not in the male. Crosby and Shephard (loc. cit.) concluded that up to 50 % of the total F excreted may appear in the sweat.

Largent (1961) has also called attention to variations among individuals with respect to the efficacy of perspiring in removing fluoride. In his experience with three subjects, sweat from one was found to contain no F, while F was present in the sweat from two others, but in only one of these was the amount increased by the ingestion of additional fluoride.

In summary, while the evidence is somewhat limited,

it does suggest that in warm climates or in hot summer months perspiration can account for the removal of appreciable fractions of the excreted fluoride. It should be pointed out that a minimal excretion of F via this route in some individuals does not constitute a hazard in the use of fluoridated water, inasmuch as in current fluoridation practices the concentration of F in the water is decreased under these environmental conditions.

VI. Fluoride and disease states

Occasionally the question has been considered of whether or not the metabolism of fluoride might be affected by the presence of disease. Greatest interest has been shown in those conditions which could be expected to alter the intake of fluoride and/or the ability of the host to excrete F.

A. Diabetes

Wagner and Muhler (1959b) induced diabetes in rats by the injection of alloxan, and supplied them thereafter with drinking water containing 1 ppm F. After 40 days the animals were sacrificed and the total carcass F determined and compared with the measured fluoride intake. A tendency toward lower retention was evident in the diabetic animals, but the difference was not significant. Wagner and Muhler (loc. cit.) suggest that retention and excretion are not affected in the alloxan-diabetic rat.

Sweeney et al. (1962) carried out a somewhat similar experiment, wherein alloxan-diabetic rats were given drinking water containing 1, 5 or 20 ppm F for 70 or 117 days. Femur concentrations of fluoride increased with increasing concentrations in the water supplies in both the normal and diabetic rats. As would be expected, water consumption was greater in the diabetic animals, relative to their controls, by a factor of 3–5. Femoral concentrations of F increased as well, but only 2–3 times over their controls, suggesting that the excretion of F in the diabetic animals had been enhanced. These results are not necessarily at variance with those just described, inasmuch as Wagner and Muhler (loc. cit.) refer to total (carcass) fluoride whereas Sweeney et al. refer to femur concentrations and sufficient data are not reported to determine the extent, if any, to which growth and femur weight might have been impaired. Evidently, a definitive experiment in this area has yet to be done.

Largent (1961) has reported balance data in one human patient diagnosed as having diabetes mellitus, intercapillary glomerulosclerosis, and hypertension. Under conditions of normal F intake this individual retained little or no F but when intake was increased by the ingestion of 2 mg F with each meal, 81.5 % of the fluoride was retained, indicating a decreased excretion of F.

B. Impaired kidney function

In view of the fact that renal excretion is a very important pathway for the removal of F from the body, considerable concern has been expressed as to whether or not the individual with damaged kidneys can successfully cope with ingested fluoride. Laboratory investigations of the problem are surprisingly few however, and usually less comprehensive than one might desire.

Yudkin et al. (1954), in a brief note, listed the results of the analyses of bloods and urines from normal subjects and nephritic patients living in an area whose water supply contained 1 ppm F, and compared these with samples from an area where the water contained 0.1 ppm F. Their data are summarized below; the numbers in parentheses refer to the number of subjects. The differences between normals and nephritis in either area, as judged by these small numbers of samples, probably are not significant. The blood F concentrations listed here are appreciably greater than would be expected on the basis of SINGER and ARMSTRONG's work (1960); however, this need not affect comparisons among the samples analyzed by YUDKIN et al., inasmuch as these were all analyzed by the same method.

Area A		Area B	
Water supply	1 ppm F	Water supply	0.1 ppm F
Normal blood (42)	1.36 ppm	Normal blood (11)	0.78 ppm
Normal urine (33)	1.02 ppm	Normal urine (10)	0.30 ppm
Nephritic blood (9)	1.70 ppm	Nephritic blood (11)	0.77 ppm
Nephritic urine (8)	0.64 ppm	Nephritic urine (10)	0.32 ppm

In a somewhat similar, small-scale study SMITH et al. (1955) measured the urinary excretion of fluoride in a series of 12 elderly normal subjects and nine nephritics when their community water supply contained approximately 0.06 ppm F, and again after the water supply had been fluoridated to a concentration of 1 ppm. In this limited series also, there were no significant differences in urinary fluoride concentrations of the normal and nephritic subjects, either before or after the addition of fluoride to the drinking water, though concentrations in both groups were increased after fluoridation.

LARGENT (1961) carried out a fluoride balance study in a patient with arteriosclerotic heart disease with mild decompensation, cardiac enlargement, essential hypertension and subnormal renal function. This subject retained 25.6 % of his normal daily intake of F; when 2 mg of F were ingested with each meal, the retention increased to 76 %. Reference has already been made to LARGENT's other subject (loc. cit.) with intercapillary glomerulosclerosis, for whom the corresponding retentions were 0 and 81.5 %.

CARLSON et al. (1960b) investigated the effect of complete nephrectomy on the tissue distribution of F^{18} in the rat. In this study F^{18} was injected after completion of the nephrectomy, and the animals were then sacrificed 80 min later. Tissue concentrations of F^{18} increased in all of the organs analyzed but not disproportionately so with respect to the increased plasma level of F^{18}; the general pattern of distribution among the various organs was unaffected. Much of that F^{18} in the nephrectomized rat which normally would have been excreted, appeared in the bone.

Unpublished data of SMITH and GARDNER (1963) showed F balance not to be significantly altered in rabbits during a two-month period following surgical removal of one kidney. Their limited data are summarized below.

	Control	Per cent of ingested F retained — Nephrectomized: normal F intake	Per cent of ingested F retained — Nephrectomized: increased F intake[1]
Range	29.4—58.9	17.9—55.4	38.0—57.8
Mean	41.6	36.6	49.0

[1] Drinking water contained 15 or 30 ppm F.

Acute renal tubular injury was induced in the rabbit by administration of uranyl nitrate and the effect noted on fluoride balance (SMITH et al., 1955). While total fluoride intake was decreased during the ten-day period of injury and repair, owing to reduced intake of food and water, the percentage of fluoride retained during this period did not differ significantly from that found prior to and after the period of injury and recovery, nor did the fraction excreted in the urine change significantly.

The renal clearance studies of CARLSON et al. (1959) have demonstrated that when urine volume is increased, tubular resorption of F decreases, indicating that diuresis enhances fluoride excretion. Renal impairment associated with tubular injury and concomitant reduction in the resorption of water would therefore be expected to increase the urinary excretion of F.

STOOKEY et al. (1963) have suggested that when the ability of the kidney to remove fluoride is impaired, fluoride concentrations in the circulating fluids are increased and the body responds to this signal by absorbing less F from the gastrointestinal tract into the circulation.

C. Vitamin deficiencies and vitamin utilization

The somewhat conflicting picture with respect to the metabolism of F in vitamin C deficiency has been commented upon earlier. MUHLER's data (1958) suggest that fluoride retention is minimal in the scorbutic guinea pig, whereas VENKATESWARLU and NARAYANA RAO (1954) found skeletal storage of F to be comparable in guinea pigs on diets deficient or adequate in vitamin C. Finally, PANDIT and RAO (1940), and WADHWANI (1952, 1955) have indicated that fluoride is more toxic in vitamin C-deficient monkeys than in animals receiving adequate levels of this vitamin. Clearly, further work on the effect of this nutritional deficiency on fluoride metabolism is indicated. Considerable clarification of the problem would be forthcoming if future experiments were designed to include measurements of fluoride intake and excretion, *i.e.* balance, and confirmatory bone analyses for F, in animals maintained on a scorbutic diet with and without supplemental vitamin C.

Fluoride deposition in vitamin D deficiency was investigated by KEMPF and NELSON (1941). In this limited study the percentage of fluoride in the tibia of rachitic rats was increased to a greater extent when the diet was supplemented with vitamin D plus fluoride than when F alone was given; the increase was proportional to the increase in ash content. ZIPKIN et al. (1959) also found fluoride deposited in the femur of rachitic rats given F in the water supply to be proportional to the ash content. In this instance the rats were rendered rachitic by means of a diet deficient in phosphorus but adequate in vitamins A and D and calcium.

From another point of view, one might enquire whether or not the metabolism of fluoride is affected by the presence of vitamins, for example as ingested in daily supplements, and also whether or not fluoride might affect the utilization of ingested vitamins. With regard to the first question, HENNON et al. (1964) fed rats 1 mg F daily with and without various commercial multivitamin preparations, and found these to be without effect on the fluoride excretion pattern or on carcass or femoral storage of F. As regards the second question, weight gains and food efficency values in rats receiving daily supplements of thiamine, riboflavin, pantothenic acid, pyridoxine and vitamin A did not differ from those seen in rats receiving the vitamin supplement plus 0.5 or 1.0 mg F per day (HARKINS et al., 1963).

D. Miscellaneous

SINGER and ARMSTRONG (1960) found the average concentration of F in plasma of 30 hospital patients to be 0.16 ppm ± 0.0095 (std. error); included were data on patients diagnosed as suffering from carcinoma, heart disease, infections, kidney diseases, and metabolic diseases. Plasma of normal subjects residing in the same community contained 0.15 ppm F ± 0.0044 (std. error).

VII. Essentiality of fluoride

Several studies have attempted to answer directly the question of whether fluoride is essential. These, together with data bearing on the question from other studies, have been reviewed in detail in several recent volumes (Hodge and Smith, in press; Underwood, 1962; Muhler, 1959) and need not be treated exhaustively here. Suffice it to say that unequivocal evidence that fluoride is required for growth, reproduction, or skeletal development, has not yet been forthcoming. Unquestionably, fluoride does improve dental health and in its absence this condition is impaired; however, the animal does not die in the absence of this optimal dentition. On the basis of present knowledge, fluoride is classed as essential by Muhler (loc. cit.) and as probably essential by Underwood (loc. cit.).

VIII. Fluoride in the treatment of disease

The use of fluorides to lower the incidence of dental caries is perhaps the best known prophylactic and therapeutic use of these compounds. Inasmuch as this has been discussed in detail by Brudevold in Chapter 4 nothing further need be said here.

A. Demineralizing diseases

The well-known effect of excess fluoride in inducing osteosclerotic changes in bone seems to have suggested to several investigators the possibility of using fluoride in the treatment of bone disease characterized by a reduction in the skeletal mass or by increased rates of bone resorption, or both. Oral doses of sodium fluoride have been used in the treatment of Paget's disease, postmenopausal osteoporosis, urticaria pigmentosa with osteoporosis, and idiopathic osteoporosis. Improvements seen included a decrease in urinary loss of Ca, increased retention of Ca, increased mineralization, increased rate of bone accretion, and a decrease in bone pain (Rich and Ensinck, 1961; Purves, 1962; Bernstein et al., 1963). Doses have ranged from 20 to 200 mg of NaF per day, and treatment has been continued for periods up to one year.

B. Bone fractures

Tam (1950) found fluoride administered in drinking water to have no effect on the healing of fractures of the fibulae in young rats, and Odell and Key (1953) could not detect any interference of water born fluoride (ca 100 ppm) on the healing of fractures of the humerus of rats.

C. Magnesium deficiency

Bunce et al. (1962) and Chiemchaisri and Phillips (1963) have reported that feeding 200–250 ppm F prevented the gross aortic lesions and soft tissue calcification customarily seen in dogs fed a Mg-deficient diet.

D. Cancer

Black and Kleiner (1947) and Black et al. (1947, 1949) have investigated sodium fluoride as one of a number of glycolytic enzyme inhibitors tested in cancer therapy. Results were not encouraging.

IX. References

AGATE, J. N., G. H. BELL, G. F. BODDIE, R. G. BOWLER, M. BUCKELL, E. A. CHEESEMAN, T. H. J. DOUGLAS, H. A. DRUETT, J. GARRAD, D. HUNTER, K. M. A. PERRY, J. D. RICHARDSON, and J. B. DE V. WEIR: Industrial fluorosis. A study of the hazard to man and animals near Fort William, Scotland. Memor. med. Res. Coun. (Lond.) **22**, 131 (1949).

ANBAR, M., and N. ERNST: A distribution study of F^{18}-labelled cationic fluorocomplexes in rats. Int. J. appl. Radiat. **13**, 47—51 (1962).

— S. GUTTMANN, and Z. LEWITUS: The accumulation of fluoroborate ions in thyroid glands of rats. Endocrinolgy **66**, 888—890 (1960).

— — — Effect of monofluorosulphonate, difluorophosphate and fluoroborate ions on the iodine uptake of the thyroid gland. Nature (Lond.) **183**, 1517—1518 (1959).

— — N. ERNST, and Z. RAMATI: A comparative study of the penetrability of various ions into the central nervous system of rats. IA-668, Israel Atomic Energy Comm., Rehovoth, Israel, August 1961.

APPELGREN, L. E., Y. ERICSSON, and S. ULLBERG: A comparison of the distribution of radioactive fluorine and calcium by use of double-isotope autoradiography. Acta physiol. scand. **53**, 339—347 (1961).

ARMSTRONG, W. D.: Mechanisms of fluoride homeostasis. Arch. oral Biol. **4**, 156—159 (1961).

— P. VENKATESWARLU, and L. SINGER: Intestinal transport of labeled fluoride, choride, and water. J. dent. Res. **40**, 727 (1961).

ASKENASY, H. M., M. ANBAR, Y. LAOR, Z. LEWITUS, I. Z. KOSARY, and S. GUTTMANN: The localization of intracranial space-occupying lesions by fluoroborate ions labelled with fluorine 18. Amer. J. Roentgenol. **88**, 350—354 (1962).

AUSKAPS, A. M., and J. H. SHAW: Hemoglobin concentration, thyroid weight, and growth rate in rats during minimum fluoride ingestion. J. Nutr. **55**, 611—621 (1955).

BELL, M. C., G. M. MERRIMAN, and D. A. GREENWOOD: Distribution and excretion of F^{18} fluoride in beef cattle. J. Nutr. **73**, 379—385 (1961).

BERCOVICI, B., I. GEDALIA, and A. BRZEZINSKI: Fluorine in human milk. Its relation to urinary fluorine levels. Obstet. and Gynec. **16**, 319—321 (1960).

BERNSTEIN, D. S., C. GURI, P. COHEN, J. J. COLLINS, and S. TAMVAKOPOULOS: The use of sodium fluoride in metabolic bone disease. J. clin. Invest. **42**, 916 (1963).

BIXLER, D., and J. C. MUHLER: Retention of fluoride in soft tissues of chickens receiving different fat diets. J. Nutr. **70**, 26—30 (1960).

— —, and W. G. SHAFER: Experimental dental caries. V. The effect of desalivation and castration on caries and fluorine storage in the rat. J. Nutr. **52**, 345—353 (1954).

BLACK, M. M., and I. S. KLEINER: The effect of inhibitors of intermediary metabolism on advanced human neoplasia. Cancer Res. **7**, 717—718 (1947).

— —, and H. BOLKER: Glycolytic enzyme inhibitor therapy in human malignant neoplasia. Cancer Res. **9**, 314—319 (1949).

— — — Energy mechanism in malignant tumors in relation to chemotherapy. Cancer Res. **7**, 818—826 (1947).

BLAKEMORE, F., T. J. BOSWORTH, and H. H. GREEN: Industrial fluorosis of farm animals in England, attributable to the manufacture of bricks, the calcining of ironstone and to enameling processes. J. comp. path. **58**, 267—301 (1948).

BLAU, M., W. NAGLER, and M. A. BENDER: Fluorine 18: a new isotope for bone scanning. J. nucl. Med. **3**, 332—334 (1962).

BODDIE, G. F.: "Fluorine alleviators." II — Trials involving rats. Vet. Rec. **69**, 48 3— 488 (1957).

BOISSEVAIN, C. H., and W. F. DREA: Spectroscopic determinations of fluorine in bones, both and other organs, in relation to fluorine in drinking water. J. dent. Res. **13**, 495—500 (1933).

BOWLER, R. G., M. BUCKELL, J. GARRAD, A. B. HILL, D. HUNTER, K. M. A. PERRY, and R. S. F. SCHILLING: The risk of fluorosis in magnesium foundries. Brit. J. industr. Med. **4**, 216 to 222 (1947).

BRIGGS, G. M., and P. H. PHILLIPS: Development of fluorine toxicosis in the rabbit. Proc. Soc. exp. Biol. (N. Y.) **80**, 30—33 (1952).

BRUDEVOLD, F., L. T. STEADMAN, and F. A. SMITH: Inorganic and organic components of tooth structure. Ann. N. Y. Acad. Sci. **85**, 110—132 (1960).

— J. W. HEIN, J. F. BONNER, R. B. NEVIN, B. G. BIBBY, and H. C. HODGE: Reaction of tooth surfaces with one ppm of fluoride as sodium fluoride. J. dent. Res. **36**, 771—779 (1957).

BRZEZINSKI, A., B. BERCOVICI, and J. GEDALIA: Fluorine in the human fetus. Obstet. and Gynec. **15**, 329—331 (1960).

— I. GEDALIA, A. DANON, and F. G. SULMAN: Fluoride metabolism in pregnant rats. Proc. Soc. exp. Biol. (N. Y.) **108**, 342—345 (1962).

BUNCE, G. E., Y. CHIEMCHAISRI, and P. H. PHILLIPS: The mineral requirements of the dog. IV. Effect of certain dietary and physiologic factors upon the magnesium deficiency syndrome. J. Nutr. **76**, 23—29 (1962).

BURNS, K. N., and R. ALLCROFT: The use of tail bone biopsy for studying skeletal deposition of fluorine in cattle. Res. Vet. Sci. **3**, 215—218 (1962).

BÜTTNER, G., and J. C. MUHLER: Fluoride placental transfer in the rat. J. dent. Res. **37**, 326—329 (1958b).

BÜTTNER, W.: Action of trace elements on the metabolism of fluoride. J. dent. Res. **42**, Part 2, 453—460 (1963).

—, and J. C. MUHLER: Effects of salivary fluoride on enamel solubility. J. dent. Res. **41**, 617 to 623 (1962).

— — The retention of fluoride by the skeleton, liver, heart and kidney as a function of dietary fat intake in the rat. J. Nutr. **65**, 259—266 (1958a).

— — The effect of fluoride administration on fluoride deposition in tissues and on serum cholesterol in the rat. J. Nutr. **63**, 263—272 (1957).

— S. SCHÜLKE, and S. SOYKA: Toxicity of fluorine-containing dentifrices. In: Caries Symposium Zürich. The present status of caries prevention by fluorine-containing dentifrices, pp. 92 to 100, ed. by H. R. MÜHLEMANN and KLAUS G. KÖNIG, Berne: Hans Huber 1961.

CALL, R. A., and D. A. GREENWOOD: The effect of atmospheric fluorides on man. Progress Rept., Sept. 1, 1957 — Aug. 31, 1958. USPHS Grant S-83, Natl. Inst. Health (1958).

CARLSON, C. H.: Retention, distribution and excretion of radiofluoride. Thesis, Univ. of Minnesota 1959.

— W. D. ARMSTRONG, and L. SINGER: Distribution and excretion of radiofluoride in the human. Proc. Soc. exp. Biol. (N. Y.) **104**, 235—239 (1960a).

— L. SINGER, and W. D. ARMSTRONG: Radiofluoride distribution in tissues of normal and nephrectomized rats. Proc. Soc. exp. Biol. (N. Y.) **103**, 418—420 (1960b).

— W. D. ARMSTRONG, and L. SINGER: Distribution, migration and binding of whole blood fluoride evaluated with radiofluoride. Amer. J. Physiol. **199**, 187—189 (1960c).

— — —, and L. B. HINSHAW: Renal excretion of radiofluoride in the dog. Amer. J. Physiol. **198**, 829—832 (1960d).

CHEN JR., P. S., F. A. SMITH, D. E. GARDNER, J. A. O'BRIEN, and H. C. HODGE: Renal clearance of fluoride. Proc. Soc. exp. Biol. (N. Y.) **92**, 879—883 (1956).

CHIEMCHAISRI, Y., and P. H. PHILLIPS: Effect of dietary fluoride upon the magnesium calcinosis syndrome. J. Nutr. **81**, 307—311 (1963).

CHOLAK, J.: Fluorides: A critical review. I. The occurrence of fluoride in air, food and water. J. occup. Med. **1**, 501—511 (1959).

COLLINGS JR., G. H., R. B. L. FLEMING, and R. MAY: Absorption and excretion of inhaled fluorides. Arch. industr. Hyg. **4**, 585—590 (1951).

COX, G. J.: The fluorine and dental caries problem. J. Amer. dent. Ass. **27**, 1107—1114 (1940).

CROSBY, N. D., and P. A. SHEPHERD: Studies on patterns of fluid intake, water balance and fluoride retention. II. Sweat as a medium for the excretion of fluoride. Med. J. Aust. **44**, 341—346 (1957).

DEEDS, F., and J. O. THOMAS: Comparative chronic toxicities of fluorine compounds. Proc. Soc. exp. Biol. (N. Y.) **31**, 824—825 (1933—1934).

DELLINGER, E.: *In vitro* studies on fluoride absorption. J. dent. Res. **40**, 725 (1961).

DERRYBERRY, O. M., M. D. BARTHOLOMEW, and R. B. L. FLEMING: Fluoride exposure and worker health. The health status of workers in a fertilizer manufacturing plant in relation to fluoride exposure. Arch. environm. Hlth. **6**, 503—514 (1963).

DUCKWORTH, R.: Urinary excretion of fluoride from a dentifrice containing stannous fluoride. J. dent. Res. **42**, 1088—1089 (1963).

DVIR, R., I. GEDALIA, and A. SULITZEANU: Relationship between dental caries activity and the fluoride level and lactobacillus count in saliva. J. dent. Res. **41**, 586—590 (1962).

ENGLE, M. B., N. R. JOSEPH, D. M. LASKIN, and H. R. CATCHPOLE: Binding of anions by connective tissues: dermis and cartilage. Amer. J. Physiol. **201**, 621—627 (1961).

ERICSSON, Y.: Fluorides in dentifrices. Investigations using radioactive fluorine. Acta odont. scand. **19**, 41—77 (1961).

— The state of fluorine in milk and its absorption and retention when administered in milk. Investigations with radioactive fluorine. Acta odont. scand. **16**, 51—77 (1958a).

— The distribution and reactions of fluoride ions in enamel-saliva environment, investigated with the radioactive fluorine isotope F^{18}. Acta odont. scand. **16**, 127—141 (1958b).

—, and CL. MALMNÄS: Placental tranfer of fluorine investigated with F^{18} in man and rabbit. Acta obstet. gynec. scand. **41**, 144—158 (1962).

—, and S. ULLBERG: Autoradiographic investigations of the distribution of F^{18} in mice and rats. Acta odont. scand. **16**, 363—374 (1958).

ERICSSON, Y., G. SANTESSON, and S. ULLBERG: Absorption and metabolism of the PO_3F ion in the animal body. Studies with F^{18}, P^{32}-labelled sodium monofluorophosphate. Arch. oral Biol. **4**, (Special Suppl.) 160—174 (1961).
— S. ULLBERG, and L.-E. APPELGREN: Autoradiographic localization of radioactive fluorine (F^{18}) in developing teeth and bones. Acta odont. scand. **18**, 253—261 (1960).
EVANS, R. J., and P. H. PHILLIPS: The fluorine content of the thyroid gland in caries of hyperthyroidism. J. Amer. med. Ass. **111**, 300—302 (1938).
FELLENBERG, T. VON: Determination of fluorine. Mitt. Lebensmitt. Hyg. **42**, 158—168 (1951).
— The importance of fluorine for the teeth. Mitt. Lebensmitt. Hyg. **39**, 124—182 (1948).
FOSTER, W. C., and J. P. RUSH: Movement of fluoride across the gastric membranes. J. dent. Res. **40**, 294 (1961).
GALLETLI, P.-M., and G. JOYET: Effect of fluorine on thyroidal iodine metabolism in hyperthyroidism. J. clin. Endocr. **18**, 1102—1110 (1958).
GARDNER, D. E., T. G. SCHARFF, F. A. SMITH, and H. C. HODGE: Investigations on the metabolism of fluoride. IV. Fluoride balance studies at high levels of intake in rabbits. J. Nutr. **61**, 207—218 (1957).
— F. A. SMITH, H. C. HODGE, D. E. OVERTON, and R. FELTMAN: The fluoride content of placental tissue as related to the fluoride content of drinking water. Science **115**, 208—209 (1952).
GDALIA, I.: Urinary fluorine levels of children and adults. J. dent. Res. **37**, 601—604 (1958).
—, and J. YARDENI: Fluorine in teeth of Israeli children in relation to fluorine in domestic waters and to dental caries prevalence. J. dent. Res. **36**, 203—207 (1957).
GEDALIA, I., A. BRZEZINSKI, and E. LAZAROV: Placental transfer of fluorine in the human fetus. Proc. Soc. exp. Biol. (N. Y.) **106**, 147—149 (1961a).
— K. A. ROSENZWEIG, and A. SADEH: Fluorine content of superficial enamel layer and its correlation with the fluorine content of saliva, tooth age, and DMFT count. J. dent. Res. **40**, 865—869 (1961b).
— J. YARDENI, and I. GERSHON: Dental caries rate and fluoride content of dental calculus and saliva. J. Amer. dent. Ass. **66**, 525—528 (1963).
— A. BRZEZINSKI, and B. BERCOVICI: Urinary fluorine levels in women during pregnancy and after delivery. J. dent. Res. **38**, 548—551 (1959).
GETTLER, A. O., and L. ELLERBROOK: Toxicology of fluorides. Amer. J. med. Sci. **197**, 625 to 638 (1939).
HAM, M. P., and M. D. SMITH: Fluorine balance studies on four infants. J. Nutr. **53**, 215—223 (1954a).
— — Fluorine balance studies on three women. J. Nutr. **53**, 225—232 (1954b).
HARDWICK, J. L.: The mechanism of fluorides in lessening susceptibility to dental caries. Brit. dent. J. **114**, 222—228 (1963).
— The fluoride content of the plaque: its possible antienzymatic action. In: Caries Symposium Zürich. The present status of caries prevention by fluorine-containing dentifrices, pp. 112 to 119. Ed. by H. R. MÜHLEMANN and K. G. KÖNIG, Berne: Hans Huber 1961.
—, and S. A. LEACH: The fluoride content of the dental plaque. In: Advances in Fluorine Research and Dental Caries Prevention, Proc. 9th Cong. of European Org. Res. on Fluorine and Dental Caries Prevention, Paris, 28—30, June, 1962, pp. 151—158. Oxford: Pergamon Press 1963.
— J. H. FREMLIN, and J. MATHIESON: The uptake, exchange and release of fluorides at the surfaces of the teeth. Rept. of preliminary investigations using the radio-active isotope F^{18}. Brit. dent. J. **104**, 47—54 (1958).
HARKINS, R. W., J. B. LONGENECKER, and H. P. SARETT: Effect of NaF on the growth of rats with varying vitamin and calcium intakes. J. Nutr. **81**, 81—86 (1963).
HARRIS, L. E., R. J. RALEIGH, M. A. MADSEN, J. L. SHUPE, J. E. BUTCHER, and D. A. GREENWOOD: Effect of various levels of fluorine, stilbestrol, and oxytetracycline, in the fattening ration of lambs. J. Animal Sci. **22**, 51—55 (1963).
HARVEY, J. M.: Chronic endemic fluorosis of Merino sheep in Queensland. Queensland Dept. Agric. Stock Div., Plant Ind. Bull. No. 60; Div. Animal Ind. Bull. No. 6, Brisbane, Australia 1952.
HATTYASY, D.: Unusually high fluorine values in the saliva of subjects free from caries. Acta med. Acad. Sci. hung. **5**, 419—420 (1954).
— J. STRAUB, and K. TOTH: The fluorine content of the saliva of caries-resistant (gypsy) individuals. Acta med. Acad. Sci. hung. **10**, 171—182 (1956).
HEIN, J. W., J. F. BONNER, F. BRUDEVOLD, F. A. SMITH, and H. C. HODGE: Distribution in the soft tissue of the rat of radioactive fluoride administered as sodium fluoride. Nature (Lond.) **178**, 1295—1296 (1956).
— F. A. SMITH, D. E. GARDNER, W. L. DOWNS, E. A. MAYNARD, and H. C. HODGE: Further studies of the caries inhibitory potential and acute toxicity of complex fluorides. J. dent. Res. **30**, 466 (1951).

HELD, H. R.: Fluoride medication and blood fluoride. Schweiz. med. Wschr. **84**, 25—1253 (1954).
— The penetration of fluorine through the placenta and its presence in milk. Schweiz. med. Wschr. **82**, 297—301 (1952).
HELLSTRÖM, I.: Fluorine retention following sodium fluoride mouthwashing. Acta odont. scand. **18**, 263—278 (1960).
HENNON, D. K., G. K. STOOKEY, and J. C. MUHLER: Fluoride retention in rats receiving various vitamin-sodium fluoride preparations. J. Pediat. **64**, 272—277 (1964).
HERMAN, J. R.: Fluorine in urinary tract calculi. Proc. Soc. exp. Biol. (N. Y.) **91**, 189—191 (1956).
—, and L. PAPADAKIS: The relationship of sodium fluoride to nephrolithiasis in rats. J. Urol. (Baltimore) **83**, 799—800 (1960).
— B. MASON, and I. LIGHT: Fluorine in urinary tract calculi. J. Urol. (Baltimore) **80**, 263—268 (1958).
HERNANDEZ-PEON, R.: Physiology of body fluids. Chapt. 40. In: Medical Physiology and Biophysics, ed. by T. C. RUCK and J. F. FULTON. Philadelphia: W. B. Saunders and Co. 1960.
HOBBS, C. S., R. P. MOORMAN JR., J. M. GRIFFITH, J. L. WEST, G. M. MERRIMAN, S. L. HANSARD, C. C. CHAMBERLAIN, W. H. MACINTIRE, and L. S. JONES: Fluorosis in cattle and sheep. Univ. Tenn. Agric. Expt. Sta. Bull. No. 235. 1954.
HODGE, H. C., and F. A. SMITH: Biological effects of inorganic fluoride. Vol. IV of Fluorine Chemistry, ed. by J. H. SIMONS. New York: Academic Press Inc. In Press.
International Commission on Radiological Protection: Recommendations of the International Commission on Radiological Protection. ICRP Pub. 2 Rept. of Comm. II on Permissible Dose for Intl. Rad. p. 151. New York: Pergamon Press 1959.
JACKSON, D., and S. M. WEIDMANN: The relationship between age and the fluorine content of human dentine and enamel: a regional survey. Brit. dent. J. **107**, 303—306 (1959).
— — Fluorine in human bone related to age and the water supply of different regions. J. Path. Bact. **76**, 451—459 (1958).
JACKSON, S. H., and D. TRAIN: The stabilization of the fluorine concentration of the total ash of rats. Canad. J. Biochem. **33**, 93—98 (1955).
JENKINS, G. N.: Theories on the mode of action of fluoride in reducing dental decay. J. dent. Res. **42**, 444—452 (1963).
KEMPF, C. A., and V. E. NELSON: The influence of sodium fluoride upon the composition of tibiae of rats partially recovering from rickets. Proc. Iowa Acad. Sci. **48**, 199—205 (1941).
— — The effect of fluorides on the teeth. Proc. Iowa Acad. Sci. **43**, 197—199 (1936).
— D. A. GREENWOOD, and V. E. NELSON: Studies relating to the toxicity of fluorine compounds. J. Lab. clin. Med. **22**, 1133—1137 (1937).
KETY, S. S.: Concepts of blood-flow distribution in the brain. In: Uptake and Distribution of Anesthetic Agents, pp. 130—139. Ed. by E. M. PAPPER, and R. J. RITZ. New York: McGraw-Hill Book Co. Inc. 1963.
KICK, C. H., R. M. BETHKE, B. H. EDGINGTON, O. H. M. WILDER, P. R. RECORD, W. WILDER, T. J. HILL, and S. W. CHASE: Fluorine in animal nutrition. Ohio Agr. Exptl. Sta. Bull. No. 558 (1935).
KNOUFF, R. A., L. F. EDWARDS, D. W. PRESTON, and P. C. KITCHIN: Permeability of placenta to fluoride. J. dent. Res. **14**, 291—294 (1935—1936).
KONIG, K. G.: Pre- and posteruptive inhibition of experimental rat caries by fluorine administered in water, milk and food. Helv. odont. Acta **4**, 66—71 (1960).
KUDAHL, J. N.: On the determination of fluoride in small samples. In: Advances in Fluorine Research and Dental Caries Prevention, Proc. 9th Cong. European Org. Res. on Fluorine and Dental Caries Prevention, Paris, pp. 53—56, 28—30 June 1962, ed. by J. L. HARDWICK, J.-P. DUSTIN, and H. R. HELD. Oxford: Pergamon Press 1963.
LARGENT, E. J.: Fluorosis. The health aspects of fluorine compounds. Columbus, Ohio: Ohio State Univ. Press 1961.
— Rates of eliminiation of fluoride stored in the tissues of man. Arch. industr. Hyg. **6**, 37—42 (1952).
— Effects of fluorides on man and animals. Proc. 1st Natl. Air Pollution Symp., Pasadena, Calif., pp. 129—134 (1951).
—, and F. F. HEYROTH: The absorption and excretion of fluorides. III. Further observations on metabolism of fluorides at high levels of intake. J. industr. Hyg. **31**, 134—138 (1949).
LAWRENZ, M., and H. H. MITCHELL: The assimilation of fluorine by rats from natural and synthetic cryolite and from cryolite-sprayed fruits. J. Nutr. **22**, 451—462 (1941a).
— — The relative assimilation of fluorine from fluorine bearing minerals and food (tea) and from water and food. J. Nutr. **22**, 621—631 (1941b).
— —, and W. A. RUTH: Adaptation of the growing rat to the ingestion of a constant concentration of fluorine in the diet. J. Nutr. **19**, 531—546 (1940).

LAWRENZ, M., H. H. MITCHELL, and W. A. RUTH: The comparative toxicity of fluorine in calcium fluoride and in cryolite. J. Nutr. **18**, 115—125 (1939a).
— — — A comparison of the toxicity of fluorine in the form of cryolite administered in water and in food. J. Nutr. **18**, 127—141 (1939b).
LEWITUS, Z., S. GUTTMANN, and M. ANBAR: Effect of thyroid-stimulating hormone (TSH) on the accumulation of perchlorate and fluoroborate ions in the thyroid glands of rats. Endocrinology **70**, 295—297 (1962).
LIKINS, R. C., I. ZIPKIN, and H. G. MCCANN: Distribution and excretion of hexafluorophosphate. Proc. Soc. exp. Biol. (N. Y.) **95**, 527—529 (1957).
LINDBERG, Z. YA.: Content of fluoride in the soil and in vegetables in the vicinity of a superphosphate factory. Vop. Pitan. **15**, 41—45 (1956).
LINDEMANN, B., u. H. PASSOW: Versuche zur Aufklärung der Beziehung zwischen Glucose. hemmung und Kaliumverlust bei der Fluoridvergiftung von Menschenerythrocyten-Pflügers Arch. ges. Physiol. **271**, 497—510 (1960).
LOVELACE, F., R. E. BLACK, Y. KUNZ, C. A. H. SMITH, E. B. BOSWORTH, C. N. WANG, L. AUSTRIA, R. L. PARK, and C. M. MCCAY: Metabolism of fluoride in old rats and hamsters. J. appl. Nutr. **12**, 142—151 (1959).
LYON, J. S.: Observations on personnel working with fluorine at a gaseous diffusion plant. J. occup. Med. **4**, 199—201 (1962).
MACHLE, W., and K. KITZMILLER: The effects of the inhalation of hydrogen fluoride. II. The response following exposure to low concentration. J. industr. Hyg. **17**, 223—229 (1935).
—, and E. J. LARGENT: The absorption and excretion of fluoride. II. The metabolism at high levels of intake. J. industr. Hyg. **25**, 112—123 (1943).
—, and E. W. SCOTT: The effects of inhalation of hydrogen fluoride. III. Fluoride storage following exposure to sub-lethal concentrations. J. industr. Hyg. **17**, 230—240 (1935).
— —, and E. J. LARGENT: The absorption and excretion of fluorides. Part I. The normal fluoride balance. J. industr. Hyg. **24**, 199—204 (1942).
— F. THAMANN, K. KATZMILLER, and J. CHOLAK: The effects of inhalation of hydrogen fluoride. I. The response following exposure to high concentrations. J. industr. Hyg. **16**, 129—145 (1934).
MAJUMDAR, B. N., and S. N. RAY: Flurine intoxication of cattle in India. II. Effect of fluorosis on mineral metabolism. Indian J. vet. Sci. **26**, 107—112 (1946a).
— — Fluorine intoxication of cattle in India. III. Effect of fluorosis on the composition of blood. Indian J. vet. Sci. **26**, 113—121 (1946b).
MAPLESDEN, D. C., I. MOTZOK, W. T. OLIVER, and H. D. BRANION: Placental transfer of fluorine to the fetus in rats and rabbits. J. Nutr. **71**, 70—76 (1960).
MARIAKULANDAI, A., and P. VENKATARAMAIAH: Biochemical study of fluorine intoxication. II. Metabolism of fluorine. Indian J. vet. Sci. **25**, 183—199 (1955).
MARTIN, D. J.: The Evanston dental caries study. I. Determination of fluorine in foods, bones and teeth. J. dent. Res. **27**, 27—33 (1948).
—, and I. N. HILL: The Evanston dental caries study. V. The fluorine content of saliva and its relationship to (A) oral lactobacillus counts and (B) the prevalence of dental caries. J. dent. Res. **29**, 291—297 (1950).
MATUURA, S., N. KOKUBU, S. WATABABE, and Y. SAMESIMA: Flourine content in animals. Menn. Fac. Sci., Kyushu Univ. Ser. C. **2**, 81—93 (1955).
MAURER, R. L., and H. G. DAY: The non-essentiality of fluorine. J. Nutr. **62**, 561—573 (1957)
MAYNARD, E. A., W. L. DOWNS, and H. C. HODGE: Oral toxicity of uranium compounds. Chapt. 20. In: Pharmacology and Toxicology of Uranium Compounds, pp. 1221—1369 Ed. by C. VOEGTLIN, and H. C. HODGE. New York: McGraw-Hill Book Co. 1949.
MCCANN, H. G., and F. A. BULLOCK: The effect of fluoride ingestion on the composition and solubility of mineralized tissues of the rat. J. dent. Res. **36**, 391—398 (1957).
MCCLURE, F. J.: Availability of fluorine in sodium fluoride vs. sodium fluosilicate. Publ. Hlth Rep. (Wash.) **65**, 1175—1186 (1950).
— Fluorine in foods-survey of recent data. Publ. Hlth Rep. **64**, 1061—1074 (1949).
— Domestic water and dental caries. III. Fluorine in human saliva. Amer. J. Dis. Child. **62**, 512—515 (1941).
— Fluorides in food and drinking water. Nat. Inst. Hlth Bull. No. 172 (1939).
—, and C. A. KINSER: Fluoride domestic waters and systemic effects. II. Fluorine content o urine in relation to fluorine in drinking water. Publ. Hlth Rep. **59**, 1575—1591 (1944).
— H. C. MCCANN, and N. C. LEONE: Excessive fluoride in water and bone chemistry (comparison of two cases). Publ. Hlth Rep. **73**, 741—746 (1958).
— H. H. MITCHELL, T. S. HAMILTON, and C. A. KINSER: Balances of fluorine ingested from various sources in food and water by five young men. Excretion of fluorine through the skin. J. industr. Hyg. **27**, 159—170 (1945).

MILLER, G. W., and J. L. SHUPE: Alkaline bone phosphatase activity as related to fluoride ingestion by dairy cattle. Amer. J. vet. Res. **23**, 24—31 (1962).
MILLER, R. F., and P. H. PHILLIPS: The effect of age on the level and metabolism of fluorine in the bones of the fluoridated rat. J. Nutr. **59**, 425—433 (1956).
— — The enhancement of the toxicity of sodium fluoride in the rat by high dietary fat. J. Nutr. **56**, 447—454 (1955).
— — The metabolism of fluorine in the bones of the fluoride-poisoned rat. J. Nutr. **51**, 273 to 281 (1953).
MINOGUCHI, G., and Y. IWAMOTO: Experimental investigation of fluorine: excretion and deposition. In: Medico-Dental Researches on Fluorides, Rept. of the Co-operative Res. Ministry of Education (Medicine), ed. by S. UTZIMO, pub. by Japan Soc. Promotion Sci., Ueno, Tokyo 1957.
MØLLER, P. F., and S. V. GUDJONSSON: Massive fluorosis of bones and ligaments. Acta radiol. (Stockh.) **13**, 269—294 (1932).
MORICHINI: Analysis of fossil teeth. Mem. mat. fis. soc. ital. sci. (Modena) **10**, Pt. I, 166 (1803).
MUHLEMANN, H. R., J. C. SOMOGYI, and G. G. PORETTI: Fluoride absorption through the enamel of human teeth after periods of various length. Bull. schweiz. Akad. med. Wiss. **11**, 386—390 (1955).
MUHLER, J. C.: Is fluorine a dietary essential. Chapt. 10. In: Fluorine and Dental Health, ed. by J. C. MUHLER and M. K. HINE. Bloomington, Indiana: Indiana Univ. Press 1959.
— Effect of vitamin C on skeletal fluoride storage in the guinea pig. J. Amer. dent. Ass. **56**, 335—340 (1958).
—, and D. A. WEDDLE: Utilizability of fluorine for storage in the rat when administered in milk. J. Nutr. **55**, 347—352 (1955a).
— — Fluorine storage in rats receiving different fluorides in the drinking water at varying pH. J. dent. Res. **34**, 895—899 (1955b).
— G. K. STOOKEY, and M. J. WAGNER: Effect of Sr^{89} on fluoride retention in the rat. Proc. Soc. exp. Biol. (N. Y.) **102**, 644—647 (1959).
MURRAY, M. M.: Maternal transference of fluorine. J. Physiol. (Lond.) **87**, 388—393 (1936).
NEUMAN, W. F., M. W. NEUMAN, E. R. MAIN, J. O'LEARY, and F. A. SMITH: The surface chemistry of bone. II. Fluoride deposition. J. biol. Chem. **187**, 655—661 (1950).
NOMMIK, H.: Fluorine in Swedish agricultural products, soil and drinking water. Acta Polytech. Chem. Met. Ser. 3, No. 7, 7—121 (1953).
ODELL, R. T., and J. A. KEY: The effect of chronic fluorine intoxication upon the healing of experimental fractures in rats. Ann. Surg. **138**, 461—466 (1953).
PANDIT, C. G., and D. NARAYANA RAO: Endemic fluorosis in South India. Experimental production of chronic fluorine intoxication in monkeys (Macaca radiata). Indian J. med. Res. **28**, 559—574 (1940).
— T. N. S. RAGHAVACHARI, D. SUBBA RAO, and V. KRISHNAMURTI: Endemic fluorosis in South India. A study of the factors involved in the production of mottled enamel in children and severe bone manifestations in adults. Indian J. med. Res. **28**, 533—558 (1940).
PERKINSON JR., J. D., I. B. WHITNEY, R. A. MONROE, W. E. LOTZ, and C. L. COMAR: Metabolism of fluorine 18 in domestic animals. Amer. J. Physiol. **182**, 383—389 (1955).
PHILLIPS, P. H., E. B. HART, and G. BOHSTEDT: The influence of fluorine ingestion upon the nutritional qualities of milk. J. biol. Chem. **105**, 123—134 (1934).
PURVES, M. J.: Some effects of administering sodium fluoride to patients with Paget's disease. Lancet 8, 1188—1189 (1962).
RANGANATHAN, S.: Studies on experimental fluorine poisoning in rats. Indian J. med. Res. **32**, 233—236 (1944).
RICH, C., and J. ENSINCK: Effect of sodium fluoride on calcium metabolism of human beings. Nature (Lond.) **191**, 184—185 (1961).
RILEY, W. F., K. S. SMITH, and R. J. FLYNN, editors: The Yearbook of Veterinary Medicine, vol. 1, p. 139. Chicago: Yearbook Medical Publishers, Inc. 1963.
ROHOLM, K.: Fluorine intoxication. A Clinical-Hygienic Study with a Review of the Literature and some Experimental Investigations, 364 pp. London: H. K. Lewis and Co. 1937.
ROSENHOLTZ, M. J., T. R. CARSON, M. H. WEEKS, F. WILINSKI, D. F. FORD, and F. W. OBERST: A toxicopathologic study in animals after brief single exposures to hydrogen fluoride. Amer. industr. Hyg. Ass. J. **24**, 253—261 (1963).
RYE, W. A.: Fluorides and phosphates-clinical observations of employees in phosphate operations. Proc. 13th Intl. Cong. on Occup. Health, July 25—29, New York, pp. 361—364 (1960).
SAVCHUCK, W. B., and W. D. ARMSTRONG: Metabolic turnover of fluoride by the skeleton of the rat. J. biol. Chem. **193**, 575—585 (1951).
SCASSELLATI-SFORZOLINI, G., and G. SCASSALLATI-SFORZOLINI: Fluorine in human eye tissue. Boll. Soc. ital. Biol. sper. **32**, 555—556 (1956).

SCHWEINSBERGER, R. A., and J. C. MUHLER: Urinary excretion of fluoride by children aged two through five years using a stannous fluoride-containing dentifrice in a natural fluoride area and a nonfluoride area. J. Pediat. **51**, 634—638 (1957).
— — Urinary fluorine levels in children following the clinical use of a stannous fluoride-containing dentifrice. J. dent. Res. **35**, 760—762 (1956).
SEPPILLI, A., A. CANDELI, and G. SCASSELLATI-SFORZOLINI: Circulation of fluorine within the body. Arch. Sci. biol. (Bologna) **45**, 414—419 (1957).
SHARPLESS, G. R.: Limitation of fluorine toxicosis in the rat with aluminum chloride. Proc. Soc. exp. Biol. (N. Y.) **34**, 562—564 (1936a).
— Prevention of fluorine toxicosis in the rat with aluminum chloride. J. Nutr. **11**, Suppl. 8—9 (1936b).
SHOURIE, K. L., J. W. HEIN, and H. C. HODGE: Preliminary studies of the caries inhibiting potential and acute toxicity of sodium monofluorophosphate. J. dent. Res. **29**, 529—533 (1950).
SHUPE, J. L., M. L. MINER, L. E. HARRIS, and D. A. GREENWOOD: Relative effects of feeding hay atmospherically contaminated by fluoride residue, normal hay plus calcium fluoride, and normal hay plus sodium fluoride to dairy heifers. Amer. J. vet. Res. **23**, 777—787 (1962).
— — D. A. GREENWOOD, L. E. HARRIS, and G. E. STODDARD: The effect of fluorine on dairy cattle. II. Clinical and pathological effects. Amer. J. vet. Res. **24**, 964—979 (1963a).
— L. E. HARRIS, D. A. GREENWOOD, J. E. BUTCHER, and H. M. NIELSEN: The effect of fluorine on dairy cattle. V. Fluorine in the urine as an estimator of fluorine intake. Amer. J. vet. Res. **24**, 300—306 (1963b).
SINGER, L., and W. D. ARMSTRONG: Comparison of fluoride contents of human dental and skeletal tissues. J. dent. Res. **41**, 154—157 (1962).
— — Regulation of human plasma fluoride concentration. J. appl. Physiol. **15**, 508—510 (1960).
SMITH, F. A., and D. E. GARDNER: Unpublished data 1963.
— — Investigations on the metabolism of fluoride. I. The determination of fluoride in blood. J. dent. Res. **30**, 182—188 (1951).
— —, and H. C. HODGE: Unpublished data 1963a.
— — — Investigations on the metabolism of fluoride. III. Effect of acute renal tubular injury on urinary excretion of fluoride by the rabbit. Arch. industr. Hlth **11**, 2—10 (1955).
— — — Age increase in fluoride content in human bone. Fed. Proc. **12**, 368 (1953).
— — — Investigations on the metabolism of fluoride. II. Fluoride content of blood and urine as a function of the fluorine in drinking water. J. dent. Res. **29**, 596—600 (1950).
— — N. C. LEONE, and H. C. HODGE: The effects of the absorption of fluoride. V. The chemical determination of fluoride in human soft tissues following prolonged ingestion of fluoride at various levels. Arch. industr. Hlth **21**, 330—332 (1960).
— — W. L. DOWNS, E. A. MAYNARD, and H. C. HODGE: Unpublished data 1963b.
— — N. C. LEONE, H. C. HODGE, and A. DUTTON: Unpublished data 1963c.
SMITH, M. C., and R. M. LEVERTON: Comparative toxicity of fluorine compounds. Industr. Eng. Chem. **26**, 791—797 (1934).
— M. VAVICH, and H. V. SMITH: Fluorine content of milk as affected by the amount of fluorine in drinking water of the cow. J. dent. Res. **20**, 286—287 (1941).
SOEJIMA, K., T. SHIMOHARA, M. EIZURU, Y. MOCHIYAMA, K. NAGOTO, K. HAGIHARA, H. KAMWAKI, E. HAMASAKI, T. MAKIZUMI, T. NOZOE, T. WATANABE, S. UJI, S. KAWASHIMA, H. KUBOTA, K. OKUNO, W. OSAKA, M. SAKO, and H. MURAOKA: Synopsis of fundamental studies on the relation between fluorides. In: Medico-Dental Researches on Fluorides. Rept. of Co-operative Res. Ministry Education (Med.), ed. by S. UTZIMO, pub. by Japan Soc. Promotion Sci., Ueno, Tokyo 1957.
SPECTOR, W. S.: Handbook of Biological Data. Table 55. Philadelphia, Penn.: W. B. Saunders Co. 1956.
SPEIRS, R. L.: The nature of surface enamel. Brit. dent. J. **107**, 209—217 (1959).
STODDARD, G. E., J. L. SHUPE, D. A. GREENWOOD, M. L. MINER, G. Q. BATEMAN, L. E. HARRIS, H. M. NIELSEN, and T. V. BISHOP: Fluorosis with dairy cows. A progress report of the first 40 months on experiment and for the first lactation. Proc. 37th Ann. Meeting Western Div. Amer. Dairy Sci. Assoc. July 16—18 (1956).
STOKINGER, H. E.: Toxicity following inhalation of fluorine and hydrogen fluoride. In: Pharmacology and Toxicology of Uranium Compounds, ed. by C. VOEGTLIN and H. C. HODGE. New York: McGraw-Hill Book Co. 1949.
STOOKEY, G. K., and J. C. MUHLER: Relationship between fluoride deposition and metastatic calcification in soft tissues of rat and guinea pig. Proc. Soc. exp. Biol. (N. Y.) **113**, 720—725 (1963).
— — Effect of molybdenum on fluoride retention in the rat. Proc. Soc. exp. Biol. (N. Y.) **109**, 268—271 (1962).

STOOKEY, G. K., and J. C. MUHLER: Effect of molybdenum on fluoride retention in the rat Proc. Soc. exp. Biol. (N. Y.) **101**, 379—380 (1959).
— D. B. CRANE, and J. C. MUHLER: Role of skeleton and kidney in fluoride absorption in rat. Proc. Soc. exp. Biol. (N. Y.) **113**, 366—370 (1963).
— — — Effect of molybdenum on fluoride absorption. Proc. Soc. exp. Biol. (N. Y.) **109**, 580—583 (1962a).
— R. A. ROBERTS, and J. C. MUHLER: Synergistic effect of molybdenum and fluoride on dental caries in rat. Proc. Soc. exp. Biol. (N. Y.) **109**, 702—705 (1962b).
— J. OSBORNE, and J. C. MUHLER: Effects of pre- and postnatal fluorides on caries. Dent. Prog. **2**, 137—139 (1962c).
SUNDVALL-HAGLAND, I., F. BRUDEVOLD, W. D. ARMSTRONG, D. E. GARDNER, and F. A. SMITH: Comparison of the increment of fluoride in enamel and the reduction in dental caries resulting from topical fluoride applications. Arch. oral Biol. **1**, 74—79 (1959).
SUTTIE, J. W., and P. H. PHILLIPS: Studies of the effects of dietary NaF on dairy cows. IV. Dental changes as the results of long-term fluorine ingestion. J. Nutr. **71**, 109—114 (1960).
— — The effect of age on the rate of fluorine deposition in the femur of the rat. Arch. Biochem. **83**, 355—359 (1959).
— —, and R. F. MILLER: Studies of the effects of dietary sodium fluoride on dairy cows. III. Skeletal and soft tissue fluorine deposition and fluorine toxicosis. J. Nutr. **65**, 293—304 (1958).
— R. F. MILLER, and P. H. PHILLIPS: Studies of the effects of dietary sodium fluoride on dairy cows. I. The physiological effects and the developmental symptoms of fluorosis. J. Nutr. **63**, 211—224 (1957).
SWEENEY, E. A., J. H. SHAW, and R. P. RUBIN: Effect of alloxan diabetes on fluoride retention and caries incidence in rats. J. dent. Res. **41**, 866—874 (1962).
TAM, J. C.: The influence of fluoride on the fracture healing process in young rats. J. dent. Res. **29**, 698 (1950).
TAYLOR, J. M., D. E. GARDNER, J. K. SCOTT, E. A. MAYNARD, W. L. DOWNS, F. A. SMITH, and H. C. HODGE: Toxic effects of fluoride on the rat kidney. II. Chronic effects. Toxicol. appl. Pharmacol. **3**, 290—314 (1961).
TOSTESON, D. C.: Halide transport in red blood cells. Acta physiol. scand. **46**, 19—41 (1959).
ULLBERG, S., L.-E. APPELGREN, C.-J. CLEMEDSON, Y. ERICSSON, B. EWALDSSON, B. SÖRBO, and R. SÖREMARK: A comparison of the distribution of some halide ions in the body. Biochem. Pharmacol. **13**, 407—412 (1964).
UNDERWOOD, E. J.: Trace Elements in Human and Animal Nutrition. Chapt. 9. 2nd edition. New York: Academic Press Inc. 1962.
VENKATARAMANAN, K., and N. KRISHNASWAMY: The amelioration of symptoms of fluorosis by aluminum salts. Indian J. med. Res. **37**, 277—282 (1949).
VENKATESWARLU, P., and D. NARAYANA RAO: An evaluation of vitamin C therapy in fluorine intoxication. Indian J. med. Res. **45**, 377—386 (1957a).
— — Distribution of fluorine in the tissues of rats. Indian J. med. Res. **45**, 387—389 (1957b).
— — Vitamin C ingestion and skeletal storage of fluorine. Indian J. med. Res. **42**, 141—146 (1954).
VOLKER, J. F., R. F. SOGNNAES, and B. G. BIBBY: Studies on the distribution of radioactive fluoride in the bones and teeth of experimental animals. Amer. J. Physiol. **132**, 707—712 (1941).
WADHWANI, T. K.: Effect of fluorine on the composition of bones: changes in the composition of bones of monkeys (Macaca radiata). Indian J. med. Res. **43**, 321—330 (1955).
— Prevention and mitigation of fluorosis (endemic). Part II. J. Indian Inst. Sci. **36**, 64—69 (1954).
— Metabolism of fluorine. Absorption, retention, distribution and elimination of fluorine, and its effect on the vitamin C content of different tissues, and on the iodine content of thyroids of rats and monkeys. J. Indian Inst. Sci. **35**, 354—362 (1953).
— Mitigation of fluorosis (experimental). Part I. Indian med. Gaz. **87**, 5—7 (1952).
WAGNER, M. J.: Absorption of fluoride by the gastric mucosa in the rat. J. dent. Res. **41**, 667—671 (1962a).
— Pattern of distribution of fluoride in young and old albino rats. J. dent. Res. **41**, 1378—1382 (1962b).
—, and J. C. MUHLER: The effect of calcium and phosphorus on fluoride absorption. J. dent. Res. **39**, 49—52 (1960).
— — The relationship between fluoride ingestion and urinary calcium. J. dent. Res. **38**, 1078—1081 (1959a).
— — Retention of aqueous fluoride by alloxandiabetic rats. J. Amer. dent. Ass. **59**, 81—83 (1959b).
— — Influence of inorganic ions on fluoride retention in the rat. Proc. Soc. exp. Biol. (N. Y.) **98**, 496—499 (1958).

WALDO, A. L., and R. E. ZIPF: The determination of fluoride in drinking water and biological materials. J. Lab. clin. Med. **40**, 601—609 (1952).

WALLACE, P. C.: The metabolism of F^{18} in normal and chronically fluorosed rats. Thesis, Univ. Calif. 1953.

WALLACE-DURBIN, P.: The metabolism of fluorine in the rat using F^{18} as a tracer. J. dent. Res. **33**, 789—800 (1954).

WEDDLE, D. A., and J. C. MUHLER: The metabolism of different fluorides in the rat. I. Comparisons between sodium fluoride, sodium silicofluoride, and stannous fluoride. J. dent. Res. **36**, 386—390 (1957).

— — Metabolism of small concentrations of fluorine in the albino rat. J. dent. Res. **34**, 900—909 (1955).

— — The effects of inorganic salts on fluorine storage in the rat. J. Nutr. **54**, 437—444 (1954).

WILLARD, H. H., and O. B. WINTER: Volumetric method for determination of fluorine. Industr. Eng. Chem. Anal. Ed. **5**, 7—10 (1933).

WILLS, J. H.: The secretion of intravenously injected fluorine in the submaxillary saliva of cats. J. dent. Res. **19**, 585—590 (1940).

WOLFF, J., and J. R. MAUREY: Thyroidal iodide transport. IV. The role of ion size. Biochim. biophys. Acta **69**, 58—67 (1963).

WUTHIER, R. E., and P. H. PHILLIPS: The effects of continued exposure to added increments of water-borne or food-borne fluoride upon the rat. J. dent. Res. **40**, 1142—1154 (1961).

— — The effects of long-time administration of small amounts of fluoride in food or water on caries-susceptible rats. J. Nutr. **67**, 581—588 (1959).

YARDENI, J., I. GEDALIA, and M. KOHN: Fluoride concentration of dental calculus, surface enamel and cementum. Arch. oral Biol. **8**, 697—701 (1963).

YUDKIN, E. P., J. CZERNIEJEWSKI, and J. R. BLAYNEY: Evanston dental caries study. XIII. Preliminary report on comparative fluorine retention in human tissues. J. dent. Res. **33**, 691—692 (1954).

ZIPKIN, I., and R. C. LIKINS: Absorption of various fluorine compounds from the gastrointestinal tract of the rat. Amer. J. Physiol. **191**, 549—550 (1957).

—, and F. J. McCLURE: Cariostatic effect and metabolism of ammonium fluosilicate. Publ. Hlth Rep. **69**, 730—733 (1954).

— — Deposition of fluorine in the bones and teeth of the growing rat. J. Nutr. **47**, 611—620 (1952).

— — Complex fluorides: caries reduction and fluorine retention in the bones and teeth of white rats. Publ. Hlth Rep. **66**, 1523—1532 (1951).

— W. A. LEE, and N. C. LEONE: Fluoride content of urinary and biliary tract calculi. Proc. Soc. exp. Biol. (N. Y.) **97**, 650—653 (1958a).

— — — Rate of urinary fluoride output in normal adults. Amer. J. Publ. Hlth **47**, 848—851 (1957).

— R. C. LIKINS, and F. J. McCLURE: Deposition of fluoride, calcium and phosphorus in experimental low-phosphorus rickets. J. Nutr. **67**, 59—68 (1959).

— — —, and A.-C. STEERE: Urinary fluoride levels associated with use of fluoridated water. Publ. Hlth Rep. **71**, 767—772 (1956).

— F. J. McCLURE, N. C. LEONE, and W. A. LEE: Fluride deposition in human bones after prolonged ingestion of fluoride in the drinking water. Publ. Hlth Rep. **73**, 732—740 (1958b).

Chapter 3

Fluoride and the Skeletal and Dental Tissues

By

J. A. WEATHERELL

With 20 Figures

I. General metabolism of fluoride

Probably all diets contain some fluoride and most water supplies possess at least traces. The concentration in food varies from sub-micro amounts to over 3 ppm. For instance, there is very little fluoride in most vegetables, citrus fruit or dairy produce (WALDBOTT 1963). Fish, on the other hand, can contain large amounts of the element and high levels of fluoride found in teeth of certain coastal populations may be due to a high consumption of fish (ELLIOTT and SMITH 1960). HARRISON (1949) suggested that about 1 mg fluoride per day might be ingested from tea; this may account for the fact that, when areas with similar water supplies are compared, skeletal fluoride levels in Britain tend to be higher than in the United States (JACKSON and WEIDMANN 1958). Seasalt is a rich source of dietary fluoride and in regions of India, where the salt is prepared by evaporation of sea water, appreciable quantities of fluoride may be consumed in this way (HADJIMARKOS 1962).

At a level of 1–20 mg fluoride per day, about half that ingested is quickly excreted in the urine and faeces, though the amount depends to some extent upon the composition of the diet. When only soluble fluoride is ingested almost the whole of it, 93–97 %, is rapidly absorbed from the gastro-intestinal tract. If the fluoride compounds are relatively insoluble, or the diet contains other substances capable of forming insoluble fluoride compounds, the gastro-intestinal absorption decreases and more fluoride is excreted via the faeces. Fluoride is absorbed more rapidly and to a greater extent from water than from milk because the calcium of the milk forms insoluble CaF_2 (ERICSSON 1958). WEDDLE and MUHLER (1957) showed that the addition of calcium to fluoridated water similarly increased the faecal excretion of fluoride in rats. Magnesium also reduces fluoride absorption whereas other dietary constituents, such as iron, molybdenum, or sulphate may increase it (STOOKEY et al. 1964).

The fluoride level of the blood reaches a maximum 30–60 min after ingestion and then decreases rapidly (HODGE 1956). WALLACE-DURBIN (1954) injected radioactive fluoride into rats and showed that the fall in the fluoride level of blood was very nearly paralleled by that of the soft tissues. Apart from occasional minor deposits in sites of ectopic calcification (CARLSON et al. 1960; ERICSSON and ULLBERG 1958; SMITH et al. 1960) the element does not accumulate in any of the soft tissues.

Thirty-five to 50 % of the fluoride absorbed is taken up by the skeleton (LARGENT and HEYROTH 1949). In rats, maximum bone-fluoride levels are reached about 4 hr after ingestion (WALLACE-DURBIN 1954). The remainder of the absorbed dose is excreted in urine within 24 hr. A proportion of the fluoride appears to be taken up by bone however small the amounts ingested, though at very low levels there seems to be a relatively greater fraction excreted in the urine (HODGE 1956; ZIPKIN and LEONE 1957).

II. Uptake of fluoride by bone

A. Distribution of fluoride in the skeleton

Numerous investigations in humans and experimental animals have been carried out to assess the concentration of fluoride in hard tissues. The situation is complicated by the fact that fluoride levels vary from one part of the skeleton to another. To some extent this is due to structural differences; cancellous bone containing higher fluoride concentrations than compact bone. For instance, trabeculae in the medullary cavity of human rib contain 1.5 to 3 times more fluoride than the adjacent cortical bone (WEATHERELL unpublished) and a similar ratio is maintained between metaphyseal cancellum and diaphyseal compacta of normal rats, rabbits and cats (WEIDMANN and WEATHERELL 1959). Bones such as human iliac crest, a predominantly cancellous structure, have a higher fluoride concentration than femur, which largely consists of compact bone (SINGER and ARMSTRONG 1962).

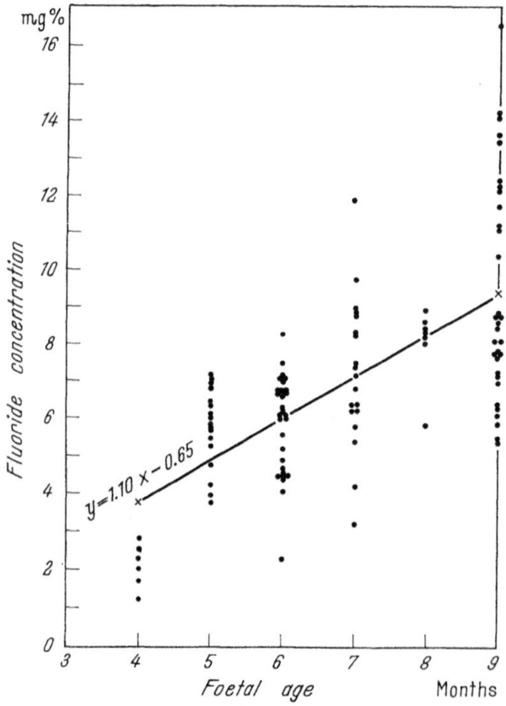

Fig. 1. Fluoride concentration in femora of foetuses from areas supplied by drinking water containing 0.5 to 0.6 ppm fluoride. (From GEDALIA et al. 1964)

Within each bone fluoride accumulates preferentially at the surface; *e.g.* endosteal and sub-periosteal regions of the long bones accumulate higher levels of fluoride than the interior of the cortex (GARDNER et al. 1959; WEIDMANN and WEATHERELL 1959).

A relationship between bone vascularity and fluoride incorporation has been repeatedly stressed but other factors, such as bone growth and mineralisation, are probably more important in governing fluoride uptake.

B. Influence of growth and mineralisation on the fluoride content of bone

The accumulation of fluoride is maximal during bone growth. In the developing skeleton of the human foetus the fluoride concentration of the femur increases appreciably from the time calcification begins until birth (Fig. 1). As they grow older, animals accumulate fluoride less rapidly; ZIPKIN and MCCLURE (1952) fed equal amounts of the element to rats of different ages and showed that bones of mature rats acquired less fluoride than those of younger animals (Fig. 2). Within individual bones highest fluoride concentration also occurs where bone growth is maximal and mineralisation is incomplete, *e.g.* in the metaphyseal regions of long bones.

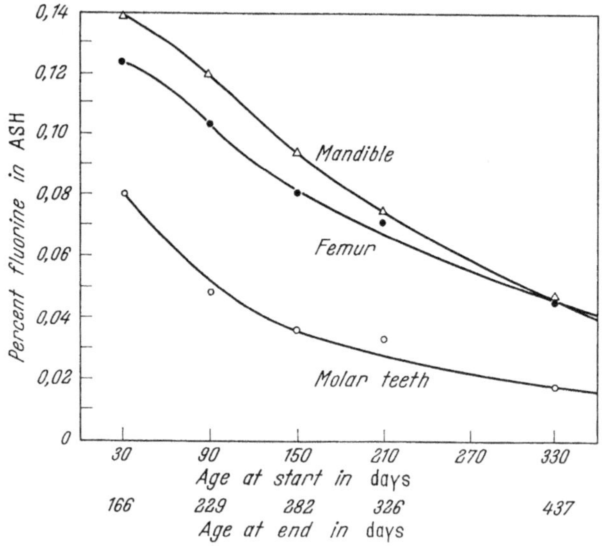

Fig. 2. Fluoride concentration in bones and teeth of growing rats receiving a total of 20 mg fluoride as NaF at different ages, with no prior exposure to fluoride. (From Zipkin and McClure 1952)

No doubt a similar relationship between growth and fluoride content holds for humans, but too few figures are available to establish fluoride levels in the bones of persons under the age of 18 years.

C. Variations in fluoride content of bone with age and duration of fluoridation

After the period of growth has ended the fluoride content of bone continues to rise, but more slowly than before. The precise relationship between the age of bone and its fluoride content is not clear, despite several investigations. The earliest study was that of Glock et al. (1941), who analysed *post mortem* specimens of human rib from two London hospitals. They showed that the level of fluoride in rib rose with age, but the scatter of the 14 results was too great to establish a more specific age-fluoride relationship.

The chief difficulty of such an investigation is to select representative specimens of bone. The pieces of rib studied by Glock et al. included variable and uncontrollable proportions of cortical and cancellous bone with widely different fluoride levels. Such heterogeneous samples are not comparable. To avoid this complication Smith et al. (1953) investigated the compact bone of rib and Jackson and Weidmann (1958) studied rib cancellum. Whereas the results of Smith et al. suggested that there was a linear increase in fluoride content with age, those of Jackson and Weidmann indicated that the fluoride level of bone did not noticeably rise after the age of about 55. More recently, Blaney et al. (1962) studied the fluoride content of iliac crest which also contained a mixture of cortical and cancellous bone. Their results supported the finding of Jackson and Weidmann (1958).

It would be very difficult to predict how the level of skeletal fluoride in man will alter after middle age. Information derived from animal studies is of little assistance, since experimental animals are relatively much younger. A gradual decrease in

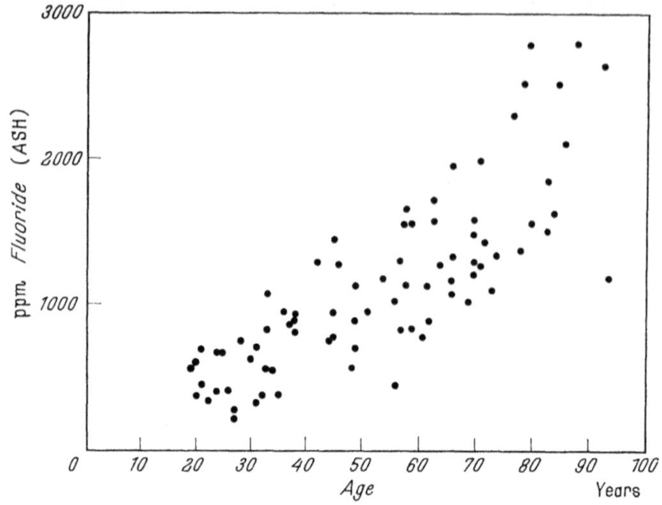

Fig. 3. Fluoride concentration in cortical bone from midshaft diaphysis of human femora of different ages from areas supplied with drinking water containing <0.5 ppm fluoride (WEATHERELL and WEIDMANN unpublished)

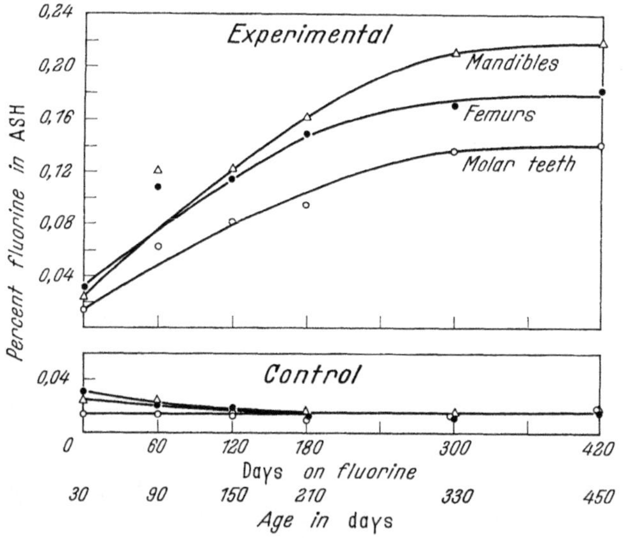

Fig. 4. Fluoride concentration in bones and teeth of growing rats receiving 10 ppm fluoride as NaF, per day, for 420 days, starting at 30 days of age. (From ZIPKIN and McCLURE 1952)

bone activity or a small rate of formation might be expected in older bone and, consequently, a reduced or slow rate of fluoride incorporation. Bone resorption apparently accelerates after the 5th decade (ATKINSON et al. 1963) and since the fluoride concentrations in older bone are high, the amounts of fluoride mobilised from the skeleton will increase after the age of about 55. It is likely, therefore, that the *total* amount of fluoride in the older human skeleton might fall. Resorption will only alter the *concentration* of bone fluoride, if the area of tissue removed contains predominantly high or especially low levels of the element. Since resorption necessarily involves bone surfaces, where fluoride tends to accumulate, it might conceivably also reduce the fluoride concentration in older bone.

These considerations would seem to favour the conclusions of the above authors, *viz.* that skeletal fluoride concentration in man will reach a plateau at about the 6th decade. The biological scatter of their results is so large, however, that a categorical statement is not justified. Recent analyses carried out on human femora, moreover, (Fig. 3) give no support to the conclusion that skeletal fluoride levels cease to rise in old age. More investigations are needed before the relation between skeletal fluoride level and age in man can be described with any certainty.

A tendency for fluoride concentration to reach a constant level in the animal skeleton was reported by ZIPKIN and McCLURE (1952). Several 30 day old rats were given 10 ppm fluoride in their drinking water for 420 days (Fig. 4). For the first 200 days the fluoride content of the rat femora increased rapidly. From the 200th to the 300th day fluoride seemed to accumulate more slowly after which there was no further increase. It is difficult to say to what extent age of bone and to what extent prolonged or increased fluoridation contributes to the development of this equilibrium state. The reduction in the rate of fluoride incorporation would be partly due to the decreased growth rate of bone as the animals became older during the 420 days of the experiment. SUTTIE and PHILLIPS (1959), however, observed the same general trend in both very young and adult rats given 500 ppm fluoride in their diet. They found that after an initial period of fluoridation the rats' bones accumulated less fluoride, irrespective of age.

The explanation is probably that fluoride levels increase more rapidly in bone which has not been previously exposed to the element. The absorption of fluoride might saturate those sites of the bone which are available to the element and thus slow down uptake. HODGE (1952) distinguished between an initial rapid uptake of fluoride followed by a slower incorporation as new sites were made available in the bone. SUTTIE and PHILLIPS (1959) explained observations made on rats in a similar way. It would seem improbable that such saturation can develop at very low levels of fluoridation, even after life-long exposure; the normal physiological processes of bone remodelling and renewal are probably sufficient to permit a steady incorporation of small amounts of fluoride.

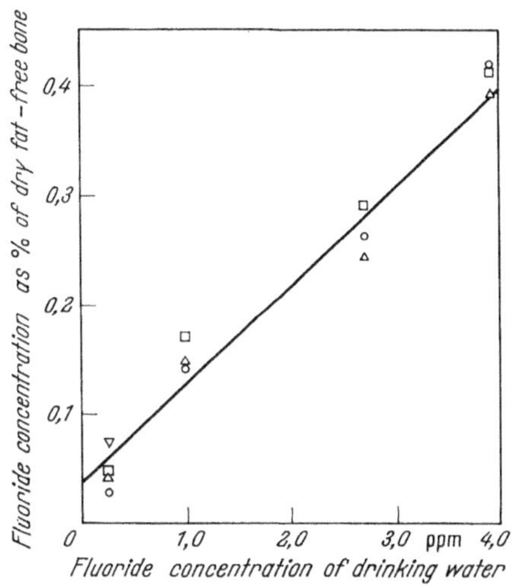

Fig. 5. Relation of fluoride concentration in human bones to fluoride concentration in drinking water. ○ Iliac crest; △ Rib; □ Vertebra; ▽ Sternum. (From ZIPKIN et al. 1958)

D. Influence of the level of fluoride ingestion on concentrations of fluoride in bone

The higher the concentration of fluoride ingested, the more rapidly it accumulates in the hard tissues. ZIPKIN (1960) found that the concentrations of fluoride in human iliac crest, rib and vertebrae were almost directly proportional to the level of fluoride in the drinking water over a range of 1 ppm to 4 ppm (Fig. 5). Steady fluoride ratios, between different types and regions of bone, are maintained so long as skeletal fluorosis does not develop.

It has been shown, however, that the persistent ingestion of high levels of fluoride causes pathological changes in the skeleton, the most obvious of which are exostotic bone formation and bone resorption. Stimulation of osteogenesis increases the uptake of fluoride and regions of exostotic bone consequently contain much higher concentrations than adjacent areas of original tissue (WEIDMANN and WEATHERELL 1959). The increased resorption, on the other hand, particularly evident in the older established tissue, will inevitably result in a mobilisation of incorporated fluoride. The net result of these opposing processes is, nevertheless, a considerable increase in the fluoride level of the skeleton.

E. Removal of fluoride by resorption of bone

The concentration of fluoride in bone is the net product of fluoride uptake and withdrawal. It is not possible to distinguish between these two factors from a study of fluoride levels, since a relatively low fluoride content could be due either to rapid removal or to slow incorporation.

When skeletal tissues are resorbed fluoride is also released. The amount of fluoride removed will depend on whether resorption occurred chiefly in a fluoride-rich region, *e.g.* bone surfaces or cancellous bone, or where the fluoride content was low, *e.g.* interior regions or compacta. Some of the fluoride removed will re-deposit locally, especially in young animals where bone is actively forming (LIKINS et al. 1959), the remainder will enter the general circulation and part of this will be excreted in the urine. Evidence that fluoride removed from the skeleton does appear in the urine comes from the work of LARGENT and HEYROTH (1949), who observed a relatively high level of fluoride excretion in a human subject even after his fluoride ingestion had been discontinued. HODGE (1961) mentioned that the urinary fluoride of persons in Bartlett, Texas remained high for two years after the fluoride content of the water supply was reduced from 8 ppm to 1 ppm. High urinary fluoride levels, in excess of intake, can only be of skeletal origin and high concentrations of fluoride in the skeleton might well increase the fluoride concentrations of urine. GEDALIA (1958) attributed the relatively low urinary fluoride levels of children to the greater capacity of young bone to absorb fluoride. His observations could equally mean, however, that the high levels of fluoride in adult urine reflect to some extent high levels of fluoride in the adult skeleton. There is little information which relates urine fluoride concentrations to age. It would be interesting to know the urine fluoride levels of aged osteoporotics in whom there is an increased resorption of high-fluoride bone.

III. Uptake of fluoride by dental tissues

A. Fluoride in enamel

Enamel contains least fluoride of all the hard tissues and although in man the concentration continues to increase throughout life, it does so at a progressively decreasing rate. JACKSON and WEIDMANN (1959) showed that at three different levels of ingestion (< 0.5, 0.8 and 1.9 ppm fluoride in drinking water) there was a consistent relationship between average enamel fluoride content and age (Fig. 6). The concentration of fluoride in enamel, at the time of tooth eruption, appeared to be approximately proportional to the level of fluoride ingested. After eruption, the level of fluoride continued to rise until a plateau was reached, after which there was little further increment. The age at which this occurred increased with the concentration of fluoride in the drinking water; at < 0.5 ppm it occurred at about 20 years; at 0.8 ppm at about 30; at 1.9 ppm, between 30 and 40 years. The maximum concentration of fluoride achieved by enamel at the three levels studied, varied with the content of fluoride in the water supply and was in each case about double the concentration in enamel at the time of eruption.

Fluoride is not uniformly distributed throughout enamel; its concentration is higher in the outer surface than in the interior. Incorporation of fluoride into inner regions occurs principally during the period of formation and mineralisation, subsequent accumulation is almost completely restricted to the tooth surface. The surface concentration of fluoride is of major interest to dentistry and there have been several attempts to measure it. JENKINS and SPEIRS (1953) found the percentage of fluoride in surface enamel was four to nine times that of the interior. BRUDEVOLD

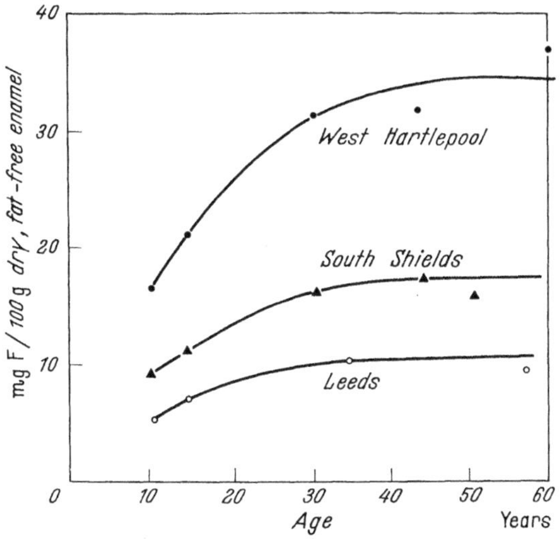

Fig. 6. Relationship between age and fluoride concentration of human premolar enamel. Fluoride in drinking water: Leeds, < 0.5 ppm; S. Shields, 0.8 ppm; W. Hartlepool, 1.9 ppm. (From JACKSON and WEIDMANN 1959)

et al. (1956) found an average thirteen-fold difference, but there was a very large variation. YOON et al. (1960a) determined differences of up to twenty times and recently an unerupted molar was found to have thirty times as much fluoride in the surface compared with the interior enamel (WEATHERELL and HARGREAVES unpublished). Appreciable biological variation in the ratio of surface to sub-surface fluoride concentration would be expected, since surface uptake is governed by many independent factors. For instance, YOON et al. (1960a) suggested that the level of fluoride in the enamel surface increases with age to a greater extent than that of the interior. Natural surface imperfections increase uptake (MYERS et al. 1952; LITTLE et al. 1962) and so does mechanical abrasion or acid etching (BRUDEVOLD et al. 1957). The above discrepancies, however, seem more likely due to sampling differences than to any true biological variation. It is clear from the work of BRUDEVOLD et al. (1956) that the gradient of fluoride concentration from surface to interior is steep. The thickness of the "surface" layer analysed will, therefore, crucially affect the result obtained. All analyses so far published have referred to pooled samples of enamel taken from many teeth of mixed age and type; the fluoride concentration of enamel at a specified depth in a single tooth was not determined. Unless this is done, it is not possible to compare accurately the surface concentration of fluoride in enamel of different teeth. A method of doing this has recently been developed. Fig. 7 shows the fluoride concentrations in thin layers of enamel from the labial surface of an upper central incisor. The layers of enamel were removed from the tooth using perchloric acid (Weatherell and Hargreaves 1965). The thickness of each layer is determinable by direct measurement of the ground section of the tooth shown in Fig. 7. The incisor shown was that of a 38 year old male, resident in a district where the fluoride content of the drinking water was < 0.5 ppm. Sufficient teeth have not yet been investigated to establish the pattern of variation in various surfaces of different teeth.

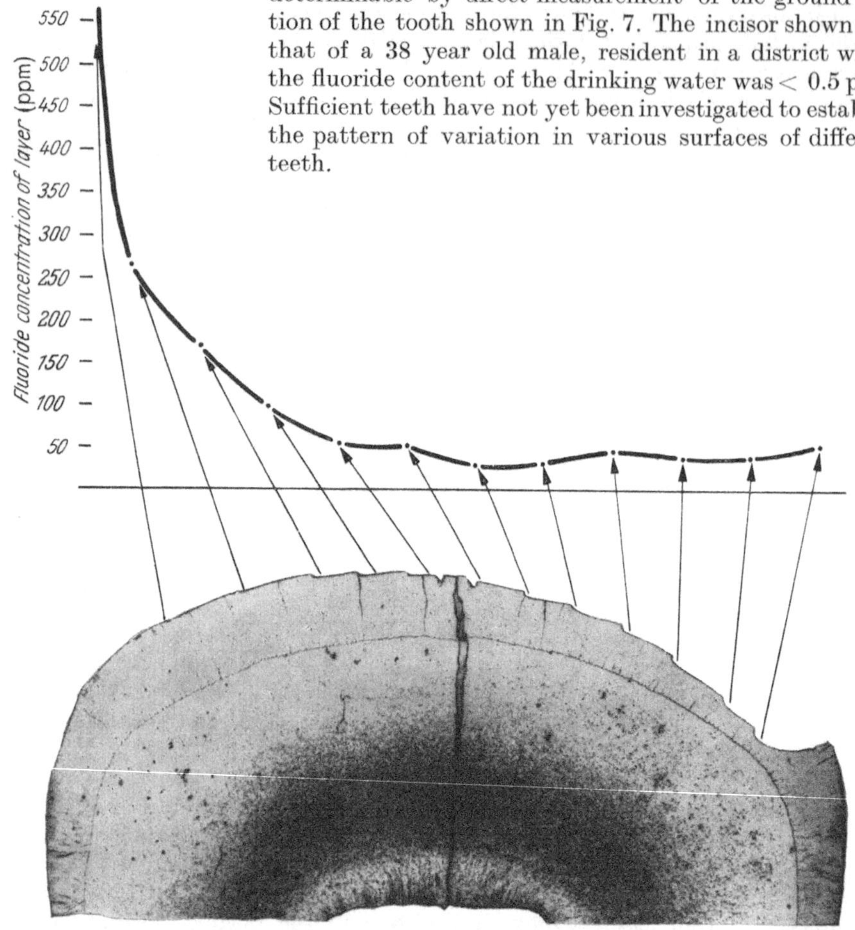

Fig. 7. Fluoride concentrations in layers of enamel removed from the buccal aspect of a human permanent incisor from a 38 year-old male. The thickness of each layer sampled is equal to the depth of the corresponding step in the ground section of the tooth shown. Fluoride content of the drinking water < 0.5 ppm. Magnification of section × 15. (From Weatherell and Hargreaves 1965)

B. Fluoride in dentine

The average concentration of fluoride in dentine is two to three times that of enamel. In permanent teeth the level of dentinal fluoride rises with age (Fig. 8), though the rate of increase gradually diminishes in a manner similar to that of enamel (Jackson and Weidmann 1959). This general trend; a rise in concentration of fluoride in the dental tissues, followed at the age of about 40 years by a reduced rate of increase; has recently been confirmed by Armstrong and Singer (1963).

In human deciduous dentine, however, an initial rise with age seems to be followed by a fall in fluoride concentration. In deciduous teeth from a district with < 0.5 ppm fluoride in the drinking water, the dentinal fluoride level rose from about 130 ppm at the age of 3, to 180 ppm at 7 years and then fell abruptly to about 110 ppm at 12 years (Fig. 9). This is apparently due to the gradual removal of high-fluoride dentine from the pulpal surface by the process of root resorption (HARGREAVES and WEATHERELL 1965).

Dentinal fluoride is not homogeneously distributed throughout the tissue, but, as in bone and enamel, tends to accumulate in surface regions (Fig. 10). The highest concentration is found closest to the pulp chamber (YOON et al. 1960a) where the systemic supply of fluoride is maximal. Thus, in the crown there is a drop in fluoride concentration from the pulpal border to the amelo-dentinal junction. This may be the reason why the gradual resorption of deciduous dentine, outwards from the pulpal region, causes such a dramatic change in the overall concentration of coronal dentinal fluoride and why secondary dentine, slowly forming in the pulp chamber, contains a

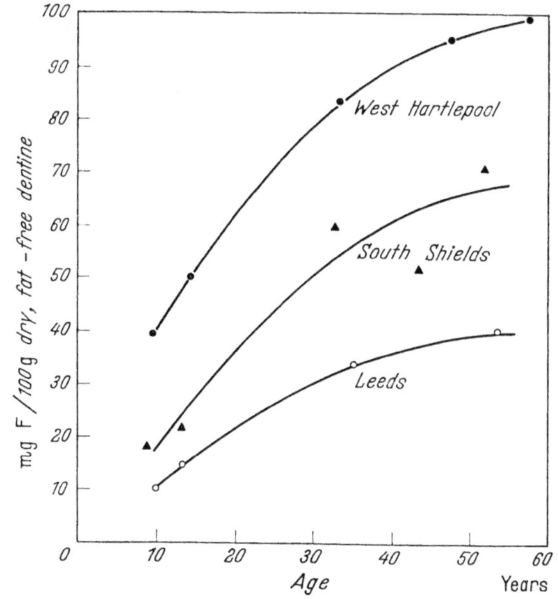

Fig. 8. Relationship between age and fluoride concentration of human premolar dentine. Fluoride in drinking water: LEEDS < 0.5 ppm; S. SHIELDS, 0.8 ppm; W. HARTLEPOOL, 1.9 ppm. (From JACKSON and WEIDMANN 1959)

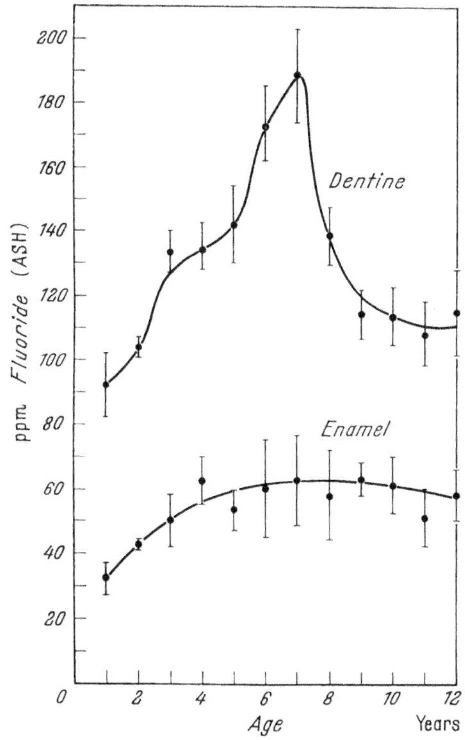

Fig. 9

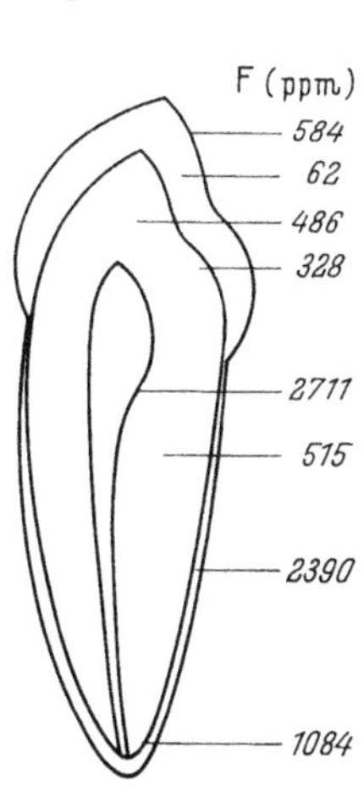

Fig. 10

Fig. 9. Relationship between age and fluoride concentration of human deciduous dentine and enamel from second molar teeth in areas supplied by drinking water containing < 0.5 ppm fluoride. Standard deviations shown in each age group. (From HARGREAVES and WEATHERELL 1965)

Fig. 10. Fluoride concentrations in portions of a tooth. (From YOON et al. 1960b) higher concentration of fluoride (JENKINS and SPEIRS 1954) than the primary structure. In the root of the permanent tooth, there is a high concentration of fluoride at the pulpal surface of dentine and at the external root surface; it is difficult at this point to distinguish between root dentine and cementum.

C. Fluoride in cementum

Cementum has been referred to as the "Cinderella" of the dental tissues; its study has been neglected, perhaps owing to sampling difficulties. From the few analyses carried out, on material which was predominantly cementum (YOON et al. 1960a; SINGER and ARMSTRONG 1962), it seemed that the tissue might contain an average level of fluoride greater than that of any other skeletal or dental structure.

Cementum, although topographically a dental tissue, is structurally more akin to bone. SINGER and ARMSTRONG (1962) investigated the fluoride content of bone and cementum from 11 male cadavers over the age of 49 and found that the fluoride content of cementum correlated well with that of the skeleton. They concluded that a knowledge of cementum fluoride concentration might be of great assistance in an assessment of skeletal levels. Further studies, particularly upon material from younger persons, would have to be carried out to confirm this tentative conclusion but, if true, cementum would provide a convenient means of estimating skeletal fluoride burdens.

Little is known about the way the concentration of cementum fluoride varies with age.

D. Influence of growth and calcification on the fluoride content of dental tissues

Dental tissues, like those of the skeleton, accumulate fluoride most rapidly during the time of formation and mineralisation. The evidence for this comes chiefly from animal experiments. WALLACE-DURBIN (1954) showed that molars of young rats absorbed radioactive fluoride (^{18}F) more readily than those of mature animals and attributed this to a difference in pulpal activity and calcification. She noticed that the incisors of the mature rats, although heavier than those of the younger ones, accumulated ^{18}F to the same extent; presumably due to the fact that rat incisors continue to grow and calcify throughout life. WEIDMANN (1962), in longer-term experiments, compared the uptake of fluoride by the teeth of half-grown cats with those of adult animals and found that the fully formed though less calcified teeth of the younger ones tended to take up more fluoride than those of the adults. The greater fluoride uptake by the teeth of the half-grown animals seemed entirely due to their incomplete mineralisation. Such a difference was not found when teeth from young, half- and fully-grown rabbits were compared; like the rat incisor, rabbit teeth continue to grow and calcify throughout life.

After the periods of growth and calcification are ended, the uptake of fluoride is almost entirely limited to tissue surfaces. In both dentine and enamel the highest level has always been found in marginal regions; *viz.* at the pulpo-dentinal junction, where the blood supply is richest, and at the surface of enamel which, when unerupted, has access to tissue fluid and, when erupted, is bathed in oral fluids. As the tooth matures, penetration to the interior becomes more difficult. The increasing density of the structure presents a diffusion barrier which hinders the passage of fluoride beyond the surface regions and fluoride, being a bone-seeking element, will be absorbed by the outer layers of the tissue. The extent to which each of these factors separately contributes to surface accumulation, is not known.

E. Influence of the level of fluoride ingestion on the fluoride content of dental tissues

The uptake of fluoride by erupted human teeth is independent of cellular function, and the overall fluoride content of the dental tissues is closely related to the level of fluoride ingestion. It was shown that fluoride concentrations in dentine and enamel from teeth of mixed age and type correlated well with the fluoride content of the water supply (McClure and Likins 1951). Though the fluoride level of dentine appears to rise more rapidly than that of enamel as the level of ingested fluoride increases, a general relationship between age of tooth and fluoride content (Figs. 6 and 8) is maintained even at different levels of intake (Jackson and Weidmann 1959).

During the period of formation relatively low levels of fluoride can effect the dentition, producing patches of mottled enamel characteristic of dental fluorosis. It has been established that such enamel contains abnormally high concentrations of fluoride, probably because the affected enamel is undermineralised and has a more open structure, allowing the element to penetrate more easily (Brudevold et al. 1956).

At very high levels of intake, tooth growth might be retarded. Bélanger et al. (1954) demonstrated this in pigs and Jackson (1956), who showed the same effect in rat incisors, found that the decrease in tooth growth reduced the rate of fluoride incorporation.

F. Removal of fluoride from dental tissues

Fluoride may be lost from teeth by resorption or by attrition. In human deciduous dentine the fluoride content rose to a maximum and then fell rapidly before the tooth exfoliated (Fig. 9). The pattern for the dentine of teeth from various sites in the mouth coincided clearly with the known chronological sequence of root resorption prior to exfoliation and the observed drop in fluoride concentration was apparently related to resorption (Hargreaves and Weatherell 1965).

Fluoride loss by attrition was clearly demonstrated by Weidmann (1962) who, after administering fluoride to rats for 30 days, withdrew the source of fluoride for periods of up to 90 days. In this period fluoride disappeared from the continuously growing rat incisors. Already after 60 days, the concentration in the roots was as low as that of the control animals and after a further 30 days it was also normal in the crowns. The loss of fluoride was in this case presumably due to attrition. There was little loss of deposited fluoride during a similar period from the permanent non-growing teeth of the cat.

IV. Mechanism of fluoride uptake and removal

In order to appreciate the factors which influence uptake and retention of fluoride, it is necessary to understand the mechanism by which it enters and accumulates in the skeleton.

Fluoride is entirely associated with the mineral of the hard tissues. It becomes part of the apatite crystal in which it is able to replace certain monovalent groups in the crystal lattice.

A. Uptake by ionic exchange

Many workers have shown that a rise in bone fluoride concentration *in vivo* is accompanied by a fall in the carbonate content of bone mineral. At the same time there appeared to be no alteration in the Ca/P ratio (McCann and Bullock 1957;

Weidmann et al. 1959). The inference was drawn that the fluoride ion is able to replace the bicarbonate group but not the phosphate of bone salt.

The above conclusion, that fluoride ion can replace bicarbonate but not phosphate, agrees with earlier *in vitro* experiments in which bicarbonate ion was shown to compete effectively with fluoride for incorporation into bone mineral (Neuman et al. 1950). Alterations in the Ca/P ratio of the solution in which the bone salt was suspended, however, did not influence fluoride uptake. It was likewise shown that

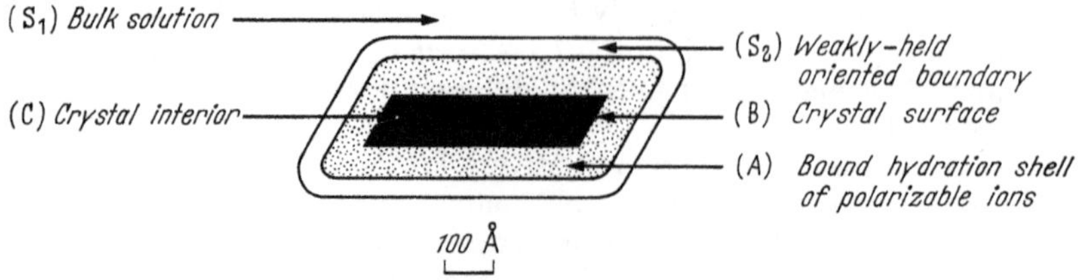

Fig. 11. A diagrammatic representation of a cross-section view of a hydroxyapatite crystal in aqueous suspension. (From Neuman and Neuman 1958)

the absorption of fluoride was influenced by the concentration of hydroxyl ion. Neuman et al. concluded that fluoride probably exchanged with the hydroxyl and bicarbonate of the bone salt crystal, but not with phosphate.

Neuman and Neuman (1958) suggested that fluoride entered the apatite crystal by a three-stage *hetero*-ionic exchange process. The hydroxyapatite of bone mineral exists in the form of extremely small crystallites surrounded by a hydration

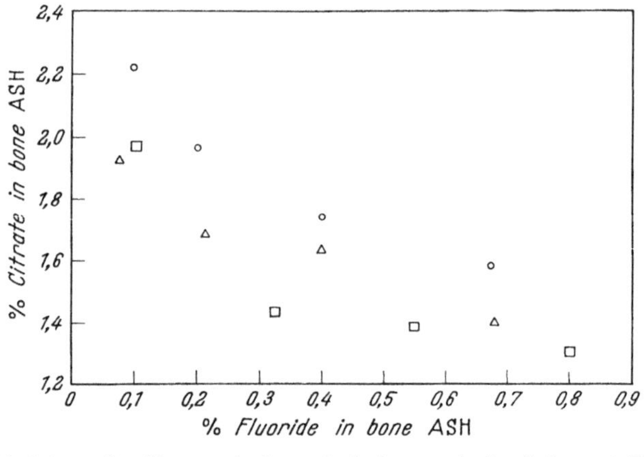

Fig. 12. Relationship between fluoride concentration and citrate concentration in bone. ○ Iliac crest; △ Rib; □ Vertebra. (From Zipkin et al. 1960)

shell (Fig. 11). Fluoride first enters the hydration shell, the ions of which are in dynamic equilibrium with those of the surrounding tissue fluids and with those of the apatite crystal surface. The second stage reaction constitutes an exchange between the fluoride of the hydration shell and a monovalent group at the surface of the apatite crystal. Once it has entered the surface of the apatite crystal, fluoride is more firmly bound. Thirdly, some of the fluoride ions may migrate still further into the apatite crystal as a result of re-crystallisation. Whereas the passage of fluoride ion from hydration shell into the crystal surface is very rapid, this further migration into the crystal interior is, presumably, slow.

An increase in the percentage of fluoride in bone mineral is accompanied by a marked reduction in the citrate content (Fig. 12). Armstrong and Singer (1956) showed *in vitro* that fluoride ions compete with citrate for entry into bone salt. Citrate appears to reside on the surface of the bone salt crystallites (HENDRICKS 1952) and would be readily available for exchange reactions. It seemed likely, therefore, that the decreased citrate content of fluoridated bone was due to its replacement by fluoride (ZIPKIN et al. 1960).

More recently, however, an alternative explanation has been proposed by POSNER et al. (1963) who have found that the X-ray diffraction pattern of bone became sharper as the fluoride content increased. They suggested that this effect was due to an improved mineral crystallinity which might indicate an increase in width and/or the degree of structural perfection of apatite crystals. Thus, the incorporation of fluoride could reduce the surface area available for exchange reactions and so decrease the uptake of citrate and other ions associated with the bone apatite crystal surface.

B. Uptake by deposition

Evidence that fluoride can deposit on the surface of apatite crystals as well as exchange with surface ions, is scanty and somewhat speculative. It has been firmly established, however, that the accumulation of fluoride is accompanied by a rise in the magnesium content of the tissue (McCANN and BULLOCK 1957; WEIDMANN et al. 1959) and it was suggested by the latter authors that this might be due to a precipitation of MgF_2 on the crystal surface. In view of the fact that the solubility of MgF_2 is considerably greater than that of CaF_2, however, which does not usually seem to be formed in fluorosed bone (NEUMAN et al. 1950; LINDEMANN 1956/57), it seems more likely that some other chemical combination occurs. Perhaps some complex form of magnesium fluoro-phosphate is deposited in the hard tissues, though there is no evidence for this.

It is generally considered that the deposition of fluorapatite is not feasible at the very low concentrations of fluoride which must appertain in tissue fluids. There is some evidence, however, from *in vitro* studies (KUYPER and KUTNERIAN 1962) that fluorapatite may precipitate even at concentrations below 3 ppm fluoride. Perhaps as a result of bone resorption, the level of fluoride in tissue fluid might occasionally rise locally to a level sufficient to produce such precipitation.

The available evidence strongly suggests that systemically absorbed fluoride is incorporated into the hard tissues largely by the process of exchange and by incorporation into the apatite lattice during mineralisation of the tissue. Deposition of systemic fluoride by precipitation reactions is probably minimal.

C. Removal of fluoride

Fluoride ions at the surface of the apatite crystal can readily pass into the hydration shell and thereby escape into the tissue fluids. There will be, for instance, rapid *iso*-ionic exchange between crystal-fluoride and the fluoride ions of the hydration shell with no net loss of fluoride from the crystal. BRUDEVOLD et al. (1957) showed that this occurred between fluoride ions present in enamel and radioactive fluoride in the solution in which the teeth were bathed. There will also be exchange between fluoride, bicarbonate and hydroxyl ions and in this way some incorporated fluoride can be lost from the hard tissues. This will be greater as the concentration of fluoride in the crystals increases relative to that in the tissue fluid.

Shortly after its incorporation in the skeleton, some of the deposited fluoride quickly appears in the urine, the remainder is apparently held more firmly by the bone. HODGE (1952) suggested that there were two phases of fluoride removal from the skeleton: (a) a rapid process of the order of weeks, probably involving an ionic exchange escape mechanism and (b) a slower removal, taking years, due not to ionic exchange but to osteoclastic resorption of bone. Plotting the logarithm of fluoride released into urine from the human skeleton against time, he obtained an almost linear relationship and it appeared that in two years about half the absorbed fluoride was removed. While, therefore, some of the incorporated fluoride was rapidly removed by *hetero*-ionic exchange, most was retained until the bone was resorbed. This clear concept of two distinct processes is very attractive, but from the little evidence available it is very difficult to be certain about the mechanism of fluoride removal. The pattern of release could be explained by the single process of osteoclastic resorption. Since the newly incorporated fluoride will remain for a short time near the surfaces of bone, it will be initially very accessible to the osteoclast. Even if osteoclasis were slow, the total fluoride appearing in the urine from all sites of resorption within the skeleton may be appreciable. As the fluoride becomes gradually buried by the subsequent accretion of mineral and by deposition of new bone, progressively less will be released. The initial rapid appearance of fluoride in urine would, thus, seem as readily explainable by cellular as by physico-chemical mechanisms. Both processes are no doubt involved, but there is not enough evidence to decide which is the predominant mechanism concerned with the initial rapid removal of fluoride.

D. Influence of growth and mineralisation on the rate of fluoride uptake

Fluoride uptake is essentially a surface reaction and the element is absorbed most readily where the available surface area of the bone mineral crystals is greatest. In areas of bone growth and mineralisation, apatite crystals tend to be small and their collective surface area correspondingly large. The extensive surface area will promote rapid uptake of fluoride by *hetero*-ionic exchange and the relatively large water content of forming bone, associated presumably with the hydration shells of the apatite crystals, will provide ions with easy access to the crystal surfaces. Both factors contribute to a rapid uptake of fluoride by *hetero*-ionic exchange.

The capacity of fluoride to replace certain ions within the crystal surface also means that the element will be incorporated in the crystal-lattice as it grows. Such inclusion of fluoride during crystal formation, unlike its incorporation by *hetero*-ionic exchange, can only take place during bone salt accretion, while the apatite crystals are forming.

Once mineralisation is complete, the uptake of fluoride is greatly diminished; the surface area of the crystals is reduced, the decrease in water content makes diffusion of the ions to crystal surfaces more difficult and there is no further uptake of fluoride by accretion of bone salt. It is not surprising, therefore, that fluoride has always been shown to react most readily in those regions undergoing growth and where mineralisation is incomplete.

V. Fluorosis

A. Skeletal changes of chronic fluorosis

When fluoride ingestion reaches a critical level the cells of the hard tissues are affected and pathological changes associated with skeletal fluorosis may develop. The most obvious features of this condition are the development of exostosis (Fig. 13) due to a stimulated osteogenesis, and increased bone resorption.

1. Formation of exostotic bone

Early reports of skeletal fluorosis in man described a condition in which ingestion of fluoride caused increased production of bone. MøLLER and GUDJONSON (1932) examined workers employed in a Danish factory who had been exposed to the dust of cryolite, a fluoride-containing aluminium ore. Radiographic examination revealed an apparent increase in the density of some of the bones together with a loss of structural detail. The radiopacity of the vertebrae at first suggested to the authors a possible diagnosis of marble bone disease but subsequent clinical examination showed that the two conditions were different. The contours of the bones were blurred and the ligaments and fibrocartilagenous attachments were the seat of extensive calcification. In extreme cases all bones were affected,

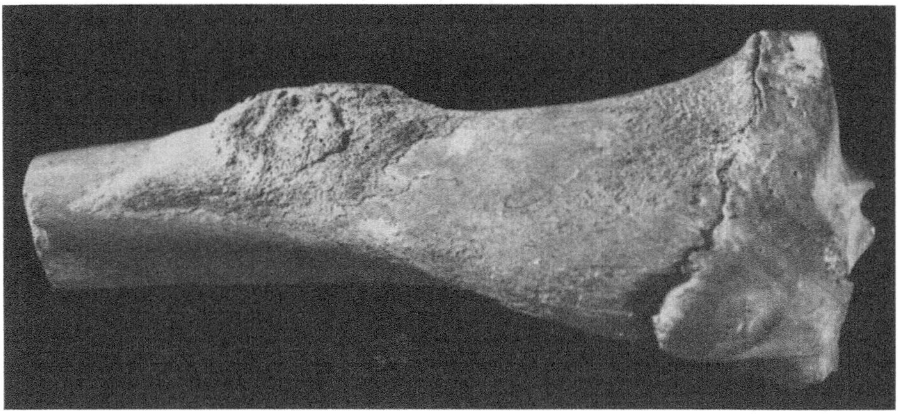

Fig. 13. Localised fluorotic exostosis in sheep tibia. (From WEATHERELL and WEIDMANN 1959)

although the most severe manifestations were always found in the vertebral column and pelvis. No analagous condition had ever arisen through the mere inhalation of silica dust and the toxic factor, it was decided, was fluoride.

ROHOLM (1937), in his classical treatise on fluoride intoxication, described *post mortem* examinations of two workers from the Danish factory. The bones were heavy and hard to saw, they were thickened by the deposition of exostotic bone and the calcification of muscle and tendon attachments. Periosteal surfaces were irregular due to extensive exostosis, the form of which varied from rounded nodules to sharp projections. SHORTT et al. (1937) made similar observations in India, describing ten cases of endemic fluorosis, which resulted from drinking water containing high levels of fluoride. The radiographic outlines of bones were roughened and curious thorn-shaped osteophytes were evident on tibia and fibula. Other descriptions of new fluorotic bone growth relate to investigations on animals subjected to experimental fluorosis and to accounts of spontaneous fluorosis found in cattle and sheep pastured on herbage contaminated with fluoride from the smoke of local factories.

The exostotic outgrowths in both human and animal fluorosis vary greatly in form and distribution. They may grow at sites of muscle and tendon attachment and several authors have attributed their distribution to the local effects of strain. PANDIT et al. (1940), for instance, described how the much used left arm and wrist of Indian basket weavers was particularly susceptible to fluorotic exostosis. There must be other factors than strain governing the distribution of lesions, since fluorotic bone may develop in the medullary cavity, where there are no muscle or tendon attachments, or may form an even layer of new tissue over the whole bone surface (SINGH et al. 1961; WEATHERELL and WEIDMANN 1959).

The new fluorotic bone is not normal; its arrangement bears little resemblance to the Haversian bone upon which it is formed and sometimes consists almost entirely of unreplaced primary bone. In the two factory workers examined *post mortem* by ROHOLM (1937), osteones had been formed but the arrangement of the Haversian systems was very irregular. The fluorotic exostoses of experimental animals, or of farm animals with spontaneous chronic fluorosis, frequently contain large tracts of woven bone with little lamellar replacement (WEATHERELL and WEIDMANN 1959). The capacity of fluoride to stimulate bone formation has, nevertheless, led to the administration of fluoride to counter the catabolic changes of osteoporosis and Paget's disease (RICH and ENSINCK 1961; PURVES 1962). Some interesting results have been obtained but the conclusions of these authors rest upon clinical data alone; it would be of advantage to know what histological alterations such treatment produced in the bones.

2. Bone resorption

Extensive production of exostotic bone is usually accompanied by increased resorption. Sometimes this feature is more obvious than the bone formation, with which it appears to be invariably associated. It has been suggested that resorption is the primary lesion and that apposition of exostotic bone is an attempt to reinforce a weakened bone (WEINMANN and SICHER 1955). This explanation is teleological and unsatisfactory; the exostotic 'reinforcement' does not always coincide with and support the regions weakened by resorption (BAUER 1945) and sometimes both bone formation and destruction proceed side by side to produce a weakened tissue as in Paget's disease. Some observations made on experimental animals showed that exostosis may occasionally develop without visible bone resorption, whereas resorption was not observed in the absence of new exostotic bone (WEATHERELL and WEIDMANN 1959). These authors, therefore, suggested that exostosis rather than bone resorption is the primary lesion of skeletal fluorosis. The sudden demand for bone mineral by the rapidly forming exostotic bone might be considerable and bone resorption the physiological response by which mineral is provided.

The balance in fluorosis between resorption and formation varies considerably. In man, the few detailed histological descriptions and the radiographic evidence suggest that the bias is more towards bone formation than destruction. This fact has given rise to such expressions as 'fluorine osteosclerosis' (WILKIE 1940). In animal studies, resorption is often more pronounced than formation, but the distinction between animals and man is not well defined and may be merely a function of age, dosage and duration of ingestion. For instance, in very young dogs, given 1 g NaF per day, KELLNER (1939) noticed periosteal apposition of new bone with rapid osteoclastic destruction of the original bone cortex advancing from the marrow cavity. In older (2–4 month) dogs resorption was less apparent, and in the oldest group osteoblastic activity seemed to predominate. BAUER (1945), experimenting upon dogs of various ages, also found that osteoclastic resorption of both cancellous and compact bone was particularly pronounced in young animals but always lagged behind the osteoblastic activity of the periosteum. In older animals resorption gave way to endosteal bone formation. It seems that fluoride-induced resorption is more pronounced in young growing bone than in the less active hard tissues of older animals. This dependence of the resorption-formation balance upon age may account for the emphasis laid upon formation in descriptions of spontaneous fluorosis in man; the majority of individuals in whom fluorotic lesions have been discovered and described have been non-growing adults.

B. Dental changes of chronic fluorosis

During tooth formation, the cells of the dental tissues, particularly the ameloblasts, are very sensitive to fluoride. At relatively low dosage, small spots of discolouration may form in the tooth surface. These spots of dental 'mottling' vary in colour from paper-white to dark brown; the staining of the fluorotic imperfections presumably depends upon conditions in the mouth. They can be so small that they are perceptible only to the eye of the trained dentist, or sufficiently pronounced to disfigure the appearance of the dentition. Teeth are more susceptible to fluoride than bone and changes in enamel are produced at levels of fluoride intake at which no skeletal effects have been recorded. Very low dosages only affect the tooth's appearance and have no detrimental effect on its form. At higher levels, however, the cells may be affected and the tooth structure severely altered. The surface of enamel is no longer smooth but thrown into the hypoplastic corrugations so frequently associated with a disturbance of amelogenesis (DIAMOND and WEINMANN 1940). These effects are only apparent when fluoride is ingested during the period of formation and calcification. After the tooth has erupted and calcification is complete any amount of fluoride may be ingested without adverse dental consequences.

Several experimental animal studies have been carried out to establish the nature of the dental reaction to fluoride. In the incisor teeth of the rat the first noticeable change is the irregular removal of the characteristic brown pigment from the labial surface. The pigment is due to the presence of iron and it was shown that its removal is associated with anaemia and increased iron excretion (PINDBORG et al. 1946). The irregularity of the changes in pigmentation and the failure of dietary supplements of iron to relieve bleaching, however, suggested that the defect lay in the ameloblasts; under the influence of fluoride they are no longer able to utilise the available iron. FLEMING (1953) presented strong evidence that fluoride interfered with cellular function. He studied the effect of fluoride upon the cells of rat teeth and of tooth germs implanted into mice and guinea pigs. The administration of relatively low levels of fluoride to the rats and to the hosts of the tooth germs caused a delay in the calcification of dentine and enamel. The walls of ameloblasts became thickened, their nuclei elongated and their orderly arrangement was disrupted. Eventually, the cytoplasm of both odontoblasts and ameloblasts disappeared and only cell walls and ruptured nuclei remained. The capacity of the ameloblasts and odontoblasts to produce a calcifiable matrix was thus destroyed.

C. Effect of fluoride on calcification

1. Evidence of interference with calcification

Most of the descriptions of human skeletal fluorosis were based upon radiographic examination. The increased radiopacity, almost invariably present in clinical radiographs, has come to be regarded as one of the main features of the condition and the term 'osteosclerosis' has, for this reason, been frequently associated with fluorosis. Unusually high skeletal mineralisation has been demonstrated in ground sections of bone from fluorotic rats (RÖCKERT 1963) and regions of very high mineral density can be seen adjacent to lowly calcified areas in the bones of rabbits with chronic skeletal fluorosis (Fig. 14). The increased density of clinical radiographs is often due, however, not to an increase in bone density or degree of mineralisation but to exostotic thickening of bone. Authors seem

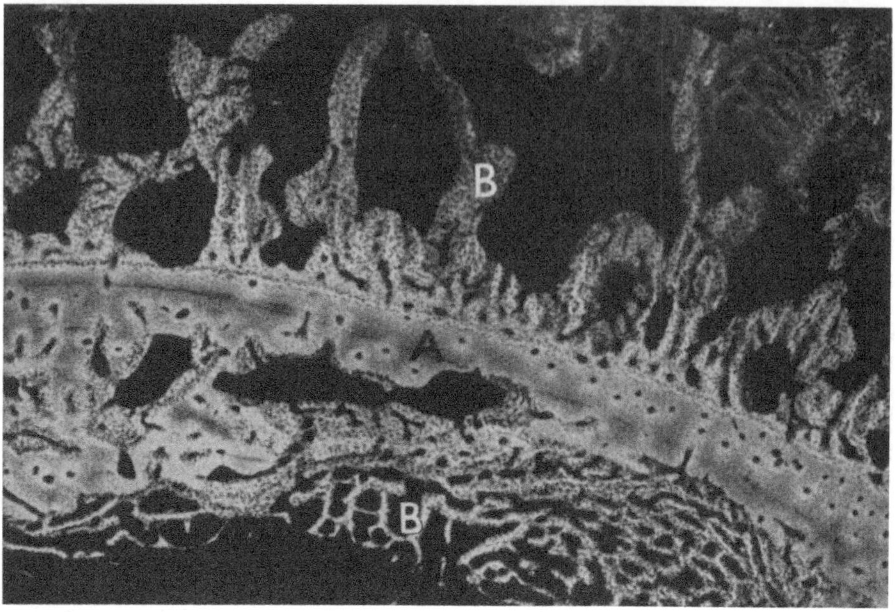

Fig. 14. Microradiograph of cross-section of midshaft tibia from rabbit with chronic skeletal fluorosis, showing adjacent areas of high and low mineralisation. Rabbit given 500 ppm fluoride in drinking water *ad libitum*, for 98 days
A = original cortex B = exostotic outgrowths Magnification × 40 (WEATHERELL unpublished).

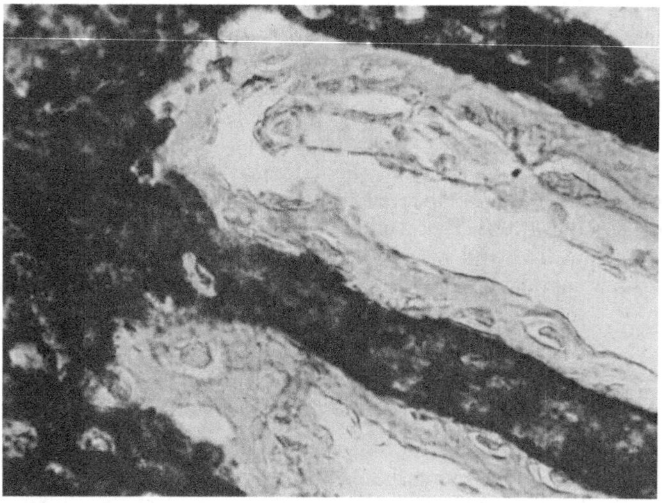

Fig. 15. Wide seams of uncalcified osteoid upon trabeculae of "woven" bone in fluorotic exostosis from sheep metatarsus. Von Kóssa stain × 270 (From WEATHERELL and WEIDMANN 1959).

occasionally to have ignored this fact and have interpreted increased radiopacity as an increase in the physical density or degree of calcification of the skeleton.

Fluorotic bone is frequently found to be less dense and less mineralised than normal (SCHWYZER 1914; WOLFF and KERR 1938; WEATHERELL and WEIDMANN 1959). This is partly due to the type of bone of which exotoses consist but there is also a good deal of evidence to show that at high levels of ingestion, fluoride may interfere with and retard mineralisation.

Several observations suggest that the pattern and process of calcification in both skeletal and in dental tissues is abnormal. For instance, numerous workers (*e.g.* KELLNER 1939; ROHOLM 1937) have described the presence of wide seams of uncalcified osteoid in fluorotic bone of animals and man (Fig. 15). In normal bone, newly formed osteoid calcifies almost immediately and unmineralised seams are rare. The wide osteoid borders of skeletal fluorosis indicate a delay in mineralisation of newly formed tissue.

Several workers have described the presence of abnormal mineral-like deposits in both calcified and decalcified sections of fluorotic bones, teeth and cartilage. There is no general agreement about their nature. It has been repeatedly suggested that they consist of or contain CaF_2 (*e.g.* SCHOUR and SMITH 1935; BÉLANGER et al. 1958). It seems improbable that the concentration of fluoride in tissue fluid could reach sufficiently high levels to precipitate CaF_2, however. ROHOLM (1937) held the opinion that fluoride produced the irregular granular deposits by affecting bone matrix, thus causing normal bone mineral to deposit in an irregular fashion. The cause and composition of these fluorotic granules remains unclear.

Developing teeth are very sensitive to fluoride and their calcification may be rapidly and markedly affected. SCHOUR and SMITH (1935) showed how less than forty-eight hours after a single injection of sodium fluoride, a line of disturbed mineralisation could be detected. Several authors (*e.g.* YAEGER and EISENMANN 1963) have shown adjacent bands of high and low mineralisation in growing teeth, each pair of bands resulting from a single injection of fluoride. FLEMING (1953. demonstrated a retardation in the calcification of rat teeth and BÉLANGER et al (1954) using an autoradiographic technique, found a disturbance of calcium deposition in the dentine of fluorosed pig incisors. Injected ^{45}Ca normally forms a smooth line of radioactivity which moves outwards from the pulp chamber towards the amelo-dentinal junction. In the fluoride-fed pigs, the band of ^{45}Ca became wavy in the dentine and progressed towards the outer border at an abnormally slow rate. The authors, very reasonably, attributed this altered pattern of ^{45}Ca incorporation to a cellular defect caused by fluoride ion. FLEMING (1953) also felt that the calcification defects were secondary to an alteration in structure and function of the odontogenic cells.

2. Mechanism of fluoride interference with calcification

There have been many suggestions as to the means whereby fluoride interferes with the normal development and calcification of the hard tissues. Large amounts of fluoride act as a general poison and some of the observed phenomena may result from a reduced growth rate and not be connected with defective calcification. For instance, a change in the orderly arrangement of cells of the epiphyseal plate (COMAR et al. 1953) might be due to a general reduction in the rate of proliferation of chondrocytes. The more slowly proliferating cells around secondary ossification centres in normal epiphyses calcify, and yet are not arranged in columns. Other changes in the fluorotic matrix are possibly more closely linked with the observed delay in calcification and the abnormalities in bone salt deposition.

a) Effect of fluoride upon the calcifiability of the organic matrix

The specific factors which confer the property of calcifiability upon a tissue are not known, but attention has been increasingly directed to the nature of the organic matrix. It is believed that some organisational or chemical characteristic of the tissue is partly responsible for its ability to calcify. Many specific suggestions have been made, some of which involve the participation of acid mucopolysaccharides, which seem to be rapidly synthesised wherever calcification takes place, or collagen, the principal fibrous protein in all hard tissues of mesodermal origin.

In attempting to explain the defective calcification of fluorotic tissues, considerable emphasis has been placed upon the possibility that the matrix produced under the influence of fluoride is abnormal. JOHNSON (1952) argued that fluorotic bone matrix did not have the visual texture of normal osteoid. It was granular and lumpy and its collagen and polysaccharide components did not stain clearly. BÉLANGER et al. (1958) reported an apparent decrease in the polysaccharide content of fluorosed skeletal tissues from young pigs. When staining with toluidine blue they found a considerable reduction in metachromasia; bone trabeculae, which are normally metachromatic, hardly stained at all and cartilage was violet-blue instead of the usual magenta colour. Osteoid had lost practically all its P.A.S. reaction. WUTHIER and IRVING (1962) showed that the ingestion of fluoride by rats induced a spreading of the zone of Sudan black B stain normally associated with calcification of hard tissues. Fluoride seemed to have inhibited the formation of the sudanophilic substance thus preventing or delaying the initiation of calcification.

It could be argued that the metachromatic and P.A.S. changes observed by BÉLANGER et al. (1958) were non-specific. Reduced metachromasia might result, for instance, merely from a decreased sulphation or a masking of the acid groups of chondroitin. P.A.S. reactions are notoriously unreliable. The diffuse sudanophilia noted by WUTHIER and IRVING (1962) could result from a change in the structure of the dentine matrix. Although the interpretation of observed staining reactions is, therefore, not clear, both groups of workers have clearly demonstrated changes in the calcifying matrices of bones and teeth associated with the ingestion of fluoride.

b) Effect of fluoride upon enzyme systems associated with calcification

Ingested fluoride might interfere with the formation and mineralisation of the hard tissues by inhibiting enzymes concerned with the extracellular calcification of the matrix, the transport of metabolites across the cell wall; or the synthesis of matrix precursors within the cell. The element has been shown *in vitro* to inhibit a large number of enzymes; probably by forming magnesium-fluoro-phosphate complexes, thus depriving the enzyme of its activating Mg^{2+} ion, or by complexing with the protein.

There have been several specific suggestions but none of them have been either proved or disproved. Alkaline phosphatase, repeatedly implicated in the many speculations about the mechanism of calcification, has received considerable attention. The evidence indicates that ingestion of high levels of fluoride for a prolonged period produces increased serum or plasma alkaline phosphatase activity (*e.g.* SHORTT et al. 1937; WEIDMANN et al. 1959).

In these studies the tacit assumption has been made that increased serum alkaline phosphatase activity reflected a stimulated osteogenesis in the fluorotic skeleton. This is not unreasonable, for in the majority of conditions involving extensive growth of hard tissues and in others, where there is extensive elaboration of connective tissue fibres, an accompanying rise in the serum or plasma activity of the enzyme has been reported. Increased serum alkaline phosphatase activity is, nevertheless, no real indication of the effect of fluoride upon the activity of the enzyme within the bone itself. DE EDS (1936) investigated 'bone phosphatase' of fluorotic rats. Here a significant reduction in activity was found. This work does not seem to have been repeated, however.

Cellular mechanisms are undoubtedly involved in calcification. The biochemical integrity of the cell seems to be an indispensible part of the process and inhibition of intracellular enzymes can reduce *in vitro* deposition of bone salt. GUTMAN and YU (1950) demonstrated that the mineralisation of mildly rachitic rat cartilage was blocked by a 1.9 ppm solution of fluoride. This was attributed to the effect of the element upon the glycolotic enzyme enolase which catalyzes the conversion of 2-P-glyceric acid to phosphopyruvic acid. Other workers (PHILLIPS et al. 1934) have indicated that the oxidase activity of certain tissues is inhibited *in vivo* by the ingestion of fluoride. Such a reaction in cartilage would affect its calcification (WHITEHEAD and WEIDMANN 1959).

The cellular activity of the hard tissues is visibly affected by high fluoride intake but it has not been conclusively demonstrated that the element inhibits their enzyme systems *in vivo*. There are two overwhelming difficulties. Firstly, the relative importance and function of enzymes present in calcifying tissues is not clear. Secondly, the concentrations of fluoride ion at the sites of mineralisation are not known. Changes in the activities of the enzyme spectrum of the skeletal tissues will only be convincing when means are found of rapidly investigating them directly in tissue removed from the fluorotic animal.

c) Effect of fluoride upon apatite crystal formation

It is known that the incorporation of fluoride into hydroxy-apatite induces slight changes in the apatite crystal and several authors have speculated upon the possible physiological significance of such alterations. The investigations of POSNER et al. (1963) suggested that the fluoridated-apatite crystals are wider and/or more perfectly formed than normal. It seems unlikely that such changes could interfere with the process of mineralisation once the crystals have been formed. It is possible, however, that the presence of fluoride in the tissue fluid from which apatite crystallises might affect the rate or extent of mineralisation. Experiments have been carried out *in vitro* to test this hypothesis. KUTNERIAN and KUYPER (1957) found that fluoride ion could inhibit the formation of apatite crystals even at a fluoride concentration as low as 0.2 ppm. TAVES and NEUMAN (1963) approached more closely to *in vivo* conditions by studying the effect of fluoride upon the mineralisation of native collagen at $Ca \cdot PO_4$ ionic products within the physiological range. They found that fluoride could either inhibit or enhance the mineralisation of collagen *in vitro*. The principal factor which decided what effect the fluoride had, was the $Ca \cdot PO_4$ product. If this was below the normal value for adult human serum, *e.g.* below 10 mg % total calcium and 4 mg % phosphate, the presence of 0.14 ppm fluoride enhanced apatite deposition. If the $Ca \cdot PO_4$ ionic product was high, however, mineralisation was inhibited. In normal *in vivo* conditions, fluoride might, therefore, act as a governer, minimising the effects of fluctuations in tissue phosphate levels. If the phosphate concentration of the tissue fluid fell, so that the $Ca \cdot PO_4$ ionic product was lowered, fluoride would enhance mineralisation, whereas if the phosphate level rose, mineralisation would be inhibited. In normal physiological circumstances, the concentration of fluoride present in adult human serum (about 0.15 ppm) would, therefore, have no net effect upon bone salt deposition. TAVES and NEUMAN (1963) suggested, however, that the abnormal mineralisation pattern of skeletal fluorosis might be explained by this dual effect of fluoride upon apatite crystal formation.

A lack of knowledge about possible fluctuations in calcium, phosphate and fluoride levels within tissue fluids prevents a full assessment of this very interesting speculation. The primary effect of excessive fluoride ingestion, however, appears to be upon the cells of the hard tissues; ameloblasts and odontoblasts are visibly defective and osteoblasts are abnormally active. It seems likely that the observed histological changes, including the calcification anomalies, seen in the fluorotic matrices of teeth and bones are principally the result of this cellular pathology. While the extra-cellular effect of fluoride upon apatite nucleation and crystallisation may account for some of the changes in tissue mineralisation, the wide seams of uncalcified osteoid present in rapidly and irregularly formed exostoses and the disorganisation in formation and mineralisation of dental tissues involves a direct interference with intra-cellular metabolism.

VI. Amounts of fluoride associated with fluorosis

A number of factors influence the sensitivity of the organism towards fluoride. Species differences, rate of growth, state of nutrition, general health and physical activity all contribute towards the individual's susceptibility to fluoride poisoning. Climatic conditions will affect the amount of food and water ingested and the composition of the diet will control the efficiency of fluoride absorption from the gastro-intestinal tract. Several of these factors have been mentioned, but nothing has been said about the dosage of fluoride likely to produce fluorosis. McCLURE (1933) felt there was such a multiplicity of variable factors that a study of comparative data was of little value. Since then, however, a vastly increased amount of information has emerged from many studies of fluoride toxicity, inspired largely by the intention of public authorities to add fluoride to the drinking water. Numerous surveys investigated the effects of different concentrations of fluoride upon the dental tissues and many radiographic studies have been made of bone changes associated with various levels of fluoride ingestion. It is now possible to draw definite broad conclusions about the concentrations of fluoride associated with fluorosis.

A. Levels of fluoride ingestion

Total intake includes both dietary and water-borne fluoride. Occasionally, investigational errors have arisen by neglecting to take into account all the sources of the element. HODGE and SMITH (1954) mention an instance where the supposedly 'normal' diet of experimental mice contained much more fluoride than the water which was intended to be the experimental fluoride source. The water contained 0.44 ppm and the 'non-fluoride' food 42 ppm. Similarly, some of the cases of human endemic fluorosis in India may well have resulted not only from the alleged concentration of fluoride in the drinking water, but by ingestion of unaccountable amounts of fluoride-containing rock dust suspended in the water and present in the diet (PANDIT et al. 1940). In America and Europe, estimates of the amount of fluoride present in the diet vary within fairly narrow ranges. In an American study, McCLURE and ZIPKIN (1958) estimated that 0.2 to 0.3 mg dietary fluoride is taken daily. HODGE (1963) puts the dietary contribution in Britain higher, at 1.3 to 1.8 mg per day; much of this being due to a high consumption of tea (LONGWELL 1957). Despite the somewhat variable background of dietary fluoride, the relationship between the level of fluoride in the drinking water and the average incidence of fluorosis is fairly clear.

1. Dental fluorosis

Dental fluorosis is only possible when fluoride is ingested while the ameloblast is active during the brief period of tooth formation. Thus, the condition can develop in man only during the first eight to ten years of life. No amount of ingested fluoride can adversely affect the dentition once the ameloblasts have ceased to function.

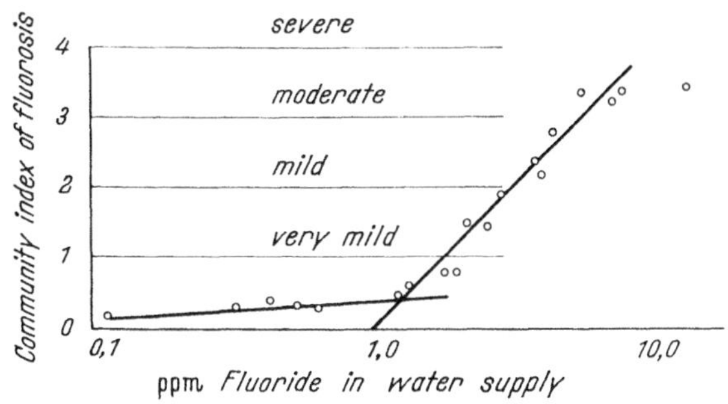

Fig. 16. Relationship between fluoride concentration of drinking water and the community index of dental fluorosis (From HODGE and SMITH 1954)

During the period of odontogenesis, teeth are affected by much lower concentrations of fluoride than bones. DEAN (1934) arbitrarily divided the appearances of dental fluorosis into seven degrees of severity. Later, a 'community index' of dental fluorosis was introduced (DEAN et al. 1935) and the distribution of fluorotic lesions has been studied in different communities.

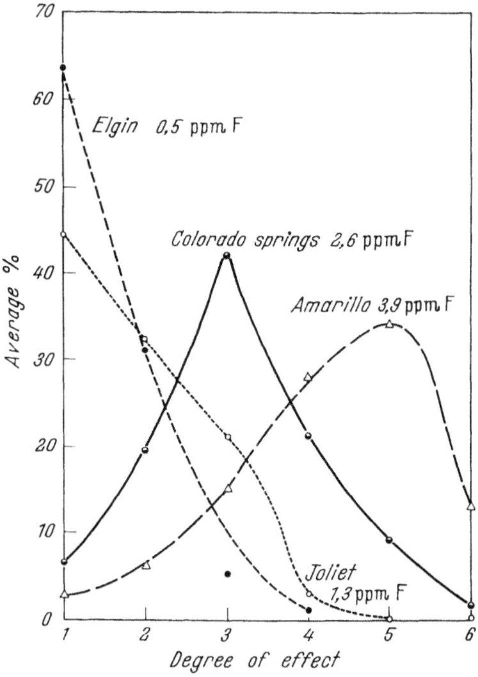

Fig. 17. Distribution of dental fluorotic lesions, of different degrees of severity, in four communities with various concentrations of fluoride in their water supply. (From HODGE and SMITH 1954)

Reviewing this work, HODGE and SMITH (1954) illustrated the precise linear relationship over a range of fluoride levels between the logarithm of water fluoride concentration and the community fluorosis index (Fig. 16). The community index clearly provides only an average assessment. A single group ingesting the same supply of high-fluoride drinking water will include some individuals with no dental lesions and others whose teeth are markedly fluorosed. HODGE and SMITH (1954) elegantly illustrated the distribution of lesions within four different communities. They pointed out how the transformation of one distribution curve into the next can be accomplished by 'lifting' the centre of the curve upwards and to the right (Fig. 17). Below 0.5 ppm fluoride no significant effects on the enamel have been usually observed, but between 0.5 and 1 ppm, 5 to 10 % of persons develop a mild form of mottling which is not aesthetically displeasing but which the trained eye can detect. Between 2 and 3 ppm fluoride, over 50 % of individuals may have defects, some developing only a slight opaqueness, others exhibiting brown mottling. Moderate to severe fluorosis, when the actual form of the teeth may be altered by marked hypoplasia and where the opaque areas and brown stains may be accompanied by severe confluent pitting of the enamel surface, does not usually occur below 2 ppm. At 4 ppm, less than 5 % of the teeth are normal; almost half have moderate or severe fluorosis and 12 % show severe symptoms. At 6 ppm no teeth are without some symptoms and over 50 % of them

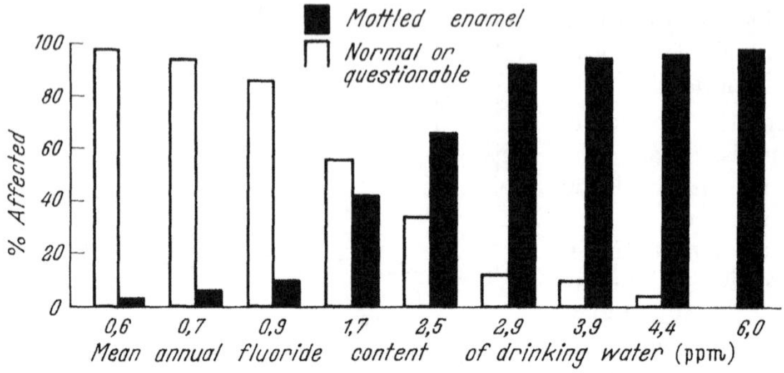

Fig. 18. Relationship between the incidence of dental fluorosis, including lesions of low severity, and the fluoride content of drinking water. (From DEAN 1936)

show a moderate to severe response. The percentage of populations affected by dental fluorosis, including persons with only very slight mottling, at different levels of water fluoridation, is shown in Fig. 18.

2. Skeletal fluorosis

There have been many investigations into the possible hazards to the skeleton of a prolonged ingestion of low concentrations of fluoride. Below 4 ppm even lifelong ingestion seems to have no deleterious effects. WEIDMANN et al. (1963) observed no evidence of skeletal fluorosis in ribs from thirty residents of West Hartlepool, where the drinking water contained 1.9 ppm fluoride. GEEVER et al. (1958) were similarly unable to discover histological differences between the bones of persons from a "non-fluoride" area and 37 individuals who had ingested 1 to 4 ppm fluoride for 36 to 90 years.

Most of the recorded evidence of skeletal fluorosis has been obtained radiographically. Changes in the radiographic appearance of the fluorotic skeleton have often been so marked that this means has been used to measure the incidence of the disease. While the radiograph lacks the sensitivity of histological examination and may well fail to detect borderline cases, the whole skeleton of large numbers of individuals can be examined. Coupled, as it usually is, with clinical studies, the radiograph provides a fairly reliable means of detecting significant adverse effects of excessive fluoride ingestion.

From 170000 radiographs of spine and pelvis, STEVENSON and WATSON (1957) reported 23 cases of skeletal fluorosis. The radiographs were mainly of persons from Texas and Oklahoma, where a large number of communities drank water containing 0.7 ppm or more fluoride. The 23 individuals were found to have ingested water with a fluoride content of 4 to 8 ppm. The fluoride content of the water supply was as low as 4 ppm in only one of these 23 cases and this seems to be the only skeletal fluorosis reported in the literature at this low level of fluorida-

Table 1. *Relationship between fluoride ingested in drinking water and the number of radiographically detectable skeletal lesions*

Locality and reference	Fluoride ingested in drinking water	Exposure (years)	No. of Persons examined	No. of Persons with skeletal lesions
Oklahoma (BLUE 1938)	1—2 ppm	—	25	0
Kempton (HODGES et al. 1941)	1.2—3 ppm	0—61	86	0
Bureau (HODGES et al. 1941)	2.5 ppm	18—68	31	0
Lubbock (MCCAULEY and MCCLURE 1954)	3.5—4.5 ppm	7—14	690	0
Amarillo (MCCAULEY and MCCLURE 1954)	3.3—6.2 ppm	7—14	591	0
Texas and Oklahoma (STEVENSON and WATSON 1957)	4—8 ppm	44—85	—	23
Bartlett (DEAN 1944)	8 ppm	—	114	13
Pampas (CAPIZZANO et al. 1940)	16 ppm	—	178	21
Southern India (PANDIT et al. 1940)	5—24 mg/day	—	1192	387

tion. MCCAULEY and MCCLURE (1954) studied the effect of drinking water containing 3.5 to 6.2 ppm fluoride upon the formation of children's wrists. They could find no radiological evidence of any effect upon calcification of the carpal bones or upon their growth and development. At 8 ppm fluoride, however, there have been several reports of radiological changes in the skeleton. LEONE et al. (1955) made a ten-year study of 116 persons in Bartlett, where the fluoride content of the water

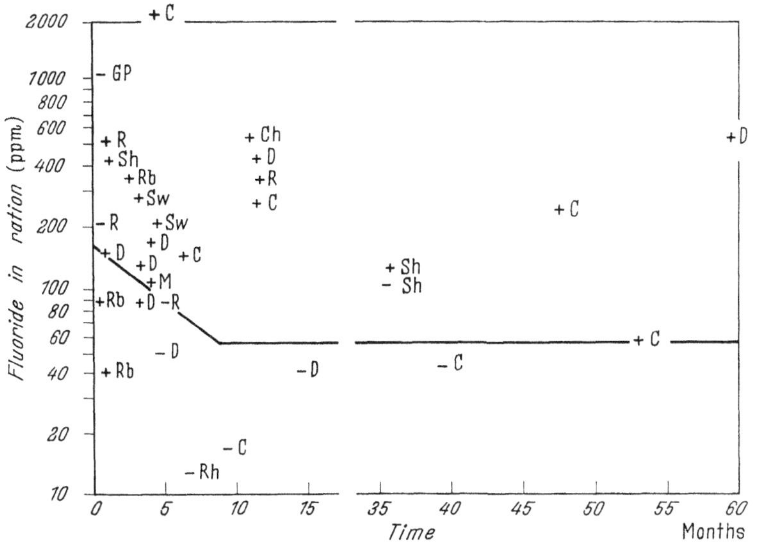

Fig. 19. Development of fluorotic symptoms in various species of animals. C, cattle; Ch, chicken; D, dog; GP, guinea pig; M, monkey; R, rat; Rb, rabbit; Sh, sheep; Sw, swine. (From HODGE and SMITH 1954)

supply was 8 ppm. They found slight bony changes in about 10 to 15 % of those exposed to fluoride. The great majority of individuals were apparently unaffected by this relatively high level of fluoride ingestion. Even at a level of 16 ppm fluoride only about 18 % of a population showed skeletal changes (CAPIZZANO et al. 1940). At higher levels than this, the ingestion of fluoride becomes a more serious problem. Table 1 gives some data relating approximate levels of fluoride ingestion to the number of recorded instances of radiographic changes.

The animal skeleton seems less sensitive than man's to fluoride. SUTTIE et al. (1964) believed that the chick was especially resistant. They estimated fluoride levels as high as 5 ppm in chick serum and suggested that the species possessed a very efficient cellular mechanism for dealing with the element. HODGE and SMITH (1954) concluded from a considerable amount of data that 50 ppm dietary fluoride was an approximate level below which skeletal changes in animals are unlikely (Fig. 19). If the duration of exposure is short, much higher levels of fluoride might be tolerated. There are, perhaps, several species differences in the reaction to fluoride (see PEIRCE 1939) but with the inadequate information about the absolute amounts of fluoride ingested, reliable comparisons of the sensitivity of different species are very difficult to make.

B. Urinary level of fluoride as an index of toxicity

MCCLURE and KINSER (1944) found that the concentration of fluoride in human urine bore a linear relationship to the fluoride content of the domestic water supply. The fluoride level in urine from over 1900 men and boys reflected the content of their drinking water with a surprising consistency (Fig. 20). These authors also showed how urinary fluoride levels corresponded almost exactly to a

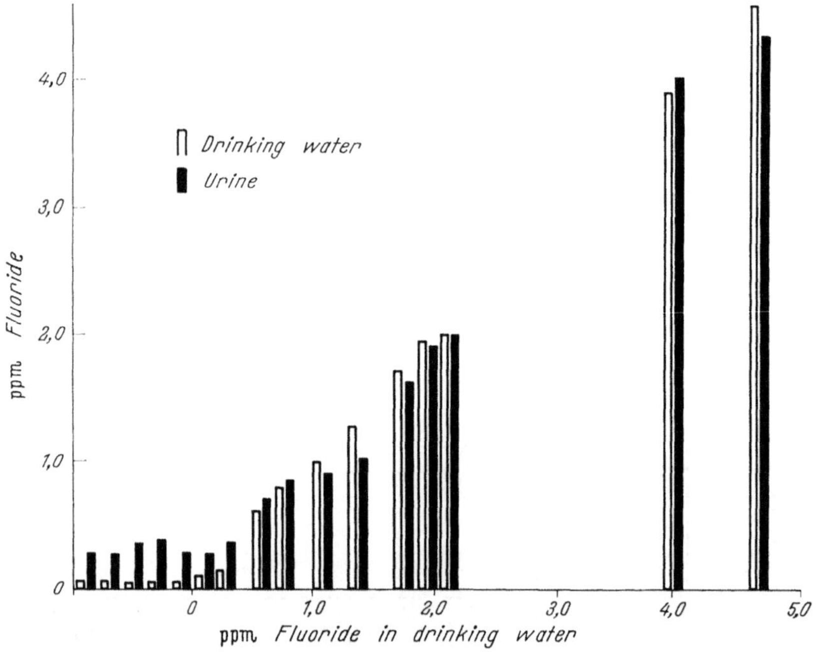

Fig. 20. Relationship between fluoride concentration of drinking water and fluoride concentration of the urine (From MCCLURE and KINSER 1944)

changing water supply as one of the authors moved from place to place (Table 2). The level of urinary fluoride thus gives an indication of the level of ingestion and its measurement provides a useful means of checking and preventing harmful levels of intake. This is unnecessary when the amounts of ingested fluoride are known but when fluoride is being inhaled as HF, or taken involuntarily as dust from fluoride containing rocks, the measurement of urinary fluoride becomes a useful and simple safeguard against the development of fluorosis Drinking water

Table 2. *Variation in the urinary fluoride concentration of one individual as he moved from place to place.* (From McClure and Kinser 1944)

Location	Date (1943)	Fluorine in drinking water (ppm)	Fluorine in urine (ppm)	Comment
Washington, D.C.	Jan. 12	0.0	0.4	24-hour collection
	Jan. 13	0	0.2	
	Jan. 14	0	0.3	
	June 29	0	0.4	
	June 30	0	0.3	
	July 1	0	0.4	
Lubbock, Tex.	July 6	3.8	3.9	First 18 hours in Lubbock
	July 7	3.8	3.9	Second 24 hours in Lubbock
	July 8	3.8	4.0	Third 24 hours in Lubbock
	July 9	3.8	3.5	Fourth 24 hours in Lubbock
	July 11	3.8	3.8	Sixth day in Lubbock, night urine
	July 13	3.8	3.5	Eighth day in Lubbock, night urine
	July 15	3.8	3.6	Tenth day in Lubbock, night urine
	July 17	3.8	3.5	Twelfth day in Lubbock, night urine
Galesburg, Ill.	Oct. 21	1.9	1.8	First day in Galesburg, night urine
	Oct. 22	1.9	1.8	Second day in Galesburg, night urine
	Oct. 23	1.9	1.3	Third day in Galesburg, night urine
	Oct. 24	1.9	2.4	Fourth day in Galesburg, night urine
Quincy, Ill.	Oct. 25	0.1	0.5	First day in Quincy, night urine
	Oct. 26	0.1	0.4	Second day in Quincy, night urine
	Oct. 27	0.1	0.5	Third day in Quincy, night urine
Galesburg, Ill.	Oct. 28	1.9	1.7	First day in Galesburg, night urine
	Oct. 31	1.9	1.1	Fourth day in Galesburg, night urine
Monmouth, Ill.	Nov. 2	1.7	1.0	Second day in Monmouth, night urine
	Nov. 3	1.7	2.1	Third day in Monmouth, night urine
Aurora, Ill.	Nov. 6	1.0	1.1	Third day in Aurora, night urine
Elgin, Ill.	Nov. 10	0.7	0.7	Fourth day in Elgin, night urine

containing less than 8 ppm fluoride is not a serious hazard, so that if the urinary concentration of fluoride is less than 8 ppm, no skeletal fluorosis would be anticipated. Irwin (*in* Hodge 1956) concluded that no fluorosis will develop in individuals whose urinary fluoride content is 5 ppm or less. Largent (1961) thought that a higher level of urinary excretion than this would usually be associated with skeletal fluorosis. He proposed that urinary fluoride levels might be used as evidence in support of roentgenological tests; an average urinary excretion of at least 8 mg fluoride per litre over a period of more than 5 years would be required to corroborate a diagnosis of skeletal fluorosis. This prediction is nicely supported by the investigations of Sankaran and Gadekar (1964), who found that the level of urinary fluoride excretion in six cases of early to advanced human skeletal fluorosis ranged between 8 and 22 ppm.

C. Concentrations of fluoride in fluorotic bone

Several analyses have been carried out on fluorotic bone. In every instance, skeletal fluorosis has been associated with abnormally high levels of bone fluoride. Attempts have, therefore, been made to discover whether there is a critical threshold of fluoride concentration in bone beyond which skeletal fluorosis is likely to occur.

Samples of bone from the two cryolite workers of Roholm (1937) had fluoride contents of 2015 to 6420 ppm and 4940 to 8515 ppm per dry, fat-free weight. Wolff and Kerr (1938) found 1800 to 2900 ppm fluoride in the long bones and 7000 ppm in a vertebral sample from a Negro with chronic fluorosis. Linsman and

McMurray (1943) describe the instance of a 22 year old soldier who exhibited signs of skeletal fluorosis. His bones contained 5000 to 5500 ppm fluoride. A recent report by Sankaran and Gadekar (1964) described six cases of human skeletal fluorosis occurring in India. The concentrations of fluoride in fat-free bone from these six individuals ranged from 6260 to 9680 ppm. The severity of fluorosis corresponded to the level of fluoride in bone.

McClure et al. (1958) suggested that the threshold level of fluoride was 5000 to 6000 ppm dry fat-free bone. This agrees well with the estimate of Jackson and Weidmann (1958), who felt that evidence from studies on both humans and animals placed the critical threshold at between 2000 and 3000 ppm fluoride in dry fat-free weight in compact bone, and 4000 to 6000 ppm in cancellous structures.

Implicit in the term "critical threshold" is the idea that the fluoride accumulated in the skeleton is in some way pathogenic. It has not been proved, however, that the mere accumulation of even very large quantities of fluoride by bone has any adverse effect. There is no evidence that the small alterations in the bone crystal have any physiological disadvantages or that the local release of fluoride from bone can cause pathological changes. Likins et al. (1963) investigated the effect of fluoride ingestion upon alveolar bone resorption in rats fed a phytate-deficient diet. The fluoride had no apparent effect and it was concluded that the changes in apatite crystallites brought about by fluoride incorporation had a negligible influence upon bone loss.

It is possible that the osteoclastic release of fluoride ion from very high fluoride bone might cause a temporary rise in the fluoride level of the surrounding tissue fluid. It is unlikely, however, that such local increases in fluoride concentrations will produce significant pathological changes. Certainly, bone can possess concentrations of fluoride at least as high as the proposed critical threshold without any visible fluorosis. Peirce (1939), in an excellent review of skeletal fluorosis occurring in a variety of species, pointed out that 10 to 15-fold increases in the fluoride content of bones and teeth apparently exerted no untoward effects upon the general health of animals and brought about no obvious morphological changes in the skeleton. Zipkin (1960) found 5640 ppm fluoride per dry, fat-free weight in human bone with no significant histological abnormalities and McCann (1960) found 6300 ppm in human rib bone with no visible skeletal lesions. Weidmann et al. (1963) similarly recorded levels of over 6000 ppm in cancellous rib bone from three persons with no visible signs of fluorosis. Hodge (1952) felt that the skeleton provided an effective detoxication mechanism. The incorporation of ingested fluoride into bone mineral and the rapid urinary excretion were together an efficient barrier against fluoride poisoning. The capacity of fluoride to cause bone changes appears to be dependent upon the dietary fluoride concentration and rate and duration of fluoride ingestion rather than upon its concentration in the skeleton.

These apparently opposite view-points: (a) that fluoride present in the bone is harmless and (b) that there exists a "skeletal threshold" of bone fluoride beyond which the pathological changes associated with fluorosis are likely, are not incompatible. Bone-fluoride content is always a rough guide to the past amount of fluoride ingested. If a bone level is achieved by a life-time's regular ingestion of small quantities of fluoride then no pathological changes will occur, whereas the same skeletal concentration, reached after a relatively short period, would be accompanied by symptoms of fluorosis. The level at which fluoride ion is absorbed is a crucial factor in deciding whether fluorosis will occur. Concentrations of fluoride in bone are a guide to the amounts of fluoride which have been ingested and the level of urinary fluoride gives an indication of the fluoride intake, but the pathogenic agent is the free fluoride ion of the tissue fluid. The dental and skeletal changes of fluorosis appear to involve some interference with cellular metabolism. There is no clear indication as to which enzyme systems are involved or even if inhibition is intra-cellular, extra-cellular or at the cell boundary. Fluoride ion inertly bound in the apatite lattice, however, is not likely to affect the cellular control or mineralisation of the hard tissues. The term "critical *index*" might be more apt than "critical *threshold*", for although the concentration of fluoride in bone mineral provides a rough indication of past history, it does not itself cause fluorosis.

References

Armstrong, W. D., and L. Singer: *In vitro* uptake and exchange of bone citrate. *In:* G. E. W. Wolstenholme and C. M. O'Connor, Eds., Ciba Found. Symp., Bone Struct. Metab., 103—116. London: J. and A. Churchill 1956.

— — Fluoride contents of enamel of sound and carious human teeth. J. dent. Res. **42**, 133—136 (1963).

Atkinson, P. J., J. A. Weatherell, and S. M. Weidmann: Changes in density of the human femoral cortex with age. J. Bone Jt. Surg. **44** B, 496—502 (1963).

Bauer, W. H.: Experimental chronic fluorine intoxication: effect on bones and teeth. Amer. J. Orthodont. **31**, 700—719 (1945).

Bélanger, L. F., W. E. Lotz, W. J. Visek, and C. L. Comar: Autoradiographic visualisation with Ca-45 of normal growth of incisor of pigs and the effect of fluoride feeding. Anat. Rec. **119**, 53—69 (1954).

— W. J. Visek, W. E. Lotz, and C. L. Comar: Rachitomimetic effects of fluoride feeding on the skeletal tissues of growing pigs. Amer. J. Path. **34**, 25—35 (1958).

Blayney, J. R., R. C. Bowers, and M. Zimmerman: Evanston dental caries study 22: A study of fluoride deposition in bone. J. dent. Res. **41**, 1037—1044 (1962).

Blue, J. A.: Mottled enamel in Oklahoma Panhandle, and its possible relations to child development. J. Okla. med. Assoc. **31**, 295—301 (1938).

Brudevold, F., D. E. Gardner, and F. A. Smith: The distribution of fluoride in human enamel. J. dent. Res. **35**, 420—429 (1956).

— J. W. Hein, J. F. Bonner, R. B. Nevin, B. G. Bibby, and H. C. Hodge: Reactions of tooth surfaces with 1 ppm fluoride as NaF. J. dent. Res. **36**, 771—779 (1957).

Capizzano, N., J. Valotta, and F. R. Megy: Osteopetrosis en el territorio de la Pampa. Rev. Med. Cienc. afin. (B. Aires) **2**, 19—33 (1940).

Carlson, C. H., L. Singer, and W. D. Armstrong: Radiofluoride distribution in tissues of normal and nephrectomised rats. Proc. Soc. exp. Biol. (N. Y.) **103**, 418—420 (1960).

Comar, C. L., W. J. Visek, W. E. Lotz, and J. H. Rust: Effects of fluorine on calcium metabolism and bone growth in pigs. Amer. J. Anat. **92**, 361—389 (1953).

Dean, H. T.: Classification of mottled enamel diagnosis. J. Amer. dent. Assoc. **21**, 1421—1426 (1934).

— Chronic endemic dental fluorosis (mottled enamel). J. Amer. med. Assoc. **107**, 1269—1272 (1936).

—, Quoted by H. C. Hodge, and F. A. Smith: *In* J. H. Shaw, Ed., Fluoridation as a Public Health Measure, 86. Washington: Amer. Assoc. Advanc. Sci. 1954 (1944).

— R. M. Dixon, and C. Cohen: Mottled enamel in Texas. Publ. Hlth Rep. (Wash.) **50**, 424—442 (1935).

Diamond, M., and J. P. Weinmann: Formation of the human organic matrix and its calcification. J. dent. Res. **19**, 302—303 (1940).

Eds, F. de: Fluorine in relation to bone and tooth development. J. Amer. dent. Ass. **23**, 568—574 (1936).

Elliott, C. G., and M. D. Smith: Dietary fluoride related to the fluoride content of teeth. J. dent. Res. **39**, 93—98 (1960).

Ericsson, Y.: The state of fluorine in milk and its absorption and retention when administered in milk. Acta odont. scand. **16**, 51—77 (1958).

—, and S. Ullberg: Autoradiographic investigations of the distribution of ^{18}F in mice and rats. Acta odont. scand. **16**, 363—374 (1958).

Fleming, H. S.: Effect of certain concentrations of fluoride on enamel and dentine as formed in transplants of tooth germs and related studies. J. dent. Res. **32**, 469—485 (1953).

Gardner, D. E., F. A. Smith, H. C. Hodge, F. Brudevold, and D. McG. Eldredge: Distribution of fluoride in the normal dog femur. J. appl. Physiol. **14**, 427—430 (1959).

GEDALIA, J.: Urinary fluoride levels of children and adults. J. dent. Res. **37**, 601—604 (1958).
— A. BRZEZINSKI, N. PORTUGUESE, and B. BERCOVICI: The fluoride content of teeth and bones of human foetuses. Arch. oral Biol. **9**, 331—340 (1964).
GEEVER, E. F., N. C. LEONE, P. GIESER, and J. E. LIEBERMAN: Pathologic studies in man after prolonged ingestion of fluoride in drinking water: II. Findings in bones in communities with water levels from 1.0—4.0 ppm fluoride. Publ. Hlth Rep. (Wash.) **73**, 721—731 (1958).
GLOCK, G. E., F. LOWATER, and M. M. MURRAY: The retention and elimination of fluorine in bones. Biochem. J. **35**, 1235—1239 (1941).
GUTMAN, A. B., and T. F. YU: A concept of the role of enzymes in endochondral calcification. *In:* E. C. REIFENSTEIN JR., Ed., Metabolic Interrelations, Trans. 2nd Conf., pp. 167—190. New York: Josiah Macy Jr. Found. 1950.
HADJIMARKOS, D. M.: The fluoride content of enamel in a group of Greek teeth. Arch. oral Biol. **7**, 651—653 (1962).
HARGREAVES, J. A., and J. A. WEATHERELL: Variation of fluoride concentration in human deciduous teeth. *In:* J. L. HARDWICK, H. R. HELD, and K. G. KÖNIG, Eds., Advances in Fluorine Research and Dental Caries Prevention **3**, pp. 247—254. Oxford: Pergamon Press Ltd. 1965.
HARRISON, M. F.: Fluorine content of teas consumed in New Zealand. Brit. J. Nutr. **3**, 162—166 (1949).
HENDRICKS, S. B.: Comments on the crystal chemistry of bone. *In:* E. C. REIFENSTEIN, JR., Ed., Metabolic Interrelations, Trans. 4th Conf., pp. 185—212. New York: Josiah Macy Jr. Found. 1952.
HODGE, H. C.: The significance of the skeletal deposition of fluoride. *In:* E. C. REIFENSTEIN, JR., Ed., Metabolic Interrelations, Trans. 4th Conf., pp. 250—260. New York: Josiah Macy Jr. Found. 1952.
— Fluoride metabolism: its significance in water fluoridation. J. Amer. dent. Assoc. **52**, 307—314 (1956).
— Metabolism of fluorides. J. Amer. med. Ass. **177**, 313—316 (1961).
— Safety factors in water fluoridation based on the toxicology of fluorides. Proc. Nutr. Soc. Engl. Scot. **22**, 111—117 (1963).
—, and F. A. SMITH: Some public health aspects of water fluoridation. *In:* J. H. SHAW, Ed., Fluoridation as a Public Health Measure, pp. 79—109. Washington. Amer. Assoc. Advanc. Sci. 1954.
HODGES, P. C., O. J. FAREED, G. RUGGY, and J. S. CHUDNOFF: Skeletal sclerosis in chronic sodium fluoride poisoning. J. Amer. med. Assoc. **117**, 1938 (1941).
JACKSON, D.: The influence of fluorine on the mineral metabolism of phosphorus in the hard tissues of the rat. D. D. S. thesis, University of Manchester, England. 1956.
—, and S. M. WEIDMANN: Fluorine in human bone related to age and the water supply of different regions. J. Path. Bact. **76**, 451—459 (1958).
— — The relationship between age and the fluorine content of human dentine and enamel: a regional survey. Brit. dent. J. **107**, 303—306 (1959).
JENKINS, G. N., and R. L. SPEIRS: Distribution of fluorine in human enamel. Proc. physiol. Soc. **121**, 21 (1953).
— — Some observations on the fluoride concentrations of dental tissues. J. dent. Res. **33**, 734 (1954).
JOHNSON, L. C.: Discussion *in* HODGE, H. C., The significance of the skeletal deposition of fluoride. *In:* E. C. REIFENSTEIN JR., Ed., Metabolic Interrelations, Trans. 4th Conf., pp. 250—260. New York: Josiah Macy jr. Found. 1952.
KELLNER, H.: Zur Histopathologie der Knochen bei chronischer experimenteller Fluorverabreichung. Naunyn-Schmiedebergs Arch. exp. Path. Pharmak. **192**, 549—569 (1939).
KUTNERIAN, K., and A. C. KUYPER: The influence of fluoride on the solubility of bone salt. J. biol. Chem. **233**, 760—763 (1957).
KUYPER, A. C., and K. KUTNERIAN: Mechanism of the incorporation of fluoride into bone salt. J. dent. Res. **41**, 345—350 (1962).
LARGENT, E. J.: Fluorosis — The Health Aspects of Fluorine Compounds. Columbus: Ohio State Univ. Press 1961.
—, and F. F. HEYROTH: Absorption and excretion of fluoride: III. Further observations on the metabolism of fluorides at high levels of intake. J. industr. Hyg. Toxicol. **31**, 134—138 (1949).
LEONE, N. C., C. A. STEVENSON, T. F. HILBISH, and M. C. SOSMAN: A roentgenologic study of a human population exposed to high-fluoride domestic water. Amer. J. Roentgenol. **74**, 874—885 (1955).
LIKINS, R. C., G. PAKIS, and F. J. MCCLURE: Effect of fluoride and tetracycline on alveolar bone resorption in the rat. J. dent. Res. **42**, 1532 (1963).
— R. O. SCOW, I. ZIPKIN, and A. C. STEERE: Deposition and retention of fluoride and radiocalcium in the growing rat. Amer. J. Physiol. **197**, 75—80 (1959).

LINDEMANN, G.: X-ray diffraction study of osseous and dental tissue from rats with experimental fluorosis. Acta odont. scand. **14**, 33—46 (1956/57).
LINSMAN, J. F., and C. A. MCMURRAY: Fluoride osteosclerosis from drinking water. Radiology **40**, 474—484 (1943).
LITTLE, M. F., J. POSEN, and L. SINGER: Chemical and physical properties of altered and sound enamel: 3. Fluoride and sodium content. J. dent. Res. **41**, 784—789 (1962).
LONGWELL, J.: Symposium on the fluoridation of public water supplies: d. Chemical and technical aspects. Roy. Soc. Prom. Hlth J. **77**, 361—370 (1957).
MCCANN, H. G.: The effects of the absorption of fluoride. Arch. industr. Hlth **21**, 336—337 (1960).
—, and F. A. BULLOCK: The effect of fluoride ingestion on the composition and solubility of mineralised tissues of the rat. J. dent. Res. **36**, 391—398 (1957).
MCCAULEY, H. B., and F. J. MCCLURE: Effect of fluoride in drinking water on the osseous development of the hand and wrist in children. Publ. Hlth Rep. (Wash.) **69**, 671—683 (1954).
MCCLURE, F. J.: A review of fluorine and its physiological effects. Physiol. Rev. **13**, 277—300 (1933).
—, and C. A. KINSER: Fluoride domestic waters and systemic effects. II. Fluorine content of urine in relation to fluorine in drinking water. Publ. Hlth Rep. (Wash.) **59**, 1575—1591 (1944).
—, and R. C. LIKINS: Fluorine in human teeth studied in relation to fluorine in the drinking water. J. dent. Res. **30**, 172—176 (1951).
— H. G. MCCANN, and N. C. LEONE: Excessive fluoride in water and bone chemistry. Publ. Hlth Rep. (Wash.) **73**, 741—746 (1958).
—, and I. ZIPKIN: Physiologic effects of fluoride as related to water fluoridation. Dent. Clin. N. Amer. **1958**, 411—458.
MØLLER, P. F., and S. V. GUDJONSSON: Massive fluorosis of bones and ligaments. Acta. Radiol. **13**, 269—294 (1932).
MYERS, H. M., J. G. HAMILTON, and H. BECKS: A tracer study of the transfer of ^{18}F to teeth by topical application. J. dent. Res. **31**, 743—750 (1952).
NEUMAN, W. F., and M. W. NEUMAN: The Chemical Dynamics of Bone Mineral. Chicago: University of Chicago Press 1958.
— — E. R. MAIN, J. O'LEARY, and F. A. SMITH: The surface chemistry of bone: II. Fluoride deposition. J. biol. Chem. **187**, 655—661 (1950).
PANDIT, C. G., T. N. S. RAGHAVACHARI, D. S. RAO, and V. KRISHNAMURTI: Endemic fluorosis in S. India. Indian J. med. Res. **28**, 533—558 (1940).
PEIRCE, A. W.: Chronic fluorine intoxication in domestic animals. Nutr. Abstr. Rev. **9**, 253—261 (1939).
PHILLIPS, P. H., F. J. STARE, and C. A. ELVEHJEM: A study of tissue respiration and certain reducing substances in chronic fluorosis and scurvy in the guinea pig. J. biol. Chem. **106**, 41—61 (1934).
PINDBORG, E. V., J. J. PINDBORG, and C. M. PLUM: Studies on incisor pigmentation in relation to liver iron and blood picture in the white rat: II. The effect of fluorine on the iron metabolism. Acta pharmacol. (Kbh.) **2**, 294—301 (1946).
POSNER, A. S., E. D. EANES, R. A. HARPER, and I. ZIPKIN: X-ray diffraction analysis of the effect of fluoride on human bone apatite. Arch. oral Biol. **8**, 549—570 (1963).
PURVES, M. J.: Some effects of administering sodium fluoride to patients with Paget's disease. Lancet **1962**, 1188—1189.
RICH, C., and J. ENSINCK: The effect of sodium fluoride on calcium metabolism of human beings. Nature (Lond.) **191**, 184—185 (1961).
RÖCKERT, H.: X-ray absorption and X-ray fluorescence microanalyses of mineralised tissue of rats which have ingested fluoridated water. Acta path. microbiol. scand. **59**, 32—38 (1963).
ROHOLM, K.: Fluorine Intoxication. London: H. K. Lewis and Co. Ltd. 1937.
SANKARAN, B., and N. G. GADEKAR: Skeletal fluorosis. *In:* H. J. J. BLACKWOOD, Ed., Bone and Tooth, 357—362. London: Pergamon Press 1964.
SCHOUR, I., and N. C. SMITH: Mottled teeth: an experimental and histologic analysis. J. Amer. dent. Assoc. **22**, 796—813 (1935).
SCHWYZER, F.: Einfluß chronischer Fluorzufuhr auf den Chlor- und Calciumstoffwechsel. Biochem. Z. **60**, 32—42 (1914).
SHORTT, H. E., G. R. MCROBERT, T. W. BARNARD, and A. S. M. NAYAR: Endemic fluorosis in the Madras Presidency. Indian J. med. Res. **25**, 553—568 (1937).
SINGER, L., and W. D. ARMSTRONG: Comparison of fluoride contents of human dental and skeletal tissues. J. dent. Res. **41**, 154—157 (1962).

SINGH, A., S. S. JOLLY, and B. C. BANSAL: Skeletal fluorosis and its neurological complications. Lancet **1961**, 197—200.
SMITH, F. A., D. E. GARDNER, and H. C. HODGE: Age increase in fluoride content in human bone. Fed. Proc. **12**, 368 (1953).
— — N. C. LEONE, and H. C. HODGE: The effects of the absorption of fluoride: V. The chemical determination of fluoride in human soft tissues following prolonged ingestion of fluoride at various levels. Arch. industr. Hlth **21**, 330—332 (1960).
STEVENSON, C. A., and A. R. WATSON: Fluorine osteosclerosis. Amer. J. Roentgenol. **78**, 13—18 (1957).
STOOKEY, G. K., D. B. CRANE, and J. C. MUHLER: Further studies on fluoride absorption. Proc. Soc. exp. Biol. (N. Y.) **115**, 295—298 (1964).
SUTTIE, J. W., and P. H. PHILLIPS: The effect of age on the rate of fluoride deposition in the femur of the rat. Arch. Biochem. **83**, 355—359 (1959).
— —, and E. C. FALTIN: Serum fluoride in the chick. Proc. Soc. exp. Biol. (N. Y.) **115**, 575—577 (1964).
TAVES, D. R., and W. F. NEUMAN: Factors controlling calcification. University of Rochester Atomic Energy Rept. UR-628. 1963.
WALDBOTT, G. L.: Fluoride in food. Amer. J. clin. Nutr. **12**, 455—462 (1963).
WALLACE-DURBIN, P.: The metabolism of fluorine in the rat using ^{18}F as a tracer. J. dent. Res. **33**, 789—800 (1954).
WEATHERELL, J. A., and J. A. HARGREAVES: The micro-sampling of enamel in thin layers by means of strong acids. Arch. oral Biol. **10**, 139—142 (1965).
— and S. M. WEIDMANN: The skeletal changes of chronic experimental fluorosis. J. Path. Bact. **78**, 233—241 (1959).
WEDDLE, D. A., and J. C. MUHLER: The metabolism of different fluorides in the rat: 1. Comparison between sodium fluoride, sodium silico-fluoride and stannous fluoride. J. dent. Res. **36**, 386—390 (1957).
WEIDMANN, S. M.: The uptake and retention of fluoride by teeth of animals under experimental fluorosis. Arch. oral Biol. **7**, 63—72 (1962).
—, and J. A. WEATHERELL: The uptake and distribution of fluorine in bones. J. Path. Bact. **78**, 243—255 (1959).
— —, and D. JACKSON: The effect of fluoride on bone. Proc. Nutr. Soc. Engl. Scot. **22**, 105—110 (1963).
— —, and R. G. WHITEHEAD: The effect of fluorine on the chemical composition and calcification of bone. J. Path. Bact. **78**, 435—445 (1959).
WEINMANN, J. P., and H. SICHER: Bone and Bones. Edn. 2. London: Henry Kimpton 1955.
WHITEHEAD, R. G., and S. M. WEIDMANN: Oxidative enzyme systems in ossifying cartilage. Biochem. J. **72**, 667—672 (1959).
WILKIE, J.: Two cases of fluorine osteosclerosis. Brit. J. Radiol. **13**, 213—217 (1940).
WOLFF, W. A., and E. G. KERR: Composition of human bone in chronic fluorine poisoning. Amer. J. med. Sci. **195**, 493—497 (1938).
WUTHIER, R. E., and J. T. IRVING: Effect of chronic fluoride ingestion on calcification patterns. Abstract of paper No. 104. Internat. Assoc. Dental Res., 40th Gen. Meeting (1962).
YAEGER, J. A., and D. R. EISENMANN: Response in rat incisor dentin to injected strontium, fluoride and parathyroid extract. J. dent. Res. **42**, 1208—1216 (1963).
YOON, S. H., F. BRUDEVOLD, D. E. GARDNER, and F. A. SMITH: Distribution of fluoride in teeth from areas of different levels of fluoride in the water supply. J. dent. Res. **39**, 845—856 (1960a).
— — F. A. SMITH, D. E. GARDNER, and N. SONI: Distribution of fluorine in teeth and alveolar bone. J. Amer. dent. Assoc. **61**, 565—570 (1960b).
ZIPKIN, I.: The effects of the absorption of fluoride: IV. The deposition of fluoride in human skeletal tissues as related to fluoride in the drinking water. Arch. industr. Hlth **21**, 329 (1960).
—, and N. C. LEONE: Rate of urinary fluoride output in normal adults. Amer. J. Publ. Hlth **47**, 848—851 (1957).
—, and F. J. MCCLURE: Deposition of fluorine in the bones and teeth of the growing rat. J. Nutr. **47**, 611—620 (1952).
— —, and W. A. LEE: Relation of the fluoride content of human bone to its chemical composition. Arch. oral Biol. **2**, 190—195 (1960).
— — N. C. LEONE, and W. A. LEE: Fluoride deposition in human bones after prolonged ingestion of fluoride in drinking water. Publ. Hlth Rep. (Wash.) **73**, 732—740 (1958).

Chapter 4

The Role of Fluorides in Tooth Chemistry and in the Prevention of Dental Caries

By

Finn Brudevold

With 11 Figures

I. Introduction

Because the relation of water fluoridation to dental caries has been so thoroughly studied and reviewed, it is not the intention of the author to discuss this subject in detail, but to present a brief outline, pertinent points and some new information. The main purpose of this discussion is to review the vast recent literature on the clinical aspects of fluoride supplementation and topically applied fluoride, and to bring up to date available basic information concerning the chemistry of fluoride and tooth mineral, and the mechanism of action of fluoride in inhibiting caries.

II. Development of controlled water fluoridation

The utilization of fluoride in the control of dental caries stems from the discovery of the relationship between fluoride ingestion and mottled enamel (Smith et al., 1931), and the specific effect on dental caries of fluoride-bearing waters (Dean, 1938). A series of epidemiological studies subsequently established that the high caries protection afforded by water-borne fluoride is very little enhanced by concentrations exceeding 1 ppm and that mottled enamel is no problem

Table 1. *Annual cumulative data for controlled fluoridation in the United States, showing numbers of communities and populations served.* U.S. Department of Health, Education and Welfare, Public Health Service, Division of Dental Public Health and Resources. Fluoridation memoranda index No. 2 and No. 8, 1962.

Year	No. of communities	Population
1945	6	231,920
1947	16	458,748
1949	49	1,062,779
1951	368	5,079,321
1953	1,007	17,666,339
1955	1,347	26,278,820
1957	1,717	36,215,208
1959	1,990	39,628,377
1961	2,197	42,201,115
1963[1]	2,455	45,000,000

[1] As of June, 1963.

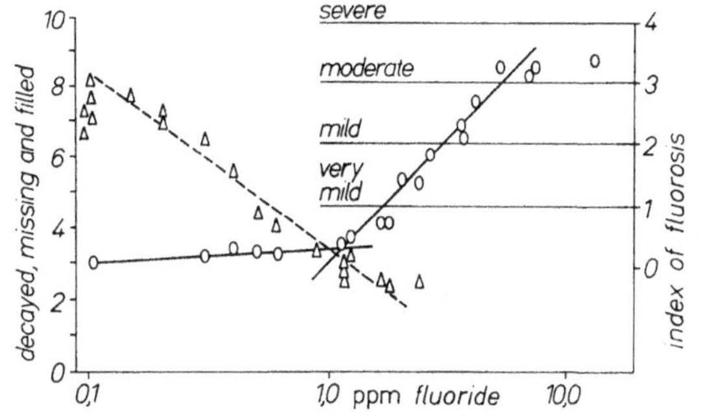

Fig. 1. Relation between water-borne fluoride, index of fluorosis and the number of decayed, missing and filled teeth (Hodge and Smith, 1954)

at this level of fluoride (Dean et al., 1941a, b; 1942). The results of these studies are summarized in Fig. 1.

Following these early observations, numerous communities initiated water fluoridation and in long range, carefully conducted studies demonstrated that 1 ppm of fluoride in the drinking water a) provides the same dental and general effects whether the fluoride occurs naturally or is added by artificial means, and b) effectively, safely and economically prevents up to 70 % of dental caries (Ast and Fitzgerald, 1962).

Table 1 shows the development of water fluoridation in the United States from 1945 to 1963. Of the entire population of nearly 187 million, 45 million were using controlled fluoridated water by June, 1963. Including the 7.3 million who have naturally fluoridated drinking water, 52.3 million or 28 % of the population consumed water containing 0.7 or more ppm of fluoride (U.S. Public Health Service, 1962). In Canada, 8.4 % of the population was living in communities with controlled fluoridation in January, 1962 (Bureau of Economic Research, 1962). Several cities in other countries have adopted water fluoridation and at least a dozen countries have experimental fluoridation programs (Leatherman, 1959).

III. Water fluoridation and dental caries

The voluminous literature dealing with water fluoridation and dental caries will be considered with regard to a) lifelong continuous fluoride exposure, b) prenatal fluoride exposure, c) pre-eruptive compared with post-eruptive exposure, and d) effects in adults.

A. Fluoride exposure throughout life

The low prevalence of dental caries in the permanent teeth of children who have used fluoridated water since birth or infancy is shown in Table 2. The data represent findings in several thousand 12–14 or 13–14-year-old children from different cities in the United States and Canada. The number of decayed, missing and filled teeth (DMFT) per child ranges from 3.2 to 4.7 in the cities with controlled fluoridation, compared to 7.5 and 12.8 DMFT per child in the two fluoride-deficient control cities included in Table 2. The reduction in caries as a result of fluoridation was calculated to range from 50 to 70 % in these children (Arnold et al., 1962; Ast and Fitzgerald, 1962; Brown et al., 1956; Hill et al., 1961). The loss of permanent teeth per child, given in the last column of Table 2, is also significantly reduced in the fluoride-exposed children. It is important to note that the children in Aurora, which has a naturally fluoridated water supply (1.2 ppm of F) have a similar caries experience and tooth loss as those from cities with controlled fluoridation. Fluoride at a concentration of about 1 ppm in the drinking water is obviously equally effective in reducing caries in permanent teeth whether it is added or occurs naturally.

One important aspect of the inhibition of caries by water-borne fluoride is that the protective effect is greater in anterior than posterior teeth. For example, Dean et al. (1942) found that the children who lived in communities with 0.6 to 2.6 ppm of fluoride in the water supply had 90 to 95 % less caries experience in the four maxillary incisors than children from fluoride-deficient areas, while the corresponding decrease for the entire dentition was 50 to 70 %. The caries reduction in different tooth types of children who had used fluoridated water all of their lives is given in Table 3 (Klein, 1948). The decrease is greatest in the mandibular anterior teeth, and least in the mandibular first and second molars.

Table 2. *Comparison of decayed, missing and filled teeth (DMFT) and missing teeth per child for specified age groups from communities with water supplies containing 1.2 ppm natural fluoride, 1.0 ppm controlled fluoride, or deficient in fluoride.* Data from AST and FITZGERALD (1962).

	F in water ppm	Age, yrs.	DMFT per child	Missing teeth per child
Aurora	1.2[1]	12—14	3.24	0.15
Grand rapids	1.0	12—14	4.26	0.29
Evanston	1.0	12—14	4.66	0.06
Brantford	1.0	12—14	3.23	0.22
Newburgh	1.0	13—14	3.73	0.10
Kingston	0.1	13—14	12.76	0.92
Sarnia	0.0	12—14	7.46	0.75

[1] Natural fluoride.

Klein suggested that the depressant effect of F on caries may be of approximately equal potential for all the different tooth types, and that the variation in per cent reduction of caries may be due to gradients in caries susceptibility. It has also been postulated that the anterior teeth come in more intimate contact with water during drinking than posterior teeth, and that they thus acquire more fluoride, and hence greater caries resistance (VOLKER and BIBBY, 1941). This concept of surface fluoride action led to the important development of topical fluoride treatments.

Table 3. *Effect of 1.3—2.2 ppm of water-borne fluoride on caries in different tooth types. Number of DMF teeth per 100 white children aged 15—19 years.* Data from KLEIN (1948).

Tooth type	Maxillary			Mandibular		
	fluoride subjects	control subjects	percentage reduction	fluoride subjects	control subjects	percentage reduction
Central incisor	7.1	47.6	85.1	0.5	6.8	92.6
Lateral incisor	8.2	52.8	84.5	0	6.0	100.0
Cuspid	2.2	11.4	80.7	0	2.4	100.0
First premolar	10.3	41.6	75.2	4.9	11.2	56.2
Second premolar	16.3	45.4	64.1	10.9	39.8	72.6
First molar	68.5	141.0	51.4	110.9	169.8	34.7
Second molar	39.7	87.0	54.3	79.3	119.2	33.5

Although the caries reducing effect of fluoridated water is less in deciduous than in permanent teeth, it is still significant. Studies from communities using water with controlled fluoride have demonstrated a decrease in caries experience of approximately 40 % in 6–8-year-old children (BROWN et al., 1956). Again the effect is similar to that observed from naturally fluoridated water. This can be seen from Fig. 2 which compares the number of carious and filled teeth per child at different ages in Grand Rapids prior to and after 7 years of fluoridation, and in Aurora which has water naturally containing 1.2 ppm of fluoride (KNUTSON, 1954).

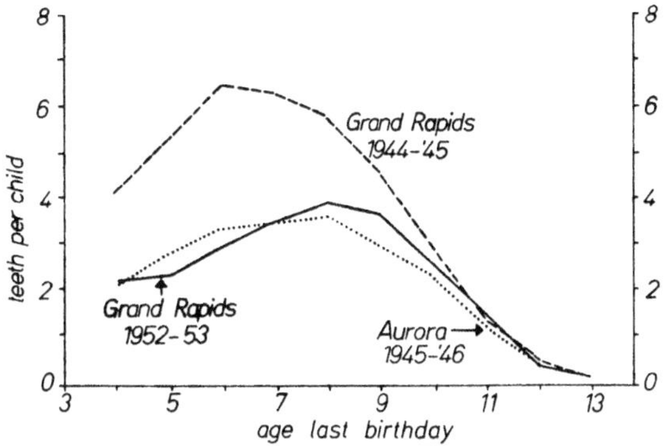

Fig. 2. Decayed or filled deciduous teeth per child for continuous residence (KNUTSON, 1954)

As a result of the depression of caries in fluoridated areas, there is diminished premature loss of deciduous teeth and of first permanent molars among young children. Early loss of teeth is particularly detrimental, not only because of impairment of proper chewing at a critical age, but because of a possible disturbance of the alignment of the permanent teeth. Five years of fluoridation increased by 20 % the number of 5- and 6-year-old children who had all their posterior deciduous teeth present and free of caries (Ast et al., 1951). Two studies have shown a decrease in malocclusion of approximately 20 % as a result of fluoridation (Hill et al., 1959; Ast et al., 1962). The marked improvement in the occlusion of 13- to 14-year-old children who were born after fluoridation began is shown in Table 4. Among these children 93 % had all first molars present, and 35 % had normal occlusion, compared to 65 and 13 %, respectively in the fluoride-deficient neighboring control city.

Table 4. *Average number of missing teeth and percentage of children with normal occlusion in communities with and without fluoridated water.* Data from Ast et al. (1962).

	Age, yrs.	No.	Missing teeth per child	Percentage children with	
				All first molars present	Normal occulusion
Newburgh[1]	13—14	160	0.1	93	35
Kingston[2]	13—14	142	0.9	65	13

[1] Fifteen years of fluoridation.
[2] Fluoride deficient.

B. Prenatal fluoride exposure

Although it is generally assumed that fluoride ingestion during pregnancy will benefit the dental health of the child (Report of Joint Committee, 1959; Blayney, 1962), convincing evidence in support of this view is lacking. The belief in the importance of prenatal fluoride exposure is usually based on the clinical observation in several studies that children born in the same years that fluoridation was initiated had a slightly greater caries experience than children of the same age group in the same community born after the water supply had been fluoridated for one or more years. However, it is obvious, since the subjects were not screened that a large percentage of the children born in the year that fluoridation started might have had their first fluoride exposure several months before or after birth, making any interpretation of pre- and postnatal effects doubtful. It should be noted that the only study reported in the literature which specifically included children whose prenatal and postnatal exposure to fluoride was known, showed no dental benefits from prenatal fluoride (Carlos et al., 1962). No difference in caries experience was observed in this study in deciduous teeth of 6-year-old children who had used fluoridated water anywhere from birth up to 3 months of age, and children of the same age who had been fluoride-exposed both pre- and postnatally. Relative to these findings mention should be made of a recent study which demonstrated that the mineralization of deciduous teeth is not as advanced

Table 5. *Extent of mineralization of deciduous teeth at birth.* Data from Reiss (1961).

	No.	Percentage of crown calcified at birth
Upper central incisors	69	36
Other incisors . . .	106	31
Cuspid	50	6
First molar	50	17
Second molar. . . .	50	5

at birth as is generally believed (REISS, 1961). The findings in this study, given in Table 5 showed that the amount of mineral present in the crowns of different deciduous tooth types at birth ranged from only 5 to 36 % of that of completely formed crowns. The deciduous molars which represent the greatest caries risk are mineralized only in the tips of the cusps in the prenatal period.

It is evident from the literature that prenatal fluoride exposure is unimportant from a dental point of view, but more data are desirable from studies carefully designed to distinguish between groups exposed to fluoride before and after birth.

C. Pre-eruptive compared to post-eruptive fluoride exposure

That appreciable resistance to caries can be derived from pre-eruptive use of fluoridated water may be deduced from the observation that children who consumed fluoride-containing water (8 ppm) during the first years of life, and then, for a period of 12 years, used a water supply which contained only traces of fluoride, had less than half the DMF teeth of children who were born and raised on fluoride-deficient water (DEAN et al. 1941a). DEATHERAGE (1943a) in a study of military servicemen from Illinois was able to confirm that use of fluoridated water during only the first 8 years of life resulted in a substantial reduction in adult caries. His findings also demonstrated an additional, but lesser reduction in caries in persons who lived continuously in fluoridated areas beyond the age of 8 years. From these findings which are summarized in Table 6, it was concluded that a significant decrease in dental caries is derived from use of fluoridated water, not only in the pre-eruptive period, but to a lesser extent also from such use after the teeth have erupted.

Table 6. *Comparison of caries experiences of 2026 white males using different water supplies continuously or for the first eight years of life.* Data from DEATHERAGE (1943a)

Fluoride in water		No. examined	Mean age, yrs.	DMF teeth av.
used continuously	used first 8 yrs. only			
Fluoride deficient (0.1 ppm or less)	—	286	23.9	10.8
—	Fluoride deficient (0.1 ppm or less)	449	25.2	10.0
0.5—0.9 ppm	—	169	25.7	7.9
—	0.5—0.9 ppm	155	26.4	8.9
1.0 ppm and over	—	454	25.3	6.2
—	1.0 ppm and over	513	26.5	7.3

Since several tooth types erupt after the age of 8 years, DEATHERAGE's evidence of post-eruptive fluoride effect is not as conclusive as that provided by KLEIN (1946) and others. From KLEIN's studies it was concluded that the largest measure of protection derived from post-eruptive fluoride exposure occurred in the youngest children, and that among the teeth present in the mouth at the beginning of the exposure to fluoride, those most recently erupted were those most protected against caries attack. The data in Table 7, taken from KLEIN's study, were obtained from children who had been drinking water containing 3 ppm of fluoride for 2 years from the age of 10 to 12. The second molars, which were erupting when the fluoride exposure began, show marked reduction in caries, but the first molars which had been erupted for 4 to 6 years before being exposed to fluoride are not benefitted.

The first permanent molar, the tooth type least protected by fluoridated water (Klein, 1946), has shown some caries inhibition after post-eruptive fluoride exposure in one study (Ast et al., 1951), while another study revealed no effect (Russell and White, 1961). In these investigations, caries was expressed in terms of DMF teeth. By using the more sensitive method of recording DMF tooth surfaces, a significant reduction in caries as a result of post-eruptive use of fluoridated water has been demonstrated in the proximal, buccal and lingual surfaces, but not in the occlusal surface (Backer Dirks, 1961). These findings which are in agreement with those of Hayes et al. (1957) are given in Table 8. Retarded growth of carious lesions was also observed by Backer Dirks in the fluoride-exposed children. From the findings of a gradient in caries inhibition in different locations of the tooth, it was suggested that the resistance to caries which develops post-eruptively is related to the accessibility of the enamel surface to external fluoride. However, a difference in the intensity of the carious attack in different surface areas may produce the same effect.

Table 7. *Effect of water containing 3 ppm fluoride used for two years on DMF of teeth initially erupted and caries-free.* Data from Klein (1946)

	Years erupted at start of F exposure	Percentage new DMF	
		F exposed	control
Second molar	0	16	47
Second bicuspid	1—2	7	10
First molar	4—6	35	38

Table 8. *Percentage reduction in caries of different surfaces of the first permanent molar after $5^1/_2$ years of fluoridation.* Data from Backer Dirks et al. (1961)

Age yrs.	Years erupted at beginning of fluoridation	F exposure in years		Percentage decrease in caries		
		pre-eruptive	post-eruptive	proximal	occlusal	buccal-lingual
13	1—2	0	$5^1/_2$	31	16	54
12	0—1	0	$5^1/_2$	49	22	71
9	0	2	$3^1/_2$	66	28	66

It is worthy of note that no significant inhibition of caries has been observed in the deciduous dentition as a result of post-eruptive use of fluoridated water (Russell and White, 1961). In Table 9 the caries experience in deciduous and permanent teeth of children who started fluoridation at different ages is compared. Only children under 2 years at the time fluoridation began showed decrease in carious deciduous teeth, while the permanent teeth benefited in all age groups studied. It is evident that fluoridated water must be used during the first year of life in order to benefit significantly the deciduous dentition.

Table 9. *Dental caries in deciduous and permanent teeth of children who began use of fluoridated water at different ages.* Data from Russell and White (1961)

Fluoridation from	Present age, yrs.	Deciduous teeth (dmf)		Permanent teeth (DMF)	
		control	F	control	F
Birth	7	4.0	2.9	1.1	0.3
Age 1 yr.	8	3.8	3.4	1.9	0.8
Age 2 yrs.	9	3.4	3.5	2.4	1.3
Age 3 yrs.	10	2.3	2.4	3.1	2.0
Age 4 yrs.	11	1.3	1.3	4.4	2.4

D. Fluoridation and dental caries in adults

The substantial reduction in caries observed in 16-year-old children living in communities with controlled fluoridation suggests that the protective effect of fluoride will extend into adult life in individuals who live continuously under this regimen. Since artificial fluoridation was introduced for the first time less than 20 years ago, evidence of fluoride effects in adult populations must be sought in areas with natural fluoride in the water. Such studies have proven beyond doubt that the dental health of adults born and reared in fluoride areas is superior to that of adults living in fluoride-deficient areas. Only one study which, incidentally, has been widely quoted, suggested that fluoride merely postponed the onset of caries (WEAVER 1944). This study was in many respects atypical and the results cannot be considered a reliable indication of fluoride effect. In contrast, McKAY (1948) concluded that the caries inhibitory effect of fluoride was permanent in natives of Colorado Springs, where the water contains 2.5 ppm of fluoride. The previously mentioned study of Deatherage showed that military selectees from communities, where the drinking water contained 0.5 or more ppm of fluoride had significantly fewer DMF teeth than those who had lived in fluoride-deficient areas (DEATHERAGE, 1943a, b). It has been found that lifelong residents in the age range of 20 to 44 years had approximately 60 % lower caries experience in Colorado Springs (2.5 ppm F) than in Boulder (traces of F) (RUSSELL and ELVOVE, 1951). The loss of teeth was also decreased materially in the fluoride-exposed group. These findings, which are summarized in Table 10, are supported by data obtained in a community with drinking water containing 0.8 to 1.6 ppm of fluoride in Hungary (ADLER, 1951). Additional confirmative data shown in Table 11, are provided by a recent study of college students who had used water containing either 0.1 or 1.2 ppm of fluoride since birth (ENGLANDER et al., 1962). In view of all the evidence, it is apparent that children raised from birth on water containing fluoride either naturally present or artificially introduced, will have lasting dental benefits in adult life.

Table 10. *Mean DMF teeth and mean number of missing teeth per person in 540 adults from Boulder and Colorado Springs Boulder Water, traces of F; Colorado Springs Water, 2.5 ppm F.* Data from RUSSELL and ELVOVE (1951)

Age/yrs	DMF teeth per person		Missing teeth per person	
	Boulder	Colorado Springs	Boulder	Colorado Springs
20—24	14.0	5.4	1.3	0.6
25—29	16.5	6.5	2.5	0.9
30—34	18.3	7.1	4.0	1.1
35—39	21.8	9.2	11.3	3.2
40—44	21.7	10.3	12.1	3.1

Table 11. *Dental caries experience for 260 native residents aged 18—19 years of Aurora and Rockford, Illinois.* Data from ENGLANDER et al. (1962)

ppm F in water supply	DMFT[1]	DMFS[2]	Percentage of caries-free persons
1.2 (Aurora)	7.3	12.2	12.5
0.1 (Rockford)	13.4	28.8	0.0

[1] Decayed, missing and filled teeth.
[2] Decayed, missing and filled tooth surfaces.

IV. Fluoride supplementation by vehicles other than communal water

Since the discovery that 1 ppm of fluoride in the water supply represents the optimal level in regard to caries inhibition, water has been considered the most suitable vehicle for fluoride supplementation. The fluoridation of a water supply is a duplication of nature's way of providing necessary fluoride. It is inexpensive, the fluoride will reach all of the people in the community, and toxic effects are excluded by the self-limiting consumption of water. However, since only a portion of the world population has communal water supplies, other means of supplying fluoride have been sought, the most important ones being supplementation through table salt, milk or by tablets or drops. In controlled water fluoridation the question of dosage need not be answered since the individual variation in water consumption involves no hazards, and the amount of fluoride ingested is known to be optimal to the population at large. In contrast, successful fluoride supplementation by other means must be based on knowledge of what constitutes the optimal dosage of fluoride in different age groups, and at what time fluoride supplementation should be initiated.

According to available evidence, the critical period for development of mottled enamel is from birth to about six years of age. The enamel of all anterior teeth and the first molars, and most of the enamel of the pre-molars calcify during this period. Therefore, since mottled enamel can form only in the early years, the dosage is not critical for older children and adults but should be carefully regulated from birth up to about six years of age. Attempts to determine the optimal dosage have been made by estimating the amounts of fluoride ingested from water containing 1 ppm fluoride. Unfortunately there is considerable uncertainty in regard to water consumption of children. We are concerned here with consumption of tap water and not with the water present in milk, carbonated beverages and solid foods, which usually contains minimal amounts of fluoride. Such a distinction has not always been made. Indeed, accurate quantitative knowledge based on measurements is greatly lacking in this very complex field of water consumption. McClure (1943) calculated the water consumption in children from available data or caloric requirements and body weight. His estimates of average daily water consumption in different age groups are given in Table 12, and have been used for determining fluoride requirements. According to these data, the daily supplement to children living in fluoride-deficient areas should be in the order of 0.5 mg for one- to three-year-old children, increasing to 1 mg in the age group 10–12 years.

Table 12. *Calculated water consumption of children.* Data from McClure (1943)

Age yrs.	Body wt. (kg)	Water consumption in ml	
		Range	Mean
1—3	8—16	390—556	470
4—6	13—24	520—745	620
7—9	16—35	650—930	790
10—12	25—54	810—1165	990

Table 13. *Daily intake of water and of milk in children aged 1—6 years.* Data from Neuman (1957)

Population fraction	Water ml	Milk ml
Upper third	618	1005
Middle third	290	840
Lower third	85	647
Mean	294	840

Data obtained from records of food and fluid intake of children show that the consumption of tap water is less and varies more than is suggested by McClure. Neuman (1957) in a study of children under 6 years of age from New York City found that the total daily fluid requirement averaged approximately 1200 ml for the 1 year and 1500 ml for the 5-year age group. Of the fluids consumed, only about 25 % was tap water, while over 70 % was dairy milk. There were marked variations in fluid intake, particularly in regard to water. This is shown in Table 13 which lists the average amounts of water and milk consumed per day by the upper, middle and lower thirds of the children.

A study from Australia (CROSBY and SHEPHERD, 1957) showed the mean volume of water intake by 3- to 5-year-old children to be 319 ml per day in the winter and 458 ml in the summer. Girls aged 12 to 15 years averaged 771 ml in the winter and 1829 ml in hot weather. Again, the water consumption varied considerably among children in the same age group. In a recent investigation which included 797 children residing in four states in the United States (Florida, Georgia, New Mexico and Michigan), the water intake proved to be consistently less than half of the total daily fluid intake in all age groups (WALKER et al., 1963). The mean daily intake of total fluids and of tap water obtained in this study for different age groups of children up to 10 years of age are plotted in Fig. 3. It is apparent that the total fluid intake increased with age, but that this increase was represented only in part by tap water. The data on water intake obtained by different investigators agree well and suggest that 0.3 to 0.4 mg of fluoride is provided per day to children up to 6 years of age from fluoridated water.

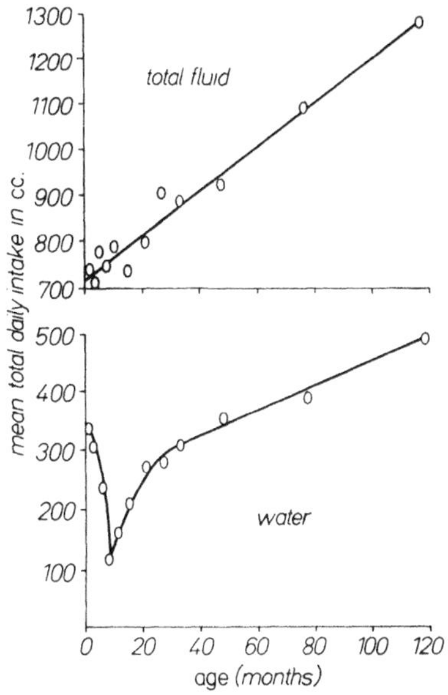

Fig. 3. Mean daily intake of total fluid and of water for children (WALKER et al., 1963)

The Council on Dental Therapeutics, of the American Dental Association (1958) has suggested use of bottled water containing 1 ppm of fluoride as most feasible for fluoride supplementation during the first 2 years of life. For children between 2 and 3 years of age, a dosage of 1 mg every other day is recommended, and for children older than 3 years, 1 mg each day. In a recent editorial in a leading pediatric journal, a daily dosage of 0.5 mg of fluoride was advocated for children up to the age of 3 years, and twice that level for children who had passed their third birthday (SCHLESINGER, 1963).

A. Fluoride pills and lozenges

In the first studies concerned with the caries-inhibiting effect of fluoride pills or lozenges, children were given from 1 to 3 mg of fluoride per day in the form of sodium fluoride or calcium fluoride. Of the six studies reported prior to 1954, two showed a caries reduction ranging from 30 to 50% (STREAN and BEAUDET, 1946; SCHMITZ, 1952) and four gave no effects (DAVENPORT and BIBBY, 1948; BIBBY and WILKINS, 1948; LARSEN, 1948 and STONES et al., 1949). In a review of these studies the validity of the findings was questioned because of the short duration of some of the experiments (less than 1 year) or because of peculiarities in the caries incidence in the groups studied (BIBBY and BRUDEVOLD, 1954).

Subsequent reports published in the period 1954 to 1961 are summarized in Table 14. In most of these studies 0.5 to 1.0 mg of fluoride per day was given to school children beginning in the first or second grade. All investigators observed a reduction in caries in the range of 20 to 40% after two or more years of fluoride ingestion.

It is worthy of note that BIBBY et al. (1955) found 30% inhibition of caries after only 1 year when the fluoride (1 mg per day) was administered in lozenges

Table 14. *Inhibition of caries by use of fluoride-containing pills. Summary of studies reported in 1954—1961*

	Initial				Length of time, yrs.	Percentage of caries reduction	Comments
	F exposed	control	Age yrs.	Fluoride mg/day			
HELD and PIGUET (1954)	105	105	5—6	0.5—1.0	3	46	F given 200 days/year
BIBBY et al. (1955)	135	50	5—14	1.0	1	0	NaF pills
	119		5—14	1.0	1	30	NaF lozenges
NIEDENTHAL (1957)	251	257	5—16	1.0	3	22	F in soluble sugar coat ing of pills
	190	186				31	After 3 yrs. on lozenge and 2 yrs. without
BINDER (1958)	565	710	7	1.0	2	35	
KESSLER and SOLTH (1958)	278	377	6—8	1.0	3	18	4 pills cont'g. 0.25 m F/day
	127	105	6—8	0.5	3	33	Pills cont'd. trace ele ments
	266	234	3—6	0.45	3	38	
	339	503	6—8	0.7—1.0	3	34	Only 1st molars
WRZODEK (1959)	8381	5335	6—9	0.3—1.0	3	21	NaF lozenges
	13,585	4975	6—9	0.3—1.0	4	22	0.3 mg F used only th 1st month
ARNOLD et al. (1960)	121		Birth-6	See text	1—15	Same as water fluoridation	Data compared wit those obtained in Grand Rapids befor and after fluoridatio
ZIEMNOWICZ-GLOWACKA (1960)	139	136	3	0.75	2	25	F given 200 days/yr.
	226	236	4	0.75	2	30	
	108	60	5	0.75	2	39	
	231	171	6	0.75	2	35	
	70	61	5	0.75	3	32	
	134	91	6	0.75	3	22	
LEONHARDT (1961)	775	532	6	1.0	2	16	
	741	408	6	1.0	3	30	
	799	398	6	1.0	4	26	
	741	665	7	1.0	2	22	
	799	429	7	1.0	3	22	
SCHUTZMANNSKY (1961)	1892		7	0.75	1	6	Given 200 days/year
	1763		7	0.75	2	8	
	1317		7	0.75	3	11	
	916		7	0.75	4	11	
	595		7	0.75	5	22	
	258		7	0.75	6	23	

which were dissolved in the mouth before swallowing, while no effect was obtained after the same period when fluoride was given in pills. These findings suggest that the local effect of supplementary fluoride on the tooth surface is of importance, and that a method of administration which permits maximal contact of the fluoride with the teeth before swallowing may be most beneficial. Some support for this view may be derived from the fact that NIEDENTHAL (1957) and ZIEMNOWICZ-GLOWACKA (1960) who instructed the children to dissolve the fluoride pills in the mouth before swallowing, appear to have obtained a greater inhibition of caries than KESSLER and SOLTH (1958) and LEONHARDT (1961) who had their subjects swallow the pills. Additional studies, designed to test this concept, are desirable.

Although more evidence is needed, investigators agree that it is advantageous to begin taking pills at the earliest possible age. Thus, ZIEMNOWICZ-GLOWACKA (1960) found 26 % reduction in caries of the deciduous teeth of kindergarten children who were given fluoride for two years from the age of three, but there was no effect in the deciduous teeth of those children who started taking pills at the age of 4 or 5 years. However, the permanent teeth of the latter group, which erupted during the study did show caries inhibition. In this study there was no difference in the caries reduction of 8-year-old children who had been given fluoride pills from the age of either 5 or 6 years (32 and 35 % reduction, respectively). WRZODEK (1959) observed caries inhibition of 27, 24 and 20 % in school children who began fluoride supplementation in first, second and third grades, respectively. LEONHARDT (1961) similarly found only slight differences in the decrease of caries in permanent teeth of 9- and 10-year-old children who had received fluoride pills from the age of either 6 or 7 years. These fndings agree well with the observation made in the previously mentioned studies concerned with water fluoridation, viz., that exposure to fluoride during and soon after tooth eruption will provide protection against caries. Only one investigator has shown a decrease in caries as a result of prenatal fluoride supplementation (FELTMAN and KOSEL, 1961). The dramatic reduction in DMF permanent teeth of from 47 to 57 % in 9- to 12-year-old children who used fluoride prenatally only, is contrary to the pattern of caries reduction obtained in water fluoridation by other investigators and must be seriously questioned. The wealth of material available concerning tooth formation and fluoride deposition precludes a caries reducing effect on permanent teeth by means of prenatal fluoride supplementation.

The effectiveness of continuous fluoride administration in the pre-eruptive as well as the post-eruptive period is demonstrated in the study of ARNOLD et al. (1960). Nearly two-thirds of the children in this study began to take fluoride tablets before their third birthday, and almost all before their sixth birthday. The number of years of ingestion of fluoride ranged from 1 to 15. No non-fluoride exposed controls were included, but comparison of the caries incidence with that found in Grand Rapids before and after fluoridation in similar age groups suggested that the fluoride pills produced a caries inhibition similar to that obtained from water fluoridation.

It may be noted from Table 14 that approximately the same caries reduction was obtained from pills supplying 0.5 mg fluoride (KESSLER and SOLTH, 1958) 0.75 mg (ZIEMNOWICZ-GLOWACKA, 1960 and SCHUTZMANNSKY, 1961), and 1 mg (NIEDENTHAL, 1957; BINDER, 1958 and LEONHARDT, 1961). However, since the comparability of these data is uncertain, and since there has been no controlled study of the relative effectiveness of different levels of fluoride intake in children residing in one community, no conclusion can be drawn in regard to the relation of dosage and caries inhibition. It is interesting that the studies in which fluoride was given to the children only on school days, that is approximately 200 days a year (HELD and PIGUET, 1954; ZIEMNOWICZ-GLOWACKA, 1960 and SCHUTZMANNSKY, 1961), showed results comparable to those in which fluoride was provided throughout the year (LEONHARDT, 1961). Again controlled studies of children from the same community must be undertaken to determine which method of administration, every day or only a limited number of days, is preferable.

No detrimental effects from the supplemental fluoride were reported in any of the studies cited. The dosage employed, from 0.5 to 1.0 mg per day must therefore be considered safe, provided of course, that the drinking water contains only traces of fluoride. The study of ARNOLD et al. (1960) is of particular interest in regard to dosage because fluoride was taken by most of the children during and following the period of formation of the permanent teeth. Infants up to 2 years of age were given fluoride by incorporating 1 ppm of fluoride in all water they consumed. This was accomplished within the family by adding 1 mg of fluoride (1 pill) to a quart of tap water. Children between 2 and 3 years swallowed 1 pill containing 1 mg of fluoride every other day, and all children older than 3 years took 1 pill every day. On this regimen one of the examiners found that 4 of 32 children had dental fluorosis, 3 instances of which were questionable, and one very mild. None of these cases was esthetically objectionable. No fluorosis was reported in the remaining children. The percentage of fluorosis in this study parallels that obersved in Grand Rapids after water fluoridation (Arnold et al., 1962). There is evidence that occurrence of non-specific and esthetically objectionable enamel opacities may be less in areas with water fluoridation (1 ppm of F) than in many low fluoride areas (Russell, 1962; Jackson, 1961), and that teeth may gain in appearance as a result of ingestion of optimal amounts of fluoride.

According to studies on water consumption, American children under 12 years of age rarely drink more than 500 ml of tap water per day (Walker et al., 1963). Although the accuracy of these data is open to question, dosages of 1 mg of fluoride per day for children over 3 years of age, employed by Arnold et al. may exceed those provided to the average child by 1 ppm of fluoride in the drinking water. Since no observable mottling takes place under this procedure, it is to be recommended. Table 15 gives a scheme for use of fluoride pills worked out by Ericsson (1959) which takes into account both age and the level of fluoride in the drinking water. Ericsson's plan has not been subjected to clinical trial and in the opinion of this writer, is too conservative. Ericsson also advises an intake of 1 mg of fluoride per day for pregnant and lactating women. However, since prenatal exposure to water-borne fluoride appears to be ineffective and since the fluoride level of human milk is maintained at a low level regardless of outside sources of fluoride, the important point would seem to be to make sure that children receive the proper amount of fluoride (0.5 mg/day) starting soon after birth.

Table 15. *Suggested usage of pills containing 0.25 mg of fluoride.* Data from Ericsson (1959)

	Recommended daily no. of pills for use with water containing		
	0—0.25 ppm F	p.25—0.50 ppm F	0.50—0.75 ppm F
Pregnancy and lactation	4	3	2
Age 0—1 yr.	1		
Age 1—6 yrs.	2	1	
Age 7—12 yrs.	3	2	1
Age over 12 yrs.	4	3	2

Considering all of the evidence, it may be concluded that supplementation of fluoride intake by pills, drops or lozenges will cause a decrease in dental caries, and that organized programs of administration in schools, beginning in kindergarten are advisable in communities which are unable to fluoridate the water supply. The use of pills in households is also advisable, but unfortunately, experience has shown that even in highly educated groups, only about one-half of the families continue giving their children pills for the necessary number of years (Arnold et al., 1960).

B. Fluoridation of kitchen salt

Fluoridated kitchen salt containing 90 mg of fluoride per kilogram of salt is used extensively in Switzerland. It was introduced in the Canton of Zurich in 1955, and in 1961 both fluoridated and fluoride-free salts were commercially available in 20 of the Cantons (WESPI, 1962). According to two progress reports, use of this salt will cause some reduction in caries of the permanent teeth of children, but the results are inferior to those obtained from water fluoridation. In one study, 58 children 8 to 9 years old who had used the fluoridated salt for 4.5 years, showed a caries reduction of 22% compared to 54 control children. Another study involving over 1200 children, showed similar results after 5.5 years' use of the fluoridated salt. Table 16 lists the percentage reduction in caries of different types of tooth surfaces obtained in the 9-year-old children in this study. Included also, is the corresponding data obtained after 5.5 years of water fluoridation in Holland. Although these findings may not be strictly comparable, they do demonstrate the greater effectiveness of water fluoridation over salt fluoridation, and suggest that the amounts of fluoride incorporated in the salt are below the optimal level. With a concentration of 90 mg of fluoride per kilogram of salt, an intake of 11 gms of salt will provide 1 mg of fluoride. The mean individual salt consumption in families with children varies in Switzerland between 3.6 and 6.8 gms per day (MARTHALER, 1961). In adults mean values of 8.4 gms per day (WESPI, 1961) and 5.6 per day (SANTESSON, 1959) have been reported. Since these data represent the amounts of purchased salt, and since there is from 20 to 30% waste of salt in the kitchen during cooking procedures, the actual intake is less than indicated by these figures (SANTESSON, 1959). It is now believed that the dosage of 90 mg fluoride per kilogram of salt should be at least doubled and that a level of 200 or 250 mg per kilogram of salt may be required to produce the inhibition of caries achieved by water fluoridation (WESPI, 1961).

Table 16. *Caries reduction in permanent tooth surfaces of nine-year-old children who used fluoridated kitchen salt or fluoridated water for 5.5 years*

	Percentage reduction in carious surfaces		
	proximal	buccal-labial	occlusal
Fluoridated salt[1]	41	32	21
Fluoridated water[2]	66	66	28

[1] From MARTHLAER and SCHENARDI (1962).
[2] From BACKER DIRKS et al. (1961).

Fluoridated kitchen salt can be manufactured and made available to the total population at low cost. This method of fluoridation, therefore, seems suitable in areas where fluoridation of the water supply is impractical. However, the optimal concentration of fluoride in the salt must be determined in long-range clinical studies before it can be seriously considered. One difficulty in determining the dosage is the considerable individual variation in salt consumption. A study in Switzerland showed that the amount of salt purchased for cooking and preparation of food for adults varied between one and fifteen gms per day. It should be noted that children use virtually no salt during the first two years of life. Since the permanent dentition is calcified for the most part after the age of 2, theoretically it could benefit as much from fluoridation of table salt as of water. This may not be true of the deciduous teeth which would receive little or no fluoride from fluoridated salt during their formation.

C. Fluoridation of milk

Milk has been suggested as a vehicle for fluoride because it is the food used most universally by infants and children during the period of tooth formation. To date only one study, involving a small group of children (65 experimental and 64 controls) has been reported in the literature (RUSOFF et al., 1962). The children were served one pint of homogenized milk fortified with 1 mg of fluoride as sodium fluoride each day at lunch, beginning at the age of six for a period of three years. There was a significant reduction in caries in the teeth which erupted during the study, the results being comparable to those which have been obtained from water fluoridation. Eighteen months after cessation of the fluoride ingestion, a significant difference in caries rate was still retained in favor of the treated group, suggesting a prolonged fluoride effect.

A study on milk fluoridation is in progress in Switzerland (ZIEGLER, 1959), but results are not yet available.

Although the caries inhibition obtained with fluoridated milk shows that the fluoride added to the milk is available for uptake by the teeth, it is of interest that fluoride in milk is absorbed at a slower rate than fluoride ingested in water (ERICSSON, 1958a). This may be because it combines with milk calcium to form the relatively insoluble calcium fluoride, or because it complexes with the organic matter, principally casein (ERICSSON, 1958a). A portion (about 25%) of the 0.2 ppm fluoride normally occurring in cows' milk is also bound to casein (EVANS and PHILLIPS, 1939). However, no sedimentation of fluoride added to milk in concentrations of 1 to 4 ppm was observed after 5 hours.

As in the case of salt fluoridation, well-controlled, long-term clinical experiments must precede serious consideration of milk as a vehicle for fluoride.

V. Topical treatment with fluoride

The observation, first made in 1942, that dental caries can be significantly reduced in children by repeated topical treatments with sodium or potassium fluoride (BIBBY, 1942; CHEYNE, 1942) has been amply substantiated. Findings published prior to 1953 have been reviewed and tabulated by several investigators (KNUTSON, 1949; BERGMAN, 1953; BIBBY and BRUDEVOLD, 1954) and will only be briefly summarized here. Of the different types of fluoride tested, aqueous solutions of sodium and potassium fluoride gave the most consistent results. The most effective procedure was found to be 3 or 4 applications per year, each lasting for 3 to 4 minutes, and the first treatment being preceded by a thorough cleaning of the teeth with an abrasive. The concentration of fluoride apparently was not critical, since levels in the range of 0.05 to 4 % gave similar results.

The duration of the fluoride exposure was more important in view of the fact that results were better with 3 or 4 than from 1 or 2 successive treatments. However, the beneficial effects were not increased by giving more than 4 repeated treatments. For example, in one representative study 2, 4 and 6 applications with 2% sodium fluoride resulted in 22, 41 and 41% decreases in caries, respectively (GALAGEN and KNUTSON, 1947). The time interval between individual treatments was not shown to be critical if care was taken to have the teeth exposed to fluoride as soon as possible after eruption (BIBBY and BRUDEVOLD, 1954). It was demonstrated that careful techniques were necessary in order to obtain maximal fluoride effects. Presence of debris on the teeth interfered with the treatment since omission of cleaning procedure prior to the first application reduced the caries inhibition effect by as much as one-half (KNUTSON et al., 1947). However, equally favorable results were obtained when supervised tooth brushing for a period of 2 weeks prior to the first fluoride treatment was substituted for the usual cleaning procedure given by a dental hygienist (CHRIETZBERG, 1951). The necessity of keeping saliva away from the teeth during the fluoride exposure was emphasized and several investigators dried the teeth with alcohol and air before applying the fluoride (BIBBY, 1942; SYRRIST, 1949d, KLINKENBERG and BIBBY, 1950; BERGMAN, 1953).

Although the advantage of thorough drying was not clearly demonstrated, it is worthy of note that the results obtained by these workers (42 to 60 % reduction) appear to be more favorable than those obtained when less careful drying procedures were used. One important observation was that some of the resistance to caries from a series of treatments persisted for more than three years (KNUTSON and ARMSTRONG, 1946; BIBBY and TURESKY, 1947). The latter findings have been confirmed in more recent work (BERGMAN, 1953; SYRRIST and KARLSEN, 1954).

Attempts in these early studies to increase the effectiveness of the fluoride solution were not successful. Contrary to expectation, acid sodium fluoride solutions, which according to solubility studies should increase the fluoride effect, failed to reduce caries (ARNOLD et al., 1944, RICKLES and BECKS, 1951; STONES et al., 1949). Although two of these trials were done on young adults, who probably are less benefitted by fluoride treatments than children, the most likely explanation for these negative findings is that the solution employed contained acetic, phthalic or hydrofluoric acid, all of which tend to dissolve tooth structure. Other types of fluoride than sodium and potassium fluoride gave variable results. Of three trials of lead fluoride, two showed no effects (GALAGEN and KNUTSON, 1947; BIBBY et al., 1947) and one gave a 40 % caries reduction (KLINKENBERG and BIBBY, 1950). A complex fluoride, sodium monofluoroborate was a failure, but sodium monofluorophosphate caused a caries inhibition of 26 % (BIBBY and BRUDEVOLD, 1954).

Much of the voluminous literature after 1953 deals with the relative efficacy of repeated applications of solutions of sodium fluoride and stannous fluoride. Findings in studies which employed three or more treatments of solutions of these and other salts are summarized in Table 17. MUHLER and co-workers have done most of the work with stannous fluoride, and claim it is superior to sodium fluoride in inhibiting caries. This view is based primarily on their findings that 4 repeated applications of stannous fluoride in a concentration of 2 % (HOWELL et al., 1955) or 4 % (McDONALD and MUHLER, 1957) gave better results than similar treatments with 2 % sodium fluoride. HOWELL et al. found reductions of 59 and 36 %, and McDONALD and MUHLER, 37 and 8 % reductions in the stannous fluoride and sodium fluoride-treated groups, respectively. Other investigators have failed to find significant differences in the effectiveness of the two compounds. McLAREN and BROWN (1955) in a two-year study, obtained a decrease in caries of 46 % compared with 39 % from stannous fluoride and sodium fluoride after one year, and 19 % compared with 18 % after two years. NEVITT et al. (1958) and LAW et al. (1961) obtained somewhat lower inhibition from stannous fluoride than from sodium fluoride, the respective reduction in figures in the two studies being 36 and 44 %, and 30 and 35 %, respectively. In view of this conflicting evidence, it seems premature to postulate a difference in the caries reducing effect of these two salts. MUHLER and co-workers have employed stannous fluoride and sodium fluoride in other studies, listed in Tables 17 and 18, but since different concentrations or application techniques were used for each agent, the findings do not provide evidence concerning their relative effectiveness.

From Table 17, it may be seen that solutions of stannous chlorofluoride and potassium fluorostannite are comparable to stannous fluoride in caries inhibiting effect (MUHLER, 1958a; GISH et al., 1959). It is worthy of note that applications of fluoride-free stannous sulfate failed to reduce caries (MUHLER, 1958a), suggesting that deposition in the enamel of tin salts without simultaneous deposition of fluoride provides no effect.

Although one or two applications of 2 % sodium fluoride, as already mentioned, are relatively ineffective in reducing caries, recent reports have shown that this

Table 17. *Summary of studies (1954—1963) of topical application of fluorides involving three or more treatments in children*

	Agent	Duration of study	Treatment		No. of subjects		Initial age yrs.	Percentage reduction in caries	Comments
			No. per year	Duration each treatment min.	Expt.	Control			
Bergman (1953)	NaF 2%	1st yr. 2nd yr. 3rd yr.	4, 3—5 mo. apart	5	114	opposite quadrant	11—13	61 54 43	No treatment 2nd and 3rd yr.
Syrrist and Karlson (1954)	NaF 2%	2 yrs.	3—4, 1 every 3—4 mo.	7	91	opposite quadrant	12	41	7 treatments, all during 1st 2 yrs. Redn. after 5 yrs. still 21%
Galagen and Vermillion (1955)	NaF 2%	1 yr.	4, 2—7 da. apart	3	282	opposite quadrant	7—16	9 not significant	0.7 ppm F in drinking water
Howell et al. (1955)	NaF 2% SnF_2 2% SnF_2 2%	2 yrs.	4, 2—6 da. apart	4	92 104 195	132	8—15	36 59 67	Applied with cotton pellets Applied with spray
McLaren and Brown (1955)	NaF 2% SnF_2 2%	2 yrs.	4, 2—7 da. apart	4	135 135	135	6—11	39, 18[1] 46, 19[2]	No treatment 2nd yr. No treatment 2nd yr.
Sundvall-Hagland (1955)	NaF 2%	1st yr. 2nd yr. 3rd yr.	4, 2—3 da. apart	4	107 104 102	opposite quadrant	2—3	19 14 9	When compared with untreated controls, reduction in caries was 34, 23 and 12% after 2 and 3 yrs
Slack (1956)	SnF_2 2%	2 yrs.	3, 7 da. apart	4	299	opposite quadrant	5.5—6.5	17	Questionable significance
McDonald and Muhler (1957)	NaF 2% SnF_2 4%	1 yr.	4, within 2 wks.	4	76 86	65	3—12	12 37	Not significant Deciduous teeth only
Muhler (1958a)	SnClF 4% $SnSO_4$ 2%	1 yr.	4 within 10 da.	4	188 189	181	6—15	37 8	1 ppm F in drinking water for 3 yrs. Not significant
Nevitt et al. (1958)	NaF 2% SnF_2 2%	16 mo.	4, 7 da. apart	3	298 290	opposite quadrant	9—14	36 44	Difference between NaF and SnF_2 not significant
Czarnoska et al. (1959)	NaF 2%	5 yrs.	7		312	119	6—11	33	Repeated annually

HARRIS (1959)	NaF 2%	5 yrs.	4, 2—7 da. apart	3	57	69	6	33	Repeated annually
GISH et al. (1959)	K fluoro-stannite 4%	1st yr. 2nd yr. 3rd yr.	4, 2—7 da. apart	4	390 319 294	411 364 342	6—15	39 39 41	No treatment 2nd and 3rd yr.
MILLER and HOBSON (1959)	NaF 1%	2 yrs.	every 2 mo.		44	43	6	none	Only 1st molars
LAW et al. (1961)	NaF 2% SnF_2 2%	1 yr.	4, 2—7 da. apart	3	269 273	opposite quadrant	7—13	35 30	
PAMEIJER et al. (1963)	NaF 2%	3—15 mo.	4 within 2 wks.	3	77	2 quad., NaF			
	NaF 2% in 0.15 M H_3PO_4					2 quad. NaF + H_3PO_4	4—10	50	In NaF + H_3PO_4 treated teeth. No untreated control

[1] 1st yr., 39; 2nd yr., 18. — [2] 1st yr., 46; 2nd yr., 19.

method of approach is more successful when more concentrated fluoride solutions are used. These findings are summarized in Table 18. Of special clinical interest are the seven studies which employed single treatments. Six of these are concerned with 8% stannous fluoride and one with a solution of 2.7% sodium fluoride in 0.1 M phosphoric acid. The results obtained from stannous fluoride vary markedly in different studies, the reported inhibition of caries ranging from 19% (BURGESS et al., 1962) to 51% (MERCER and MUHLER, 1961). The results obtained with solutions of phosphate fluoride (WELLOCK and BRUDEVOLD, 1963) give promise of an improvement in topical treatment. A single application gave 70% reduction, and in another study listed in Table 17, caries reduction was 50% greater in the teeth given four treatments of the phosphate fluoride solution than in teeth given four treatments of sodium fluoride solution. These findings, which need to be confirmed in other trials, suggest that acid fluoride-phosphate solutions may be potent anti-caries agents. These solutions have important advantages over stannous fluoride. They are stable, and are therefore easier to handle than the highly unstable stannous fluoride. They have an acceptable taste, and are well tolerated by patients. The obnoxious taste of stannous fluoride causes profuse salivation which may interfere with the treatment procedure (WEISZ, 1962). More important, fluoride-phosphoric acid solutions do not affect the appearance of teeth, while the majority of patients treated with stannous fluoride develop discoloration which forms as a brownish pigment, probably consisting of stannous sulfide (BACKER DIRKS, 1961; ISAAC and BRUDEVOLD, 1957). The discoloration is particularly prevalent in carious lesions and margins of faulty fillings, but may develop in other areas (HINE et al., 1957).

Topical fluoride treatments in adults have given variable results. Available reports, summarized in Table 19, show contradictory results with only 4 of 9 studies giving significant caries reduction.

Table 18. *Summary of studies (1954—1963) of topical applications of fluorides involving one or two treatments in children*

	Agent	Duration of study	Treatment: No. per year	Treatment: Duration each treatment min.	No. of subjects: expt.	No. of subjects: control	Initial age yrs.	Percentage reduction in caries	Comments
HAWES et al. (1954)	KF 10%	1 yr.	2, 6 mo. apart	3	117	opposite quadrant	8—12	30	
PETERSEN and JORDAN (1957)	Na_2SiF_6 0.9%	1st yr. 2nd yr.	2, within 4 da.	4	211 199	opposite quadrant	13—14	13 16	No treatment 2nd yr.
ABDUL-GHAFFER and MUHLER (1959)	NaF 4% SnF_2 8% SnF_2 8%	1 yr.	1 ea. agent 1 da. apart 2, 1 da. apart	4 4	199 211	192	6—15	61 78	Differences between 2 groups not significant
MUHLER (1960)	SnF_2 8%	1st yr. 2nd yr. 30 mo.	2, 1 every 6 mo.	4	199 134 78	196 124 70	6—17	31 35 49	1 ppm F in water supply for past 6 yrs. 2 treatments each year
MUHLER (1961)	SnF_2 8%	1 yr. 2nd yr. 3rd yr.	2, 1 every 6 mo.	4	230 199 156	220 193 158		58 55 63	2 treatments ea. yr., and also brushing with SnF_2 toothpaste
COMPTON and GRAINGER (1959)	SnF_2 8%	1 yr.	1	4	112	92	2—4	28	
JORDAN et al. (1959)	SnF_2 8%	1st yr 2nd yr.	1 every yr.	4	234 209	238 211	12—13	14 49	Combined for 2 yrs., 38%
LAW et al. (1961)	SnF_2 8%	1 yr.	1	3	281	opposite quadrant	7—13	24	Not significant
MERCER and MUHLER (1961)	NaF 2% SnF_2 8% SnF_2 8%	1 yr.	1 1 2, a few days apart	4 4 4	201 201 201	199	6—14	none 51 53	
BURGESS et al. (1962)	SnF_2 8%	1st yr. 2nd yr.	1 every yr.	4	122	122	2—4	19 29	
GISH et al. (1962)	SnF_2 8% NaF 2%	1st yr. 2nd yr. 3rd yr. 4th yr. 5th yr.	1 every yr. 4, 2—7 da. apart, every 3rd yr.	4 4	934 862 586 SnF_2 364 157	922 875 646 NaF 387 170	8	38 32 31 28 35	No untreated controls
WELLOCK and BRUDEVOLD (1963)	NaF 2.7% in 0.1 M H_3PO_4	1st yr. 2nd yr.	1 every yr.	4	115	113	9—11	71 70	

Table 19. *Summary of studies of topical application of fluorides in adults*

	Agent	Duration of study	Treatment		No. of subjects		Initial age yrs.	Percentage reduction in caries	Comments
			No. per yr.	Duration each treatment min.	expt.	control			
Arnold et al. (1944)	NaF 1.1% in acetate buffer pH 4	1 yr.	1	5	94	94	17—22	none	
Klinkenberg and Bibby (1950)	NaF 1% PbF_2 0.06%	14 mo.	4, 3 mo. apart	5	139	opposite quadrant	18—40	57 40	Upper or lower quadrant treated with NaF and PbF_2, respectively
Rickles and Becks (1951)	NaF 2% (pH 7) NaF 2% in phthalate HCl buffer pH 3.5	2 yrs.	4, 3 mo. apart	4	25 22	opposite quadrant	22—34 22—34	50 —33	The acidulated solution increased caries
Kutler and Ireland (1953)	NaF 2%	13 mos.	4, 2 da. apart	4	147	opposite quadrant	20—42	none	
Carter et al. (1955)	NaF 2%	8—14 mos.	1 to 4, mostly 3 or 4	5	60	88	19—39	9	Not significant
Muhler (1958b)	SnF_2 10%	1 yr.	1	4	228	207	17—38	16	Not significant
Protheroe (1961)	SnF_2 10%	1 yr.	1	4	83	opposite quadrant	17—21	42	Treated teeth isolated with rubber dam

Table 20. *Summary of studies of effectiveness of tooth brushing or mouth rinsing with fluoride solutions*

	Agent	Duration of study	Treatment: No. per year	Treatment: Duration each treatment min.	No. of subjects: expt.	No. of subjects: control	Initial age yrs.	Percentage reduction in caries	Comments
Berggren and Welander (1960)	NaF 1%	2 yrs.	5 brushings, 1st yr. 4 brushings, 2nd yr.		568	1116	3—8	30	Children brushed teeth with soln. under supervision
Weisz (1961)	NaF 0.25%	2—10 yrs.	daily rinsings		37	60	5—6 and 8—9	80—90	The concn. of F too high for routine use in homes
Torell and Siberg (1962)	NaF 0.2% NaF 0.2%	1 yr.	rinse once per mo.	3	150 912	337 1019	9		Significant red'n. in caries of incisors. No data on remaining teeth. Effect in only 3*rd* grade not 1*st* and 2*nd* grade children
	KF 0.2%	1 yr.	rinse once per mo.		520	508	9	no effect	

More work is clearly needed to determine the benefits of topical fluoride in adult populations.

A recent report from Sweden demonstrates that a few supervised brushings with a solution of sodium fluoride can produce worth-while caries reduction in children (Berggren and Welander, 1960). The purpose of this study was to develop a less time-consuming method of applying fluoride than the conventional topical treatment procedure. Using school hours, groups of children brushed their teeth for four minutes with 1% sodium fluoride. As can be seen from Table 20, five repeated brushings during the first year, and 4 during the second year, resulted in a decrease in caries of 25 to 30%. It was possible to treat 200 children per school day with this procedure, compared to 30 with topical applications. Also listed in Table 20 are findings from studies concerned with fluoride mouth rinses. Although work in this field is still preliminary, the results indicate that supervised rinsing with fluoride solutions may be a practical method for exposing the teeth of large groups of children to fluoride.

VI. Fluoride dentifrices

Only a brief summary will be given of the present status of fluoride dentifrices. The many variables and uncertainties which relate to clinical studies concerning the effectiveness of these products (Bartelstone et al., 1961) and the conflicting reports in the literature concerning their usefulness preclude a detailed report. The use of fluoride dentifrices has become widespread in the United States since the

American Dental Association's Council on Dental Therapeutics in 1960 recognized a stannous fluoride pyrophosphate dentifrice as "an effective anti-carious dentifrice that can be of significant value when used in a conscientiously applied program of oral hygiene and regular professional care." (Council on Dental Therapeutics, 1960). It was classified in Group B, which includes products lacking sufficient evidence to justify present acceptance in Group A, but for which there is reasonable evidence of usefulness and safety. This dentifrice has now been classified in Group A, and two additional stannous fluoride dentifrices have been classified in Group B. One group of workers which has conducted the majority of the clinical studies on this dentifrice has reported statistically significant reductions in caries among children after both unsupervised and supervised brushing with it (MUHLER, 1955; 1958c; MUHLER et al., 1955; PEFFLY and MUHLER, 1960), and among adults after unsupervised brushing (MUHLER and RADIKE, 1957). Other investigators have not been able to demonstrate significant reduction in caries from use of this dentifrice by children brushing with supervision (FINN and JAMISON, 1963) or without supervision (JORDAN and PETERSON, 1959; HILL, 1959; WELLOCK, personal communication), or among adults (KYES et al., 1961). Recently it has been reported that use of dentifrices containing approximately 0.1 % fluoride combined with certain amines (MARTHALER, 1963) e.g bis(hydroxyethyl)aminopropyl-N-hydroxyethyloctadecylaminedi-HF and cetylamine-HF, or fluoride as sodium monofluorophosphate, significantly reduced caries in children. These findings have not as yet been confirmed in other studies.

A number of factors may contribute to the variable results obtained in the testing of dentifrices by different workers. The thoroughness and frequency of brushing appear to be important. For example, it has been shown that children brushing three or more times per day had from 14 to 29 % less caries than those brushing 2 or less times per day (MUHLER et al., 1956). As important may be the fact that it has been difficult to stabilize the stannous fluoride pyrophosphate dentifrice. As a result the concentrations of stannous and fluoride ions available for reaction with the teeth have been reported to decrease markedly after 10 or more weeks (MANLY, 1961). Presumably more stable products will become available.

The past failure of sodium fluoride dentifrices to reduce caries can be attributed to the use of ingredients which combined with fluoride and rendered it inactive. Commonly employed abrasives such as calcium carbonate and calcium phosphate react with fluoride to form relatively insoluble calcium fluoride. The availability of fluoride in different dentifrice formulations has been investigated in 3 recent studies (MANLY, 1961; ERICSSON, 1961, 1962). It is interesting that several fluoride pastes now on the market have eliminated calcium salts in the formulation and utilize insoluble sodium metaphosphate as an abrasive. These dentifrices have a high percentage of available fluoride, but although theoretically they should be effective caries-reducing agents, their effectiveness against caries has not yet been established in clinical studies.

VII. Mechanism of action of fluoride in inhibiting caries

A. Introduction

In order to discuss the mechanism of action of fluoride in inhibiting caries it is desirable to consider briefly the chemistry of enamel and dentin. The highly calcified enamel has approximately 96 % by weight of mineral, 1 % organic matter and 3 % water (LEICESTER, 1949). Corresponding figures for dentin are 69, 20 and 11 % (ARMSTRONG and BREKHUS, 1937). The nature of the organic matter in the two tissues has been reviewed elsewhere (BRUDEVOLD, 1962a) and will not be dealt with here because, although the organic matter may serve to facilitate penetration of fluoride into enamel and dentin, it is not as far as is known, involved in fluoride reactions. Physiologically, fluoride is a hard tissue seeker because of its great affinity for bone and tooth mineral. Only traces of fluoride are present in soft tissues, (LAWRENZ et al., 1940; ERICSSON and ULLBERG, 1958) and no fluoride has been detected in the organic matter of dental tissues (PECKHAM et al., 1956). Furthermore, of the two phases of the carious process, viz. demineralization and lysis of the organic matter, fluoride affects only the former, according to available evidence. Since demineralization precedes proteolysis in caries of both enamel and dentin (BRUDEVOLD, 1962a) interference with this process will prevent or arrest tissue destruction.

Theoretically fluoride could inhibit demineralization by preventing bacterial production of demineralizing agents, or by decreasing the solubility of the tooth mineral, or promoting mineral formation, *i.e.*, remineralization. Regardless of which of these mechanisms is operating it is evident that deposition of fluoride in the tooth mineral is of primary importance. This is demonstrated by the clinical observation that exposure to water-borne fluoride even when it occurs only during the early years of life, and topical application of fluoride will both provide prolonged caries resistance. The nature of the tooth mineral and the uptake by teeth of ingested and topically applied fluoride will therefore be considered first, and then the effect of fluoride on bacterial acid production and on solubility and formation of tooth mineral will be examined.

B. The mineral phase of enamel and dentin

The concentrations of the principal mineral components in enamel and dentin on a dry weight basis, as obtained from a survey of the literature are listed in Table 21. Although the considerable ranges in concentrations may, to some extent, reflect the use of different chemical and sampling procedures, there is a real and sometimes marked variation in the composition of mineral from different teeth, and as will be shown later, in surface and subsurface material from the same tooth.

Table 21. *Percentage composition of enamel and dentin, dry weight basis*

	Enamel		Dentin	
	Range	Mean	Range	Mean
Inorganic	98.9—99.8	99.2	76.0—82.0	80.0
Ca	34.0—39.0	36.0	25.0—29.0	27.0
P	17.0—18.0	17.5	12.0—14.0	13.0
Ca/P	1.95—2.17	2.08	1.92—2.10	2.07
CO_2	1.95—3.00	2.50	3.00—3.57	3.30
Na	0.68—0.90	0.77	—	0.30
Mg	0.25—0.56	0.42	0.73—0.96	0.84
Cl	0.19—0.30	0.25	—	Traces
Organic	0.2 —1.1	0.8	18.0—24.0	20.0

These differences are not surprising considering the nature of the tooth mineral. X-Ray and electron microscope studies have shown the mineral to be crystalline, and to have a diffraction pattern similar to that of apatite. The crystals are rod shaped and vary greatly in size. Enamel crystals, which are the largest and best developed, measure on the average 3000 to 5000 Å in length, and 500 to 1200 Å in width (FRANK et al., 1960) according to observations with the electron microscope.

Corresponding figures obtained by x-ray diffraction are 1000 to 2700 Å and 370 to 450 Å (GLAS and OMNELL, 1960). The smaller crystals in dentin approximate the size of those in bone, averaging 200 to 300 Å in length (maximum 1000 Å) and only 20 to 75 Å in width (FRANK et al., 1960; JOHANSEN and PARKS, 1960, 1962). The smallest repeating unit in the crystals, the unit cell, contains 10 Ca^{++}, 6 $PO_4^{\equiv}$ and 2 OH^-, each ion occupying a definite position in relation to the others.

The apatite crystals have two characteristics of fundamental importance: 1) Ca^{++}, $PO_4^{\equiv}$ and OH^- can be replaced by other ionic species, and 2) these ionic exchange reactions are facilitated by the large total surface area of the apatite, resulting from the minute size of the individual crystals.

Because of the large surface area, apatite crystals will attract water, and hydrated or polarized ions such as Ca^{++} and $HPO_4^{=}$ (JOHANSEN and PARKS, 1962). Apparently electrical assymetry on the crystal surface sets up a powerful electrical field which pulls charged ions and water molecules toward it. Radioactive studies have shown that the layer of water adjacent to the crystal, termed the hydration shell, must be considered part of the crystal from a chemical point of view, and that exchange of ions between the crystal and the surrounding fluids may involve 1) only the hydration shell, 2) the crystal surface and 3) the body of the crystal (NEUMAN and NEUMAN, 1958).

This versatile system permits the presence in the mineral of teeth and bone of a great number of ionic species in addition to Ca^{++} and $PO_4^{\equiv}$ and explains largely the variation in the composition of the inorganic phase of enamel and dentin shown in Table 21. The exact location of many of the substituting ions in the crystal system is still uncertain. For example, carbonate has been postulated to be located inside the crystal, as part of the lattice (McCONNELL, 1952) and according to another theory, on the surface of the crystal (NEUMAN et al., 1956; CARLSTROM, 1955). Recent evidence suggests that it may be present in both interior and surface positions (TRAUTZ, 1960). Presumably many ionic species can be located in the hydration shell. Fewer ions, including sodium, strontium, magnesium, citrate and fluoride can be located on the crystal surface. Internal substitutions are restricted to ions such as fluoride and strontium, which have the proper size to fit into the lattice (NEUMAN et al., 1956).

C. The chemistry of fluoride and tooth mineral as related to water fluoridation

Two different salts, fluorapatite and calcium fluoride may be precipitated from solutions of calcium, phosphate and fluoride, or formed when hydroxyapatite is exposed to fluoride. The formation of fluorapatite in aqueous solutions containing low concentrations of fluoride has been observed by a number of investigators (MACINTIRE et al., 1937; MONTEL and CHAUDRON, 1952; GIESECKE and RATHJE, 1941). Calcium fluoride, being more soluble at neutral pH can only precipitate at the relatively high concentrations of fluoride required to exceed its solubility product (Ksp, 3.2×10^{-11}). Presence of fluoride as fluorapatite in normal as well as fluorosed teeth is suggested by x-ray diffraction analysis which showed only the pattern of apatite and not that of calcium fluoride (GEROULD, 1945). Since the concentration of fluoride in body fluids is little influenced by the amount of fluoride ingested (ARMSTRONG, 1961) and rarely exceeds 0.3 ppm (SMITH et al., 1950; SINGER and ARMSTRONG, 1960) and since the level of ionic calcium is only of the order of 1.2 mM in serum (WALSER, 1961) and 0.5 mM in saliva (VOGEL et al., 1965) even the several ppm of fluoride which may be present in drinking water will not exceed the solubility product of calcium fluoride. Therefore, this salt cannot precipitate and has not been observed under physiological conditions.

The reaction between hydroxyapatite and low concentrations of fluoride has been postulated to be an ionic exchange in which fluoride replaces and assumes the positions of the hydroxyl ions in the crystal lattice without otherwise disturbing the lattice structure (NEUMAN et al., 1950). The equation expresses these reactions:

$$Ca_{10}(PO_4)_6(OH)_2 + 2\,F^- \rightarrow Ca_{10}(PO_4)_6F_2 + 2\,OH^- .$$

In addition to this exchange, it was also suggested that fluoride could replace carbonate, since the amount of fluoride taken up by bone mineral was inversely related to the concentrations of both OH^- and HCO_3^- in the solution. However, it was unrelated to the concentrations of solution calcium and phosphate, thus indicating that these ions were not involved in the fluoride reaction. In addition, radioactive studies showed that presence of fluoride in bone mineral did not significantly affect the exchange of calcium and phosphate between the mineral and the solution (NEUMAN et al., 1950). Other investigators found a slightly lowered rate of exchange of phosphate in fluorosed dentin which was considered due to the lower solubility of the fluoride exposed mineral (McCANN and FATH, 1958). It was also shown in the latter study that presence of low levels of fluoride in the solution increased the rate of exchange of phosphate (contrary to the effect of fluoride in the solid phase), suggesting that uptake of fluoride by hydroxyapatite was associated with recrystallization. This has been confirmed in a recent study with radioactive isotopes, in which it was demonstrated that presence of fluoride in the solution (2 to 10 ppm) caused dissolution of calcium and phosphate from hydroxyapatite and reprecipitation of these ions with fluoride as fluorapatite (KUYPER and KUTNERIAN, 1962). Two mechanisms for fluoride uptake by hydroxyapatite have thus been demonstrated: 1) replacement of hydroxyl, carbonate and incidentally also of citrate ions (*cf.* ARMSTRONG and SINGER, 1956) with fluoride, while maintaining the integrity of the crystal lattice, and 2) recrystallization, involving dissolution of the hydroxyapatite and precipitation of fluorapatite.

Additional evidence that fluoride substitutes for hydroxyl groups in the apatite lattice is the finding by x-ray diffraction that the unit cell of bone mineral decreases in size from that of hydroxyapatite toward that of fluorapatite in fluoride-exposed bone (0.7 % or more of fluoride) (POSNER and EANES, 1963). X-ray diffraction studies have also shown increased resolution of x-ray reflections from certain crystalline planes of the apatite in human and rat bone as a result of fluoride ingestion (ZIPKIN et al., 1962; SCHRAER et al., 1962). These observations on bone, which by analogy should apply to the mineral of dental tissues, show that presence of fluoride in the lattice structure either increases the size of the crystals, or corrects lattice imperfections thus improving the crystallinity of the enamel.

D. Fluoride in enamel and dentin

Having discussed the mechanism of fluoride fixation, the next step is to consider to what extent fluoride fixation in enamel and dentin occurs under physiological conditions. In the first studies in this field, fluoride was determined in total tissues, and analyses of teeth from different communities showed that there generally was an increase in fluoride concentrations in both enamel and dentin with an increase in the fluoride level of the drinking water (McCLURE and LIKINS, 1951). In addition, enamel consistently contained lower levels of fluoride than dentin from the same tooth, a fact ascribed to the larger crystal size in the enamel and smaller accessible internal subsurface (McCLURE and LIKINS, 1951; ARMSTRONG and BREKHUS, 1938). Some of these findings are summarized in Table 22.

The correlation between the mean fluoride levels of the different tooth groups and the concentrations of fluoride in respective drinking waters, is remarkable in view of the climatic and environmental differences of the communities from which the teeth originated. From these and other findings (Boissevain and Drea, 1933; Bowes and Murray, 1936; Ockerse, 1943; Harrison, 1949) it is evident that drinking water is the main source of fluoride in human dietaries. The wide range in the concentrations of fluoride in teeth from the same community is likely to reflect differences in age and fluoride ingestion (water consumption).

Table 22. *Fluoride in enamel and dentin (ppm of ash weight) of teeth from geographical areas with different levels of fluoride in the water supply.* Data from McClure and Likins (1951)

No. of individuals	Geographical area and tooth description	F in drinking water (ppm)	ppm fluoride in ash					
			Enamel			Dentin		
			min	max	av.	min	max	av.
9	McDuffie County, Ga.	0.1						
	16 non-carious teeth		51	220	86	99	480	216
	13 carious teeth		40	193	97	143	544	186
33	Washington, D.C. and vicinity	0.0—0.4						
	224 non-carious teeth		46	203	102	113	482	240
	202 carious teeth		42	220	98	86	517	297
9	Oslo, Norway	0.2—0.4						
	27 non-carious teeth		25	178	79	50	126	86
31	Aurora, Illinois age 8—25	1.1—1.2						
	36 non-carious and carious teeth		64	253	135	125	702	360
12	Age 25—45, 35 non-carious and carious teeth		48	221	142	316	632	361
17	Age over 45, 30 non-carious and carious teeth		96	200	140	253	706	440
—	West Texas Panhandle area	2.5—5.0						
	20 non-carious and carious teeth		149	564	345	550	1033	762
12	Compagnano di Roma, Italy	3.5						
	12 non-carious and carious teeth		386	772	599	1123	2139	1589
—	Chetopa, Kansas	7.6						
	7 non-carious teeth		384	1059	658	809	1812	1277

1. Distribution of fluoride in enamel

It will be noted from Table 22 that there is only a slight difference in the mean fluoride level of enamel from areas with mere traces of fluoride and 1 ppm of fluoride in the drinking water (100 and 135 ppm, respectively). The difficulty of relating this minute difference in concentrations to the reduction in caries experience from water fluoridation has been resolved by the finding that fluoride accumulates in the outermost enamel in several times greater concentrations than those found by analysis of the total tissue (Jenkins and Speirs, 1953; Brudevold et al., 1956a; Yoon et al., 1960a) and that water-borne fluoride markedly increases the deposition of fluoride in the enamel surface (Isaac et al., 1958b; Speirs, 1958; Yoon et al., 1960b).

The distribution of fluoride from the surface toward the dentin in teeth of differently aged residents from a low fluoride area (0.1 ppm fluoride in the water supply) is given in Table 23 (BRUDEVOLD et al., 1956a). Four or more successive layers were ground and pooled from groups of teeth; each layer was only $^1/_{20}$ to $^1/_{10}$ mm thick. It will be noted that fluoride begins to accumulate in the surface enamel after calcification before the tooth erupts, and that it builds up in the outer portion of the enamel throughout the life of the tooth. The deposition of fluoride in the enamel undoubtedly occurs in the following three stages (BRUDEVOLD et al., 1956a):

a) Low concentrations reflecting the low levels of fluoride present in tissue fluids (SMITH et al, 1950) are incorporated in the apatite crystals during their formation. These concentrations deposited during the period of calcification correspond to those found in the inner layers of the enamel.

Table 23. *Parts per million of fluoride in successive layers of enamel ash of teeth from a low fluoride area.* Data from BRUDEVOLD et al. (1956a)

Layer no.	Deciduous	Unerupted		Erupted			
		I[1]	II[2]	under 20 yrs.	20—29 yrs.	30—39 yrs.	over 50 yrs.
1	448	331	528	571	1205	1070	1247
2	126	101	232	269	531	553	667
3	43	57	150	113	324	368	404
4	56	33	96	172	190	233	315
5				48	180		176
6					77		147
7					67		97
8					77		58
9					105		

[1] Not fully formed from Buffalo, N. Y.
[2] Fully formed from Buffalo, N. Y.

b) After calcification is complete, but before eruption, more fluoride is taken up by the external enamel which contacts tissue fluids. There is only slight penetration of fluoride into the underlying enamel, which is virtually blocked off, due to high mineralization (minute intercrystalline spaces).

c) After eruption and throughout life, the surface enamel continues to take up fluoride from the oral environments. It is evident from the low concentrations of fluoride in the innermost portion of the enamel (layers 8 and 9) that there is no significant diffusion of fluoride from the pulp via the dentin.

Table 24. *Parts per million of fluoride in successive layers of ashed enamel of persons under 20 years of age and living in communities with 0.1, 1.0 or 5.0 ppm fluoride in the water supply.* Data from ISAAC et al. (1958b)

Enamel layer	0.1 ppm F (BUFFALO, N. Y.)	1.0 ppm F (MCKINNEY, Texas)	5.0 ppm F (POST, Texas)
1	499	889	3370
2	162	363	1710
3	108	255	1124
4	63	171	926
5	76	133	811
6	42	129	570

It will be seen from Table 23 that the distribution of fluoride in deciduous enamel is the same as that of permanent enamel, but that the concentrations are lower. This may seem a paradox in view of the fact that deciduous enamel acquires fluoride more readily than permanent enamel (BRUDEVOLD et al., 1962). The low fluoride level in deciduous teeth is explained by the short life span and hence the short period of fluoride exposure of these teeth. The formative and functional life of these teeth total only 6 to 8 years, or a period similar to the pre-eruptive period of permanent teeth.

The previously mentioned marked increase in the deposition of fluoride in the surface enamel with increased fluoride exposure is shown in Table 24 (ISAAC et al., 1958b). As the level of fluoride in the water supply increases from 0.1 ppm to 1.0 and 5.0 ppm, the fluoride concentrations in the surface enamel increase from 499 ppm to 889 and 3370 ppm respectively, and that of the sixth layer which in this case is approximately in the middle of the enamel, from 42 ppm to 129 and 570 ppm, respectively.

Since caries begins on the enamel surface, the rate of fluoride uptake by surface enamel is of obvious importance. The data obtained in one laboratory from analyses of a great number of teeth of different ages, and obtained from geographical areas with 0.1, 1.0, 3.0 and 5.0 ppm of fluoride in the water supply (BRUDEVOLD et al., 1960) are summarized in Fig 4. The uptake by the surface enamel is rapid during the first years following enamel formation and prior to eruption, and then tapers off at a level closely governed by the concentration of fluoride in the drinking water. The initial rate of fluoride deposition is greater at high than at low levels in the water. At 5 ppm in the water the surface enamel has acquired at the time of eruption almost as great concentrations as those found in teeth of old persons, while at lower water levels the pre-eruptive uptake is less, and there is a significant post-eruptive increase in deposited fluoride with age.

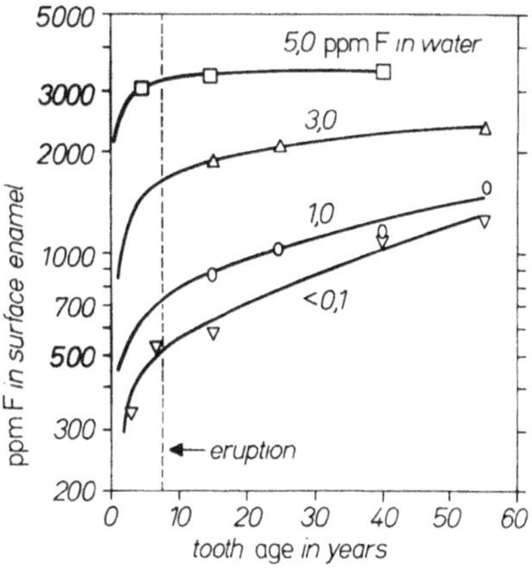

Fig. 4. Parts per million of fluoride in ash of surface enamel of teeth from areas with different levels of fluoride in the water supply. The dotted vertical line respresents the time of eruption (BRUDEVOLD et al., 1960)

The inhibition in caries resulting from water fluoridation (1 ppm) must be related to the 200 to 300 ppm greater fluoride concentrations in the surface enamel over those found in surface enamel from low fluoride areas. The surface enamel of teeth from areas with 1 ppm in the drinking water is obviously not fluoride saturated during the 10 years following tooth eruption which are most critical in regard to caries, since additional fluoride is acquired in subsequent years. However, sufficient amounts of fluoride occupy accessible positions at the surface of those crystals which are exposed to the oral environment, with the net effect of reinforcing the total structure. This point will be discussed later, but it should be emphasized here that the higher concentrations of fluoride in surface enamel of teeth from areas with 3 or more ppm of fluoride in the water may be associated with mottling or softening of the enamel due to faulty calcification (NEWBRUN, 1960; NEWBRUN and BRUDEVOLD, 1960). The immunity to caries expected from the high surface level of fluoride in these teeth may thus be partly impaired by structural imperfections.

2. Distribution of fluoride in crown dentin

Like enamel, crown dentin is exposed to fluid on one side (the side facing pulp), but unlike enamel, this dentinal surface is continuously renewed because of appositional dentin formation. For this reason, and because of the presence of dentinal tubuli which facilitate ionic diffusion, the accumulation of fluoride extends further into subsurface material in dentin than in enamel (Yoon et al., 1960a, 1960b; Brudevold et al., 1960). A comparison of the distribution of fluoride in enamel and dentin of teeth from areas with 0.1 and 2.9 ppm of fluoride in the water supply is given in Fig. 5. Going from the enamel across the dentino-enamel junction into the dentin there is a sharp rise in concentration reflecting the difference in fluoride levels in the two tissues. As the pulp is approached there is an additional increase to a maximum at the pulpal surface. The marked increase in fluoride levels in both enamel and dentin with increase in fluoride in the drinking water is also seen in Fig. 5.

There is no change with age in the fluoride level of crown dentin except in the portions approaching the pulp, which show a marked increase. For example, the distribution curves of fluoride in the crown dentin of teeth from a community with 3 ppm of fluoride in the water, given in Fig. 6, show that the junction and middle portions of the dentin contain concentrations of fluoride ranging from 700 to 1200 ppm whereas the pulpal portion of dentin of teeth

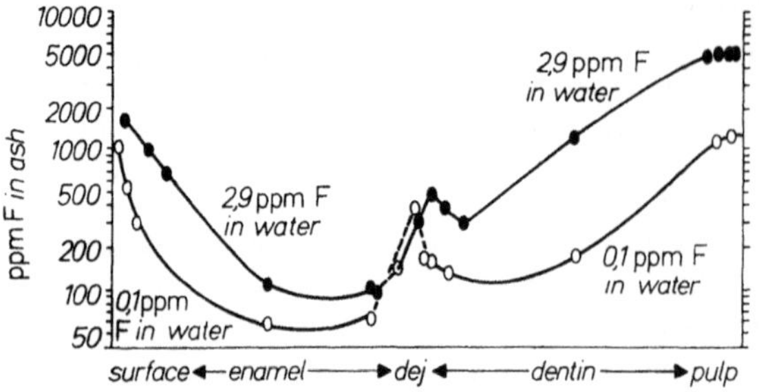

Fig. 5. Distribution of fluoride in enamel, from the surface through the coronal dentin to the pulp. Teeth were obtained from persons over 50 years of age residing in communities with 0.1 or 2.9 ppm of fluoride in the water supply

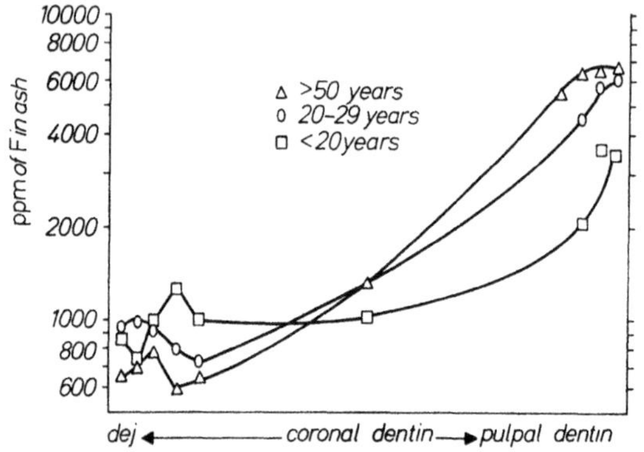

Fig. 6. Increase of fluoride in coronal dentin with age. Successive layers were removed by grinding from the dentinoenamel junction (DEJ) to the pulp in teeth of individuals aged under 20, 20—29, and over 50 years and living in a community with 3 ppm of fluoride in the drinking water (Yoon et al., 1960b)

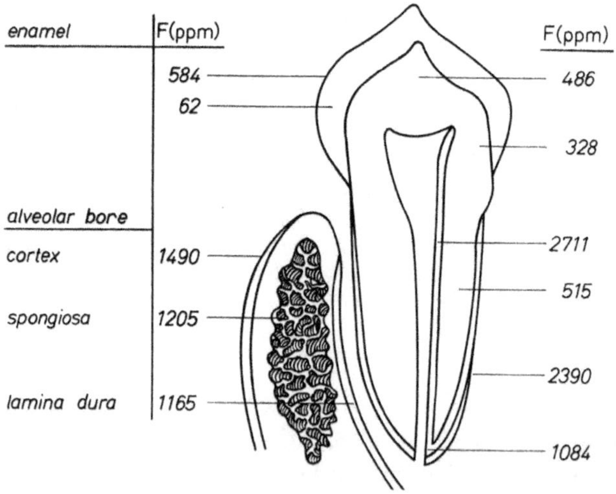

Fig. 7. Parts per million of fluoride in the ash of layers of enamel, coronal dentin, the apical portion, and the alveolar bone of a 90-year-old person of unknown history (Yoon et al., 1960a)

under 20 years of age contain 3400 ppm and that of teeth over 50 years old, 6600 ppm (Yoon et al., 1960a).

Although only the fluoride present in the enamel and dentin is of interest in regard to dental caries, the distribution of fluoride in the entire tooth will be considered briefly in order to give a more complete picture of the dental aspects of fluoride deposition. It can be seen from Fig. 7 that fluoride accumulates in all surface structures. The findings were obtained from analyses of pooled layer samples prepared from several teeth and the adjacent bone of a 90-year-old person of unknown history (Yoon et al., 1960a). The greatest concentrations of fluoride occurred in the surface layer of dentin adjacent to the pulp (2718 ppm), followed by the surface of the root (2390 ppm), the apical portion (1084 ppm) and the surface of the enamel (584 ppm). The latter value is unusually low due to marked attrition of the teeth and loss of fluoride-rich surface enamel. The lowest fluoride level observed was in the inner portion of the enamel (62 ppm). Although concentrations as mentioned may vary markedly in teeth of different persons it is notable that the levels may differ by a factor of at least 40 in different portions of single teeth.

E. Changes in composition of bone and tooth mineral associated with fluoride deposition

Increase in the fluoride content of bone and tooth mineral has been reported to effect changes in the concentrations of magnesium, carbonate and citrate in the mineral phase. The mechanism involved, and the significance of these changes in regard to caries is not clear, but since the effect of fluoride on the physical properties of the mineral may in part be mediated through these secondary compositional changes, the literature in this area is reviewed.

1. Magnesium

Several workers have observed that increased fluoride deposition in bone and teeth is accompanied by an increase in magnesium (Kick et al., 1935; McCann and Bullock, 1957; Weidmann et al., 1959; Zipkin et al., 1960). It will be noted from Table 25 that ingestion of 100 ppm of fluoride in the drinking water significantly increased the concentrations of magnesium in enamel and dentin of rat teeth (McCann and Bullock, 1957). This was particularly true in the growing incisor which was renewed during the test period, but it was also noticeable in the molars which were almost fully developed at the beginning of the experiment. Human bone of persons using drinking water containing 1 ppm or more of fluoride also showed higher magnesium than similar bone obtained from low fluoride areas (Zipkin et al., 1960). However, enamel and dentin from high and low fluoride areas failed to show differences in magnesium (Bowes and Murray, 1936; Ockerse, 1943). This latter work should be repeated with the improved methods

Table 25. *Fluoride and magnesium in enamel and dentin of rats given drinking water containing 100 ppm of fluoride for 100 days from weaning.* Data from McCann and Bullock (1957)

	Percentage of F[1]		Percentage of Mg[1]	
	exp.	control	exp.	control
Incisor enamel	0.197	0.002	0.66	0.25
Molar enamel	0.077	0.004	0.37	0.32
Incisor dentin	0.521	0.004	1.92	1.49
Molar dentin	0.480	0.009	0.44	0.37

[1] Dry weight basis.

of analysis now available. The mechanism of magnesium fixation has been attributed to formation of a magnesium fluoride complex of unknown composition (McCann and Bullock, 1957).

2. Carbonate

There is general agreement that deposition of fluoride in bone causes a decrease in mineral carbonate (Kick et al., 1935; McCann and Bullock, 1957; Weidmann et al., 1959; Zipkin et al., 1960). Although a similar relationship may be expected in tooth mineral, findings in the literature are contradictory and preclude final conclusions. For example, mottled enamel has been reported to have higher levels of carbonate than normal enamel (Bowes and Murray, 1936), while in pig teeth no relation was found between fluoride and carbonate concentrations (Kick et al., 1935). Likewise, enamel and dentin exposed to fluorides *in vitro* showed no decrease in carbonate with increased fluoride deposition (Leach, 1959a). In contrast, it has been reported that fluoride and bicarbonate compete for surface positions on the apatite crystal (Neuman etal., 1950), and more recently, analyses of enamel of deciduous teeth from areas with 0.1, 1.0 and 1.6 ppm fluoride in the drinking water have shown that with increased fluoride concentrations there is a decrease in carbonate (Nikiforuk, 1961). These findings are summarized in Table 26.

Table 26. *Percentages of carbonate and of fluoride in enamel from primary non-carious teeth from areas with 0.1, 1.0 and 1.6 ppm of fluoride in the water supply.* Data from Nikiforuk (1961)

ppm F in water supply	Enamel		
	ppm F	% CO_3	
0.1	48	3.70	Total enamel
1.6	134	3.43	
0.1	136	2.08	Outer enamel
1.0	357	1.90	

It was found in the latter study (Nikiforuk, 1961) that the CO_2/F ratio of surface enamel was higher in carious than in caries-free teeth, and it was postulated that resistance to caries resulted from a combination of high fluoride and low carbonate levels. In this connection, it should be noted that the outermost portion of the enamel of human teeth is always high in fluoride (Brudevold et al., 1960) and low in carbonate (Little and Brudevold, 1958) compared to subsurface enamel and that surface enamel is also naturally more resistant to caries than subsurface enamel (Brudevold, 1962b). Ingestion of water-borne fluoride simply increases this effect by the dual mechanism of increasing the deposition of fluoride and decreasing the deposition of carbonate, according to the above mentioned study.

It should be emphasized here that the role of carbonate in tooth mineral in relation to caries is by no means as clear as that of fluoride. Theoretically, presence of carbonate should weaken the mineral, since x-ray diffraction studies have shown that it interferes with crystallization (Trautz and Zapanta, 1961) and other studies have shown that it increases the solubility of hydroxyapatite (Grøn et al., 1963). In accordance with these findings it has been shown that a decrease in the level of carbonate in rat teeth was associated with decreased caries (Sobel et al., 1960), but other studies have failed to corroborate these results (Wynn et al., 1956, 1957; McClure and McCann, 1960). It is evident that the relationship between fluoride and carbonate in tooth mineral, and the role of carbonate in the carious process need to be further clarified.

3. Citrate

A similar relationship has been found between fluoride and citrate in bone as exists between fluoride and carbonate. Analyses of bone of groups of individuals who had been drinking water containing 4 ppm and only traces of fluoride respectively, showed 30 % less citrate in the former (ZIPKIN et al., 1960). Although citrate is readily acquired by hydroxyapatite, and fluoride and citrate compete for crystal surface positions (ARMSTRONG and SINGER, 1956), the decrease in bone citrate is much greater as a result of fluoride deposition than can be accounted for from stoichiometrical considerations (ZIPKIN et al., 1960). It has been suggested that fluoride reduces the number of locations available for citrate at the bone crystal surface by improving the crystallinity of the mineral (ZIPKIN et al., 1962). However, the fluoride-citrate relationship may be more complex, since a portion of the citrate in bone, and in dentin as well, is organically bound (HARTLES, 1961).

The concentration of citrate in enamel (0.1 %) is much lower than that of dentin and bone (1 %) (STACK, 1955), and its distribution in the enamel, which is similar to that of the organic material (BRUDEVOLD et al., 1960) suggests that it is mainly organically bound. The solubilizing effect which has been attributed to the citrate present in bone (HARTLES, 1961) is therefore unlikely to apply to enamel. Since the relation between fluoride and citrate in enamel and dentin remains to be established, the possible significance of this relationship to caries is purely speculative and in need of study.

VIII. The chemistry of topically applied fluoride

It is generally assumed that the effectiveness of topical fluoride treatment of teeth is proportional to the amount of fluoride deposited, or in the case of stannous fluoride to the amounts of tin and fluoride deposited. The problem has been therefore to find solutions of fluoride which will provide maximal uptake by the enamel within a few minutes of exposure. In order to accomplish this, highly concentrated solutions (> 0.5 % fluoride) have been employed. At these concentrations the solubility product of calcium fluoride is likely to be exceeded, and this salt may form in addition to fluorapatite. The reactions involved are expressed by the following equations:

$$Ca_{10}(PO_4)_6(OH)_2 + 2\ F^- \rightarrow Ca_{10}(PO_4)_6F_2 + 2\ OH^- \quad (1)$$

$$Ca_{10}(PO_4)_6(OH)_2 + 20\ F^- \rightarrow 10\ CaF_2 + 6\ PO_4^{\equiv} + 2\ OH^- \quad (2)$$

Since the caries reduction obtained from drinking fluoridated water, as previously mentioned, is associated with formation of fluorapatite, the formation of this salt is desirable in topical treatments. The significance of the presence of calcium fluoride in enamel is on the other hand, uncertain. There is no evidence that deposition in teeth of calcium fluoride per se will reduce caries. It has been proposed that calcium fluoride deposited in the enamel will dissolve and provide low concentrations of fluoride for formation of fluorapatite. However, this reaction has been reported to be slow at body temperature (KNAPPWORST, 1949), and hence may be of little significance. Since the formation of calcium fluoride is associated with decomposition of the tooth mineral (equation 2 above), it may actually be detrimental and offset the beneficial effects derived from the fluoride deposited as fluorapatite. Until more is known about the role of calcium fluoride in providing caries resistance, it is important to learn not only about the factors which influence deposition of fluoride in enamel and dentin, but also about the extent to which fluorapatite and calcium fluoride are formed under different conditions. In reviewing the literature on reactions between high concentrations of fluoride and tooth mineral, the latter problem will be dealt with in conjunction with a consideration of the effect of the concentration of fluoride on fluoride uptake. Additional factors influencing the acquisition of fluoride, including the exposure time, pH, solution cations and temperature will then be discussed. Finally attention will be given to the deposition of fluoride from solutions employed clinically.

A. Fluoride uptake by tooth mineral

1. Effect of concentration

The formation of calcium fluoride from high concentrations of fluoride has been demonstrated with x-ray and electron diffraction methods (GEROULD, 1945; SCOTT et al., 1950; FISCHER and MUHLER, 1952; FISCHER et al., 1954a, b) and by determining the amount of phosphate dissolved during the fluoride exposure (SOBEL et al., 1953; McCANN, 1953; McCANN and BULLOCK, 1955; LEACH, 1959a; MALAOWALLA and MYERS, 1962). It has been shown that calcium fluoride will form in increasing amounts with an increase in fluoride concentration and a decrease in pH (McCANN and BULLOCK, 1955; LEACH, 1959a; MALAOWALLA and MYERS, 1962), and that less calcium fluoride is formed when intact enamel is fluoride exposed than when powdered enamel is similarly treated (FISCHER and MUHLER, 1952). These findings are not surprising, since the rate of dissolution of calcium from hydroxyapatite increases with fall in pH and is less from intact than from powdered enamel.

In a study of powdered enamel and dentin it was concluded that at neutral pH, fluorapatite is formed almost exclusively up to a concentration of 100 ppm and that the increasing amounts deposited with further increase in the concentrations of fluoride is derived primarily from formation of increasing amounts of calcium fluoride and to a lesser extent, magnesium fluoride (McCANN and BULLOCK, 1955). In a similar investigation it was concluded that fluorapatite was the sole reaction product below 75 ppm of fluoride, and that calcium fluoride as well as fluorapatite were formed in increasing amounts at higher concentrations (LEACH, 1959a). The latter findings are given in Table 27.

Table 27. *Uptake of fluoride by 1 g of powdered enamel or dentin from 100 ml of solutions containing various concentrations of fluoride as NaF. Estimate of amounts of fluorapatite and CaF_2 formed.* Calculated from data of LEACH (1959a)

ppm F initially in soln.	F in enamel ppm F taken up as			F in dentin ppm F taken up as		
	total	fluorapatite	CaF_2	total	fluorapatite	CaF_2
10	665	665	0	703	703	0
25	1615	1650	0	1900	1900	0
100	4370	3610	760	5320	4180	1140
5000	11970	6840	5130	19000	11020	7980
18000	26980	7980	19000	36290	15010	21280

These findings show that the concentration of fluoride is critical in regard to calcium fluoride formation. However, the composition of the tooth mineral appears to be of equal importance. In synthetic hydroxyapatites the extent of calcium fluoride formation has been reported to be influenced by the Ca/P ratio of the material. Fluorapatite formation was favored in nearly pure hydroxyapatite (Ca/P ratio approaching 1.67) while calcium fluoride formed readily in calcium-deficient hydroxyapatite (McCANN, 1953). For example, at fluoride concentrations of 0.1 to 0.2 % little or no fluorapatite was formed until the Ca/P ratio exceeded 1.62. These findings which were derived from chemical analyses, have been substantiated by x-ray diffraction (TRAUTZ and ZAPANTA, 1961). Only traces of calcium fluoride were detected in well-crystallized hydroxyapatite (Ca/P ratio 1.67) after one month's exposure to a solution of 2 % sodium fluoride, while appreciable amounts were formed from a material with Ca/P ratio of 1.5 and large amounts from brushite (Ca/P ratio 1.0). Calcium carbonate was also rapidly converted to calcium fluoride, suggesting that the carbonate content in teeth, as well as the Ca/P ratio of the mineral will influence the reaction products from fluoride exposures.

2. Period of fluoride exposure

In the above mentioned studies the period of exposure to fluoride extended over several weeks. The important question, still unanswered, is the extent to which calcium fluoride forms during the few minutes of fluoride exposure employed in topical treatments. Since calcium fluoride tends to form supersaturated solutions (Tovborg-Jensen, 1937) its solubility product may well be considerably exceeded before spontaneous precipitation occurs. It is notable that x-ray diffraction studies of teeth which were exposed for 20 min to a strong solution of sodium fluoride and extracted one week later suggested presence of fluorapatite rather than calcium fluoride (Syrrist, 1949b). However, minute amounts of calcium fluoride have been detected by electron diffraction on ground enamel surfaces after only 3 min exposure to 2 % sodium fluoride (Scott et al., 1950), but were dissolved or washed away after 90 min subsequent exposure to water.

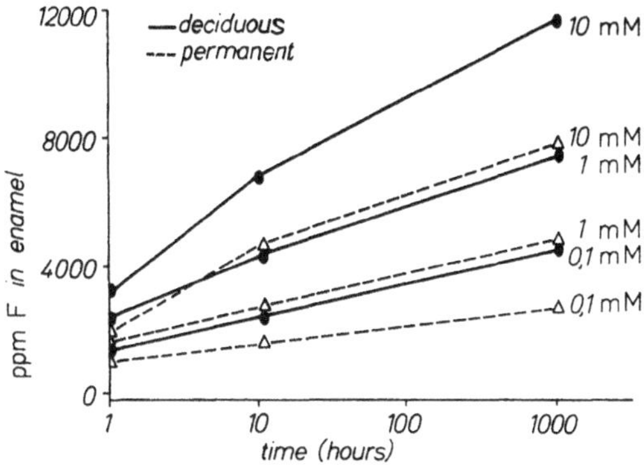

Fig. 8. Uptake of fluoride by powdered permanent and deciduous enamel exposed for periods of 1—1000 hrs to 0.1, 1.0 and 10.0 mM of NaF at pH 7.0 (Brudevold et al., 1962)

The rate of uptake of fluoride by tooth mineral is initially high and then gradually tapers off. For example, a radioactive study which employed intact teeth and solutions containing 1 ppm of fluoride showed that of the fluoride taken up in 20 min, 28 % was acquired during the first minute, 41 % during the first 3, and 93 % during the first 9 min of exposure (Brudevold et al., 1957b). In powdered enamel and dentin it has been noted that 50 % of the uptake at six hours occurred within the first minute of contact (Leach, 1959a).

The effect of the period of exposure on deposition of fluoride in deciduous and permanent powdered enamel from NaF solutions with initial concentrations of from 0.1 to 10 mM are shown in Fig. 8 (Brudevold et al., 1962). At low concentrations the uptake is linear with the logarithm of time of exposure. The break in the curves at higher concentrations is likely due to CaF_2 formation. The greater uptake of fluoride by deciduous than by permanent enamel seen in Fig. 8 is likely due to the higher organic content in deciduous enamel (Savory and Brudevold, 1959), which is believed to facilitate ionic diffusion.

It has been postulated that the uptake of fluoride from low fluoride solutions proceeds in 3 phases: 1) diffusion into and exchange with anions in the tightly held water layer adjacent to the crystal; 2) fixation in the surface of the hydroxyapatite crystal by replacing surface bound hydroxyl, bicarbonate or citrate ions; 3) migration into the body of the crystal and incorporation in the interior lattice (Neuman and NEUMAN, 1958). The study which demonstrated these steps employed radioactive phosphate, but the results apply by analogy to fluoride which because of the short half-life of F^{18} could not be studied by the method used. According to these findings, the first step is very rapid, the second is slower and the third step is exceedingly slow. The plateauing of fluoride uptake with time reflects the slow rate of the third phase. The further fluoride gets into the crystal body, the slower is the process of acquisitoin.

This concept of fluoride fixation explains the extreme rapidity with which fluoride reacts with bone and tooth mineral (BRUDEVOLD et al., 1957b; NEUMAN and NEUMAN, 1958). It also explains the fact that concentrations of fluoride in teeth and bone, even of individuals who live in high fluoride areas, are far below the levels of saturation. If all hydroxyl groups in tooth mineral were replaced by fluoride, the concentration would be about 3.8 %, while under physiological conditions concentrations exceeding 0.3 % in the enamel and 0.6 % in dentin are rarely seen. The time required by fluoride to fill surface positions of hydroxyapatite crystals at pH 7 is indicated in Fig. 9. The data were calculated on the premise that crystal surface positions were filled before exchange occurred in the interior lattice structure. The surface was considered to consist of one layer of unit cells. Working with a synthetic hydroxyapatite of known surface area, and assuming that two hydroxyl ions of each unit cell could be replaced by fluoride, it was calculated that some surface positions were still unfilled after 1000 hours exposure to 0.1 mM fluoride, while the surface became fluoride saturated after 100 hours exposure to 1 mM of fluoride. Since the concentrations of fluoride in body fluids generally are less than 0.01 mM and ions competing with fluoride for lattice positions, including hydroxyl, bicarbonate and citrate ions, are present in appreciable concentrations, and considering in addition the limited accessability of the majority of tooth and bone crystals, it is not surprising that relatively low concentrations of fluoride are found physiologically, even in old individuals. It is evident from the data presented that the uptake of fluoride can be greatly increased in topical fluoride treatments by employing highly concentrated solutions.

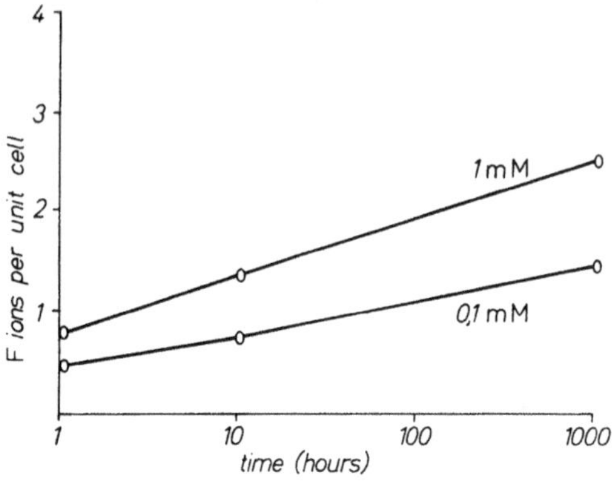

Fig. 9. The number of fluoride ions deposited per surface unit cell of hydroxyapatite after exposure to 0.1 or 1.0 mM NaF at pH 7.0 for periods of 1—1000 hrs (BRUDEVOLD et al., 1962)

3. Effect of pH

There is a marked increase in uptake of fluoride by hydroxyapatite with decrease in pH (ADLER et al., 1950; NEUMAN et al., 1950; MEGERIAN, 1951; MCCANN, 1953; BRUDEVOLD et al., 1956b, 1957a, 1963; SPINELLI et al., 1963) as would be expected, since fluoride competes with hydroxyl ions for lattice positions. In one study the acquisition of F was about 50 % greater at pH 6 than at pH 7, and at pH 5, it was double that obtained at pH 7 (SPINELLI et al., 1963). Different types of acid have been used to acidify the fluoride solution, including lactic, acetic, aspartic and orthophosphoric acid (NEUMAN et al., 1950; MEGERIAN, 1951; MCCANN,

1953; BRUDEVOLD et al., 1957a, 1963; SPINELLI et al., 1963). There is some evidence that less fluoride is deposited in enamel from solutions of aspartate than from equivalent solutions of acetate and orthophosphate (BRUDEVOLD et al., 1963), but anion effects have not been adequately studied. Increasing the concentration of orthophosphoric acid from 6 to 60 mM slightly decreased the F uptake, probably as a result of increase in ionic strength (SPINELLI et al., 1963). The deposition of fluoride in powdered enamel from phosphate buffers at different pH levels and containing different concentrations of fluoride is shown in Table 28.

Table 28. *Parts per million of fluoride taken up by 200 mg of enamel treated for 6 min in 600 ml of 0.1 M phosphate buffer varying in pH and fluoride concentration.* BRUDEVOLD et al. (1963)

ppm F in soln.	ppm F in enamel exposed to phosphate soln. of		
	pH 4.5	pH 5.5	pH 8.0
0	144	107	175
1	514	450	193
10	869	579	296
100	1194	992	418
1000	1980	1785	811

4. Cation effect

Because of the current use of stannous fluoride in topical treatments, it is of interest that less fluoride is taken up from solutions of this salt than from neutral NaF (BRUDEVOLD et al., 1956c; SMITH et al., 1957; COOLEY, 1961). A comparison of fluoride acquisition by enamel from 0.1 M fluoride as stannous and sodium fluoride is shown in Fig. 10. The limited uptake from stannous fluoride needs to be explained in view of the low pH of stannous fluoride solutions (pH 3 or less), which should favor fluoride acquisition. Two factors are known to be involved: 1) Hydrolysis of stannous fluoride causes formation of an insoluble fluoride-containing precipitate, thus reducing the fluoride available for reaction with the enamel (SMITH et al., 1957). 2) The stannous ion reacts quickly with surface enamel to form a coating (SMITH et al., 1957) consisting primarily of hydrated stannous oxide (SCOTT, 1960). This coating retards diffusion of fluoride into the enamel. Contrary to the cited findings, stannous fluoride has been reported to deposit greater amounts of fluoride in enamel than NaF (MUHLER et al., 1952; HATTON et al., 1955). However, in these studies fluoride precipitated from the solution as a result of hydrolysis of stannous fluoride was assumed to be acquired by the enamel mineral, thus giving misleading results.

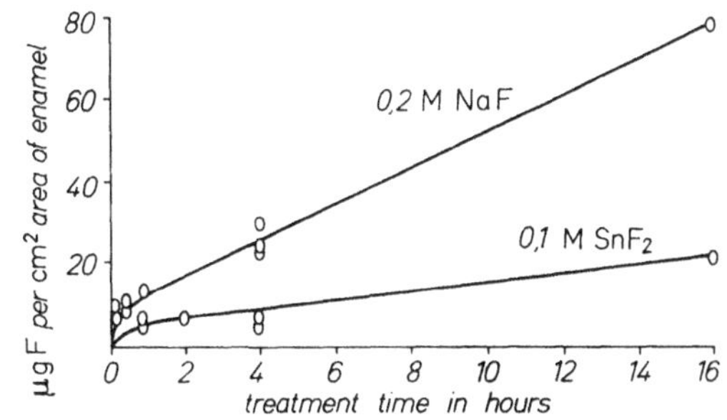

Fig. 10. Deposition of fluoride on acid etched enamel from solutions of SnF_2 (pH 2.8) and NaF (pH 6—7). Samples were treated by brushing at room temperature in unbuffered solution (COOLEY, 1961)

5. Effect of temperature

The uptake of fluoride by synthetic hydroxyapatite has been reported to be greater at 100° C than at 37° C (McCANN, 1953). In another study the acquisition of fluoride was increased by factors of 2 and 4 when the temperature was increased from 24 to 50 and 75° C, respectively (BRUDEVOLD et al., 1962). The marked effect of temperature on fluoride deposition is shown in Table 29 taken from the latter study. The results are in accord with the findings that the rate of recrystallization of hydroxyapatite increases with increasing temperatures (NEUMAN and MULRYAN, 1951). Sweeping the tooth surface with a high frequency vibrating instrument during fluoride exposure greatly increases the uptake of fluoride (BRUDEVOLD et al., 1962). This effect was due to the heat generated by the instrument since the vibrations failed to increase fluoride deposition when the temperature was controlled. In view of the fact that temperatures of about 50° C are well tolerated in the mouth, clinical utilization of the increased uptake of fluoride at elevated temperatures seems worthy of investigation.

Table 29. *Uptake of fluoride by hydroxyapatite. Effect of temperature and time.* Data from BRUDEVOLD et al. (1962)

Time hrs	ppm F taken up at			
	3° C	24° C	50° C	75° C
1	1288	1852	2386	3546
5	1688	2244	4730	8057
25	2303	3367	7885	15053
50	2599	4100	10637	18262

Solution contained 100 mg hydroxyapatite/500 ml, 5 ppm F, pH 7.0 and ionic strength μ 0.16.

6. Electrophoresis

Electrophoresis has been advocated as a means of promoting fluoride deposition. However, *in vitro* and *in vivo* tests have shown this procedure to be ineffective, probably because of the large resistance of enamel to the passage of electric current (ERICSSON, 1958b).

7. Topical application — mechanism of fluoride uptake

According to the foregoing discussion, fluoride uptake from topically applied fluoride should be favored by the use of high concentrations and long exposure time. However, as can be seen from Table 30, which lists the results of several studies on fluoride uptake by intact enamel, exposure to 2 % neutral sodium fluoride for a total of 80 min caused an increment of fluoride of only 610 ppm in the outer enamel. After shorter periods of exposure, ranging from 16 to 20 min, the fluoride increments varied from 50 to 500 ppm. The modest uptake of fluoride is consistent with the theory that the crystal surface, and not the bulk of the crystal reacts with the fluoride. The increment is confined to the outermost enamel which includes not more than 0.1 to 0.2 mm of the surface layer. For example, in the fourth and fifth studies listed in Table 30, two successive extremely thin layers of enamel were

Table 30. *Uptake of fluoride by intact enamel treated with different fluoride solutions*

Solution	No.	Time (min)	Enamel analyzed	ppm F in ash		Reference
				exptl.	control[4]	
NaF 2%	8	10	Outer enamel	950	340	HORD and ELLES (1951)
NaF 2%	4	5	Outer portion	620[1]	430	SYRRIST (1949a)
NaF 4%	4	10	Outer portion	1001[1]	570	SYRRIST (1949a)
NaF 1%	1	20	1*st* outer layer	1440[2]	924	BRUDEVOLD et al. (1956b)
			2*nd* outer layer	561	400	
NaF 0.02%	1	20	1*st* outer layer	968[2]	777	BRUDEVOLD et al. (1956b)
			2*nd* outer layer	508	445	
NaF 2%	4	4	1*st* outer layer	165[3]	110	SUNDVALL-HAGLAND et al. (1959)
			2*nd* outer layer	60	50	

[1] Fluoride exposure *in situ* once a week.
[2] Fluoride exposure *in vitro.*
[3] Fluoride exposure *in situ* within a week.
[4] Untreated.

analyzed and the fluoride increase in the second layer was only a fraction of that of the first layer.

The penetration of fluoride into the enamel must be mediated through hydrated spaces, since there is no diffusion through the apatite crystals. Cracks and lamellae will readily permit diffusion, but the slight penetration consistently found in fluoride-exposed enamel cannot be dependent on the presence of defects. Diffusion could occur through the interprismatic substance and the striae of Retzius, or involve the prisms as well. In either case, it must take place between individual enamel crystals in the water spaces which in fully calcified enamel, approach atomic dimensions. Highly charged ions such as fluoride, do not readily pass through, presumably because they tend to be trapped by electrostatic forces on the surfaces of the crystals. The narrower the spaces, *i.e.* the more highly calcified the enamel, the stronger will be the electrostatic field, and the more unlikely the passage of the fluoride ions.

In the partly decalcified enamel of initial carious lesions, spaces between the crystals are augmented as has been demonstrated by polarizing microscopy (Darling, 1961). The increased hydration of carious enamel (Little et al., 1962) will facilitate diffusion of fluoride, a fact verified by radioactive studies (Myers et al., 1952; Brudevold et al., 1957b; Nevin et al., 1957). But, even when there is appreciable penetration of fluoride, the reactions involved must be limited to the surface of the crystals. The fact then, that fluoride acts somewhat as a coating agent explains how the slight increments of fluoride provided by topical applications can furnish partial protection against dental caries.

Topical applications of stannous fluoride involve reactions of stannous as well as the fluoride ion. Table 31 shows that appreciable concentrations of tin are acquired by intact enamel surfaces, and that there is a slight penetration of tin into the enamel. Tin deposits rapidly in enamel probably in the form of tin phosphates and oxides (Cooley, 1961). In addition, a loose fluoride-containing precipitate (Smith et al., 1957) forms on the enamel surface as a result of hydrolysis of the stannous fluoride. The protection which is provided to the enamel surface by topical application of stannous fluoride is unlikely to be due to this easily removable complex, but probably results from impregnation of the surface enamel with fluoride and possibly tin. The deposition of tin is actually of doubtful significance in regard to caries, since topical application of a fluoride-free tin salt has been reported to be ineffective (Muhler, 1958a). The usefulness of the stannous ion rather may be to decrease dissolution of enamel by the acid stannous fluoride solution (pH 3) during the treatment procedure and permit reaction of fluoride with the enamel at low pH without undue detrimental effects. It is possible that the combination of limited dissolution of the enamel (limited release of Ca^{++}) and low pH promotes formation of fluorapatite since in one study no calcium fluoride was detected even after one week's exposure to stannous fluoride solution (Fischer

Table 31. *Concentrations of tin and fluoride in the external enamel after exposing for 20 min to solutions containing NaF (1%), SnF_2 (1.86%) or SnClF (4.12%).* From Brudevold (1956c)

Test agent	pH	Per cent in test soln.		Enamel			
				ppm Sn in		ppm F in	
		tin	fluoride	layer 1	layer 2	layer 1	layer 2
NaF	5.6	0.0	0.452	25	5.6	1440	561
SnF_2	2.9	1.41	0.452	600	250	1200	580
SnClF	1.6	2.82	0.452	640	300	1031	570
Control	—	0.0	0.0	15	10	924	400

et al., 1954b). The decrease in fluoride deposition from stannous fluoride compared to sodium fluoride, discussed earlier and also seen in Table 31, may thus be offset by the fact that fluorapatite is the main fluoride reaction product. However, this point is by no means conclusively proven. The yellowish brown discoloration noted in teeth following stannous fluoride treatments is probably due to the formation of insoluble stannous sulfide, since *in vitro* experiments have demonstrated that this compound will readily form in stannous fluoride-treated enamel in the presence of sulfide (ISAAC and BRUDEVOLD, 1957).

The limiting effect of the stannous ion on fluoride uptake by enamel can be clearly seen from the data given in Table 32 (BRUDEVOLD et al., 1963). Here teeth were exposed to solutions of either stannous fluoride or sodium fluoride dissolved in 0.1 M phosphoric acid. The solutions contained the same concentrations of fluoride and had a similar pH. Analyses of two consecutive thin layers ground off the fluoride-exposed teeth, showed approximately 3 times greater uptake and a much greater penetration of fluoride into the enamel in the case of the teeth treated with the phosphate-fluoride solution. The effectiveness of the phosphate-fluoride solution, demonstrated in 4 clinical studies (WELLOCK and BRUDEVOLD, 1963; PAMEIJER et al., 1963; WELLOCK et al., 1965; BIBBY, personal communication), may be due to the dual effects of 1) deposition of relatively large amounts of fluoride in the enamel, and 2) formation of fluorapatite rather than calcium fluoride. This is suggested by one experiment in which teeth were kept for 115 days without visible demineralization in a solution of 2% sodium fluoride and 0.1 M sodium phosphate, final pH 4.3. The x-ray diffraction pattern of chips of enamel from these teeth was characteristic of apatite, and no diffraction lines of calcium fluoride were found. Evidently phosphate in solution has the combined effect of depressing enamel dissolution and formation of calcium fluoride as may be expected, since both processes are associated with release of mineral phosphate. A slight loss in CO_2 was also observed in enamel exposed to acid fluoride phosphate solutions. This effect, which may be partly due to a displacement of enamel carbonate with phosphate, may add to the caries resistance provided by the fluoride in the solution.

Table 32. *Concentrations of fluoride in the surface enamel of permanent teeth exposed 20 min to 1.6% fluoride as NaF in 0.1 M phosphate buffer at pH 2.8, and to 1.6% fluoride as SnF_2 at pH 2.6.* From BRUDEVOLD et al. (1963)

Enamel layer	NaF P buffer ppm	SnF_2 ppm	Control ppm
1	2229	650	582
2	1254	370	316
1	2813	1066	881
2	987	623	451

It is of considerable interest that the capacity to take up fluoride varies in different teeth. Experiments in the author's laboratory showed that among teeth that had received the same cleaning with an abrasive, some teeth picked up as much as 10 times more fluoride than other teeth after a 3-minute exposure to 0.1% sodium fluoride solution. By electron microscopy of ground enamel surfaces, a difference in reactivity to fluoride has been observed both in different teeth, and in different areas on the same tooth (SCOTT et al., 1950).

The reason for this difference in reactivity is not known. It is possible that tooth age may be a contributing factor, as is suggested by the observation that water fluoridation is effective in teeth first fluoride-exposed 1 or 2 years after eruption, but apparently not in teeth erupted for several years before the first fluoride exposure. Because of the concentrated solutions of fluoride used, topical treatment can benefit even teeth of adults, but differences in structural or chemical characteristics of the surface enamel affect the fluoride uptake in a way which is not understood.

B. Loss of fluoride from tooth mineral

Once fluoride is acquired by hydroxyapatite it is not readily removed. Megerian found no loss of fluoride from fluoride-exposed ashed bone after shaking for 4 days in solutions having a final pH of 6.7–8.9, suggesting that the exchange of F^- and OH^- is not reversible in this pH range (MEGERIAN, 1951). MCCANN and BULLOCK (1957) observed that the rate of desorption of fluoride from bone and tooth mineral by 1 N KOH depended on the period of exposure to fluoride. For example, of the fluoride acquired by dentin after 1 day's exposure to 2 ppm of fluoride at 37° C, 68 % could be removed in 1 to 7 days, while only 34 % was removed of that acquired after 1 week's exposure. Apparently surface-bound fluoride is removed more readily than fluoride which has penetrated into the crystal. These workers found that fluoride was removed more readily from enamel than from dentin. The reason for this is not clear.

The slow rate of displacement of F^- by OH^- is shown in Table 33 from a study by BRUDEVOLD et al. (1962a). Virtually no fluoride was removed from hydroxyapatite which had been heated to 450° C, probably because fluoride was incorporated in the interior lattice in this material. Leach observed that repeated washing of enamel or dentin exposed to high levels of fluoride caused a 100–200-fold fall in fluoride concentrations (LEACH, 1959a). This was considered to be loss of excess fluoride present in the liquid accompanying the enamel. Subsequently, there was a slower release of fluoride and loss in concentrations (in the washings) of 8 to 10 ppm which was attributed to loss of calcium fluoride. No further amounts of fluoride and calcium were released on prolonged shaking, suggesting that the fluoride present as fluorapatite was firmly bound. It is of interest that only traces of the fluoride present in enamel are removed during acid etching at pH 4 or 5 (ISAAC et al., 1958a), consistent with the concept that fluoride fixation is favored by low pH.

Radioactive studies have shown that fluoride-exposed enamel surfaces lose from 10 to 50 % of the acquired fluoride if brushed immediately in running water for 3 min (BRUDEVOLD et al., 1957b). The loss is great during the first minute and decreases rapidly thereafter. Evidently a portion of the fluoride taken up by the enamel is loosely bound and a certain amount of time is required to allow maximal fixation. According to these findings it would be advisable to postpone mouth rinsing, brushing or eating as long as possible after topical treatments, in order to minimize removal of fluoride and allow maximal time for reaction with the surface enamel.

Table 33. *Removal of fluoride from 100 mg of fluoridated hydroxyapatite upon exposure for 1—50 hours to 500 ml of KOH at pH 10.2.* Data from BRUDEVOLD et al. (1962a)

Time	ppm fluoride remaining on enamel			
	pre-exposed at 24° C		pre-exposed at 50° C	
	air dried	dried 450°	air dried	dried 450°
0	4100	4235	10,637	10,656
1	4224	4374	8960	10,968
5	3213	4612	9731	10,028
25	3341	4480	9851	10,828
50	3452	4170	9823	9947

The hydroxyapatite was initially fluoridated by exposure to a solution containing 5 ppm F at pH 7.0 and then air dried or dried at 450° C.

It should be mentioned that since fluoride uptake occurs only in a superficial layer of the enamel, it is obvious that using abrasives under heavy pressure will cause loss of fluoride along with a portion of the enamel. For example, 50 % of the acquired fluoride was removed from enamel surfaces after 2 seconds of heavy pumicing, 80 % after 10 seconds, and nearly 100 % after 50 seconds (BRUDEVOLD et al., 1957b). We would hope that such heavy pumicing does not occur under ordinary conditions in the dental office.

It has been mentioned previously that the concentrations of fluoride in the surface enamel tend to increase with age, even in teeth of persons who live in low fluoride areas. Apparently the levels of fluoride present in saliva, food and water are sufficient to maintain positive fluoride balance. Two studies have shown that fluoride applied to the tooth surface by topical treatment will remain in the enamel for a long period of time. HELD et al. (1951) found that there was only an insiguificant loss of fluoride in teeth extracted 22 months after fluoride treatments. More recently analyses of the surface enamel of deciduous teeth subjected to topical treatments showed no decrease in the acquired fluoride over a period of 7 years (SUNDVALL-HAGLAND et al., 1959). These findings are summarized in Table 34. In this study, carried out in a community with only traces of fluoride in the water supply, the children received four sodium fluoride applications at the age of three years. The teeth, exfoliated as the children grew older, had consistently more fluoride in the surface enamel than the untreated controls.

Table 34. *Parts per million of fluoride in the ash of outer portions of deciduous enamel three to seven years after receiving four topical applications of 2% NaF.*
Data from SUNDVALL-HAGLAND et al. (1959)

	Interval after fluoride treatment									
	3 years		4 years				5 years		6—7 years	
	treated	control	treated	control	treated	control	treated	control	treated	control
No. of teeth	16	16	29	23	39	41	22	29	23	18
Surface enamel, ppm F, ash wt.	151	95	143	81	165	125	155	110	185	130

The mineral of carious enamel (DOWSE and JENKINS, 1957) and carious dentin (JOHANSEN and NORDBACK, 1962) has been found to be higher in fluoride than the mineral of adjacent normal enamel and dentin. This increase in concentration, which must be due to both the porosity and the low pH which frequently accompany carious lesions and favor acquisition rather than loss of fluoride, demonstrate the unique ability of fluoride to concentrate in and reinforce those areas of the tooth which are subjected to the carious attack.

IX. Inhibition of bacterial acid production

The clinical observation that water-borne fluoride exerts its major caries reducing effect when incorporated in the enamel prior to and immediately after tooth eruption suggests that it is the fluoride which is built into the tooth which is primarily effective against caries, and that the fluoride present in dental plaque or in saliva has little or no effect. The caries inhibition obtained from topically applied fluoride also points to the importance of impregnating the enamel with fluoride.

Although fluoride decreases the solubility of enamel in proportion to the levels present, it has been postulated that fluoride may be released from the enamel surface at low pH in sufficient concentrations to interfere with glycolytic enzymes and prevent further increase in hydrogen ion concentration (JENKINS, 1958). Available evidence does not support this view. Fluoride uptake by hydroxyapatite is favored by low pH, and consequently, higher concentrations of free fluoride would not be expected adjacent to the enamel surface at low pH. Thus, only minute concentrations of fluoride are released into acid buffers from enamel or dentin at low pH (ISAAC et al., 1958a). For example, buffers equilibrated at pH 4.7 with dentin having fluoride levels of 0.19 and 0.53% contained only 0.02 and 0.8 ppm of F respectively (Table 35). Since the concentration of fluoride in surface enamel increases with age in spite of frequently being exposed to acids formed from carbohydrate fermentation, and since in addition the tooth mineral from carious lesions contains higher concentrations of fluoride than that of intact tooth structure, it is evident that *in vivo* dissolution of fluoride deposited in enamel or dentin must be minimal and reversible. Much larger concentrations than those which can be dissolved from teeth are needed to stop bacterial growth (250 ppm) (BIBBY and VAN KESTEREN, 1940). The level of fluoride required to inhibit acid production varies depending on the growth rate of the bacteria and the pH, and presence of Ca, P, Mg and other ionic species in the medium. Thus, the first detectable inhibition has been found at concentrations of fluoride ranging from 1 ppm to 30 to 40 ppm (LILIENTHAL, 1940). Conversion of glucose to lactic acid by bacterial suspensions of *L. casei* in micro-incubation cells was inhibited in the presence of enamel with a history of fluoride exposure (BRINER, 1961). However, in *in vivo* experiments the inhibition was found to decrease sharply 24 hours after the topical fluoride treatment, and to disappear completely after 7 days (ZWEMER, 1957). The rapid diminution with time in the degree of inhibition may be attributed to early dissolution of loosely bound fluoride in the enamel and to an increasing unavailability of the retained fluoride. The latter finding seems related to the *in vitro* observation that powdered enamel, synthetic hydroxyapatite and naturally occurring fluorapatite had no effect on the rate of acid formation by salivary sediment, whereas materials exposed to 2% NaF solutions, and thus containing CaF_2, inhibited acid production to a degree similar to that caused by pure CaF_2 (LILIENTHAL and MARTIN, 1956). These studies suggest that the fluoride present in the surface enamel does not significantly prevent acid production.

Table 35. *Calcium and fluoride released from fluoridated dentin by shaking in water followed by shaking in 0.2 M acetic acid buffer at pH 4.7 (1 g dentin/100 ml of wash solution).* From LEACH (1959b)

Dentin	Water wash		Buffer wash	
	mg Ca	mg F	mg Ca	mg F
0.19% F	0.43	0.05	120.0	0.002
0.53% F	0.43	0.08	58.0	0.08
3.7% F	1.04	1.06	29.8	0.13
1.5% F, washed free of CaF_2 prior to washing with buffer	0.4	0.05	31.0	0.12

1 mg/100 ml = 10 ppm of Ca or F.

The concentrations of fluoride present in saliva are too low to effect bacterial metabolism. Although radioactive studies have shown that fluoride readily appears in salivary glands or in saliva (WILLS, 1940; VOLKER et al., 1941; WALLACE, 1953; HEIN et al., 1956), the level rarely exceeds 0.1 or 0.2 ppm (MCCLURE, 1941a, b; GEDALIA et al., 1961). In addition the salivary fluoride was found to be similar in areas with only traces and up to 3 ppm of fluoride in the drinking water (MCCLURE, 1941a, b). This observation is supported by radioactive fluoride experiments which showed that the salivary level is little influenced by fluoride ingestion (CARLSON et al., 1960). Thus there appears to be no relation between the reduction in caries found in fluoride areas and the presence of fluoride in saliva.

In contrast to saliva, appreciable amounts of fluoride may accumulate in dental plaque. A recent study showed mean concentrations of 6 ppm (wet weight) and maximal concentrations of 60 ppm (HARDWICK, 1961). Although it is not known in what form this fluoride is present, there are good reasons for believing that only a minor fraction is ionized. Calcium and phosphate are known to accumulate rapidly in plaque material (ALLAN and NEVOR, 1957; DAWES and JENKINS, 1962) and to form inorganic salts in increasing concentrations with time (SCHROEDER, 1963). The latter author found 41% dry weight inorganic material, probably present as hydroxyapatite, in 2-day-old plaque and 65% in 12-day-old plaque samples. In artifically produced plaque, mineral formation has been shown to increase linearly with time (VON DER FEHR and BRUDEVOLD, 1960). In view of these findings it is likely that the level of fluoride in plaque material is related to the amount of mineral present, as is true in biological material in general, and that it occurs primarily as fluorapatite.

The interest in the antienzymatic action of fluoride has been revitalized recently by the observation that the inhibiting effect on salivary acid production is greater at acid than at neutral pH (JENKINS, 1959). However, regardless of whether fluoride is added to glucose-saliva mixtures at an initial pH of 7.5 or 5.0, there was little difference in the final pH after 4 hours of incubation at fluoride levels below 6 ppm. Since less than 1 ppm of fluoride will cause rapid precipitation of fluorapatite from such high concentrations of calcium and phosphate as are present in plaque (BRUDEVOLD and MESSER, 1961) it is unlikely that fluoride inhibition of bacterial acid production in plaque is of any significance.

It has been suggested that the relatively high concentrations of fluoride introduced into the mouth through mouth washes or dentifrices could significantly inhibit acid production. Although there is a decrease in lactic acid formation in saliva collected shortly after rinsing the mouth with a solution of 0.5% NaF, the effect disappears after 20 to 30 min (ERICSSON and HELLSTROM, 1952), and the effect of rinsing with 0.1% NaF lasts only for 10 to 15 min (HELLSTROM, 1960). Stannous fluoride has been reported to have a greater inhibitory effect on bacterial acid production than NaF, presumably due to the powerful anti-enzymatic action of the stannous ion (LILIENTHAL, 1958a, b; JENKINS, 1961). There is no evidence showing that this effect of stannous fluoride has any clinical significance.

X. Solubility

In considering the dissolution of tooth mineral associated with the carious process it should be realized that saliva, as secreted from the salivary gland, is supersaturated in respect to hydroxyapatite (SCHMIDT-NIELSEN, 1946; ERICSSON, 1949). Dissolution can therefore take place only if Ca-complexing agents are formed at the site of the lesion, or if there is a fall in pH sufficient to increase the solubility of the tooth mineral beyond the activity product of salivary Ca and P. Available evidence overwhelmingly favors dissolution by acid as being the primary mechanism. Calcium complexing substances are without doubt, produced in dental plaque. For example, some of the intermediate products of carbohydrate metabolism are powerful chelators. However, until it is demonstrated that chelators are present in carious lesions in significant concentrations, it must be assumed that acid decalcification is the main mechanism of demineralization.

It is well known that F incorporated into the crystal lattice will reduce the solubility of hydroxyapatite (RATHJE, 1952; MCCANN and BULLOCK, 1957). The data in Table 36, which illustrate this point, were obtained on synthetic hydroxyapatite fluoridated under conditions which favored formation of fluorapatite and excluded formation of CaF_2. These precautions have not been taken in most solubility studies. The high concentrations frequently used in exposing tooth mineral to fluoride will deposit fluoride as calcium fluoride and fluorapatite. At low pH tooth mineral is more soluble than CaF_2 (ERICSSON, 1950). As pH values increase, the solubility of tooth mineral decreases and at neutral pH CaF_2 is more soluble than tooth mineral (LEACH, 1959b). In the case of fluorapatite the solubility is a function of the fluoride concentration, and is less than hydroxyapatite containing a smaller concentration of fluoride (RATHJE, 1952; McCANN and BULLOCK, 1957; LEACH, 1959b).

Table 36. *Solubility in water of synthetic hydroxyapatite containing increasing proportions of fluorapatite.* Recalculated from RATHJE (1952)

ppm F in hydroxyapatite	Calcium, phosphorus and fluoride in solution		
	ppm Ca	ppm P	ppm F
0	2.14	0.87	0
1900	0.71	0.43	0.002
3800	0.71	0.22	0.003
7600	0.36	0.09	0.003

CaF_2 appears to have little effect on the solubility of hydroxyapatite at low pH, because at equilibrium the large concentration of dissolved calcium depresses dissolution of fluoride as would be expected according to the mass law (McCANN and BULLOCK, 1957). The effect of CaF_2 on the rate of dissolution of hydroxyapatite has not been established.

Several factors make it almost impossible to quantitate the solubility reducing effect of fluoride. For example, the solubility of hydroxyapatite increases with an increase in solid-solution ratio, both at neutral (NEUMAN and NEUMAN, 1958) and acid pH (LEACH, 1959b). Although the dependence of the solubility on the solid-solution ratio is decreased by presence of fluoride (LEACH, 1959b), it is still marked at the fluoride concentrations found in dental tissues under physiological conditions. Another consideration is that the solubility of hydroxyapatite increases with increase in the molarity of acid buffers (LEACH, 1959b). In addition, a number of constituents in the tooth affect its solubility, including, CO_2, Zn and Mg. The interionic action which may occur between these ions and Ca and P, thus modifying the process of dissolution, is poorly understood (*e.g.* complex formation between Mg^{++}, F^-, Ca^{++} and $PO_4^{\equiv}$). It is evident therefore that the solubility reducing effect of fluoride on dental tissues can be expressed only in general terms.

There is abundant evidence that fluoride increases the resistance of enamel and dentin to acid. For example, decalcification in 0.0025 M HCl of powdered, fluoride-exposed enamel ceased at pH 4.8 compared to 5.7 for untreated enamel (ERICSSON, 1950). In order to dissolve like quantities of enamel, a pH approximately 0.5 unit lower was required in the case of fluoride-treated enamel (KOVALIV and HELD, 1947; SUESS and FOSDICK, 1951). Even in strong buffers (0.4 M acetate) the pH at equilibrium was consistently lower as a result of fluoride exposing the enamel. This pH effect is secondary to a marked reduction in dissolution of Ca and P, as can be seen from Table 37. The solubility reducing effect of fluoride is pH dependent, and disappears at the low pH of strong mineral acids (McCLURE and LIKINS, 1949) due to formation of undissociated hydrofluoric acid (pK = 3.45). However, fluoride is effective in the pH range of dental plaques and carious lesions (pH 4—8).

An interesting aspect of decalcification of powdered tooth material is that the rate is always high during the first minutes of acid exposure and decreases rapidly (LEACH, 1959a, b; MANLY and HARRINGTON, 1959). It has been suggested that rapid dissolution of the smaller particles may contribute to this effect. In addition, as decalcification proceeds, increasing amounts of Ca and P in the buffer will retard dissolution, due to common ion effects. However, these factors are not the only ones, because the leveling off of dissolution may occur in the presence of excess acid and undissolved tooth mineral (LEACH, 1959a, b; MANLY and HARRINGTON, 1959). For example, in the experiment referred to in Table 37, the buffers used were capable of dissolving additional amounts of fresh enamel, and the acid-exposed enamel was dissolved further in fresh buffer. Apparently the conditions responsible for decreasing the rate of dissolution involve changes in both the solid and the solution. Studies indicate that fluoride present in the tooth material is one factor concerned in this phenomenon, with other tooth constituents playing an as yet undetermined role.

During acid decalcification virtually all the fluoride which is being dissolved will redeposit on the residual solid, leaving only traces in solution (LEACH, 1959b; ISAAC et al., 1958a). It is known that minute concentrations of fluoride (less than 0.5 ppm) will accelerate precipitation of calcium phosphate, and that fluorapatite probably is formed in this process (BRUDEVOLD and MESSER, 1961). Once a protective layer has been laid down on the surface of the tooth material, equilibrium conditions can develop at a pH level far below that tolerated by pure hydroxyapatite (see Table 37) provided that certain concentrations of fluoride, calcium and phosphate are present in the solution.

Table 37. *pH change and calcium and phosphorus release from one gram of normal or fluoridated enamel shaken in 100 ml of 0.4 M acetate buffer*. Data from LEACH (1959b)

Enamel	Inital pH	Final pH	mg Ca/100 ml	mg P/100 ml
Normal enamel	3.54	4.00	170	77
	4.00	4.20	132	55
	4.70	4.80	85	35
	5.74	5.86	20	8
Enamel containing 1.8% fluoride	3.54	3.76	67	29
	4.00	4.06	47	21
	4.70	4.72	27	10
	5.74	5.74	12	4

From the foregoing, one would expect powdered enamel of teeth from fluoride areas to be more resistant to acid dissolution than samples of enamel originating from low fluoride areas. Findings do not always bear out this view. In two studies no difference was found in the rates of dissolution of mildly fluorosed and of normal enamel, but the fluoride level of the respective enamel samples was not determined (VOLKER, 1940; JENKINS et al., 1952). In a third study enamel containing 618 to 909 ppm F was shown to be more slowly dissolved in a number of organic acids than non-fluorosed enamel (containing 111 ppm F) (MCCLURE and LIKINS, 1949). In addition, deciduous enamel from Newburgh, New York (1 ppm F in water supply) has been shown to dissolve at a slower rate than comparable enamel from Rochester, New York (0.09 ppm F in water supply) (FINN and DEMARCO, 1956). These experiments employed the total enamel of the respective teeth which, in contrast to surface enamel, differ relatively little in fluoride concentrations.

Figure 11 shows that surface enamel resists acid more than underlying enamel (ISAAC et al., 1958a). Here, the loss in weight resulting from acid etching of layer samples has been plotted against the depth from the surface. The acid resistance of the surface is a consistent finding, attributable to differences in the composition of surface and subsurface enamel. Since the relative acid resistance of the surface enamel was maintained after the organic material in the enamel had been extracted with ethylene diamine, it must be due to differences in composition of the mineral of surface and subsurface enamel. A relationship was shown to exist between the concentrations of F in the layer samples and the rate of acid dissolution (ISAAC et al., 1958a). This relationship was consistent in regard to surface-subsurface enamel from the same tooth groups, but did not always apply when different tooth groups were compared. Mottled enamel with its high fluoride content was more acid resistant than the teeth from low fluoride areas, and deciduous enamel which has lower levels of fluoride than permanent enamel, was less resistant. On the other hand, enamel of teeth from different areas may be similar in respect to fluoride content, and yet have different solubility rates. That factors other than fluoride are contributing to the acid resistance of enamel is clearly shown from the data in Table 38. Here powdered enamel was exposed in solutions containing from 1 to 1000 ppm of fluoride, 0.1 M orthophosphate, and having a pH pf 4.5, 5.5 or 8.0. Following the treatment the enamel was etched in acetate buffer at pH 4.5 for 30 min. Enamel samples treated at the same pH levels show the expected decrease in dissolution with increase in F content, but among samples with similar fluoride concentrations, those pretreated with phosphate at low pH are consistently more resistant to acid dissolution than samples pretreated at pH 8 or with water (no phosphate). These findings are not fully understood, but there is some evidence that the decrease in dissolution caused by the acid phosphate treatment may be caused by a combination of displacement of CO_2 in the enamel with phosphate, and recrystallization of the enamel with formation of fluorapatite (BRUDEVOLD et al., 1963).

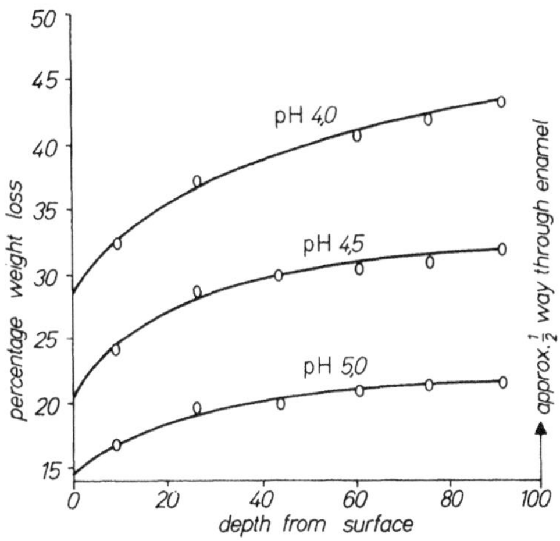

Fig. 11. Weight loss of successive layers of enamel of permanent teeth after exposure for one hour to acetate buffers. Enamel from permanent teeth of persons under 20 years of age (ISAAC et al., 1958a)

Although the solubility-reducing effect of fluoride upon powdered enamel has been well established, the effect upon intact enamel surfaces is less well defined. In view of the obvious differences existing between powdered enamel and the intact enamel surface, the same fluoride effect could not be expected. In addition to a much greater surface area, the powdered enamel particles have previously unexposed surfaces. This type of enamel has been found to pick up fluoride at a greater rate than the intact surface enamel (VOLKER et al., 1940). Therefore, a smaller fluoride effect is to be expected on the intact enamel surface than on powdered enamel.

Table 38. *Weight loss of fluoridated enamel upon exposure for 30 min to acetate buffer at pH 4.5. Enamel was fluoridated by treatment with fluoride-containing 0.1 M phosphate buffer at pH 4.5, 5.5 or 8.0.* Data from BRUDEVOLD et al. (1963)

ppm F in enamel	Wt. loss of 50 mg of enamel in 10 ml acetate buffer			
	pH of fluoridating buffer			fluoridated without buffer
	pH 4.5 mg	pH 5.5 mg	pH 8.0 mg	
100—199	13.8	13.5	19.5	23.4
200—399			17.5	18.5
400—599	11.5	11.9	18.5	17.0
800—999	10.3	11.2	13.9	15.0
1200	10.3			
2000	8.1			

Because of the variation in dissolution rate from tooth to tooth, and even from place to place or area to area on the same tooth, it is difficult to establish a quantitative effect of fluoride on enamel surface acid solubility (Brudevold, 1948). However, workers in this field agree that fluoride does have a solubility reducing effect on the majority of the teeth (Ericsson, 1950; Jenkins et al., 1952; Brudevold and Little, 1951; Massler et al., 1951). Of particular interest is a study on the rate of dissolution of phosphate from standard areas of deciduous teeth from geographic areas with 0.25, 1.4 and 2.0 ppm of fluoride in the drinking water, respectively (Jenkins et al., 1952). While less phosphate leached away from the teeth originating from fluoride areas, the difference was significant only in the 2 ppm group. The same trend was found in permanent teeth, but the difference was not significant.

It is of interest that the solubility reducing effect of fluoride is more pronounced on surfaces that have been etched with acid before being exposed to the fluoride solution, than on untreated surfaces (Brudevold and Little, 1951). This is in accordance with the observation of increased uptake of fluoride by acid-etched or carious enamel (Dowse and Jenkins, 1957; Myers et al., 1952).

It has also been reported that in teeth from high fluoride areas the enamel of initial carious lesions is less soluble in acid than similar enamel from low fluoride areas (Dowse and Jenkins, 1957). These findings suggest that one effect of fluoride is to lower the solubility of the mineral matter in initial carious lesions and thus slow down their progress.

A number of anions and cations, including oxalate, tin, zinc, lead and indium have been reported to decrease the rate of dissolution of powdered enamel Muhler and van Huysen, 1947; Manly and Bibby, 1949). In these and many other studies the extent of decalcification was measured by weight loss after exposure of the enamel to an acid buffer, ignoring the fact that many of the salts with which the enamel was pretreated would partly decompose the enamel and form insoluble decomposition products of Ca or P, or hydrolyze to form insoluble precipitates (*e.g.*, Pb^{++} and Sn^{++}). The weight of the new compounds, which was not accounted for, could in some instances materially affect the results. In addition, the significance of a decrease in decalcification before equilibrium has been established is open to question (Leach, 1959b). Although an extraneous precipitate on the enamel may form a barrier against ionic diffusion and thus slow down the rate of acid dissolution, it may not decrease the amount of enamel dissolved after equilibrium has been reached.The extent to which such precipitates will be retained in the surface of the tooth *in vivo* has not been determined, nor is there any convincing evidence that they can produce caries inhibition. Fluoride appears to be unique in that it reinforces the tooth mineral by being incorporated in the crystal lattice without significantly altering the microstructures normally present.

XI. Remineralization

Since saliva is supersaturated in respect to tooth mineral (Schmidt-Nielsen, 1946; Ericsson, 1949), it is not surprising that mineralization can take place in the mouth, as is evidenced by calculus formation. There is some indication that deposition of mineral in the enamel surface will continue after tooth eruption. For example, in unerupted teeth the uptake of P^{32} was remarkably high throughout the enamel, reflecting active calcification (Sognnaes et al., 1955). Teeth in the process of erupting acquired P^{32} from the saliva, but the uptake was limited primarily to the outer enamel because underlying enamel was highly calcified and relatively impermeable to the isotope. In functional teeth the uptake by the surface enamel was less than in erupting teeth, presumably due to increased mineralization. Replica studies of partly demineralized enamel also suggest that mineralization, or in this case, remineralization, can take place in the mouth (WOLF and NEUWIRTH, 1941; MANNERBERG, 1960), but because attrition as well as mineral deposition can alter the appearance of etched enamel surfaces this method of approach does not offer conclusive evidence. However, *in vitro* experiments have demonstrated irrefutably that remineralization of enamel or dentin can occur. For example enamel partly demineralized in weak organic acids will increase in hardness upon being exposed to saliva (HEAD, 1912) or calcifying solutions (KOULOURIDES et al., 1961; KOULOURIDES, 1962; SEINS and KOULOURIDES, 1963). In addition, remineralization has been demonstrated by polarizing microscopy and microradiography (JOHANSSON, 1965). Dentin has been studied less than enamel, but appears to acquire mineral as readily *in vitro*. For example, completely demineralized dentin will mineralize in a calcifying solution (SOLOMONS et al., 1960).

In view of these findings it seems justified to conclude that remineralization of dental tissues may occur in the mouth, and that deposition of mineral from saliva is important, not only in the process of posteruptive maturation of the enamel, but also in counteracting decalcification in carious lesions. It is notable that presence of fluoride in the calcifying solution will greatly accelerate remineralization of slightly etched enamel (KOULOURIDES et al., 1961; KOULOURIDES, 1962; SEINS and KOULOURIDES, 1963). Concentrations of only 1 ppm increase the rate of rehardening of acid-etched enamel surfaces by a factor of about 5. Apparently the metastability of the calcifying solution is increased by low levels of fluoride, since as little as 0.2 ppm of fluoride significantly increases the rate of precipitation of hydroxyapatite from supersaturated solutions of calcium and phosphate in the pH range of 6.2–7.4 (BRUDEVOLD and MESSER, 1961; BRUDEVOLD et al., 1961).

In regard to carious lesions, it is well known that pH may fluctuate over a wide scale, and that both dissolution and precipitation of mineral may take place, depending on the existing acidity. Considering in addition, the ability of enamel and dentin to remineralize before spontaneous precipitation occurs, it is reasonable to assume that the dissolution of mineral associated with caries is reversible, and that the progress of the carious lesions is determined by the balance between the processes of dissolution and formation of mineral. According to the evidence presented here, fluoride may promote mineral precipitation in the carious lesion, and thus retard mineral dissolution. This action of fluoride and its influence on posteruptive calcification of the surface enamel are difficult to evaluate, but are likely to be important.

XII. Concluding remarks

It has been concluded in this review that the caries reducing effect of fluoride is related to its presence in the tooth mineral, and that the mechanism of action has to do with the several ways in which low concentrations of fluoride can influence the mineral.

Fluoride 1) reduces lattice dimensions, *i.e.*, increases interionic forces in the apatite crystal by replacing hydroxyl groups in the crystal lattice;

2) improves the crystallinity of the mineral, either by relieving internal stress, thus reducing lattice imperfections, or by increasing the size of the apatite crystals;

3) reduces the solubility of tooth mineral, both at neutral and acid pH;

4) accelerates precipitation of calcium phosphate, and appears to favor formation of apatite crystals, when other crystalline species, such as brushite or octacalcium phosphate would otherwise form; and

5) it can alter the composition of the mineral, *i.e.*, increase the concentrations of magnesium and decrease the concentrations of carbonate and citrate.

All these effects are likely to be different facets of one basic mechanism, the tendency of fluoride to combine with calcium and phosphate to form the well crystallized and only slightly soluble fluorapatite. Since most of the fluoride present in bone and tooth mineral is located in the surface of the crystals its effect on crystallinity is readily detectable in the tiny crystals of bone which have a significant number of their unit cells located in the surface, but change in crystallinity has not so far been noted in the much larger crystals of enamel which have a small surface area and the majority of unit cells located in the interior structure. But by analogy the observations on bone mineral should also apply to enamel. Therefore, it is permissible to speculate on the relative roles of the different facets of the fluoride effects on tooth mineral in regard to caries. It is quite possible that pre-eruptive and post-eruptive effects of fluoride are different in importance. The pre-eruptive effect of water fluoridation may be one of improving the crystallinity of the mineral, particularly that portion located in the enamel surface which acquires the greatest concentrations of fluoride. This effect could extend to the first years after eruption when mineral deposition in the surface enamel is believed to take place primarily from saliva. On the other hand, topically applied fluoride may serve to impregnate accessible crystal surfaces with fluoride, as does waterborne fluoride, but without materially affecting crystallinity. The penetration of fluoride into surface imperfections may be facilitated by the use of high concentrations in the treatment solution. In the carious lesion, where dissolution of mineral is a predominant feature, the combined effects of fluoride, viz., of resisting dissolution and of accelerating precipitation of fluorapatite will tend to preserve the mineral and thus retard growth of the lesion. To assess the relative importance of the different biological effects of fluoride on enamel and dentin and learn how best to take advantage of them is a challenging task. As far as is known the unique role of fluoride in the calcium-phosphate system of tooth mineral is not shared by any other ionic species, and the caries inhibiting effect of fluoride must be viewed in this light.

References

ABDUL-GHAFFAR, H., and J. C. MUHLER: Pretreatment of teeth with sodium fluoride application in children. J. dent. Res. **38**, 901—904 (1959).

ADLER, P.: Der Kariesschutz bei Erwachsenen durch natürlich fluorhaltiges Trinkwasser. Dtsch. Zahn-, Mund- u. Kieferheilk. **15**, 24—30 (1951).

— J. STRAUB, and M. PROPOVIES: Intra vital uptake of fluorides in the teeth under various conditions. J. dent. Res. **29**, 549—555 (1950).

ALLAN, W., and B. W. NEVOR: Calcium content of plaque and saliva. Intl. Assoc. Dental Res. 35th Genl. Meeting Abstr. No. 108 (1957).

ARMSTRONG, W. D.: Mechanism of fluoride homeostasis. Arch. oral Biol. Suppl. **4**, 156—159 (1961).

—, and P. J. BREKHUS: Chemical constitution of enamel and dentin. Principal components. J. biol. Chem. **120**, 677—687 (1937).

— — Possible relationship between the fluorine content of enamel and resistance to dental caries. J. dent. Res. **17**, 393—397 (1938).

—, and L. SINGER: In vitro uptake and exchange of bone citrate. Ciba Symp. on Bone Structure and Metabolism, pp. 103—116. Boston: Little, Brown 1956.

ARNOLD, F. A. JR., F. J. MCCLURE, and C. L. WHITE: Sodium fluoride for children. Dent. Progr. **1**, 12—16 (1960).

—, H. T. DEAN, and D. W. SINGLETON JR.: The effect on caries incidence of a single topical application of a fluoride solution to the teeth of young adult males of a military population. J. dent. Res. **23**, 155—162 (1944).

— R. C. LIKINS, A. L. RUSSELL, and D. B. SCOTT: Fifteenth year of the Grand Rapids fluoridation study. J. Amer. dent. Ass. **65**, 780—785 (1962).

AST, D. B., and B. FITZGERALD: Effectiveness of water fluoridation. J. Amer. dent. Ass. **65**, 581—587 (1962).

— N. ALLAWAY, and H. L. DRAKER: Prevalence of malocclusion, related to dental caries and lost first molars, in a fluoridated city, and a fluoride deficient city. Amer. J. Orthop. **48**, 106—113 (1962).

— S. B. FINN, and H. C. CHASE: Newburgh-Kingston caries fluorine study. III. Further analyses of dental findings including the permanent and deciduous dentitions after four years of water fluoridation. J. Amer. dent. Ass. **42**, 189—195 (1951).

BACKER DIRKS, O.: Bias in clinical testing of caries-preventive dentifrices. In: Caries Symp., Zurich, pp. 37—47. Berne and Stuttgart: Hans Huber 1961.

— B. HOUWINK, and G. W. KWANT: Some special features of the caries preventive effect of water fluoridation. Arch. oral Biol. **4**, 187—192 (1961).

BARTELSTONE, H. J., I. D. MANDEL, and N. W. CHILTON: Critical evaluation of clinical studies with stannous fluoride dentifrices. Caries Symp., Zurich, ed. by H. R. MÜHLEMANN, and K. G. KÖNIG, pp. 27—36. Berne and Stuttgart: Hans Huber 1961.

BERGGREN, H., and E. WELANDER: Supervised tooth brushing with a sodium fluoride solution in 5,000 Swedish school children. Acta odont. scand. **18**, 209—234 (1960).

BERGMAN, G.: The caries inhibiting action of sodium fluoride. Acta odont. scand. **11**, Suppl. 12, 1—112 (1953).

BIBBY, B. G.: A new approach to caries prophylaxis. Tufts. dent. Outlook **15**, 4—8 (1942).

—, and F. BRUDEVOLD: The action of fluorides and other agents on the teeth in the prevention of dental decay. In: Fluoridation as a Public Health Measure. Amer. Ass. Advancement Sci., pp. 148—178. Washington, D.C. 1954.

—, and S. S. TURESKY: A note on the duration of caries inhibition produced by fluoride applications. J. dent. Res. **26**, 105—108 (1947).

—, and M. VAN KESTEREN: The effect of fluorine on mouth bacteria. J. dent. Res. **19**, 391—402 (1940).

—, and E. WILKINS: Unpublished report (1948).

— E. DEROCHE, and E. WILKINS: The effect of topical applications of lead fluoride on dental caries. J. dent. Res. **26**, 446 (1947).

— E. WILKINS, and E. WITOL: A preliminary study of the effects of fluoride lozenges and pills on dental caries. Oral Surg. **8**, 213—216 (1955).

BINDER, K.: Vorläufiger Bericht über die bisherigen Erfahrungen und Resultate der Fluortablettenverabfolgung an Wiener Schulkinder. Öst. Z. Stomat. **55**, 653—657 (1958).

BLAYNEY, J. R.: Economy of water fluoridation. J. Amer. dent. Ass. **65**, 595—597 (1962).

BOISSEVAIN, C. H., and W. F. DREA: Spectroscopie determination of fluorine in bones, teeth and other organs, in relations to fluorine in drinking water. J. dent. Res. **13**, 495—500 (1933).

BOWES, J. H., and M. M. MURRAY: A chemical study of "mottled teeth" from Maldon, Essex. Brit. dent. J. **60**, 556—562 (1936).

BRINER, W. W.: The effect of enamel fluoride on acid production by lactobacillus casei. J. dent. Res. **40**, 667 (1961).

BROWN, H. K., H. R. MCLAREN, G. H. JOSIE, and B. J. STEWART: The Brantford-Sarnia-Stratford fluoridation caries study — 1955 report. J. Canad. dent. Ass. **22**, 207—216 (1956).

BRUDEVOLD, F.: Study of the phosphate solubility of the human enamel surface. J. dent. Res. **27**, 320—329 (1948).

— Chemical composition of the teeth in relation to caries. Chapt. 1 in, Chemistry and Prevention of Dental Caries, R. F. SOGNNAES, ed. Springfield, Ill.: Chas. C. Thomas Springfield, Ill. 1962a.

— Dental tissue factors in dental caries. Int. dent. J. **12**, 496—508 (1962b).

—, and M. LITTLE: Chemical studies of the human enamel surface. J. dent. Res. **30**, 477 (1951).

—, and A. C. MESSER: Seeding effect of hydroxyapatite in calcifying solutions containing different amounts of fluoride. J. dent. Res. **40**, 728 (1961).

— B. H. AMDUR, and A. C. MESSER: Factors involved in remineralization of carious lesions. Arch. oral Biol. **6**, 304 (1961).

— D. E. GARDNER, and F. A. SMITH: The distribution of fluoride in human enamel. J. dent. Res. **35**, 420—429 (1956a).

— R. B. NEVIN, and J. BONNER: Effect of concentration and pH on fluoride uptake by intact enamel. Int'l. Assoc. Dental Res., 34th Genl. Meeting, Abstr. No. 156 (1956b).

— A. SAVORY, and L. BOWMAN: The effec of fluoride in phosphate buffers on enamel. Int'l. Assoc. Dental Res. 35th Genl. Meetingt Abstr. No. 27 (1957a).

— L. T. STEADMAN, and F. A. SMITH: Inorganic and organic components of tooth structure. Ann. N. Y. Acad. Sci. **85**, 110—132 (1960).

— P. GRØN, R. SPEIRS, M. SPINELLI, and D. E. GARDNER: Acquisition of fluoride. Int'l. Assoc. Dental Res. 40th Genl. Meeting Abstr. No. 123 (1962).

BRUDEVOLD, F., J. W. HEIN, J. R. BONNER, R. B. NEVIN, H. C. HODGE, and B. G. BIBBY: Reaction of tooth surfaces with 1 ppm of fluoride as sodium fluoride. J. dent. Res. **36**, 771—779 (1957b),

— A. SAVORY, D. E. GARDNER: M. SPINELLI, and R. SPEIRS: A study of acidulated fluoride solutions. I. In vitro effects on enamel. Arch. oral Biol. 8, 167—177 (1963).

— L. T. STEADMAN, D. E. GARDNER, J. ROWLEY, and M. F. LITTLE: Uptake of tin and fluoride in intact enamel. J. Amer. dent. Ass. **53**, 159—164 (1956c).

Bureau of Economic Research: Fluori dation in Canada 1962. J. Canad. dent. Ass. 28, 520—524 (1962).

BURGESS, R. C., T. G. MONDROW, G. NIKIFORUK, and F. H. COMPTON: Topical stannous fluoride as a caries preventive for pre-sc hool children. J. Canad. dent. Ass. 28, 312 (1962).

CARLOS, J. P., A. M. GITTELSOHN, and W. HADDON: Caries in deciduous teeth in relation to maternal ingestio n of fluoride. Publ. Hlth Rept. **77**, 658—660 (1962).

CARLSON, C. H., W. D. ARMSTRONG, and L. SINGER: Distribution and excretion of radio fluoride in the human. Proc. Soc. exp. Biol. (N. Y.) **104**, 235—239 (1960).

CARLSTROM, D.: X-ray crystallographic studies on the apatite and calcified structures. Acta radiol. (Stockh.) Suppl. **121** (1955).

CARTER, W. J., P. JAY, I. L. SHKLAIR, and L. H. DANIEL: The effect of topical fluoride on dental caries experience in adult females of a military population. J. dent. Res. **94**, 73—76 (1955).

CHEYNE, V. D.: Human dental caries and topically applied fluorine. A preliminary report. J. Amer. dent. Ass. **29**, 804—807 (1942).

CHRIETZBERG, J. E.: Tooth brushing as a substitute for quick cleansing in the topical fluoride technic. J. Amer. dent. Ass. **42**, 435—438 (1951).

COOLEY, W. E.: Reactions of tin (II) and fluoride ions with etched enamel. J. dent. Res. **40**. 1199—1210 (1961).

COMPTON, F. H., and R. M. GRAINGER: The Riversid epre-school Dental Project. J. Canad. dent. Ass. **25**, 478—488 (1959).

Council on Dental Therapeutics: Prescribing supplement of dietary fluoride. J. Amer. dent. Ass. **56**, 589—591 (1958).

Council on Dental Therapeutics: Evaluation of Crest toothpaste. Amer. dent. Ass. J. **61**, 272—274 (1960).

CROSBY, N. D., and P. A. SHEPHERD: Studies on patterns of fluid intake, water balance and fluoride retention. Part I. Patterns of fluid intake in relation to the ingestion of plain water. Med. J. Australia **44**, 305—311 (1957).

CZARNOSKA, R., A. DOBRZONSKA, M. SZPRINGER, and E. I. JACHIMCSAK: Effect of the topical application of an aqueous sodium fluoride solution on the caries incidence in Polish children. Czas. stomat. **12**, 699—706 (1959).

DARLING, A. I.: The structure of the enamel revealed in dental disease. Arch. oral Biol. **4**, 80—85 (1961).

DAVENPORT, R. R., and B. G. BIBBY: Unpublished report (1948).

DAWES, C., and G. N. JENKINS: Some inorganic constituents of dental plaque and their relationship to early calculus formation and caries. Arch. oral Biol. **71**, 161 (1962).

DEAN, H. T.: Endemic fluorosis and its relation to dental caries. Publ. Hlth Rept. **53**, 1443—1452 (1938).

— F. A. ARNOLD, and E. ELVOVE: Domestic water and dental caries. V. Additional studies of the relation of fluoride domestic waters to dental caries experience in 4425 white children, aged 12 to 14 years, of 13 cities in 4 states. Publ. Hlth Rept. **57**, 1155—1179 (1942).

— P. JAY, F. A. ARNOLD JR., and E. ELVOVE: Domestic water and dental caries. I. A dental caries study, including L. acidophilus estimations of a population severely affected by mottled enamel and which for the past 12 years has used a fluoride-free water. Publ. Hlth Rept. **56**, 365—381 (1941a).

— — — — Domestic water and dental caries. II. A study of 2832 white children aged 12 to 14 years, of eight suburban Chicago communities, including L. acidophilus studies of 1761 children. Publ. Hlth Rept. **56**, 761—792 (1941b).

DEATHERAGE, C. F.: Fluoride domestic waters and dental caries experience in 2026 white Illinois selective service men. J. dent. Res. **22**, 129—137 (1943a).

— A study of fluoride domestic waters and dental caries experience in 263 white Illinois selective service men living in fluoride areas following the period of calcification of the permanent teeth. J. dent. Res. **22**, 173—180 (1943b).

DOWSE, C. M., and G. N. JENKINS: Fluoride uptake in vivo in enamel defects and its significance. J. dent. Res. **36**, 816 (1957).

ENGLANDER, H. R., R. DE PALMA, and R. G. KESEL: The Aurora-Rockford, Illinois study. I. Effects of water having naturally occurring fluoride on dental health of young adults. J. Amer. dent. Ass. **65**, 614—621 (1962).

ERICSSON, Y.: Enamel-apatite solubility. Acta odont. scand. 8, Suppl. 3, 1—131 (1949).
— Reduction of the solubility of enamel surfaces. Acta odont. scand. 9, 60—83 (1950).
— The state of fluorine in milk and its absorption and retention when administered in milk. Acta odont. scand. 16, 51—77 (1958a).
— The distribution and reactions of fluoride ions in enamel-saliva environment, investigated with the radioactive fluorine isotope F^{18}. Acta odont. scand. 16, 127—141 (1958b).
— Karies profylax genom fluortabletter. Meddelanden frau Kungl Medicinalstyrelsen Stockholm 1959.
— Fluoride in dentifrices. Investigations using radioactive fluorine. Acta odont. scand. 19, 31—77 (1961).
— Aluminum compounds in fluorinated toothpastes and dental prophylaxis pastes. Acta odont. scand. 20, 441—451 (1962).
—, and I. HELLSTROM: The lactic acid content of the saliva after carbohydrate ingestion. II. Source of the salivary lactic acid and inhibition of its formation. Acta odont. scand. 10, 118—133 (1952).
—, and S. ULLBERG: Autoradiographic investigations of the distribution of F^{18} in mice and rats. Acta odont. scand. 16, 363—374 (1958).
EVANS, R. J., and P. H. PHILLIPS: The fluorine content of various fractions of milk and commercial caseins. J. Dairy Sci. 22, 621—622 (1939).
VON DER FEHR, F., and F. BRUDEVOLD: In vitro calculus formation. J. dent. Res. 39, 1041—1048 (1960).
FELTMAN, R., and G. KOSEL: Prenatal and postnatal ingestion of fluorides — fourteen years of investigation — final report. J. dent. Med. 16, 190—199 (1961).
FINN, S. B., and C. DEMARCO: The effect of artificial water fluoridation on the solubility of tooth enamel. J. dent. Res. 35, 185—188 (1956).
—, and H. C. JAMISON: A comparative clinical study of three dentifrices. J. Dent. Child. 30, 17—25 (1963).
FISCHER, R. B.,N. H. ELSHEINER, and J. C. MUHLER: The effect of several fluoride reagents on the structure of whole teeth. J. dent. Res. 33, 538—541 (1954b).
—, and J. C. MUHLER: The effect of sodium fluoride upon the surface structure of powdered dental enamel. J. dent. Res. 31, 751—755 (1952).
— —, and C. J. WUST: The effects of several fluoride reagents upon the structure of powdered dental enamel. J. dent. Res. 33, 50—54 (1954a).
FRANK, R., R. F. SOGNNAES, and R. STERN: Dental aspects of mineralization with special reference in the metastructural pattern of enamel. In: Calcification in Biological Systems, pp. 163—202, ed. by R. F. SOGNNAES, Amer. Ass. Advancement Sci., Washington, D. C. (1960).
GALAGEN, D. J., and J. W. KNUTSON: The effect of topically applied fluorides on dental caries experience. V. Report of findings with two, four and six applications of sodium fluoride and of lead fluoride. Publ. Hlth Rept. 62, 1477—1483 (1947).
—, and J. VERMILLION: Effect of topical fluorides on teeth matured on fluoride-bearing water. Publ. Hlth Rept. 70, 1114—1115 (1955).
GEDALIA, I., K. A. ROSENZWEIG, and A. SADEH: Fluorine content of superficial enamel layer and its correlation with the fluorine content of saliva, tooth ages and DMFT count. J. dent. Res. 40, 865—869 (1961).
GEROULD, C. H.: Electron microscope study of the mechanism of fluoride deposition in teeth. J. dent. Res. 24, 223—233 (1945).
GIESECKE, F., and W. RATHJE: The phosphates. III. Hydroxyl fluorapatite, the mineral of raw phosphate. Berichte 74B, 349—356 (1941).
GISH, C. W., J. C. MUHLER, and C. L. HOWELL: The effect of topically applied fluorostannite on the dental caries experience in children. III. Results at the end of three years. J. dent. Res. 38, 881—882 (1959).
— — — A new approach to the application of fluorides for the reduction of dental caries in children. Results at the end of five years. J. Dent. Child. 29, 65—71 (1962).
GLAS, J. E., and K. A. OMNELL: Studies on the ultra structure of dental enamel. I. Size and shape of the apatite crystallites as deduced from x-ray diffraction data. J. Ultrastruct. Res. 3, 334—344 (1960).
GRØN, P., M. A. SPINELLI, O. R. TRAUTZ, and F. BRUDEVOLD: The effect of carbonate on the solubility of hydroxyapatite. Arch. oral Biol. 8, 251—263 (1963).
HARDWICK, J. L.: The fluoride content of plaque: Its possible antienzymatic action. Caries Symp., Zürich, ed. by H. R. Mühlemann and K. G. König, pp. 112—119. Berne and Stuttgart: Hans Huber (1961).
HARRIS, R.: Observations on the effect of topical sodium fluoride on caries incidence in children. Australia dent. J. 4, 257—260 (1959).
HARRISON, M. F.: Fluorine content of New Zealand teeth. N. Z. dent. J. 45, 2—27 (1949).
HARTLES, R. L.: The role of citric acid in mineralized tissues. Brit. dent. J. 111, 52—56 (1961).

HATTON, W. E., W. H. NEBERGALL, and J. C. MUHLER: The removal of fluorine from dilute solutions of sodium fluoride and stannous fluoride by powdered dental enamel. J. dent. Res. **34**, 350—357 (1955).

HAWES, R. R., S. SANNES, and F. BRUDEVOLD: Pilot studies of three topical fluoride application procedures. J. dent. Res. **33**, 661 (1954).

HAYES, R. L., N. W. LITTLETON, and C. L. WHITE: Posteruptive effects of fluoridation on first permanent molars of children in Grand Rapids, Michigan. Amer. J. Publ. Hlth **47**, 192—199 (1957).

HEAD, J.: A study on saliva and its action on tooth enamel in reference to its hardening and softening. J. Amer. med. Ass. **59**, 2118—2122 (1912).

HEIN, J. W., J. F. BONNER, F. BRUDEVOLD, F. A. SMITH, and H. C. HODGE: Distribution in the soft tissue of the rat of radioactive fluoride administered as sodium fluoride. Nature (Lond.) **178**, 1295—1296 (1956).

HELD, A. J., u. F. PIGUET: Kariesprophylaxe mit Fluortabletten. Stoma (Heidelb.) **7**, 213—215 (1954).

— —, et L. ROSEGEN: Imprégnation fluorique des dents temporaires. Bull. schweiz. Akad. med. Wiss. **7**, 343—501 (1951).

HELLSTROM, I.: Fluorine retention following sodium fluoride mouth washing. Acta odont. scand. **18**, 263—278 (1960).

HILL, I. N., J. R. BLAYNEY, and W. WOLF: Evanston dental caries study. XIX. Prevalence of malocclusion of children in a fluoridated and control area. J. dent. Res. **38**, 782—794 (1959).

— — — Evanston fluoridation study. Twelve years later. Dent. Progr. **1**, 95—99 (1961).

HILL, T. J.: Fluoride dentifrices. J. Amer. dent. Ass. **59**, 1121—1127 (1959).

HINE, J., M. SWARTZ, and R. W. PHILLIPS: Staining of resin and silicate restorations by topically applied solutions of stannous fluoride. J. Periodont. **28**, 138—144 (1957).

HODGE, H. C., and F. A. SMITH: Some public health aspects of water fluoridation. In: Fluoridation as a Public Health Measure. ed. by R. F. SOGNNAES. Amer. Ass. Advancement Sci., Washington, D. C. (1954).

HORD, H. B., and R. G. ELLES: The effect of topical application of sodium fluoride on the CaF_2 content of vital teeth. J. dent. Res. **30**, 360—362 (1951).

HOWELL, C. L., C. W. GISH, R. D. SMILEY, and J. C. MUHLER: Effect of topically applied stannous fluoride on dental caries experience in children. J. Amer. dent. Ass. **50**, 14—17 (1955).

ISAAC, S., and F. BRUDEVOLD: Discoloration of teeth by metallic ions. J. dent. Res. **36**, 753 — 758 (1957).

— — F. A. SMITH, and D. E. GARDNER: Solubility rate and natural fluoride content of surface and subsurface enamel. J. dent. Res. **37**, 254—263 (1958a).

— — — — The relation of fluoride in the drinking water to the distribution of fluoride in the enamel. J. dent. Res. **37**, 318—325 (1958b).

JACKSON, D.: A clinical study of non-endemic mottling of enamel. Arch. oral Biol. **5**, 212—223 (1961).

JENKINS, G. N.: A note on the possible mode of action of fluoride in dental caries. Brit. dent. J. **104**, 54—55 (1958).

— The effect of pH on the fluoride inhibition of salivary acid production. Arch. oral Biol. **1**, 33—41 (1959).

— Anti-caries mechanism of fluorides in dentifrices. Caries Symp., Zurich, ed. by H. R. MÜHLEMANN, and K. G. KÖNIG, pp. 104—111. Berne and Stuttgart: Hans Huber (1961).

—, and R. L. SPEIRS: Distribution of fluorine in human enamel. J. Physiol. (Lond.) **121**, 21 (1953).

— P. A. ARMSTRONG, and R. L. SPEIRS: Laboratory investigations on the relation of fluorine to dental caries on Tyneside and district. Proc. roy. Soc. Med. **45**, 517—525 (1952).

JOHANSEN, E., and L. G. NORDBACK: The chemistry of carious lesions. III. The fluoride content of carious dentin. Int'l. Assoc. Dental Res. 40th Genl. Meeting, Abstr. No. 143, 1962.

—, and H. F. PARKS: Electron microscopic observations on the three-dimensional morphology of apatite crystallites of human dentin and bone. J. biophys. biochem. Cytol. **7**, 743—746 (1960).

— — Electron microscopic observations on sound human dentin. Arch. oral Biol. **7**, 185—193 (1962).

JOHANSSON, B.: Remineralization of slightly decalcified enamel studied by polarized light microscopy. J. dent. Res. **44**,64—70, (1965).

JORDAN, W. A., and J. K. PETERSON: Caries inhibiting value of a dentifrice containing stannous fluoride. Final report of a two year study. J. Amer. dent. Ass. **58**, 42—46 (1959).

— J. R. SNYDER, and U. WILSON: A study of a single application of 8 per cent SnF_2. J. Dent. Child. **26**, 355—359 (1959).

KESSLER, W., u. K. SOLTH: Ergebnisse der Zahnkaries-Prophylaxe durch interne Fluorgaben. Stoma (Heidelb.) **11**, 14—20 (1958).
KICK, C. H., R. M. BETHKE, R. H. EDGINGTON, O. H. M. WILDER, P. R. RECORD, W. WILDER, T. J. HILL, and S. W. CHASE: Fluorine in animal nutrition. Bull. 558, Ohio Agric. Expt. Sta. 1935.
KLEIN, H.: Dental caries (DMF) experience in relocated children exposed to water containing fluorine. II. J. Amer. dent. Ass. **33**, 1136—1141 (1946).
— Dental effects of community waters accidentally fluoridated for nineteen years. II. Differences in the extent of caries reduction among the different types of permanent teeth. Publ. Hlth Rept. **63**, 563—573 (1948).
KLINKENBERG, E., and B. G. BIBBY: The effect of topical applications of fluorides on dental caries in young adults. J. dent. Res. **29**, 4—7 (1950).
KNAPPWORST, A.: Physikalisch-chemische Grundlagen einer lokalen Kariestherapie des Dentins mit Fluorionen. Dtsch. zahnärztl. Z. **4**, 553—567 (1949).
KNUTSON, J. W.: Evaluation of the use of fluorine as a caries control measure. The effect of topically applied fluorides. J. Amer. dent. Ass. **38**, 204—212 (1949).
— An evaluation of the Grand Rapids water fluoridation project. J. Mich. med. Soc. **53**, 1001—1006 (1954).
—, and W. D. ARMSTRONG: The effect of topically applied sodium fluoride on dental caries experience. Publ. Hlth Rept. **58**, 1701—1715 (1943).
— — Effect of topically applied sodium fluoride on dental caries experience. III. Report of findings for the third study year. Publ. Hlth Rept. **61**, 1683—1689 (1946).
— —, and F. M. FELDMAN: The effect of topically applied sodium fluoride on dental caries experience. IV. Report of findings with two, four and six applications. Publ. Hlth Rept. **62**, 425—430 (1947).
KOULOURIDES, T.: Remineralization of enamel and dentin. Dental Clin. No. Am., July, 485—487 (1962).
— H. CUETO, and W. PIGMAN: Rehardening of softened enamel surfaces of human teeth by solutions of calcium phosphates. Nature (Lond.) **189**, 226—227 (1961).
KOVALIV, P., et A. J. HELD: Influence de fluor sur la résistance de l'émail dentaire. Schweiz. Mschr. Zahnheilk. **57**, 305—332 (1947).
KUTLER, B., and R. L. IRELAND: The effect of sodium fluoride application on the dental caries experience in adults. J. dent. Res. **32**, 458—462 (1953).
KUYPER, A. C., and K. KUTNERIAN: Mechanism of incorporation of fluoride into bone salt. J. dent. Res. **41**, 345—350 (1962).
KYES, F. M., N. J. OVERTON, and T. W. MCKEAN: Clinical trials of caries inhibitory dentifrices. J. Amer. dent. Ass. **63**, 189—193 (1961).
LARSEN, N. P.: Tooth decay in relation to diet and general health. J. Amer. med. Ass. **137**, 832—837 (1948).
LAW, F. E., M. H. JEFFREY, and H. C. SHEARY: Topical applications of fluoride solutions in dental caries control. Publ. Hlth Rept. **76**, 287—290 (1961).
LAWRENZ, M., H. H. MITCHELL, and W. A. RUTH: Adaptation of the growing rat to the ingestion of a constant concentration of fluorine in the diet. J. Nutr. **19**, 531—546 (1940).
LEACH, S. A.: Reaction of fluoride with powdered enamel and dentin. Brit. dent. J. **106**, 133 by 142 (1959a).
— Some notes on the solubility of enamel and dentin in acid. Arch. oral Biol. **1**, 218—232 (1959b).
LEATHERMAN, G. H.: Fluoridation around the world. Int. dent. J. **9**, 517—535 (1959).
LEICESTER, H. M.: Biochemistry of the Teeth. C. V. Mosby Co., St. Louis, Mo. 1949.
LEONHARDT, H.: Ergebnisse der Fluortablettenzufuhr bei Salzburger Schulkindern im Alter von 6—10 Jahren, 4 Jahre nach Beginn der Aktion. Arch. oral Biol. Spec. Suppl. **6**, 17—26 (1961).
LILIENTHAL, B.: The effect of fluoride on acid formation by salivary sediment. J. dent. Res. **35**, 197—204 (1940).
— Inhibition of acid formation from carbohydrates by stannous fluoride and stannous chlorofluoride. Australian dent. J. **3**, 165—173 (1958a).
— The effect of a stannous fluoride mouth wash on acid formation in the mouth and some observations on the mechanism of inhibition. Australian dent. J. **3**, 221—227 (1958b).
—, and N. D. MARTIN: Investigations of the anti-enzymatic action of fluoride at the enamel surface. J. dent. Res. **35**, 189—196 (1956).
LITTLE, M. F., and F. BRUDEVOLD: A study of inorganic carbon dioxide in intact human enamel. J. dent. Res. **37**, 991—1000 (1958).
— E. S. CUETO, and J. ROWLEY: Chemical and physical properties of altered and sound enamel. I. Ash: Ca, P, CO_2, N, water, microradiolucency and density. Arch. oral Biol. **7**, 173—184 (1962).

MacIntire, W. H., L. J. Hardin, F. D. Oldham, and J. W. Hammond: Development of P_2O_5 insolubility in phosphate mixtures. The formation of fluorapatite as its cause. Industr. Eng. Chem. **29**, 758 (1937).
Malaowalla, A., and H. M. Myers: Interaction of sodium fluoride and synthetic apatite. J. dent. Res. **41**, 413—419 (1962).
Manly, R. S.: Stability of stannous fluoride dentifrices. Caries Symp., Zurich, ed. by H. R. Mühlemann, and K. G. König, pp. 70—79. Berne, Stuttgart: Hans Huber (1961).
—, and B. G. Bibby: Substances capable of decreasing the solubility of tooth enamel. J. dent. Res. **28**, 160—171 (1949).
—, and D. P. Harrington: Solution rate of tooth enamel in acetate buffer. J. dent. Res. **38**, 910—919 (1959).
Mannerberg, F.: Appearance of tooth surface, as observed in shadowed replicas in various age groups, in long-time studies, after tooth-brushing in cases of erosion and after exposure to citrus fruit juice. Odont. Revy **11**, Supp. 6 (1960).
Marthaler, T. M.: Zur Frage des Fluorvollsalzes: erste klinische Resultate. Schweiz. Mschr. Zahnheilk. **71**, 671—682 (1961).
— Die Wirkung aminfluoridhaltiger Zahnpasten auf den Karieszuwachs bei Kindern während drei Jahren überwachten Gebrauches. Schweiz. Mschr. Zahnheilk. **73**, 390—409 (1963).
—, and C. Schenardi: Inhibition of caries in children after $5^1/_2$ years of fluoridated table salt. Helv. odont. Acta **6**, 1—6 (1962).
Massler, M., C. Tapia, and E. Zwemer: Action of acid on topically fluoridized intact enamel surfaces. J. dent. Res. **30**, 515 (1951).
McCann, H. G.: Reaction of fluoride ion with hydroxyapatite. J. biol. Chem. **201**, 247—259 (1953).
—, and F. A. Bullock: Reactions of fluoride ion with powdered enamel and dentin. J. dent. Res. **34**, 59—67 (1955).
— — The effect of fluoride ingestion on the composition and solubility of mineralized tissues of the rat. J. dent. Res. **36**, 391—398 (1957).
—, and E. H. Fath: Phosphate exchange in hydroxyapatite enamel, dentin and bone. II. Effect of fluoride on the exchange. J. biol. Chem. **231**, 869—872 (1958).
McClure, F. J.: Domestic water and dental caries. Fluorine in human saliva. Amer. J. Dis. Child. **62**, 512—515 (1941a).
— Domestic water and dental caries. III. Fluorine in human saliva. J. dent. Res. **20**, 283 (1941b).
— Ingestion of fluoride and dental caries. Quantitative relations based on food and water requirements of children 1 to 12 years old. Amer. J. Dis. Child. **66**, 362—369 (1943).
—, and R. C. Likins: The effect of fluoride on the solubility of human enamel. J. dent. Res. **28**, 636 (1949).
— — Fluorine in human teeth studied in relation to fluorine in the drinking water. J. dent. Res. **30**, 172—176 (1951).
—, and H. G. McCann: Dental caries and composition of bones and teeth of white rats: Effect of dietary mineral supplements. Arch. oral Biol. **2**, 151—161 (1960).
McConnell, D.: Crystal chemistry of carbonate apatites and their relationship to the composition of calcified tissues. J. dent. Res. **31**, 35—63 (1952).
McDonald, R. E., and J. C. Muhler: The superiority of topical applications of stannous fluoride on primary teeth. J. Dent. Child. **24**, 84 (1957).
McKay, F. S.: Mass control of dental caries through the use of domestic water supplies containing fluoride. Amer. J. Publ. Hlth **38**, 828—832 (1948).
McLaren, H. R., and H. K. Brown: A study of the use of a topically applied stannous fluoride solution in prevention of dental caries. Canad. J. Publ. Hlth **46**, 387—395 (1955).
Megerian, D.: The deposition of fluorine in glycol-ashed bone. Univ. Rochester Atomic Energy Project Rept. No. UR-168, 1951.
Mercer, V. H., and J. C. Muhler: Comparison of a single application of stannous fluoride with a single application of sodium fluoride or two applications of stannous fluoride. J. Dent. Child. **28**, 84—86 (1961).
Miller, J., and P. Hobson: Silver nitrate and sodium fluoride on enamel caries. Brit. dent. J. **106**, 246—249 (1959).
Montel, G., and G. Chaudron: The action of tricalcium phosphate and hydrated dicalcium phosphate on calcium fluoride suspensions in water. C. R. Acad. Sci. (Paris) **234**, 839 (1952).
Muhler, J. C.: Effect of a stannous fluoride containing dentifrice on caries reduction in children. II. Caries experience after one year. J. Amer. dent. Ass. **50**, 163—166 (1955).
— Effects of fluoride and non-fluoride containing tin salts on the dental caries experience in children. J. dent. Res. **37**, 422—426 (1958a).
— The effect of a single topical application of stannous fluoride on the incidence of dental caries in adults. J. dent. Res. **37**, 415—416 (1958b).

MUHLER, J. C.: The effect of a modified stannous fluoride-calcium pyrophosphate dentifrice on dental caries in children. J. dent. Res. **37**, 448—450 (1958c).
— The anticariogenic effectiveness of a single application of stannous fluoride in children residing in an optimal communal fluoride area. Results at the end of 30 months. J. Amer. dent. Ass. **61**, 431—438 (1960).
— A practical method for reducing dental caries in children not receiving the established benefits of communal fluoridation. J. Dent. Child. **28**, 5—12 (1961).
—, and A. W. RADIKE: Effect of a dentifrice containing stannous fluoride on dental caries in adults. II. Results at the end of two years of unsupervised use. J. Amer. dent. Ass. **55**, 196—198 (1957).
—, and G. VAN HUYSEN: Solubility of enamel protected by sodium fluoride and other compounds. J. dent. Res. **26**, 119—128 (1947).
— H. G. DAY, and W. H. NEBERGALL: Relationship between pH, age, and concentration of solutions of stannous fluoride and sodium fluoride in decreasing enamel solubility and affecting the uptake of fluoride. J. dent. Res. **31**, 756—760 (1952).
— A. W. RADIKE, W. H. NEBERGALL, and H. G. A. DAY: Comparison between the anti- cariogenic effects of dentifrices containing SnF_2 and NaF. J. Amer. dent. Ass. **51**, 556—559 (1955).
— — — — The effect of a stannous fluoride-containing dentifrice on dental caries in adults. J. dent. Res. **35**, 49—53 (1956).
MYERS, H. M., J. G. HAMILTON, and H. BECKS: A tracer study of the transfer of F^{18} to teeth by topical application. J. dent. Res. **31**, 743—750 (1952).
NEUMAN, H. H.: The milk and water intakes of small children. A survey of drinking habits. Arch. Pediat. **74**, 456—462 (1957).
NEUMAN, W. F., and B. J. MULRYAN: The surface chemistry of bone. IV. Further data on recrystallization. J. biol. Chem. **193**, 237—241 (1951).
—, and M. W. NEUMAN: The chemical dynamics of bone mineral. Chicago, Ill.: Univ. Chicago Press 1958.
— T. Y. TORIBARA, and B. J. MULRYAN: Surface chemistry of bone. IX. Carbonate-phosphate exchange. J. Amer. chem. Soc. **78**, 4263—4266 (1956).
— M. W. NEUMAN, E. R. MAIN, J. O'LEARY, and F. A. SMITH: The surface chemistry of bone. II. Fluoride deposition. J. biol. Chem. **187**, 655—661 (1950).
NEVIN, R. B., F. BRUDEVOLD, and M. F. LITTLE: Uptake and loss of F^{18} from intact enamel. Int'l. Assoc. Dental Res. 35th Genl. Meeting, Abstr. No. 1261 (1957).
NEVITT, G. A., D. H. WITTER, and W. D. BOWMAN: Topical applications of sodium fluoride and stannous fluoride. Publ. Hlth Rept. **73**, 847—850 (1958).
NEWBRUN, E.: Studies on the physical properties of fluorosed enamel. II. Microhardness. Arch. oral Biol. **2**, 21—27 (1960).
—, and F. BRUDEVOLD: Studies on the physical properties of fluorosed enamel. I. Microradiographic studies. Arch. oral Biol. **2**, 15—20, 38—674 (1960).
NIEDENTHAL, A.: Kariesprophylaxe mit Natriumfluorid-Dragees bei Offenbacher Schulkindern. Zahnärztl. Mitt. **45**, 576—578; 648—650 (1957).
NIKIFORUK, G.: Carbonates and fluorides as chemical determinants of tooth susceptibility to caries. Caries Symp., Zurich, ed. by H. R. MÜHLEMANN, and K. G. KÖNIG, pp. 62—69. Berne and Stuttgart: Hans Huber (1961).
OCKERSE, T.: The chemical composition of enamel and dentin in high and low caries areas in South Africa. J. dent. Res. **22**, 441—446 (1943).
PAMEIJER, J. H. N., F. BRUDEVOLD, and E. E. HUNT JR.: A study of acidulated fluoride solutions. III. The cariostatic effect of repeated topical sodium fluoride applications with and without phosphate: A pilot study. Arch. oral Biol. 8, 183—185 (1963).
PECKHAM, S. C., R. S. LEOPOLD, and W. C. HESS: Determination of fluoride in organic and inorganic factors of dentin and enamel. J. dent. Res. **75**, 205—209 (1956).
PEFFLEY, G. E., and J. C. MUHLER: The effect of a commercial stannous fluoride dentifrice under controlled brushing habits on dental caries incidence in children. Preliminary report. J. dent. Res. **39**, 870—874 (1960).
PETERSON, J. K., and W. H. JORDAN: Relative caries inhibiting values of topically applied sodium silico fluoride and sodium fluoride. J. dent. Res. **36**, 124—128 (1957).
POSNER, A. S., and E. D. EANES: Fluoride in bone and teeth. Norelco Reptr **10**, 71—75 (1963).
PROTHEROE, D. H.: A study to determine the effect of topical application of stannous fluoride on dental caries in young adults. Preliminary report. Roy. Canad. dent. Corps Quart. **1**, No. 4, 18—23 (1961).
RATHJE, W.: The formation of hydroxyfluor-apatite in tooth enamel under influence of drinking water containing fluoride. J. dent. Res. **31**, 761—766 (1952).
REISS, L. Z.: Strontium 90 absorption by deciduous teeth. Science **134**, 1669—1673 (1961).
Report of Joint Committee of American Academy of Pediatrics and American Society of Dentistry for Children: Pediatrics **23**, 400—407 (1959).

RICKLES, N. H., and H. BECKS: The effects of an acid and a neutral solution of sodium fluoride on the incidence of dental caries in young adults. J. dent. Res. **30**, 757—765 (1951).

RUSOFF, L. L., B. S. KONIKOFF, J. B. FRYE, J. E. JOHNSTON, and W. W. FRYE: Fluoride addition to milk and its effect on dental caries in school children. Amer. J. clin. Nutr. **11**, 91—101 (1962).

RUSSELL, A. L.: Dental fluorosis in Grand Rapids during the seventeenth year of fluoridation. J. Amer. dent. Ass. **65**, 608—612 (1962).

—, and E. ELVOVE: Domestic water and dental caries. VI. A study of the fluoride-dental caries relationship in an adult population. Publ. Hlth Rept. **66**, 1389—1401 (1951).

—, and C. L. WHITE: Dental caries in Maryland children after seven years of fluoridation. Publ. Hlth Rept. **76**, 1087—1093 (1961).

SANTESSON, G.: Aspects of salt fluoridation II: Observations on the consumption of table salt by adult. Presented at 6th ORCA Congress, Pavia 1959.

SAVORY, A., and F. BRUDEVOLD: The distribution of nitrogen in human enamel. J. dent. Res. **38**, 436—442 (1959).

SCHLESINGER, E. R.: Dental caries and the pediatrician. Amer. J. Dis. Child. **105**, 1—4 (1963).

SCHMIDT-NIELSEN, B.: The solubility of tooth substances in relation to the composition of saliva. Acta odont. scand. **7**, Suppl. 2, 1—88 (1946).

SCHMITZ, W.: Zahnschutzhärtung durch Fluorpinselung. Dtsch. zahnärztl. Z. **7**, 204—208 (1952).

SCHRAER, H., A. S. POSNER, R. SCHRAER, and I. ZIPKIN: Effect of fluoride on bone crystallinity in the growing rat. Biochim. biophys. Acta **64**, 565—567 (1962).

SCHROEDER, H. E.: Inorganic content and histology of early dental calculus in man. Helv. odont. Acta **7**, 17—30 (1963).

SCHUTZMANNSKY, G.: Sechs Jahre Kariesprophylaxe durch Fluortablettengaben. Arch. oral Biol. Spec. Suppl. **6**, 27—32 (1961).

SCOTT, D. B.: Electron microscope evidence of fluoride-enamel reactions. J. dent. Res. **39**, 1117 (1960).

— R. G. PICARD, and W. G. WYCKOFF: Studies of the action of sodium fluoride on human enamel by electron microscopy and electron diffraction. Publ. Hlth Rept. **65**, 43—56 (1950)

SEINS, R. M., and T. KOULOURIDES: Effects of intermittent treatments with calcifying solutions on the softening of teeth. Int'l. Assoc. Dental Res. 41st Genl. Meeting, Abstr. 285 (1963).

SINGER, L., and W. D. ARMSTRONG: Regulation of human plasma fluoride concentrations. J. appl. Physiol. **15**, 508—510 (1960).

SLACK, G. L.: The effect of topical application of stannous fluoride on the incidence of dental caries in 6 year old children. Brit. dent. J. **101**, 7—11 (1956).

SMITH, F. A., D. E. GARDNER, and H. C. HODGE: Investigations on the metabolism of fluoride. II. Fluoride content of blood and urine as a function of the fluorine in drinking water. J. dent. Res. **29**, 596—600 (1950).

— — S. A. LEACH, and H. C. HODGE: Fluoride removal by powdered dental enamel from solutions of stannous or sodium fluoride. Nature (Lond.) **180**, 1421—1422 (1957).

SMITH, M. C., E. M. LANZ, and H. V. SMITH: The cause of mottled enamel. Science **74**, 244 (1931).

SOBEL, A. E., A. HANOK, H. A. KIRSHNER, and I. FANKUCHEN: Calcification of teeth. II. Comparison of some properties of human and rat teeth. J. dent. Res. **28**, 61—67 (1953).

— J. H. SHAW, A. HANOK, and S. NOBEL: Calcification XXVI. Caries susceptibility in relation to composition of teeth and diet. J. dent. Res. **39**, 462—472 (1960).

SOGNNAES, R. F., J. H. SHAW, and R. BAGORACH: Radio tracer studies on bone, cementum, dentin and enamel of Rhesus monkeys. Amer. J. Physiol. **180**, 408—420 (1955).

SOLOMONS, C. C., J. T. IRVING, and W. F. NEUMAN: Calcification of the dentin matrix. In: Calcification in Biological Systems, ed. by R. F. SOGNNAES, Amer. Ass. Advancement Sci., pp. 203—216, Washington, D. C. (1960).

SPEIRS, R. L.: The uptake, exchange and release of fluoride at the surface of teeth. Brit. dent. J. **104**, 347—348 (1958).

SPINELLI, M. A., J. J. VOGEL, and F. BRUDEVOLD: Effect of pH and phosphate concentrations on uptake of fluoride by hydroxyapatite from aqueous solutions and saliva. Int'l. Assoc. Dental Res. 41st Genl. Meeting, Abstr. No. 330 (1963).

STACK, M. V.: The chemical nature of the organic matrix of bone, dentin and enamel. Ann. N. Y. Acad. Sci. **60**, 585—595 (1955).

STONES, H. H., F. E. LAWTON, E. R. BRANSBY, and H. D. HARTLEY: Effect of topical application of potassium fluoride and of the ingestion of tablets containing sodium fluoride on the incidence of dental caries. Brit. dent. J. **86**, 263—271 (1949).

STREAN, L. P., and J. D. BEAUDET: Dental caries inhibited by fluoride vitamin tables. Dent. Surv. **22**, 689—691 (1946).

SUESS, P. H., and L. S. FOSDICK: Solubility of normal and fluoridized enamel. J. dent. Res. **30**, 177—181 (1951).

SUNDVALL-HAGLAND, I.: Sodium fluoride application to the deciduous dentition. A clinical study. Acta odont. scand. **13**, 5—131 (1955).

— F. BRUDEVOLD, W. D. ARMSTRONG, D. E. GARDNER, and F. A. SMITH: A comparison of the increment of fluoride in enamel and the reduction in dental caries resulting from topical fluoride applications. Arch. oral Biol. **1**, 74—79 (1959).

SYRRIST, A.: A study of the increment of fluorine content of enamel following topical applications of sodium fluoride to human teeth in vitro. Odont. T. **57**, 381—394 (1949a).

— Histological studies on the effect of sodium fluoride on human dental enamel. Odont. T. **57**, 395—408 (1949b).

— E Klinisk studie av effekten av lokale behandlinger med natriumfluorid som kariesprofylaktisk middel. Odont. T. **57**, 511 (1949d).

—, and K. KARLSEN: A five year report on the effect of topical applications of sodium fluoride on dental caries experience. Brit. dent. J. **97**, 1—6 (1954).

TORELL, P., and H. SIBERG: Mouth wash with sodium fluoride and potassium fluoride. Odont. Revy **13**, 62—72 (1962).

TOVBORG-JENSEN, A.: Über die Ausscheidung von CaF_2 und übersättigten Lösungen. Z. phys. Chem. A **180**, 93—116 (1937).

TRAUTZ, O. R.: Crystallographic studies of calcium carbonate phosphate. Ann. N. Y. Acad. Sci. **85**, 145—160 (1960).

—, and R. R. ZAPANTA: Experiments with calcium carbonate phosphates and the effect of topical application of sodium fluoride. Arch. oral Biol. Spec. Suppl. **4**, 122—133 (1961).

U.S. Public Health Service: Fluoridation memoranda. Index No. 2 and No. 8. (1962).

VOGEL, J. J., R. NAUJOKS, and F. BRUDEVOLD: The effective concentrations of calcium and inorganic orthophosphate in salivary secretions. Arch. oral Biol. **10**, 523—535 (1965).

VOLKER, J. F.: Solubility of fluorosed enamel and dentin. Proc. Soc. exp. Biol. and Med. (N. Y.) **43**, 643—645 (1940).

—, and B. G. BIBBY: The action of fluorine in limiting dental caries. Medicine **20**, 211—227 (1941).

— R. F. SOGNNAES, and B. G. BIBBY: Studies on the distribution of radioactive fluoride in the bones and teeth of experimental animals. Amer. J. Physiol. **132**, 707—712 (1941).

WALKER, J. S., F. J. MARGOLISM, H. L. TEATE, M. L. WEIL, and H. L. WILSON: Water intake of normal children. Science **140**, 890—891 (1963).

WALLACE, P. C.: The metabolism of F^{18} in normal and chronically fluorosed rats. Univ. California Rept. UCRL-2196, 119 pp., Berkeley, Calif. (1953).

WALSER, M.: Ion association. VI. Interaction between calcium, magnesium, inorganic phosphates, citrate and protein in normal human plasma. J. clin. Invest. **40**, 723—730 (1961).

WEAVER, R.: Fluorine and dental caries. Further investigations on Tyneside and in Sunderland. Brit. dent. J. **77**, 185—193 (1944).

WEIDMANN, S. M., J. A. WEATHERELL, and R. G. WHITEHEAD: The effect of fluorine on the chemical composition and calcification of bone. J. Path. Bact. **78**, 435—445 (1959).

WEISZ, W. S.: Reduction of dental caries through use of sodium fluoride mouth wash. J. Amer. dent. Ass. **60**, 438—456 (1961).

— A comparison of the relative effects of sodium and stannous fluoride when applied topically. J. Dent. Child. **29**, 22—35 (1962).

WELLOCK, W. D., and F. BRUDEVOLD: A study of acidulated fluoride solutions. II. The caries inhibiting effect of single annual topical applications of an acidic fluoride and phosphate solution. A two year's experience. Arch. oral Biol. 8, 179—182 (1963).

— A. MAITLAND, and F. BRUDEVOLD: Caries increments, tooth discoloration, and state of oral hygiene in children given single annual applications of acid phosphate-fluoride and stannous fluoride. Arch. oral Biol. **10**, 453—460 (1965).

WESPI, H. J.: Experiences and problems of fluoridated cooking salt in Switzerland. Arch. oral Biol. **6**, 33—39 (1961).

— Entwicklung und gegenwärtiger Stand der Kariesbekämpfung mit „Fluor-Vollsalz" in der Schweiz. Schweiz. Mschr. Zahnheilk. **72**, 323—331 (1962).

WILLS, J. H.: The secretion of intravenously ingested fluorine in the submaxillary saliva of cats. J. dent. Res. **19**, 585—590 (1940).

WOLF, J., u. F. NEUWIRTH: Reparative Vorgänge an der Oberfläche natürlicher und künstlich hervorgerufener Schmelzdefekte. Z. Zahn-, Mund- u. Kieferheilk. 8, 222—349 (1941).

WRZODEK, G.: Ist eine Kariesprophylaxe mit Fluordragees erfolgversprechend? Zahnärztl. Mitt. **47**, 258—262 (1959).

WYNN, W., J. HALDI, K. D. BENTLEY, and M. L. LAW: Dental caries in the albino rat in relation to the chemical composition of the teeth and of the diet. II. Variations in the Ca/P ratio of the diet induced by changing the phosphorus content. J. Nutr. **58**, 325—334 (1956).

— — — — Dental caries in the albino rat in relation to the chemical composition of the teeth and of the diet. III. Composition of incisor teeth of animals fed diets with different Ca/P ratios. J. Nutr. **63**, 57—64 (1957).

YOON, S. H., F. BRUDEVOLD, F. A. SMITH, D. E. GARDNER, and N. SONI: Distribution of fluorine in teeth and alveolar bone. J. Amer. dent. Ass. **61**, 565—570 (1960a).

— — D. E. GARDNER, and F. A. SMITH: Distribution of fluoride in teeth from areas with different levels of fluoride in the water supply. J. dent. Res. **39**, 845—856 (1960b).

ZIEGLER, E.: Grundlagen der Milchfluorierung in Winterthur. Schweiz. Mschr. Zahnheilk. **69**, 111—114 (1959).

ZIEMNOWICZ-GLOWACKA, W.: Prevention of caries with "Fluordar" tablets. Czas. stomat. **13**, 719—728 (1960).

ZIPKIN, I., F. J. MCCLURE, and W. A. LEE: Relation of the fluoride content of human bone to its chemical composition. Arch. oral Biol. **2**, 190—195 (1960).

— A. S. POSNER, and E. C. EANES: The effect of fluoride on the x-ray diffraction pattern of the apatite of human bone. Biochim. biophys. Acta (Amst.) **59**, 255—258 (1962).

ZWEMER, J. D.: Lactic acid formation by lactobacilli exposed to fluoridized enamel. J. dent. Res. **36**, 182—191 (1957).

Chapter 5

The Effects of Fluoride on Plants

By

MOYER D. THOMAS[1] and ERNEST W. ALTHER[2]

With 23 Figures and 3 Plates

The role of fluorine in plant physiology has assumed great importance in recent years, stemming primarily from its toxic properties when absorbed by or deposited on plants as gases or solids emitted by certain industries such as aluminum, steel, ceramics and phosphate fertilizers, as reviewed by SEMRAU (1957). Fluorine compounds are present in the raw materials or are used in the manufacturing processes of these industries. The great expansion of some of these industries in the past 20–30 years has drawn attention to their fluoride emanations as air pollutants capable of doing substantial damage to both plants and animals. The necessity for remedial measures has also been recognized and at least partially achieved. Fluoride damage to animals is due largely to ingestion of fodder containing 30 to 50 ppm or more fluorine. ALTHER (1961) has recently reviewed this subject.

I. Industrial sources of fluorine

Plant damage due to gaseous fluorine compounds, principally hydrogen fluoride and silicon tetrafluoride, has been observed and studied in Western Europe for over a century, but such studies in North America are largely confined to the past 20 to 30 years. The greatest damage has been caused by the electrolytic aluminum and phosphate fertilizer industries. Many other industries, such as copper smelting, steel and ceramics, emit fluorides in relatively small amount, at high temperatures, and usually from tall stacks. As a consequence, they have done only limited plant damage which has not been widespread in distribution. However, some steel factories have smelted ores rich in fluoride which has caused extensive plant damage.

Fluoride damage, particularly in North America, increased substantially during and immediately following the second World War, due primarily to extensive expansion of the aluminum industry. Table 1 gives worldwide data for aluminum production which indicates the potential fluoride air pollution production near aluminum factories. The industry was very small in 1900, then increased to 67,000 tons in 1912 and to 148,000 tons in 1918. After a post-war decline output of the metal increased to about 300,000 tons in 1930, then nearly tripled by 1940 due to the second World War. Production continued to expand in North America but not in Europe during the War to a maximum of 2.1 million tons in 1943, then fell off to about half of 1943 production in 1945, and increased again to over 1.6 million tons in 1950. FRARY (1943) states that there was a seven-fold wartime

[1] Air Pollution Research Center, University of California, Riverside, California.

[2] Consulting member: Fluorine Commission, Swiss Academy of Medical Sciences, Berne, Switzerland. Present address: Cantonal Agricultural College, Flawil, St. Gallen, Switzerland.

Table 1. *Aluminum production as an indicator of the potential production of fluoride air pollution near aluminum factories* (WALLACE, 1937; U.S. Bureau of Mines' Minerals Yearbooks)

	Aluminum production (thousands of short tons)						
	Western Europe	Russia	Japan	Canada	United States	Other	Total
1900	4.5				3.5		8
1912	38			9	20		67
1918	69			17	62		148
1920	59			13	69		141
1921	48			9	27		84
1930	141			37	114	1	293
1933	89	5		18	42	1	155
1935	167	27	4	23	60	3	284
1935[1]	182[2]	30	4	26	100	—	347
1940	427	66	35	109	206	25	868
1943	483	69	126	496	920	61	2155
1945	119	86	6	216	495	22	944
1950	265	209	27	395	719	16	1631
1960	1120	745	264	761	2015	105	5010

[1] Data compiled by R. K. STRONG, Editor, Kingzeits' Chemical Encyclopedia, pp. 94. 1946.
[2] France-26; Italy-16; Germany-93; United Kingdom-16; Switzerland-16; Norway-15.

expansion in the United States to over one million tons of aluminum per year. Since 1950, there has been a further three-fold expansion, world-wide. There was also an expansion of phosphate production in the United States, mainly in Florida, from 3.5 million tons in 1945 to 11.1 million tons in 1950.

This great industrial activity caused substantial fluoride damage to plants and animals and provoked a number of lawsuits which, in turn, stimulated a great deal of world-wide research related not only to the immediate animal and plant damage problems but also to all phases of fluorine chemistry in physiology and agriculture. It is of great interest that the post-war expansion of aluminum production has been attended by a decrease, rather than an increase, in fluorine damage due to the design and installation of effective devices for collecting and dispersing the fluorides. In the aluminum industry, remedial measures include better hooding for the electrolytic cells, water scrubbing and filtering the gases, and the construction of tall stacks up to 500 feet in height to improve dispersion of the pollutants. MÜLLER et al. (1959) have discussed these engineering developments. In the steel industry many fluoride problems have been solved by such measures as selection and/or beneficiation of ores to secure charges of low fluoride content and the use of electric precipitators on the stack gases with or without the dispersing of lime dust into the flue gases to convert gaseous fluorides to calcium fluoride for collection.

Table 2. *Range of fluoride in vegetation as affected by distance from the source and use of collecting equipment in the factory* (WILLIAMS, 1956)

Product	Collectors	Fluoride in vegetation at distance (miles)					Claims or complaints
		0—0.5 ppm	1 ppm	2 ppm	4 ppm	6 ppm	
Fertilizer	Full	3—21	6—14	0—15	3—24	6—21	None
Fertilizer	Partial	81—153	39—120	16—81	14—47	6—44	None
Fertilizer	Partial	52—285	35—177	19—41	9—48	6—17	None
Fertilizer	Partial	130—845	78—327	100—223	64—114	—	Some claims
Phosphorus[1]	—	62—495	20—316	26—212	8—140	12—110	Some claims
Aluminum[1]	—	160—1600	95—1000	36—380	8—135	4—87	Some claims

[1] Average several factories.

The effect of full or partial removal of the fluorides from the effluent gases from fertilizer factories on the uptake of fluorine by vegetation within six miles of the plants is shown by the data of WILLIAMS (1956) in Table 2. With full removal of fluoride, the vegetation had normal fluoride content and there were no complaints of damages. With only partial removal of fluoride, elevated levels were found in some vegetation samples, especially near the factory, and claims for damage were made against one plant which evidently emitted an appreciable amount of fluoride. The phosphorus and aluminum factories which operated without controls produced still higher concentrations in the vegetation and also provoked damage claims.

The European experience with industrial fluoride damage is summarized in books and monographs by SCHROEDER and REUSS (1883), REUSS (1896), HASELHOFF and LINDAU (1903), WILLE (1922), HASELHOFF (1932), HASELHOFF et al. (1932), ROHOLM (1937, 1938), BOREI (1945), TRUHAUT (1948), BREDEMANN (1951, 1956), BERGE (1958), and an extensive literature. BURGI (1927) discussed all the halogens in HEFFTER-HEUBNER *Handbuch der experimentellen Pharmakologie*. GARBER (1960, 1962) published an extensive review of the recent literature of smoke, dusts and gases, including various fluorides.

II. Field observations in Europe

SCHROEDER and REUSS (1883) described fluoride injury to vegetation near a copper smelter and classified the severity of the damage as "mild," "medium," and "heavy acute." REUSS (1896) discussed "acute" and "chronic" forms of damage, the former causing immediate foliar necrosis due to high concentrations of hydrogen fluoride, the latter showing gradually developing symptoms due to lower concentrations. The author recommended that the diagnosis should be confirmed by leaf analysis for fluorine. RHODE (1895) employed the same methods to diagnose fluorine damage in a rye field near a superphosphate factory emitting hydrogen fluoride. MAYRHOFER (1891) also observed fluorine damage in the vicinity of a superphosphate factory, while OST (1907) attributed the destruction of forest trees to fluorine effluents extending to a distance of 800 meters from glass and fertilizer factories. WISLICENUS (1898, 1901) concluded that hydrogen fluoride from a superphosphate factory, like sulfur dioxide, damages pine during active assimilation. Leaf analysis was needed to confirm the cause of injury. QUANJER et al. (1906) observed injury in parks and gardens in the Netherlands due to fluoride from neighboring glass factories. FRESENIUS (1902) found much more fluorine in a branch of an apple tree growing near an industrial source of hydrogen fluoride than in corresponding tissue in an area free of industrial effluents. HAMMIG et al. (1913) found fluorine damage on pines and spruce near a brick works.

KOTTE (1929) described symptoms attributed to fluoride on the leaves and fruit of plum trees growing near a brick works. The leaves had brown margins and spots of necrotic tissue. The fruit had coffee-brown, sharply defined spots. Beneath these spots, the fruit flesh was brown in color and woody in texture. There was also marginal injury on the leaves of hornbeam, oak, lime, chestnut, walnut and wine grape, but not on acacia, maple, blackberry, apple and cherry. Possibly the plums were injured at an early stage of development.

BREDEMANN and RADELOFF (1937) observed that the green bark of twigs, but not the underlying wood, could take up appreciable amounts of fluoride from the atmosphere, but very little from the soil. As there was no translocation of the absorbed fluorine, analysis of the bark served to diagnose fluoride fumigations.

Marotta et al. (1938) analyzed plant samples to a distance of three kilometers from an aluminum factory, provided with good control equipment, at Mori, Italy. The leaf tissues showed 2 to 73 ppm fluorine and the surface dust on the leaves, 12 ppm fluorine.

Agate et al. (1949) found 270 to 25 pptm total fluoride and 140 to 9 pptm gaseous fluoride in the atmosphere from 100 to 1700 meters downwind from an aluminum factory in Scotland. Vegetation samples had 1000 to 5 ppm fluoride. Damage to vegetation, if any, was not reported.

Lindberg (1956) found 1950 and 135 ppm fluorine in the surface 2.5 cm of soil at 400 meters and 2000 meters, respectively, from a superphosphate plant in Latvia, whereas the corresponding 15-cm layer of soil had 120 and 6 ppm. Vegetables and hay grown in the area had increased fluoride levels, as did also the milk of dairy cattle given these feeds. The fluorine content of the milk of human mothers who worked in the factory (1 to 2 ppm) or lived within 1000 to 1500 meters was measurably greater (0.5 ppm) than the controls (0.2 ppm).

Bovay (1954, 1958) observed that an aluminum factory emitting fluorides and a soda ash factory emitting hydrogen chloride, both operated near a fruit-growing district, caused leaf lesions on the trees year after year. Leaf analyses during several seasons indicated that the fluorine levels exceeded 100 ppm at times and the chlorine levels, which were extremely variable, reached 2000 ppm. In 1957, the aluminum factory was out of operation while the soda ash plant operated normally. No leaf lesions were found that season. Fluorine levels in the leaves barely reached 25 ppm while the chloride ranged from 213 to 1130 ppm. It appeared, therefore, that the leaf lesions were caused by the aluminum factory. However, a synergism between fluoride and chloride was not ruled out; further, the maximum chloride concentration in 1957 was only about half the maximum for other years.

Bovay (1958) found a range of 5 to 1852 ppm fluorine in the leaves of apple, apricot, cherry, pear, poplar, grape and strawberry near industrial sources of fluoride compared with a range of 2 to 42 ppm in control plants outside the industrial area.

III. Early fumigation studies

Most of the foregoing observations of plant damage are essentially qualitative because reliable determinations were not made of the atmospheric fluoride concentrations. Fumigation experiments were carried out by Schmitz-Dumont (1896) using 33 and 100 ppm hydrogen fluoride applied for 1 to 5 hours daily to three-year-old pine and Norway maple until leaf damage was produced, requiring about three to four weeks at the lower concentration and one to two days at the higher level. The leaves developed yellow margins which gradually assumed a dark-brown shade. Ost (1896) evaporated a 39 % solution of hydrofluoric acid in a fumigation chamber containing mayflowers. A two-to-three-hour exposure in an estimated concentration of 100 ppm was required to cause leaf damage. Haselhoff and Lindau (1903) produced fluoride damage on the leaves of plum, cherry, fir, oak and chestnut by evaporating hydrofluoric acid in the open atmosphere. The air concentrations were not determined but 1890 to 2990 ppm fluorine was found in the leaves of the oak and chestnut. Wislicenus (1913) fumigated conifers with silicon tetrafluoride, causing injury with concentrations of 5 to 10 ppm. Sertz (1921) caused browning of the needles of pine and fir by a one-hour fumigation with 100 ppm hydrogen fluoride or silicon tetrafluoride. At 4 ppm, daily fumigations of three hours or less, for one week to one month, were required to cause plant damage.

The high concentrations of hydrogen fluoride calculated in the foregoing fumigation experiments are unrealistic because the gas is avidly absorbed by all surfaces, resulting in a very rapid decrease in concentration unless the air-gas mixture is continuously renewed at a very rapid rate. The calculated concentrations may be 1 to 3 orders of magnitude too high as suggested by fumigation experiments described later. The analyses of the vegetation for fluorine are also somewhat questionable.

IV. Determination of fluorine in vegetation

A. Willard and Winter method

The method of analysis for fluorine in vegetation that has found general acceptance in North America and elsewhere is based on the WILLARD and WINTER (1933) steam distillation procedure, as described by REMMERT et al. (1953), ROWLEY et al. (1953) and NICHOL et al. (1957). The Boyce Thompson method (GWIRTSMAN et al., 1957) is also essentially similar.

1. Sample preparation and combustion

In the initial preparation of the sample it is usually advisable to wash the fresh leaves with distilled water, with or without a detergent, rubbing gently with absorbent cotton. If the value of the surface fluoride is desired the washed and unwashed leaves can be determined separately, or the washings can be also analyzed. There is evidence that an appreciable amount of fluoride can be extracted from the interior of the leaves if the washing process is prolonged or is too vigorous.

A dry pulverized sample (5 to 10 g) or a fresh sample, comminuted with water in a "blendor," is mixed with a suspension of fluorine-free lime sufficient to render the mixture alkaline, and evaporated to dryness in a platinum, nickel or Inconel dish or crucible. The residue is charred on a hot plate or under infrared lamps and heated in a furnace for about one hour at 600° C until white. The ash is fused over a low burner with 5 g sodium hydroxide.

2. Steam distillation and fluoride estimation

The fusion is transferred with water to a distilling flask where it is acidified with about 35 ml excess perchloric acid plus silver perchlorate, and steam distilled at 135° C, collecting 500 ml distillate. The distillate is adjusted to pH 3.0 by pH meter or by adding monochloroacetate buffer solution and aliquot portions are titrated with thorium nitrate (equivalent to 10 or 100 μg fluorine per milliliter, depending on the amount of fluoride in the sample) using sodium alizarin sulfonate as indicator. Chrome azurol S at pH 3.3 is also a satisfactory indicator. The SPADNS indicator (BELLACK and SCHOUBOE, 1958), sodium-2-(p-sulfophenylazo)-1,8-dihydroxynaphthalene-3,6-disulfonate-zirconium lake, may be employed to read directly the amount of fluorine in the distillate, using a spectrophotometer or colorimeter. Eriochrome cyanine R is also an excellent indicator. An accuracy of 0.02 mg per liter is claimed for readings in the range from 0.00 to 1.40 mg fluorine per liter.

3. Statistical evaluation

Boyce Thompson Institute (GWIRTSMAN et al., 1957) carried out cooperative analyses with 15 laboratories on composite samples of corn, apple and tea leaves. The average fluorine values and their statistics from the 15 different analysts are given in Table 3, which indicates that the coefficient of variability ranged from 6.2 to 7.5 %.

Benedict et al. (private communication, 1963) at Stanford Research Institute prepared large, wellmixed samples, each sufficient for about 1000 replicate analyses, of 35 different types of vegetation. The Institute made 30 random analyses of each of these large samples by the foregoing method and sent random portions to many other laboratories for analyses. Table 4 gives the results for six samples, together with a statistical treatment of the data. Evidently a high degree of agreement was reached between the different laboratories. The coefficient of variability did not exceed 11 %, except with the alfalfa sample which had a low fluoride level.

Table 3. *Fluorine content of dried, well-mixed, leaf samples of corn, apple and tea as determined by 15 laboratories* (Adapted from Gwirtsman et al., 1957)

	Corn	Apple	Tea
Average F, ppm	81.0	38.0	100.0
σ	6.1	2.8	6.2
Coefficient of variability, %	7.5	7.4	6.2

Table 4. *Standard deviation and coefficient of variability of fluoride content of six dried, well-mixed samples of pasture grass, alfalfa leaves and pine needles analyzed by Stanford Research Institute and many cooperating laboratories* (Benedict, private communication, 1963)

	Pasture grass		Alfalfa		Pine needles	
	SRI	Others	SRI	Others	SRI	Others
Concentration $\pm \sigma$, ppm	221 ± 25[1]	231 ± 24	39 ± 2[1]	42 ± 4	116 ± 6[1]	119 ± 8
Coefficient of variation, %	11	10	5	9	5	7
Concentration $\pm \sigma$, ppm	56 ± 3[1]	58 ± 6	13 ± 3[1]	11 ± 3	44 ± 3[1]	45 ± 3
Coefficient of variation, %	6	11	21	26	6	7

[1] 30 replicate analyses.

B. Modifications of the Willard-Winter method

Many other similar methods, which differ only in detail from the foregoing, have been proposed. For example, Hoskins and Ferris (1936) analyzed the distillate by titrating the fluoride with thorium nitrate in 50 % alcohol which gives a sharp endpoint with the sodium alizarin sulfonate indicator. Adams and Koppe (1956) recommended titrating at pH 2.9 in the presence of added sodium chloride. Ballczo and Kaufmann (1952) recommended heating the ash with powdered magnesium metal after the initial combustion with calcium acetate. Distillation was done in a jacketed still, heated to 146° by boiling tetrachloroethane. Fabre et al. (1955) incinerated 5 to 10 g samples with magnesium acetate at 600°; steam distilled with 50 % sulfuric acid at 146° using tetrachloroethane to control the distillation temperature; and titrated with thorium nitrate sodium alizarin sulfonate at pH 3.5. No fusion with sodium hydroxide was carried out. Mavrodineanu and Gwirtsman (1956) carried out the combustion of vegetation samples with sodium peroxide and potassium perchlorate in the Parr bomb. Time required was about 30 min, compared with six hours for the standard ashing procedure. Excellent agreement was obtained by the two methods.

Oelschläger and Kirchgessner (1960) recommended 450° as the optimum temperature for ashing. The use of lime proved unnecessary for their raw fodder and feed samples. Uptake of fluorine from the refractories in the furnace was observed and the crucibles were therefore placed in closed (but not air-tight) metal containers during the ashing process. The need for fusion with sodium hydroxide of samples high in silica was confirmed.

Nielsen (1958) proposed a method of concentrating the fluoride in the Willard-Winter distillate to facilitate the determination of microgram quantities of fluorine. A glass tube, 9 mm in diameter by 30 cm, with a 6 mm tube at one end, was charged with a 2—2.5 cm column length of 200—400 mesh ion exchange resin Dowex-1-X-8. This was first treated with normal sodium acetate to convert it to the acetate form. After removing excess acetate, aliquots of the distillate were allowed to flow through the resin at 6—12 drops per minute. Fluoride was absorbed by the resin to its capacity of 6—8 μg, then displaced by successive 10 ml portions of 0.1, 0.2 and 0.3 N sodium acetate. Fluoride was determined spectrophotometrically at 527.5 mμ, using zirconium Eriochrome Cyanine R lake.

C. Rapid semi-quantitative methods

A number of other methods have been proposed which have been used principally for diagnostic purposes. These are largely qualitative or semi-quantitative procedures.

1. Lipase method

Amberg and Loevenhart (1908) employed the inhibiting action of fluoride on the enzyme lipase. The method was applied to biological fluids such as milk and beer, also to meat extracts. Presumably, it can also be applied to extracts of leaf tissue, *etc.*

A solution of lipase was prepared as follows: Grind up 10 grams of pig's liver and extract with successive portions of water to a final volume of 100 ml. Add 1 ml toluene, stopper, mix and incubate at 35—40° for 24 to 36 hours. Filter portions as needed. The unfiltered solution keeps well at room temperature. The fluoride solution should contain at least 1 ppm fluorine. Mix 1 to 4 ml with 1 ml lipase in a test tube, add 0.2 ml ethylbutyrate and 4 drops of toluene. Dilute to 5 ml. Prepare a blank with water and reagents. Stopper, shake and incubate in a thermostat at 35—40° for 14 to 18 hours. Remove the tubes, add litmus solution and titrate with 0.05 N sodium hydroxide. The titer is reduced according to the amount of fluoride present. Prepare a curve with known fluoride additions versus titers.

2. Silico-fluoride — Silico-molybdate methods

Bredemann and Radeloff (1933) have used a method in which the fluoride is volatilized as silicon tetrafluoride, collected in a drop of liquid and identified as hexagonal crystals of sodium silicofluoride (Na_2SiF_6), or as the blue silicomolybdate according to Feigl and Krumholz (1929). Place 3.0 g of comminuted, fresh or air-dry plant sample, mixed with fine ignited quartz sand, in a low glass cylinder. Add concentrated sulfuric acid to wet the mass, insert a plug of glass wool and cover with a watch glass wet on lower surface with a drop of 5 % sodium nitrate solution. Warm the cylinder to volatilize silicon tetrafluoride which is absorbed in the liquid on the watch glass and forms characteristic crystals of Na_2SiF_6.

Identification of the fluoride can also be accomplished by the method of Feigl and Krumholz (1929). The silicon tetrafluoride is collected in a drop of water on the watch glass and transferred to 1 ml of 0.2 to 0.5 N nitric acid. Add 2 drops of acid ammonium molybdate (100 ml 15 % molybdate + 100 ml 35 % nitric acid). Warm to boiling, cool, add 1—2 drops of 0.25 % benzidine or benzidine chlorohydrate in 10 % acetic acid, and finally, add an equal volume of saturated sodium acetate solution. A blue color or blue precipitate indicates silica and therefore, silicon tetrafluoride. The color can be intensified by extracting with amyl alcohol. Neither of these procedures can give an unequivocal indication of the natural fluoride level in vegetation in the range from 1 to 5 ppm. A positive test, however, was considered to be proof of a harmful concentration in sensitive plants. KRUGER (1941) preferred the Na_2SiF_6 method. It did not fail to show harmful concentrations of fluoride in several hundred analyses in which fluoride-damaged leaves were analyzed. BIRAGHI (1938) used this procedure also. On the other hand, the method was criticised by MUHLSTEPH (1942) who insisted that smoke damage could only be established by analyses of soil, air, rain and leaves and observations on the plant lesions.

Ross et al. (1963) proposed a semi-quantitative procedure by which vegetation samples can be analyzed rapidly to determine whether excessive concentrations of fluorine (30 to 40 ppm or more) are present. Such information, if readily available, would be useful in the diagnosis of suspected fluoride damage to the plants. Neither drying, combustion, fusion, nor distillation processes are required.

Two grams of fresh plant material are macerated in a Pyrex mortar with the aid of finely ground, ignited silica sand, and 4 ml of water. The slurry is transferred to a 25 mm test tube having a small hole in the bottom covered by a layer of paper pulp. Forced filtration of the liquid is accomplished by means of a rubber stopper mounted on the end of a glass tube. The large end of the stopper fits snugly against the inside wall of the test tube and when pushed down, applies pressure on the liquid to force it through the paper pulp. One or two drops of clear liquid are placed in a depression of a spot plate; one drop of sodium acetate-acetic acid buffer (7.5 g of each per liter, pH 4.0 to 4.5); one drop pink 0.001 M alizarin complexan solution, 3-di(carboxymethyl)aminomethyl-1-2-dehydroxy-anthaquinone, and with immediate stirring, one drop of 0.002 M cerous III nitrate or lanthanum nitrate, are added. A definite blue color indicates about 40 ppm fluorine. The deeper the blue, the higher the fluorine, to a limit of about 200 ppm. The complexan solution is prepared by dissolving in water 192.5 mg complexan reagent, by addition of the minimum amount of 10 % sodium hydroxide, adjusting to a red color at pH 5 with dilute hydrochloric acid and making up to 500 ml (BELCHER et al., 1959).

3. Oxygen combustion-diffusion method

Two new techniques have been described which are suitable for microgram and submicrogram amounts of fluorine in plants which cannot be handled satisfactorily by the macro-procedure.

Combustion of small samples can be instantaneously accomplished in a 125 or 250 ml separatory funnel or glass-stoppered flask filled with oxygen (SCHONIGER, 1955; SOEP, 1961; WADE et al., 1964). A solution of the fluoride sample is dried on a piece of filter paper (area about 6—10 square centimeters) which is then mounted below a thin strip of filter paper to serve as a fuse, on a platinum wire attached to the ground glass stopper of the funnel or flask. The fuse is ignited with a flame just before the sample and stopper are thrust into the momentarily opened funnel or flask. Weighed strips of dried leaves can be mounted on the wire and similarly burned. Pulverized plant samples (50 to 100 mg) can be ignited in a small platinum boat attached to the stopper. A coil of fine platinum wire is mounted immediately underneath the boat with heavy leads extending to and through the stopper. The coil is heated electrically to ignite the sample in oxygen. Combustion is usually complete. The fluoride from the combustion is collected in 5 ml water, preferably by use of a mechanical shaker.

The distillation method can be replaced by a diffusion technique (SINGER and ARMSTRONG, 1954, 1959; HALL, 1960, 1963; WHARTON, 1962). The fluoride solution

(1 ml) plus 2 ml 70 % perchloric acid, is placed in either a 20 ml polyethylene bottle (HALL, 1960), a three-compartment polypropylene Conway dish (WHARTON, 1962), or a plastic petri dish (ADAMS, 1963). A piece of sodium succinate-impregnated filter paper is attached to the screw-cap cover of the polyethylene bottle; a solution of 1.3 N sodium hydroxide is placed in the center well of the Conway dish; or about 0.2 ml 3 N sodium hydroxide is placed on the undersurface of the petri dish cover by spotting many tiny droplets with a fine-tipped pipet. The closed assembly is maintained at 60° for about 24 hours to transfer the hydrogen fluoride by diffusion to the collecting surface from which it can be readily dissolved and determined colorimetrically or spectrophotometrically using SPADNS or the lanthanum alizarin complexan reagent of BELCHER et al. (1959) and GREENHALGH and RILEY (1961).

V. Determination of fluoride in the atmosphere

A. Field methods

A knowledge of the fluoride content of the atmosphere is important in the appraisal of industrial plant damage. Since average fluoride levels in the field do not, in general, exceed 1 pphm except perhaps very close to a source, large air samples are usually required for the conventional methods of analysis (ADAMS et al., 1952; BREWER et al., 1960a, b; MAVRODINEANU et al., 1962).

Large GREENBURG-SMITH impingers are often employed for sampling at about 30 liters per minute for 3 to 24 hours, using up to 500 ml distilled water as absorbent to allow for evaporation. The analysis is completed by a Willard-Winter steam distillation or an ion-exchange separation for concentration of the fluoride (NIELSEN, 1958), followed by thorium nitrate titration or one of the photometric procedures. PACK et al. (1959) describe methods of distinguishing between gaseous and particulate fluorides, using aluminum or sodium bicarbonate coated tubes to absorb gaseous fluoride.

B. Automatic methods

Two continuous automatic recorders are now available for atmospheric fluoride analysis.

The "Mini-Adak" recorder of ADAMS et al. (ADAMS and KOPPE, 1959; ADAMS et al., 1961; ADAMS, 1960) absorbs continuously the fluoride from a large volume of air (30 liters per minute) in 15 ml of liquid maintained at constant volume by controlled automatic addition of water. Two colorimetric reagents, zirconium-eriochrome-cyanine R and ferron, the ferric salt of 7-iodo-8-hydroxy-5-quinoline sulfonic acid, are used for different concentration ranges. The color is recorded continuously and the absorbing solution is replaced with fresh solution at definite time intervals or when a selected color change has been attained. Sensitivity with the eriochrome reagent is 20 μg F^- full scale, and with the quinoline reagent, 4 mg F^- full scale.

The Stanford Research Institute fluoride recorder (THOMAS et al., 1958) employs the quenching by hydrogen fluoride of the fluorescence of magnesium 8-hydroquinoline impregnated in a filter-paper tape. The analysis is not sensitive to other fluorides without pyrohydrolysis. Two aliquot, six-liter-per-minute air samples, one deprived of hydrogen fluoride by passing through a glass tube having the inside surface coated with a thin layer of sodium bicarbonate, the other passing through a similar clean glass tube, are drawn through adjacent areas of the paper tape illuminated with near-ultra-violet light. The beams of visible light emitted from the two areas are compared by two photomultiplier tubes. At 30-minute intervals, the tape is automatically advanced to place unexposed areas in the two air lines and the tubes are balanced for a zero reading on a recorder. As fluoride is absorbed, fluorescence of one area of the tape is progressively quenched and the recording indicates the changes in current required to maintain the phototubes in balance. Sensitivity of recorder response may be 1 pptm full scale up to 15 pptm full scale in 30 min, depending on the setting of a range selector switch.

C. Lime paper method

Hydrogen fluoride in the atmosphere is readily absorbed on filter paper impregnated with lime, prepared by dipping 11 cm sheets of quantitative paper in a one per cent lime suspension, and allowing them to drain and dry. The papers are hung in louvered boxes mounted on poles at least 2.5 meters above the ground, usually for periods of one month, followed by fluoride analysis of the disks. Rate of fluoride uptake is a function of the fluoride concentration and wind speed. ADAMS (1957, 1961) found a similar pattern of uptake of fluoride by the papers and by the leaves of nearby plants (Fig. 1), indicating that the method would be useful for surveying a location to find the relative distribution of the gas in the area with relation to its source. In a controlled experiment, uptake of fluoride was 7.6 μg F^-/dm^2(paper)/day/μg F/m^3 (in air).

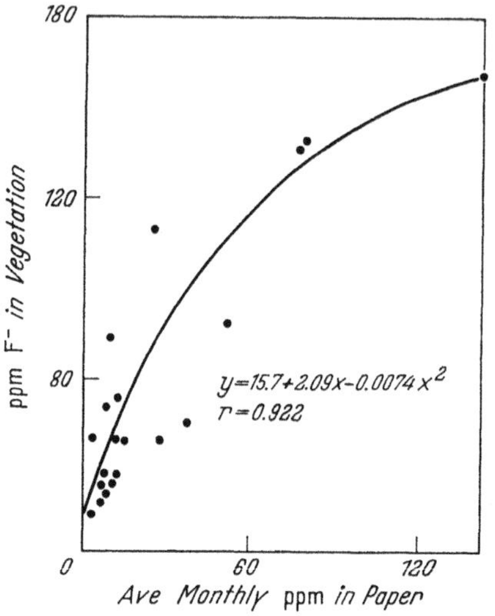

Fig. 1. Curvilinear relationship between fluoride concentrations in limed paper and nearby vegetation at 20 exposure sites in 1954 (ADAMS, 1957)

VI. Fluorine in minerals and soils

Fluorine is classified among the "minor," non-essential elements in plant physiology although it is rather abundant in many soil-forming minerals and in practically all soils. Its abundance in the earth's crust is about 0.1 % and about 0.06 % in igneous rocks (CLARK, 1911; MELLOR, 1956). Its occurrence in minerals and soils has been studied by MCCAUGHEY and FRY (1913) who found biotite (trace to 4.23 % F) and tourmaline (0.06 to 1.19 % F) in 21 of 25 American soils examined. Muscovite (0.12 to 1.25 % F) was present in 20 soils; apatite (1.31 to 3.86 % F) in 12, and fluorite (49 % F) in 4 of these soils. STEINKOENIG (1919) found an average fluorine content of 300 ppm in 9 soils, maximum 1500 ppm. GEMMEL (1946) reported a range of 68 to 540 ppm fluorine in 23 New Zealand soils. ROBINSON and EDGINGTON (1946) analyzed the profiles of 30 soils in the United States, 137 samples in all. The surface layer (0 to 2 or three inches) ranged from 20 to 500 ppm with a mean of 190 ppm. The surface zero to twelve inch layer ranged from 20 to 1620 ppm with a mean of 292 ppm. In 24 of the 30 profiles the concentration increased with depth; in 6, it decreased. One soil from Idaho had 1620 ppm in the surface foot and 3870 in the second foot. The 25 to 40 inch layer of the Maury silt loam in the phosphate area of Tennessee had 7070 ppm.

Phosphate rock always contains fluoride. Continental deposits usually have 3 to 5 % and sea island deposits, 2 % or less. Sea island deposits used extensively by feed producers include those from Christmas Island (1.5 % F) and Curacao Island (0.5 % F). Evidently, this association of fluoride with phosphate is the end product of a geochemical process often related initially to volcanic action. Volcanic gases may be rich in gaseous fluorides, having as much as 3 to 6 % fluoride. The association with phosphate is finally stabilized by the formation of insoluble apatite. The low solubility of fluorine compounds in the soil generally precludes any expression of fluoride toxicity in plants due to excessive uptake of the element.

VII. Fluorine in normal plants

Because of the virtually universal presence of fluorine in soils, detectable amounts of the element can be found in all plants. Reports of fluorine-free plants in the early literature are probably due to inadequate analytical methods. Concentrations usually range from about 1 to 15 ppm in the leaves. Higher levels generally denote uptake of gaseous compounds or deposition of solids from the atmosphere. Translocation of this absorbed fluorine in the plant is slight and the roots do not show elevated concentrations. If, as sometimes happens, the soil contains soluble fluoride, similar high levels may be found in the leaves, but in this case, still higher concentrations are found in the roots. A criterion is thus available to decide whether the fluorine in a plant came from the atmosphere or the soil, as discussed by BRENNAN et al. (1950) (see Fig. 4, page 254).

JAULMES, quoted by TRUHAUT (1955) found 4 to 6 ppm fluorine in grasses. GERICKE and KURMIES (1955) noted that the fluorine content of different species of plants varied considerably. The observed range in cereal grains was 0.2 to 7.1 ppm; in grain straw 2.0 to 7.0 ppm; in potatoes, 0.2 to 2.9 ppm; in beet, 0.2 to 0.6 ppm; in spinach, 0.4 to 6.4 ppm; and in hay, 0.2 to 3.3 ppm. In pot cultures, the addition to the soil of 70—80 ppm fluoride was required to cause a noticeable increase in the fluorine content of the plants; while in the field 200 kg fluoride per hectare raised the fluorine content of the potatoes but not of rye, wheat, corn or beans. VON POLHEIM and DIETRICH (1955) analyzed 171 samples of vegetation from the Württemberg-Baden area in Germany and found an average of 6.3 ppm fluorine for the "natural" fluorine content. Near factories emitting hydrogen fluoride, over 50 ppm was found without visible plant damage. FABRE et al. (1955) found 15 to 19 ppm in oats, wheat and barley. Many factors influence the uptake of fluoride from the soil by plants, such as soil texture, pH, phosphate, calcium and nitrogen content, *etc.* These are discussed later.

Some species of plants normally accumulate from the soil relatively high concentrations of fluorine in their leaves while other plants in the same environment take up very little. The camellia family furnishes outstanding examples of "accumulator" plants. WANG et al. (1949) found 57 to 355 ppm fluorine in commercial tea leaves, the oldest leaves having the most fluorine. McCLENDON and GERSHON-COHEN (1955) reported that camellias growing in a field fertilized with phosphate slag had 121 to 1370 ppm in their leaves. ZIMMERMAN et al. (1956, 1957) analyzed young camellia leaves in the greenhouse which had 67 ppm fluorine while old leaves had 3062 ppm and tea leaves in the same greenhouse had 1530 ppm fluorine. A flowering shrub, Deutzia, contained 75 ppm while another shrub, Weigela, growing nearby, had 6 ppm. Two comparable samples of gifblaar from Africa absorbed 38 and 116 ppm fluorine in the greenhouse.

A. Is fluorine an essential element?

MITCHELL and EDMAN (1945) reviewed the literature on fluorine in soils, plants and animals, and concluded that the element is non-essential for plants and animals, although it plays an important role in preventing dental caries. Further, its uptake by plants or animals in excessive amounts from soils or water is improbable except in exceptional circumstances. Local atmospheric contamination from industry needs careful consideration in some places.

A number of attempts have been made to determine whether or not fluorine is an essential element for plants. SALM-HORSTMAR (1861) observed stimulation of growth of barley due to the presence of small amounts of fluorine, and concluded that the element is essential for the full development of the plant. AMPOLA (1904) recorded increased growth of plants, due to addition of calcium fluoride to soils from Mt. Vesuvius. BERTRAND (1903) considered fluorine to be an essential element. MAZE (1915) decided that fluorine at 2 ppm in a nutrient solution is necessary for the growth of corn.

Aso (1904, 1906) observed a stimulating effect of small concentrations of sodium fluoride on the germination and growth of a number of plants. In pots to which 20 mg of the fluoride was added, flowers appeared earlier than in the controls, but there was little difference in the size of the blooms in the treated and untreated pots. Soil containing 2.5 ppm sodium fluoride gave an increased yield of some species but not of others. However, 25 ppm had no effect. Calcium fluoride gave some stimulation also. Evidently, the low levels of sodium fluoride were precipitated as calcium fluoride and the stimulating agent was really the latter. Higher concentrations of sodium fluoride which could not be completely converted to calcium fluoride by the soil were either without effect or were toxic.

WOBER (1920) compared the toxicities of arsenic, antimony and fluorine compounds to a number of plants. Beans and peas were more sensitive than the cereal grain plants to these poisons. In water cultures, arsenite at 10 mg As_2O_3 per liter, was strongly toxic while 100 mg per liter was fatal to all plants. Antimonites were much less toxic. Sodium fluoride at 100 mg per liter was definitely harmful. Sodium fluoride at about 0.5 % in the soil, or a 1 % solution sprayed on the leaves, was required to cause plant damage.

BARTHOLOMEW (1935) grew cowpeas in nutrient solutions to which sodium fluoride and sodium fluorosilicate were added in concentrations up to 10 ppm fluorine and calcium fluoride up to 7.7 ppm fluorine. Growth data were variable, but did not suggest that dry matter production was materially affected by the fluoride which accumulated primarily in the roots in concentrations up to 1000 to 2000 ppm. The tops had less than 64 ppm fluorine, except with 10 ppm fluorosilicate which contributed 450 ppm fluorine.

Sudan grass was grown in silt loam soil in 10 kg jars with various additions of calcium phosphates and pulverized rock-phosphates from a number of different sources together with fluorine salts up to 10 ppm fluoride (Table 5). Neither added fluorides nor fluorosilicates had any significant effect on the yield of two cuttings of grass when no phosphate, or when phosphates as calcium salts were added. However, the use of rock phosphate or basic slag gave yields that were inversely proportional to the fluoride content of the rock. Possibly the fluoride interfered with the availability of phosphate to the plants. GERICKE (1949) also observed that the fluoride in rock phosphate inhibited the growth of cabbage and panic grass.

BOUYER and COLLOT (1952) added singly, many trace elements including fluoride, to the peanut soils of Senegal. The addition of 6–10 kg per acre of sodium fluoride was definitely toxic to peanuts in Bambey but not in Louga.

A possible explanation of some of the stimulating effects of small additions of fluoride is suggested by the work of LEROUX (1941) who added "trace elements" to a soil in which peas were subsequently grown from April through June. Nitrogen fixation was increased by each of the nine elements added at the rate of either 2 or 5 mg per kilogram soil. This fixation for the different elements ranged from

Table 5. *Yield of Sudan grass grown in Clarksville silt loam with various phosphorus and fluorine treatments* (BARTHOLOMEW, 1935)

Source of P	Source of F	No. of treatments	Conc. of F in soil, ppm	Yield (Dry Wt.) in grams		
				First cutting	Second cutting	Total
None	None	1	—	2.3	9.7	12.0
None	CaF_2	4	1—10	2.2	8.7	10.9
None	NaF	4	1—10	2.1	8.8	10.9
None	$BaSiF_6$	2	1.5 & 3.0	2.3	8.1	10.4
None	Na_2SiF_6	1	3	2.5	7.6	10.1
None	Na_3AlF_6	1	3	2.4	8.2	10.6
$CaH_4(PO_4)_2H_2O$ . . .	None	1	0	23.3	21.3	44.6
$CaH_4(PO_4)_2H_2O$ . . .	CaF_2	4	1—10	24.5	21.9	46.4
$CaH_4(PO_4)_2H_2O$ . . .	NaF	1	10	26.0	23.7	49.7
$Ca_3(PO_4)_2$	None	1	0	21.6	21.3	41.9
$Ca_3(PO_4)_2$	CaF_2	4	1—10	23.0	21.3	43.3
$Ca_3(PO_4)_2$	NaF	4	1—10	21.3	22.4	43.7
Phosphate Rock A . .		1	0.3	21.7	23.4	45.1
Phosphate Rock B . .		1	0.5	19.6	20.4	40.0
Phosphate Rock C . .		1	1.0	16.2	19.4	35.4
Phosphate Rock D . .		1	1.6	14.7	23.6	38.3
Phosphate Rock E . .		1	2.2	8.2	23.5	31.6
Phosphate Rock F . .		1	3.4	10.0	20.6	30.6
Fluorspar basic slag .		1	3.5	6.4	16.1	22.5

1.3 to 4.9 % of the total nitrogen in the system. The increases of nitrogen fixation associated with the two levels of fluorine were 2.9 and 4.0 %, respectively. The increases of the nitrogen values in the fluorine-treated plants were 9 and 11 % of their total nitrogen, respectively.

Fluorine does not appear to be an essential element in plants but rigidly controlled experiments to furnish unquestionable proof have not yet been carried out.

B. Effect of fluorine on water relations in plants

WILSON (1933) investigated the effects of halogen salts on tobacco, extending the work done on chlorine to bromine and fluorine. It is common field practice to add up to about 2 % of chloride to tobacco fertilizers. GARNER et al. (1930) had found a 10 % increase in yield due to chloride which was ascribed to increased solubility of magnesium and to an increased water content of the tissues that enabled the plant to better withstand periods of drought. An excess of chloride caused dwarfing of the plants. The leaves became thick and brittle with upcurled margins. Their water content was abnormally high and interference with carbohydrate metabolism caused engorgement with starch.

WILSON (1933) noted that bromide and fluoride salts behaved similarly to chlorides. Thickening of the leaves was caused by an enlargement of all cells. Elongation of the palisade cells was particularly noticeable with fluoride. Excessive amounts of fluoride caused more pronounced inhibition of growth than did equivalent amounts of the other halides. Thickening was also marked with fluorides but upward rolling of the leaf margins occurred only with ammonium fluoride. Leaf sap from sodium fluoride-treated plants had a somewhat greater freezing point depression (+ 0.15° C) than from the tap water control plants and smaller depression (up to 0.3° C) than sap from the chloride and bromide treatments (except ammonium bromide). In most cases, the sodium fluoride-treated plants had appreciably more "bound" water than did the others. It is suggested that fluoride toxicity may have interfered with absorption of water, increasing the "bound" water as in drought. In fact, the plant appeared to be in a state of physiological drought.

C. Effect of fluorine on germination

This subject has been investigated repeatedly. Bokorny (1913) found that a solution of 10 ppm hydrofluoric acid stimulated, and 100 ppm inhibited, the germination of cress, barley, pea, lentil and bean seeds. Sodium fluoride at 1000 ppm inhibited germination of the cress seeds only. Riehm (1927) obtained no inhibition of germination when barley and oats were soaked for 20 to 260 min in 1000 ppm solutions of sodium or potassium fluoride or sodium or copper fluorosilicate. Wheat was inhibited by the potassium fluoride and also by a 500 ppm solution of hydrogen fluoride applied for one hour. Scharrer and Schropp (1932) found that the addition of 600 ppm of potassium fluoride to soil slightly inhibited germination and early growth of wheat, oats, rye and barley. The effect was greater with acid than with alkaline soils. Nommik (1953) made similar observations on sodium fluoride. A concentration of the latter in sandy soil which inhibited germination of wheat 90 % was without effect in a loam soil. Calcium fluoride did not inhibit germination in either soil. Inhibition was also greater in acid than in neutral soils. Gisiger (1931) observed no inhibition of germination of wheat and rye by solutions of 50 ppm sodium fluoride, cryolite, or ammonium ferric fluoride. Germination was reduced by 1000 ppm and completely inhibited by 2000 ppm. A short exposure of corn to 3300 ppm sodium fluoride speeded up germination.

Bartholomew (1935) observed the effect of fluorides on the germination of Sudan grass, cowpeas, soybeans, red clover and Dutch white clover, by placing the seeds on germination pads wet either with water, or with solutions of sodium fluoride or sodium fluorosilicate ranging from 0.25 to 50 ppm fluorine. Solutions of calcium fluoride ranging from 0.25 to 7.7 ppm fluorine were also used. Practically all the tests showed the same germination rates as in fluorine-free water within allowable variations and suggested very little, if any, harmful effect on the germination of these seeds. Sodium fluorosilicate increased germination of white Dutch clover from 39.0 % with 0.25 ppm fluorine to 48.3 % as the average of six tests with 0.5 to 50 ppm fluorine.

Table 6. *Germination of corn as affected by hydrogen, sodium and calcium fluoride solutions* (Morse, 1935)

Fluoride solution	Conc F ppm	pH	Percentage germination		Time days
			Polar Dent	Picketts Dent	
None	0	—	98	99	2.3
HF	100	2.88	49	70	2.2
HF	200	2.66	9	22	3.0
HF	300	2.49	0	9	4.0
HF	400	2.40	0	0	—
NaF	100	5.47	61	72	2.0
NaF	200	5.57	10	65	2.4
NaF	300	5.61	12	23	3.0
NaF	400	5.63	0	0	—
CaF_2 (Solid)	—	—	98	99	2.3

Morse (1935) tested the influence of fluoride in solution and in phosphate fertilizers on the germination of corn. In one experiment, 100 seeds were wrapped in moist cloths (the so-called "ragdoll") and placed in 1.5 liter jars containing 400 ml of well aerated sodium fluoride solutions ranging in concentration from 0 to 400 ppm fluorine. Data in Table 6 show that 100 ppm reduced germination by 30 to 50 % and 300–400 ppm inhibited germination completely. Time for germination was increased from 2 to

Table 7. *Effect of mixing superphosphate fertilizers with soil on the germination of corn* (MORSE, 1935)

Fertilizer	Tons acre	Per cent germination in soil					
		Brookstown loam		Miami silt loam		Fox sandy loam	
		Contact	Mixed	Contact	Mixed	Contact	Mixed
None	—	100	98	98	100	98	98
Superphosphate 20%	3.1	90	—	80	—	—	—
	6.3	46	98	50	98	100	100
	12.5	0	98	12	98	100	100
	50.0	—	100	0	98	98	98
Superphosphate 44% A	1.4	98	—	96	—	—	—
	2.8	78	96	84	98	98	100
	5.7	16	100	52	100	100	98
	11.4	0	100	0	100	100	100
	22.8	0	100	0	94	8	6
Superphosphate 44% B	1.4	74	—	86	—	—	—
	2.8	56	100	44	98	100	100
	5.7	6	98	18	96	98	98
	11.2	0	98	0	98	100	98
	22.8	—	94	—	92	2	0
	pH	7.1		5.2		6.5	5.1

3–4 days. Hydrofluoric acid interfered with germination to a greater extent than did sodium fluoride, and Polar Dent seed was more sensitive to fluoride than Picketts' Dent.

The superphosphate fertilizers (Table 7) also inhibited germination if they were spread out on the soil and came into direct contact with seed, especially with the embryo. This inhibition was substantially reduced if the contact was with the endosperm rather than with the embryo. Contact inhibition was more effective in the heavier soils. There was practically no inhibition if the fertilizer was mixed with the soil, except with the heaviest application of the 44 % superphosphates in the sandy soil. Evidently, this soil had a more limited capacity for lowering the fluoride concentration below the toxic level than did the loam soils.

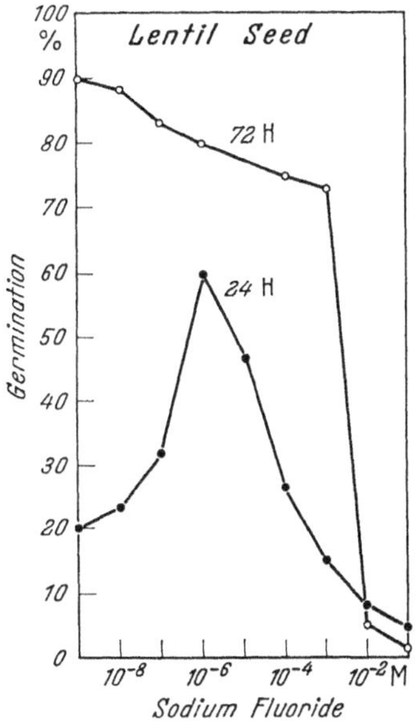

Fig. 2. Effect of sodium fluoride on the germination of lentil seed (PILET, 1964)

PILET (1963) has observed the germination of lentil seeds after first soaking them with deionized water in the dark at 25° for four hours, then placing them in petri dishes on filter paper moistened with solutions of sodium fluoride for 24 and 72 hours. The data are presented in Fig. 2. The 24-hour germination reached a peak of about 60 % with 10^{-6} M fluoride, whereas with both weaker and stronger fluoride solutions germination was substantially less. After 72 hours the germination ranged from 90 % at 10^{-9} M to 75 % at 10^{-3} M. Higher fluoride concentrations (10^{-2} M) reduced the germination to less than 5 %. Evidently, the rate of germination of lentil seeds was reduced appreciably by dilute fluoride solutions but the total germination was not greatly affected if the fluoride concentration did not exceed 10^{-3} M.

VIII. Local studies of fluoride effects

A. Pot and field experiments in France

GAUTIER and CLAUSMANN described the effects of fluoride on vegetation in a series of papers from 1915 to 1919. They found fluorine in every one of 63 plants that they analyzed, ranging from 0.6 to 139 ppm with an average of 26.5 ppm (GAUTIER, 1915). The element was most abundant in the leaves. There was about ten times as much fluorine in the peel as in the pulp of apples and bananas. A trace of fluorine in the nutrient solution usually favored growth, flowering and seed production. Sometimes its influence was doubtful, and in a few cases, it appeared to be harmful.

In a pot experiment using specially purified carbon to support the plants, 13 species were studied in complete nutrient culture with and without the addition of sufficient fluoride to raise the fluoride content from 4 to 300 mg per pot. A fertile garden soil was used for comparison. Of the 13 species, 7 (garden cress, cabbage, poppy, spinach, blue thistle, corn spurry and hemp) grew best with the fluoride treatments. Three (morning glory, onion and rye) showed no difference in growth with or without added fluoride, and three (chick pea, sweet pea and a composite "petite centaures") grew best in the soil.

The authors carried out a field experiment at Lainville, near Paris, in which they treated a slightly calcareous silicious clay soil containing 88 ppm fluorine with amorphous calcium fluoride prepared by reacting calcium carbonate with hydrogen fluoride. The field was divided into 18 pairs of plots, ranging in size from 31 to 153 square meters per plot. In 1916, enough fluoride was added to one plot of each pair to raise the top 25 cm of the soil to 188 ppm fluorine. An equivalent amount of powdered calcium carbonate was added to the control plots.

Table 8. *Effect of adding amorphous calcium fluoride to the soil on the growth of field crops* (GAUTIER and CLAUSMANN, 1919)

Crop	Portion Weighed	1916			1917		
		—F Kg.	+F Kg.	Change %	—F Kg.	+F Kg.	Change %
Wheat	Grain	23.5	27.5	+17.0	10.8	10.3	— 5.0
Wheat	Straw	46.6	53.5	+15.0	34.7	34.0	— 2.0
Oats	Grain	26.4	27.8	+ 5.0	14.0	15.5	+11.0
Oats	Straw	64.6	74.2	+15.0	30.0	26.0	—13.0
Barley	Grain	—	—	—	18.4	18.2	— 1.0
Barley	Straw	—	—	—	36.2	37.8	+ 4.0
Carrots	Roots	305.5	360.2	+18.0	154.1	189.0	+23.0
Potatoes	Roots	69.4	70.2	+ 1.0	10.1	16.0	+59.0
Beets	Roots	212.5	198.2	— 7.0	120.0	105.5	—12.0
Peas	Seed	10.5	11.1	+ 6.0	4.5	5.0	+12.0
Kidney beans	Seed	10.2	9.7	— 5.0	6.3	6.8	+ 8.0
Beans	Seed	—	—	—	3.0	4.4	+47.0
Cabbage	Total plant	91.4	92.7	+ 1.0	105.7[1]	85.6[1]	—19.0
Turnip	Roots	—	—	—	64.7	54.0	—16.0
Poppy	Seed	0.250	0.285	+14.0	—	—	—
Mustard	Seed	—	—	—	2.3	2.3	0
Leek	500 Leeks	—	—	—	62.5	63.4	+ 1.4

[1] 125 heads.

Each pair of plots was cropped with a different crop in 1916. In 1917, the pairs of plots were planted to the same or different crops, but no more fluoride was added. Table 8 summarizes the results. Wheat and oats were somewhat stimulated in growth the first year by fluoride but in the second year, growth was practically the same in both plots of each pair. Possibly, the solubility of the added fluoride was reduced by contact with the soil for a year.

By contrast, potatoes, peas and beans showed little effect of the fluorides the first year, but the relative growth was distinctly better the second year in the calcium fluoride plots. Carrots improved both years with the fluoride treatment. Beet, mustard, leek, turnip and cabbage gave zero, or negative, response both years.

Only cabbage was used in both the pot and the field experiments. There was improved growth in the fluoride-treated carbon, but not in the field. However, the two experiments were not strictly comparable because the field soil control plots had appreciably more fluorine than did the carbon controls.

B. Tennessee studies

Extensive studies have been carried out at the University of Tennessee in cooperation with the Tennessee Valley Authority on the fate of fluoride in soils, its uptake by plants, its reactions with phosphate, its presence in the atmosphere and analytical methods. These studies have been published by MacIntire, Hardin and associates in over 40 papers since 1935. Resumes of this work appeared in 1949, 1952, 1955 and 1957.

1. Lysimeter experiments

One of the first of these studies (MacIntire et al., 1935) was a four-year lysimeter experiment starting in 1929 to determine the fate of barium fluosilicate in soil. Applications of this chemical at the rate of 1500 pounds per acre had been recommended for the control of the larvae of the Japanese beetle on golf greens.

The lysimeter tanks were 67 cm in diameter and 30 cm deep. They held 45 kg soil to a depth of 19 cm (7.5 inches). Seven hundred and fifty ppm of the barium salt, equivalent to 300 ppm fluorine, was incorporated into the soil with and without 2000 ppm of 100-mesh limestone or dolomite. The tanks were exposed to an average annual rainfall of 49 inches for four years. The incorporation of 750 ppm barium fluosilicate was repeated annually in some of the lysimeters. Analysis of drainage water and soil showed substantial retention of sulfate and practically complete retention of barium. Fluoride analyses made in the fourth year when the Willard-Winter method first became available, (1933), indicated that leaching losses three to four years after a single application were about two percent of the fluorine added and eight percent after four annual incorporations. Limestone and dolomite reduced the fluoride losses.

2. Phosphate-fluoride relationships

Close attention was given to the fluorine problems associated with the phosphate industry in central Tennessee (Maury County) and also with the aluminum industry in eastern Tennessee (Blount County). An important question was raised concerning the reduced availability of phosphate in mixed fertilizers and it was demonstrated that reversion of superphosphate to insoluble fluoroapatite (MacIntire et al., 1937) occurred when large piles of processed fertilizers were aged, especially when the superphosphates were ammoniated and/or dolomite was incorporated. Reduced solubility of phosphate did not occur in fluoride-free mixtures. Evidently, similar apatite formation is possible in the soil, as has been found in the Broadbalk plots at Rothamsted, England, which have been fertilized with superphosphate for over 100 years. Apatite was isolated from the soil and identified by its X-ray pattern by NAGELSMITH and NIXON (1944).

Other important findings in Tennessee may be listed as follows:

(1) Fluoride added to the soil with rock phosphates or superphosphates or associated with high levels of phosphate in the soils of phosphate-rich areas, was generally very insoluble and was not taken up significantly by vegetation (MACINTIRE et al., 1948). Even 45 to 60 inches of rainfall did not leach out an appreciable amount of this fluoride. Leaching was not affected appreciably by the addition of lime to some of the soils unless the soil was acid, in which case fluoride solubility was reduced. In 10-year lysimeter experiments, nine variously phosphated soils showed about 98 % retention of 2400 pounds of fluorine per acre added over several years as calcium fluoride and the percolate from the soil contained only about 0.1 to 1 ppm fluoride.

Table 9. *Yield and F content of three successive crops on two soils with three annual additions of 100, 125 and 100 ppm fluoride from various fluorine sources* (MACINTIRE et al., 1951a)

Incorporation	Soybeans		Lespedeza		Oats		Total yield
	Yield grams	F ppm	Yield grams	F ppm	Yield grams	F ppm	
			Clarksville silt loam[1]				
None	398	7	316	7	139	5	853
Cryolite	411	8	388	8	148	5	947
Rock phosphate	121	8	338	9	113	6	572
MgF_2	395	6	367	10	141	5	903
NaF	383	7	381	9	159	4	923
Na_2SiF_6	405	7	383	7	139	4	927
			Hartsells fine sandy loam[2]				
None	408	7	333	7	100	4	841
Cryolite	415	7	397	6	135	5	947
Rock phosphate	155	7	319	8	66	6	540
MgF_2	428	7	361	8	107	5	896
NaF	408	7	424	7	122	5	954
Na_2SiF_6	409	7	384	6	118	5	911

[1] pH 6.1—6.4.
[2] pH 5.1—6.1.

(2) Addition of quenched calcium silicate slag, containing 3.2 % fluorine and 1.2 % phosphate, resulted in a relatively high rate of leaching of the fluoride (MACINTIRE et al., 1948). A 1280-pound-per-acre input of fluoride in 20 tons of quenched slag, gave 14 times greater outgo of fluoride in six years than a 2400-pound input as calcium fluoride in ten years. The slag percolate contained up to 72 ppm fluoride, plus solvated silica. However, passage of this percolate through a shallow layer of subsoil reduced the fluoride concentration by about 80 %. It is suggested that the subsoil could render innocuous the fluoride from large additions of slag. The 20-ton slag addition in this experiment was intentionally excessive.

(3) Fluoride (MACINTIRE et al., 1951a) as sodium fluoride, sodium fluorosilicate, magnesium fluoride, cryolite and rock phosphate was added to fine sandy loam and silt loam soils at the rate of 300 pounds per acre to a nine-inch depth. A three-year succession of crops — soybeans, lespedeza and spring oats — was grown with the addition of 375 pounds of fluorine before the lespedeza and another

300 pounds before the oats (Table 9). The dry weight of the plants was unaffected or slightly increased by all treatments except rock phosphate which gave poor growth with soybeans and oats. The fluoride content of the plants ranged from 4 to 10 ppm, indicating only slight uptake of fluorine. Evidently, the fluorine was rendered insoluble in the soil.

(4) Hydrofluoric acid additions (MacIntire et al., 1951b) to Hartsells fine sandy loam and Clarksville silt loam to the extent of 100 or 400 pounds per acre had only a slight effect on growth or fluorine content of red clover if the soils were limestoned with two or four tons per acre before adding the acid. At 800 pounds hydrofluoric acid per acre, there was a 10–20 % reduction in growth and a 1.2 to 7-fold increase in the fluorine content of the plants. If no limestone was added the yield was slightly reduced and the fluoride level slightly raised by 100 pounds per acre of acid. Four hundred pounds hydrogen fluoride caused 40–90 % reduction in yield and fivefold increase in leaf fluoride while 800 pounds practically inhibited growth. pH was also reduced. It was concluded that the reaction of the soil and its fertility would not be impaired significantly by air-borne hydrogen fluoride except possibly very close to the source since it was noted that 100 pounds per acre represents 50 times the annual fluoride increment from rain water.

(5) MacIntire et al. (1954) grew red clover, rye grass and Sudan grass in pots outdoors at Knoxville for six weeks. Then, some of the plants were taken to Columbia, in Maury County, near the phosphate fertilizer factories, for three weeks. Some were placed outdoors, with and without protection from the rain; others were grown in the washed atmosphere of a closed chamber. Analyses of the plants for fluorine were made at the beginning of the exposure at Columbia and three weeks later at both Knoxville and Columbia. Table 10 gives the values for the outdoor exposures; due probably to washing by rain, all of the Knoxville values and the "washed air" exposure at Columbia were approximately equal. Evidently, increments of 16 to 34 ppm in the various samples were due to absorption from the atmosphere at Columbia.

Table 10. *Fluorine content of red clover, rye grass, and Sudan grass grown at Knoxville and Columbia, Tennessee* (Data from MacIntire et al., 1954)

		6 Initial weeks at Knoxville	3 Additional weeks at			Difference under tree
			Knoxville	Columbia		
				Open field	Under tree	
		ppm	ppm	ppm	ppm	ppm
May 1952	Red clover . . .	7	5	18	23	16
May 1952	Rye grass . . .	10	11	20	31	20
June 1953	Sudan grass . .	4	—	—	37	33
Sept 1953	Sudan grass . .	13	—	—	47	34

Analysis of Spanish moss exposed three months in both east and central Tennessee showed very high fluorine values (1200–2400 ppm) near the pot room of the aluminum factory in Blount County. The concentration fell rapidly with distance from this source. Samples in Maury County ranged from 100 to 600 ppm near the phosphate industry.

C. New Jersey studies

Daines and associates (1952) in New Jersey investigated the uptake of fluoride by plants through the roots and through the leaves as influenced by the concentration not only of the fluoride but also three principal plant nutrients: nitrogen, calcium and phosphorus.

1. Effect of fluoride concentration in nutrient solution

Peach seedlings, tomato and buckwheat (Leone et al., 1948) were grown in quartz sand in glazed crocks using a complete fluoride-free nutrient solution applied by the continous drip method for circulating the liquid. After about three to six weeks, sodium fluoride was added to the nutrient solution in concentrations ranging from 1 to 400 ppm fluoride. Buckwheat and peach showed incipient injury in 1 to 13 days, depending on the fluoride concentration. The tomatoes required 2 to over 48 days for injury. Leaves, stems and roots were analyzed for fluoride.

Table 11. *Effect of uptake of sodium fluoride from the nutrient solution on peach, tomato and buckwheat* (Leone et al., 1948)

Conc F in solution ppm	Exposure to cause injury days	Injury to		Fluorine uptake by	
		leaves (Marginal)	roots	leaves (Dry basis) ppm	stems (Dry basis) ppm
Peach seedlings					
0	No injury	None	None	6	0
10	10	Slight	Majority dead	220	5
25	10	Slight	Majority dead	261	52
100	3	Dead	Dead	550	144
400	1	Dead	Dead	1442	1286
Tomato					
0	—	None	None	10	12
10	No injury	None	None	82	15
25	48	Slight	Brown	277	9
100	18	Moderate	Small roots brown	499	28
200	5	Dead	Small roots brown	1824	127
400	2	Dead	Very small roots dead	2129	—
Buckwheat					
0	No injury	None	None	16	—
10	No injury	None	None	101	—
25	13		Moderate	533	—
50	4		Moderate	580	—
100	3	Majority dead	Dead	506	—
400	2	Dead	Dead	1920	—

Table 11 gives typical data. The peach seedlings in the 10 ppm nutrient required 10 days to build up sufficient fluoride (220 ppm) in the leaves to cause slight injury. The tomatoes required 48 days in the 25 ppm fluoride solution for a slightly greater build-up (277 ppm) in the leaves which caused slight marginal "scorch." Buckwheat was uninjured after 21 days at 10 ppm and absorption of 101 ppm. At 25 ppm for 13 days and with absorption of 533 ppm, buckwheat was moderately injured. Evidently, a treatment for incipient slight injury lies between these two. Fluoride concentrations of 100 ppm in the nutrient solution were very toxic to peach and buckwheat in three days, but tomato required 18 days for moderate injury. At 400 ppm for one to two days all the plants were killed.

Leone et al. (1956) gave tomato and corn plants three fumigation treatments described as "long-low" (513 hours at 5 parts per thousand million); "intermediate" (26 hours at 100 pptm); and "short-high" (4.2 hours at 650 pptm),

Fig. 3. The time-concentration product was approximately the same in the three fumigations. The results are summarized as follows:

a) The short-high concentration caused the most injury.

b) Corn was more sensitive than tomato.

c) Tomato absorbed twice as much fluoride as did corn.

d) The older leaves accumulated more fluoride than did the younger leaves, whether applied to old and young leaves on a single plant, corresponding leaves on old and young plants, or mature and young portions of a single leaf.

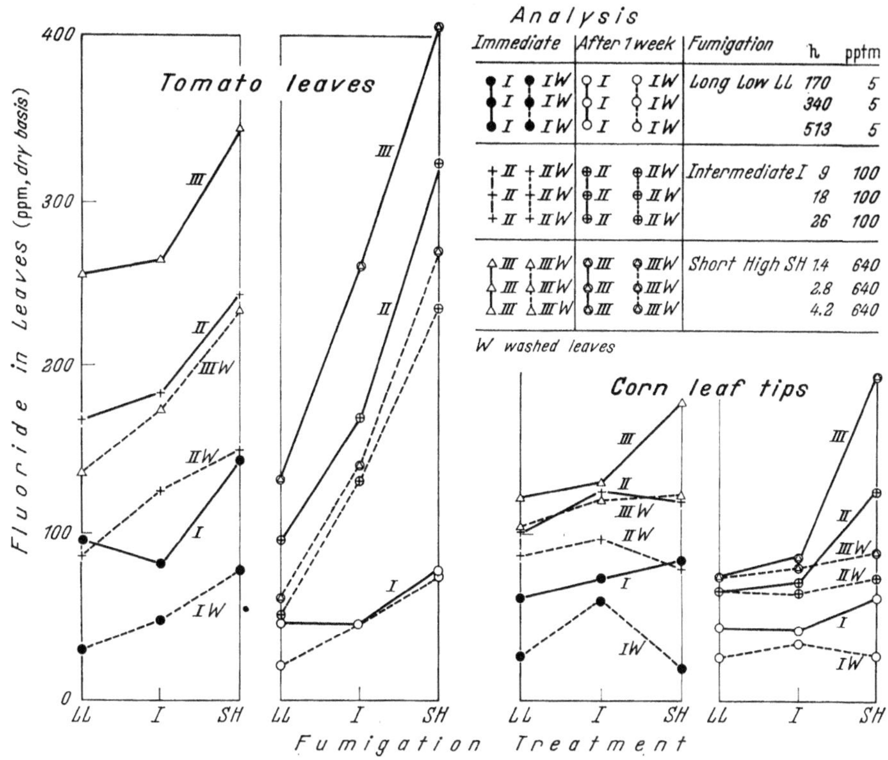

Fig. 3. Uptake of fluoride by tomato leaves and the tips of corn leaves following three fumigation treatments having the same time-concentration product. Some samples were removed after one-third and two-thirds of the full allotted time for each treatment. Some plants were analyzed immediately after the fumigations; others, after standing one week, with and without washing the leaves with water (LEONE et al., 1956)

e) Fluoride retention in the leaves was greatest with the "short-high" fumigation treatment. A considerable amount of fluoride present on the leaf surface was lost by volatilization after the fumigation or could be washed off with water.

PRINCE et al. (1949) carried out similar studies with buckwheat and tomatoes in sandy loam and loam soils, at different pH levels. Buckwheat was not injured by 180 ppm fluorine in sandy loam when the pH was above 5.5. At 360 ppm, injury occurred at pH 6.5. Large increases of the fluorine content of buckwheat were found at pH 4.5 with 180 and 360 ppm fluorine in the soil. Uptake was reduced by 85 % by adding lime to bring the soil pH to 5.5 and uptake fell to a very low level at pH 6.5. Phosphate reduced the fluoride uptake in some cases but not in others.

Tomatoes (Table 12) were injured on sandy loam soil at 360 ppm fluorine and pH 6.5. On loam the toxic point was between 360 and 720 ppm fluorine. Toxicity

Table 12. *Growth and fluorine content of tomato grown on sandy loam and loam at different pH and added hydrofluoric acid levels* (PRINCE et al., 1949)

F in soil	pH 6.3		pH 5.5		pH 4.5	
ppm	Wt. grams	F ppm	Wt. grams	F ppm	Wt. grams	F ppm
			Sassafras sandy loam			
0	34	5	18	22	10	20
90	23	19	17	33	5	56
180	26	42	8	134	1	66
360	17	242	3	327	0	—
720	1	678	—	—	0	—
			Sassafras loam			
0	55	7	45	15	43	23
90	49	8	50	27	16	78
180	53	16	32	89	3	190
360	46	91	2	480	1	1008
720	5	276	0	—	0	—

increased at lower pH on both soils. Hydrofluoric acid was somewhat more toxic than sodium fluoride. On loam, toxicity due to 180 ppm would be completely prevented by lime and fairly effective control was had at 260 ppm. Growth fell off rapidly above 360 ppm. On sandy loam at 180 ppm, there was no injury at pH 6.5, but growth fell off above 180 ppm. Extra phosphate was useful below 180 ppm.

Tomato leaves ranged from 23 ppm to 1009 ppm fluorine, when 0–360 ppm fluorine was added to the soil at low pH. Intermediate pH gave 15–480 ppm fluorine and high pH, 7–91 ppm fluorine in the leaves.

2. Effect of a major nutrient upon uptake of fluoride

BRENNAN et al. (1950) observed fluorine effects on tomato, as influenced by the principal plant nutrients. Two weeks after germination tomato seedlings were transplanted into 48 crocks of silica sand where they grew for three weeks in complete nutrient solution. Then the solution was modified so as to give four levels of one of the major nutrients, for example, nitrogen, in 16 crocks without changing the other nutrients. Four levels of calcium and four levels of phosphorus were similarly established in the other two groups of 16 crocks. Each of the 12 different nutrient treatments produced plants of characteristic color, growth-habit and rate of growth.

Four fluoride treatments were applied to four groups of 12 crocks, each of which represented the 12 nutrient treatments. Series A received 50 ppm fluorine as sodium fluoride in the nutrient solution for 13 days; Series B received 50 ppm fluorine until the plants in each individual crock either showed injury or were exposed for 31 days; Series C received a 4.5-hour fumigation with 48 pptm hydrogen fluoride; Series D received a 3.5-hour fumigation with 470 pptm hydrogen fluoride. One fumigated plant of each treatment was harvested at the completion of the treatment and the remainder, seven days later. No plant damage was seen in Series C.

Table 13 presents data for Series A and Series B, and Table 14 for Series C and Series D. Figure 4 depicts Series D and Series A. Typical symptoms of injury were the same whether the plants received the fluorine through the leaves or

Table 13. *Effect of 50 ppm fluorine as sodium fluoride in the nutrient solution on tomato plants grown with different levels of nitrogen, calcium, and phosphorus in the nutrient solution. Other nutrients optimal in each case* (BRENNAN et al., 1950)

Nutrient treatment	Series A (13 Days treatment)			Series B			
	Degree of injury	F in tissue		Degree of injury	Days of treatment	F in tissue	
		leaves	roots			leaves	roots
ppm		ppm	ppm			ppm	ppm
N 14	None	74	280	None	31	250	1310
N 56	None	96	3010	Moderate	24	1000	3440
N 112	Moderate	540	2000	Moderate	13	500	1185
N 448	None	160	1800	None	31	430	1220
Ca 10	None	170	460	None	31	435	480
Ca 40	Moderate	950	1290	Moderate	6	1000	750
Ca 80	None	116	3610	Moderate	8	850	1300
Ca 240	None	62	4360	None	31	161	3945
P 0	Trace	274	2739	Trace	31	421	6565
P 0.8	Slight	480	2305	Slight	31	620	2305
P 15.5	Slight	464	1050	Moderate	13	890	2080
P 62	Moderate	1010	970	Severe	13	672	1340

Table 14. *Effect of fumigation with hydrogen fluoride on tomato plants grown in different levels of nitrogen, calcium and phosphorus in the nutrient solution. Other nutrients optimal in each case* (BRENNAN et al., 1950)

Nutrient treatment	Series C-48 pptm HF—4.5 Hrs.			Series D-470 pptm HF—3.5 Hrs.		
	F in leaves[1] after		F in roots after	F in leaves after		F in roots after
	1 day	7 days	1- & 7-day	1 day	7 days	1- & 7-day
ppm	ppm	ppm	Avg., ppm	ppm	ppm	Avg., ppm
N 14	40	53	18	375	415[2]	19
N 56	43	40	13	655	360[3]	13
N 112	35	32	23	500	465[4]	22
N 448	47	30	15	540	360[2]	16
Ca 10	45	50	14	460	355[2]	15
Ca 40	55	30	22	435	405[4]	32
Ca 80	40	40	18	550	255[3]	25
Ca 240	45	30	14	405	255[2]	27
P 0	43	40	30	385	420[2]	13
P 0.8	40	40	11	375	365[2]	32
P 15.5	23	28	10	470	420[3]	17
P 62	40	35	14	575	280[4]	16
Average	41	37		477	363	

[1] No leaf injury in Series C.
[2] Slight leaf injury.
[3] Moderate leaf injury.
[4] Severe leaf injury.

through the roots. The fluoride levels in the leaves that showed injury were about the same from both sources.

Medium levels of nitrogen, calcium and phosphorus favored absorption and translocation of fluorine from both sources. These were approximately 112 ppm N; 40 ppm Ca and 62 ppm P. Lower levels of the three nutrients and higher levels of nitrogen and calcium reduced uptake and injury due to fluorine. A luxury level of phosphorus was not attained, if one exists. Excess calcium tends to precipitate insoluble fluorine compounds in and around the roots.

The fumigated plants showed high fluorine in the leaves and practically normal fluorine in the roots, indicating little or no translocation downward. The reverse was true of the fluorine from the nutrient solution. Although appreciable translocation upward occurred, the fluorine in the roots was much higher than that in the leaves. A criterion is thus afforded to distinguish between uptake from the soil and the atmosphere, as mentioned earlier.

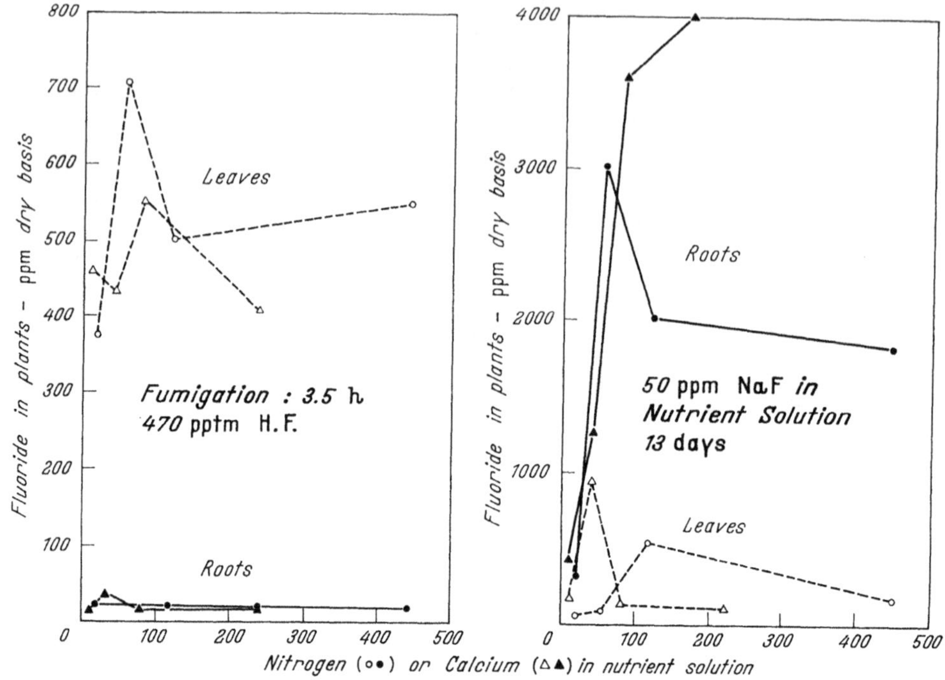

Fig. 4. Fluoride content of tomato leaves and roots grown in nutrient solutions having various levels of calcium or nitrogen. Fluoride added as 470 ppm hydrogen fluoride for 3.5 hours or as 50 ppm sodium fluoride in the nutrient solution for 13 days (BRENNAN et al., 1950)

D. Boyce Thompson studies with radioactive fluorine, F^{18}

LEDBETTER et al. (1960) have used the radioactive isotope F^{18} as well as the stable isotope, F^{19}, to study the uptake and distribution of the element in tomato plants, after addition of hydrogen fluoride via the atmosphere or one percent sodium fluoride in the soil. A two-hour fumigation experiment with HF^{18} was carried out in which the soil container was covered so that no hydrogen fluoride could come into direct contact with the roots or crown. Distribution of the element was determined by radioautographs and by counting. The autographs showed the principal accumulation in the margins of the leaves and in small glands along the stems. The stems themselves, the petioles and the roots were nearly free of activity.

The Geiger counter (Fig. 5) showed that the main stem ranged from 310 to 1500 counts per minute per milligram dry matter, starting just above the pot and extending to the tip leaves, while the protected roots had only 6 cpm. The lowest leaf, which was much smaller than the others, had 24,000 cpm per milligram; the next three leaves averaged 15,000; the next two, 9300; the next three, 6700; and the top cluster of emerging leaves, 3800 cpm per milligram. Evidently, the gas absorbing facilities of all the leaves was in course of development with the oldest leaf having six times the absorptive capacity of the youngest.

Using NaF^{19} in the nutrient solution the gross distribution was: Roots > lower leaves > upper leaves > stems. Fractionation of leaf structures after long-term F^- accumulation from the air or from the soil showed cell walls > chloroplasts > soluble proteins > mitochondria > microsomes. The fluorine in the chloroplasts was largely associated with the proteins; the pigments and lipids had only traces of fluorine.

Regardless of mode of entry, 68 % of the absorbed fluorine could be washed off or out of the leaves with distilled water and 83 %, with a detergent.

Experiments with Sedum spectabile fumigated for 30 min with HF^{18} showed about 80 % of the fluorine in the stripped epidermis of the leaves and the remainder in the mesophyll, either immediately or three hours after the treatment. A fumigation of one week's duration with 10 ppb HF^{19} showed a 70–30 % distribution between epidermis and mesophyll immediately after fumigation; an 80 to 20 % distribution one week later and 92–8 % two weeks later.

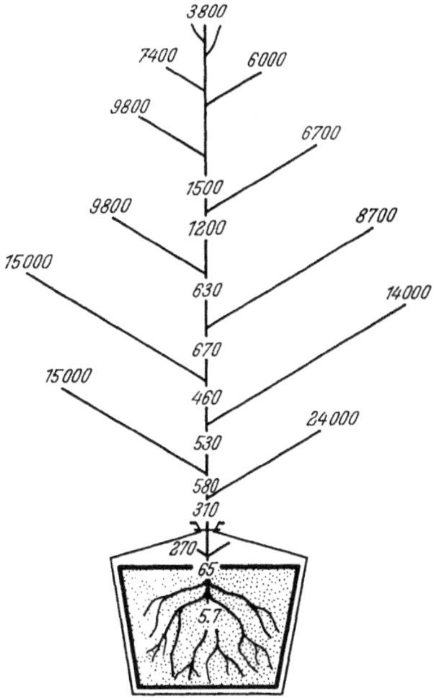

Fig. 5. Distribution of radioactive fluoride in a tomato plant after a two-hour fumigation with HF^{18}. Values in counts F^{18} per minute per mg. (Gas excluded from roots) (LEDBETTER et al., 1960)

E. Stanford Research Institute fumigation studies

Table 15 (BENEDICT et al., 1964) gives the distribution of fluorine in fumigated

Table 15. *Fluoride content of different parts of alfalfa and orchard grass plants with and without fumigation with hydrogen fluoride* (BENEDICT et al., 1964)

Fumigation: Duration days	Fumigation: Concentration μg/M³	Plant part	Fluoride content ppm: Control	Fluoride content ppm: Fumigation
		Alfalfa		
60	50	Leaves (marked)	25[1]	2580
60	50	Leaves (not marked)	25	2202
60	50	Petioles	22	1280
60	50	Stems	10	455
35	0.8	Leaves, top	2	51
35	0.8	Leaves, middle	5	121
35	0.8	Leaves, bottom	23	324
		Orchard grass		
60	50	Tip 2 inches	62	3571
60	50	Second 2 inches	12	2028
60	50	Third 2 inches	9	1491
60	50	Fourth 2 inches	6	1004
60	50	Fifth 2 inches	5	427
60	50	Sixth 2 inches	4	136
35	0.8	Tip 2 inches	86	415
35	0.8	Second 2 inches	10	31
35	0.8	Third 2 inches	5	11
35	0.8	Remainder	7	7

[1] Not marked.

and control leaves and stems of alfalfa and blades of orchard grass, according to the position of the leaf or leaf section on the plant. Two fumigation treatments were applied: 50 μg HF/M^3 for two months and 0.8 μg HF/M^3 for five weeks. The more severe fumigation contributed twice as much fluorine to the alfalfa leaves as to the petioles and five times the amount in the stems. There was a 20-fold gradient from the top to the bottom of the blades of orchard grass with 3520 ppm in the tip two inches. After the lighter fumigation there was six times as much fluorine in the old lower leaves as in the young top leaves of alfalfa. In the orchard grass, there was a 40-fold gradient in the top six inches of the blades similar to the gradient often observed in gladiolus. The control blades also had a substantial accumulation in the tips.

F. Fluorides in Florida

Large phosphate deposits are located in a 500-square-mile area centered at Bartow, Florida. Mining began here in 1890 and has expanded to the present annual output of over 10 million long tons of rock phosphate. This represents about three-fourths of the nation's supply and one-third of the world's supply of phosphate. The mineral is principally apatite, containing about four percent of fluorine. Most of the mined phosphate was shipped elsewhere for processing until the second World War, when a number of companies began making superphosphate and minor amounts of other phosphorus compounds. Between 1945 and 1952, rock phosphate production increased from 3.8 to 9.2 million tons. Eight different companies are now operating in an area of 100 square miles and two others are located just outside this area. According to HENDRICKSON (1961) a considerable amount of plant damage has been caused by fluorides emitted in this concentrated district, principally to citrus, due to treatment of the ores with sulfuric and phosphoric acids. A large amount of fluoride-bearing dust is also emitted. HENDRICKSON states, "As much as eight tons of gaseous hydrogen fluoride per day may be discharged into the atmosphere in this area" . . . although ". . . most of the manufacturers involved are making rapid strides toward bringing their fluoride emissions under further control." Claimed damage to citrus trees includes defoliation, reduction of growth and yield, leaf "burn" and severe chlorosis. Concentrations of 300 to 350 ppm fluorine in the leaves have been reported. Further west, near the coast, is an area devoted to truck crops and gladiolus. The latter is a multi-million dollar industry which has suffered a considerable amount of plant damage. Fluoride concentrations above 175 ppm have been reported in the leaves. The growers have made a practice of clipping off the necrotic areas of the leaf blades before marketing the flowers. Truck crops are visibly injured only with much greater difficulty than gladiolus. However, damage claims for tomatoes have been made, based on alleged reduced yields, although experimental proof of such reduction is lacking.

G. Fluorine studies in Western United States

During the second World War there was a great expansion of the aluminum industry in the United States and Canada. FRARY (1943) called attention to the fact that this increase was seven-fold to over one million tons of metal per year (Table 1, page 232). A substantial part of this increase was represented by new industries in the West. Further, two large steel plants which later encountered fluorine problems were built in Southern California and Utah at this time. Three aluminum plants were operated along the lower Columbia River, one in Oregon and two in Washington; a fourth was located at Tacoma, Washington; a fifth at

Wenatchee and a sixth north of Spokane, near Mead. A seventh plant has recently been built on the Columbia River at The Dalles, and a new aluminum industry has also been constructed in British Columbia.

An aluminum factory in the Central Valley of California was operated for two years until it was shut down in August, 1944. Severe damage to apricot orchards, and also to figs and walnuts, was observed in 1943 and 1944. DE ONG (1946) described this apricot damage as a marginal bleach on the leaves leading to a considerable amount of defoliation and loss of fruit. There was also gumming of the young twigs which is now associated with boron toxicity rather than with fluoride damage. Lesions were most severe near the plant, but could be traced for eight miles downwind. Chemical analysis of the leaves indicated a high fluorine content. When the plant was shut down, evidence of leaf lesions soon disappeared but the 1945 crop was only about 50% of normal, due presumably to the defoliation of the previous year.

JOHNSON et al. (1947) and MILLER et al. (1948) described similar symptoms on Italian prune trees near the aluminum factories of southwestern Washington. This injury also began as a "marginal scorch of the leaves with necrotic areas appearing in the center of the lamina, . . . followed by severe leaf drop in midsummer." The fluorine content of the leaves ranged from 1400 ppm down to 18 ppm within a 20-mile radius of the factories, whereas at greater distances the range was 6 to 15 ppm fluorine.

1. Citrus and grapes in Southern California

Studies of the effects of fluorides on citrus in Southern California have been in progress during the past ten years. A preliminary survey by KAUDY et al. (1955) in 130 citrus groves showed a moderate accumulation (20–60 ppm) of fluoride in citrus leaves in an industrial area of Los Angeles county, and a much larger accumulation (up to 211 ppm) in San Bernardino county near a steel factory at Fontana. Maximum accumulation occurred in the summer and autumn months before the winter rains began. Elsewhere, the fluoride levels in the leaves were about 1–3 ppm except in the immediate vicinity of ceramic factories or other sources of fluoride. Definite leaf lesions on citrus, attributable to fluorine, were seldom seen although wine-grapes near the Fontana factory exhibited appreciable marginal necrosis. Possibly, some of the chlorotic and necrotic lesions on citrus were caused by fluorine but they were indistinguishable from the chlorosis due to manganese deficiency or necrosis due to excess boron. Chemical analysis of the leaves is necessary to establish the fluoride etiology. WANDER and MCBRIDE (1956) attributed similar chlorotic effects on citrus to fluoride from nearby triple-superphosphate factories in Florida. The leaves contained 48–470 ppm fluorine.

a) Fluoride from the nutrient solution

BREWER and associates (1959, 1960) have studied the effects, on large bearing citrus trees, of fluoride added to the roots in the nutrient solution, or to the leaves as hydrogen fluoride or fluoride salt spray.

In the nutrient solution experiment (BREWER et al., 1959) 12 four-year-old bearing Washington Navel orange trees were grown for two years in complete nutrient cultures in 100 liter tile tanks, then transferred to 700 liter tanks having 0, 25 and 100 ppm hydrogen fluoride added to the nutrient solution at pH 4.0. The four trees in the 100 ppm culture wilted within 24 hours and soon shed their leaves. They had to be discarded. The roots were found to be covered with a gelatinous film of calcium fluorophosphate.

The experiment with the 0 and 25 ppm fluoride cultures was continued for 18 months, although two of the latter trees were lost by temporary failure of the system used for aerating the solutions. Top growth in the 25 ppm culture was reduced 36 % and total growth, 18 %. The fluoride-treated roots were coarse, brown, and matted while the control roots were white and well branched. Fluoride in the active leaves was only about 40 to 50 ppm. Two crops of fruit were harvested. The 25 ppm fluoride treatment reduced the total number of fruit by about one-third and the weight of fruit by about one-half, compared with the control. The taste of the fluoride-treated fruit was described as "fair" in the first crop and "poor" in the second, while the control fruit was said to be "excellent" and "good," respectively.

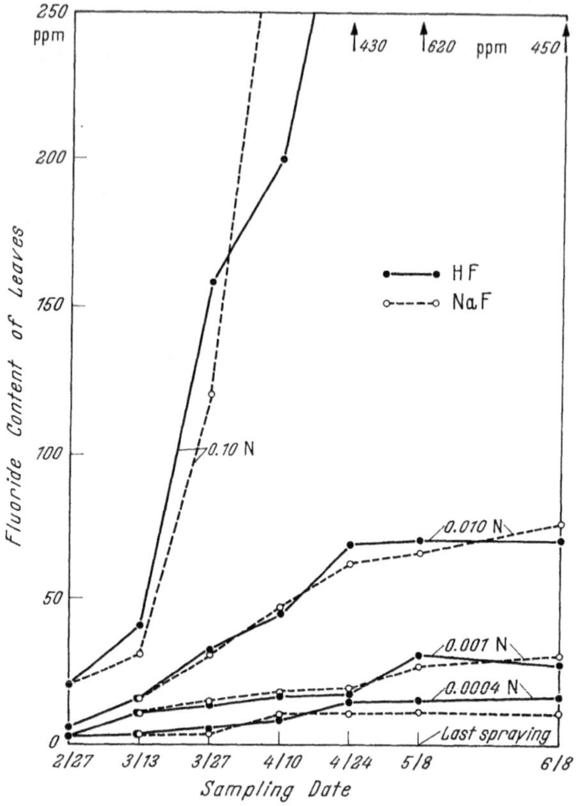

Fig. 6. Uptake of fluoride by the leaves of young navel orange trees sprayed with solutions of sodium fluoride and hydrofluoric acid at two-week intervals. Surface fluoride removed by washing (Brewer et al., 1960c)

b) Fluoride sprays on citrus

Spraying of citrus trees in a grove with fluoride salts was considered to be a more convenient experimental means of introducing fluoride into the leaves than covering many trees with transparent canopies and fumigating with hydrogen fluoride, in order to determine the fluoride effect on yield and quality of fruit. A sufficient number of trees could thus be readily treated to give statistically significant yield and quality data.

Brewer et al. (1960c) sprayed five-year-old Washington Navel orange trees growing in a commercial grove with 0.10, 0.01, 0.001 and 0.0004 N solutions of HF, NaF, NH_4F and H_2SiF_6; also, 0.0004 N CaF_2 (saturated). HF and NaF were the compounds most readily absorbed at the three highest concentrations, and HF and H_2SiF_6, at the lowest concentration (Fig. 6). Differences in uptake of the different compounds was ascribed to differences in the size of the cation. Average uptakes per spray determined by leaf analysis were 90, 12, 5 and 1.5 ppm fluorine in the leaves for the four sprays, respectively. The spray method has been extensively applied but the results are yet not available.

c) Fumigation of seven citrus varieties

Brewer et al. (1960a) fumigated seven varieties of potted citrus trees with hydrogen fluoride in two air-conditioned greenhouses supplied with carbon-filtered air.

Four one-year-old trees of each variety, all field-grown budded scions on rough lemon root stock, were placed in each house on December 4, 1956. Air flow, temperature and humidity were maintained as nearly the same as possible in the two houses. Approximate hydrogen fluoride concentrations in one of the houses were as follows: Dec. 1956 to Feb. 1957, 12 pptm; Feb. 1957 to Jan. 1958, 7 pptm; Jan. 1958 to June 23, 1958, 3–5 pptm. The hydrogen fluoride in the air was determined by bubbling an air sample at 28 liters per minute through water for three hours, then automatically emptying the solution into a polyethylene cup on a turntable, recharging the absorber and resuming the aspirating. A modification of the spectrophotometric method of Megregian was used to evaluate the fluoride.

The initial hydrogen fluoride concentration was evidently too high for a long fumigation treatment because the mature leaves acquired over 250 ppm fluorine within two months. In March 1957, new growth on the fumigated trees was less vigorous and the new leaves smaller and more chlorotic than on the controls. In May and June 1957, acute injury appeared as a collapse and necrosis on the tips of many immature leaves which contained about 185 ppm fluorine, whereas chlorotic, chronically injured mature leaves had over 300 ppm fluorine. Excessive branching occurred when the injured immature leaves were abscissed and the axillary buds produced many weak spindly shoots which caused greater total stem elongation than on the control trees. In May and June 1958, after the hydrogen fluoride concentration had been reduced to 3–5 ppm, since January, the new spring flush leaves accumulated 188 to 262 ppm fluorine on six of the seven varieties, while Valencia orange leaves accumulated 419 ppm. Detailed measurements on the trees at the end of the experiment indicated that the average trunk diameter, leaf size and top weight of fumigated trees were 8, 37 and 15 % smaller, respectively, than the controls, while linear growth was 123 % greater.

Table 16 gives the relative response of the seven citrus varieties to the fluoride treatments as indicated by gross growth, leaf size and chlorosis. The seven varieties are arranged in order of degree of response to each criterion. Increasing response is indicated by numbers 1 to 7. The two grapefruit varieties and Temple oranges were somewhat more resistant than the others in all criteria. The lemons showed the most chlorosis while the oranges were most retarded in growth and leaf size.

Table 16. *Relative response of seven citrus varieties to hydrogen fluoride fumigation.* A rating of 7 indicates maximum sensitivity (Brewer et al., 1960a)

Variety	Criteria			
	Gross growth	Leaf size	Chlorosis	Total score
Lisbon lemon	4	5	7	16
Eureka lemon	5	3	6	14
Red grapefruit	3	1	5	9
March grapefruit	2	2	4	8
Temple orange	1	4	1	6
Navel orange	7	7	2	16
Valencia orange	6	6	3	15

d) Fumigation of large bearing orange trees

Brewer et al. (1960b) carried out a two-year fumigation treatment on bearing Washington Navel orange trees growing on Troyer Citrange root stock. In May, 1955, four one-year-old trees were transplanted to each of two 3 × 6 m greenhouses provided with an imported, fertile, sandy-loam soil, to a depth of 1.6 m. After June, 1956, the trees were supplied with cooled, thermostated, carbon-filtered air for the remainder of the experiment. In October, 1956, treatment of one of the houses with 3–5 pptm hydrogen fluoride was started and continued until March, 1957. At that time, the concentration was reduced to 2.0 pptm until January, 1958, and finally to 1.0–1.5 pptm until January, 1959, when the experiment was terminated and the trees removed. Samples of leaves, fruit, twigs, wood and roots were then taken for fluoride analysis. Tree and trunk dimensions were recorded monthly and after removal of the trees complete weight data were taken. Yield and quality of the fruit were determined each year. Table 17 summarizes the fumigation, growth, yield and fruit quality data.

Table 17. *Growth, yield and fruit quality data for orange trees after 13 or 26 months continuous fumigation with 1—5 pptm hydrogen fluoride* (BREWER et al., 1960b)

	Date	Fumigated[1]	Control	Difference	Difference %
Trunk diameter, cm . . .	Dec 1958	8.1	8.6	—0.5	6
Tree volume m³	Dec 1958	8.8	11.9	—3.1	26
Area of leaf, cm²	Dec 1957	26	42	—16	38
Area of leaf, cm²	Dec 1958	37	42	—5	12
Linear growth, m	Jan 1959	242 ± 8[2]	295 ± 13[2]	-53 ± 15[3]	18 ± 5
Green Wt., Leaves, Kg. .	Jan 1959	8.6 ± 0.3[2]	9.6 ± 0.3[2]	-1.0 ± 0.4[3]	10 ± 4
Green Wt., Tops, Kg . .	Jan 1959	18.4 ± 0.6[2]	22.1 ± 1.5[2]	-3.7 ± 1.6[3]	17 ± 7
F Content Leaves, ppm .	July 1957	150[4]—75[5]			
	Mar 1958	200[5]			
	Jan 1959	118	2	+116	98
F Content, All wood, ppm	Jan 1959	3	2	+1	30
No. Fruit per tree	Jan 1958	18	35	—17	49
No. Fruit per tree	Jan 1959	26	72	—46	63
Avg Wt/Fruit, g	Jan 1958	158	206	—48	23
Avg Wt/Fruit, g	Jan 1959	218	215	+3	2
Juice, %	Jan 1959	50	57	—7	12
Sol. Solids, %	Jan 1959	11.9	12.4	—0.5	4
Vitamin C mg/100 ml . .	Jan 1959	35.8	38.5	—2.7	7

[1] Fumigation treatment: Oct 1956 to Mar 1957: 3—5 pptm HF; Mar 1957 to Jan 1958: 2.0 pptm HF; Jan 1958 to Jan 1959: 1.0—1.5 pptm HF.
[2] Standard error.
[3] Standard error of difference.
[4] Leaves formed Fall 1956.
[5] Leaves formed Mar 1957.

In March, 1957, it was noted that the fluoride-treated trees had less vigorous shoot growth, smaller leaves, delayed blossoming and decreased fruit set as compared with the control trees. In May and June 1957, there was considerable chlorosis and some necrosis on the mature treated leaves. Some of the symptoms resembled those due to manganese deficiency or excess boron, but no such symptoms appeared on the control trees which had an identical environment except for the fluoride fumigation. June leaf drop was greater on the treated trees. In July, the old fall-flush leaves had 150 ppm fluorine and the young April-flush leaves, 75–80 ppm. The latter increased steadily to about 200 ppm in March, 1958.

The fumigated trees were smaller than the controls by about the same amount both years, but the fumigated leaves were much smaller the first year than the second. This may have been due to the higher hydrogen fluoride concentrations the first year. The weight differences between control and treated trees amounted to about 17 % and are statistically significant. The yield and quality data suggest strongly that the fumigation had a detrimental effect on both factors.

The foregoing trees were replaced by a different type of four-year-old Washington Navel orange on a rough lemon root stock (BREWER, personal communication, 1963). Four trees were fumigated at 1 pptm from May 1959 to August, 1961, when the experiment was terminated earlier than originally intended because the trees were found to be an unsatisfactory variety. The control trees appeared more vigorous and deeper green in color and had larger leaves than the fumigated trees. In the spring of 1961, the control trees blossomed profusely and set a heavy crop of fruit. The fumigated trees blossomed lightly and abscissed most of the blooms. Only two individual fruit were set on the four trees. These dropped off later. Linear growth was greater on the fumigated trees due to the production of many small branches instead of a few larger ones. Overall reduction in growth was about the same as in the earlier experiment, confirming the deleterious effect of prolonged continuous exposure of citrus to hydrogen fluoride in the 1–5 pptm range. The cause of the blossom abscission is not clear. Probably, other factors beside or in addition to fluoride are involved. It has recently been found that blossom abscission can often be avoided by a temporary girdling of the tree at peak bloom. A cut is made through the bark around the trunk, using a sharp knife. The wound heals in about two weeks and the blossoms are largely retained.

It should be pointed out that continuous day and night exposure to a toxicant is seldom a realistic treatment by which to assess an industrial exposure. In the latter, there are always periods of zero or trace exposure during which the system has an opportunity to dispose of accumulated toxicants or products of their reactions and return to more normal function. Injury is possible at very low concentration levels with continuous fumigation, whereas higher concentrations are required to cause injury if the fumigations are intermittent.

e) Effects on wine grapes

Wine grapes are an important crop in Southern California. There is a large acreage near the Fontana steel factory. The different varieties show a wide range of sensitivity to hydrogen fluoride. The principal varieties grown in this area are Mission, Zinfandel and Grenache, which range in their reaction to fluoride from sensitive to resistant, in that order. The leaves show the typical reddish-brown marginal collapse characteristic of fluoride lesions on broadleaf plants, but the reddish color soon fades to tan.

BREWER et al. (1957) collected leaf samples of the Palomino and Zinfandel varieties on June 9 and September 1, 1955, at various distances and directions from the steel factory. Fruit samples were also collected on September 1. A visual estimate was made of leaf injury which was designated "injury index" on a scale of 0 to 5, each number representing a range of percentage of leaves having markings from any cause. Fluorine analyses were carried out also.

Table 18 summarizes the results. On the earlier date, all but four leaf samples had low fluoride levels and showed no leaf injury; however, the sample in the prevailing wind direction two miles northeast of the factory had 159 ppm fluorine and an injury index of 3. There was a substantial increase in the amount of fluoride in the leaves between June 9 and September 1. The different directions had different concentrations and gradients. The fluoride levels decreased with distance in each direction. Comparable samples of two varieties (Palomino and Zinfandel) showed approximately the same amount of fluoride at one sampling station but at other stations, Zinfandel absorbed more fluoride with less injury than did Palomino. Not all the injury was due to fluoride. Hot weather, drought, and smog played a part. For example, in the seven-mile, southwest samples with

Table 18. *Fluoride content and injury index of the leaves and fruit of Palomino (P) and Zinfandel (Z) wine grapes at various distances from an industrial emission of hydrogen fluoride* (BREWER et al., 1957)

Variety	Distance-miles and direction from source	Leaves				Fruit
		June 9		Sept 1		
		F ppm[1]	Injury index[3]	F ppm[1]	Injury index[3]	F ppm[2]
P	2.0 NE	159	3	462	5	2.7
Z	3.0 NE	36	1	233	5	1.3
P	9.0 NE	19	0	92	4	0.8
Z	9.0 NE	24	0	114	4	0.7
P	5.0 SE	13	0	55	3	0.3
Z	5.0 SE	12	0	70	3	0.5
P	1.5 W	27	0	97	3	0.6
Z	2.0 W	49	2	98	4	0.6
P	5.0 WSW	35	1	75	3	0.5
Z	5.0 WSW	16	0	109	4	0.5
P	6.0 NW	21	0	71	4	0.3
Z	6.5 NW	22	0	46	3	0.5
P	7.0 SW	8	0	32	2	0.1
Z	7.0 SW	2	0	31	2	0.4

[1] Dry basis.
[2] Fresh basis.
[3] 0 = no visible injury; 1 = < 10% of leaf area injured; 2 = 10—25% injured; 3=25, to 50% injured; 4 = 50—75% injured; 5 = > 75% injured.

only 31—32 ppm fluorine, the injury index of 2, or 10—25 % of the leaves showing some injury, was probably practically all due to weather and smog. Fluoride lesions could not be distinguished from weather injury, although ozone stipple, to which grapes are very susceptible and which is often present in the area, is quite different from fluoride injury.

The fruit ranged from 0.1 to 2.7 ppm fluorine on a fresh-weight basis. Evidently, these levels are too low to affect the wine. No yield data were reported. The authors conclude: "The effects, if any, of elevated fluoride concentrations and subsequent marginal necrosis on grape production cannot be determined from the information now available."

2. Gladiolus and pine in the Northwest

a) Gladiolus

COMPTON and REMMERT (1960) studied fluoride damage to mature gladiolus plants located at different distances and directions from an aluminum factory in Oregon. The fourth leaf was cut into three-inch sections which were analyzed separately. Table 19 shows that the highest fluoride concentrations occurred near the factory, indicating this was the principal source in the area. The large concentration gradient from the tip to the base of the blade, which reached 100-fold in one plant, is characteristic of fumigated gladiolus leaves. Four different varieties of gladiolus having the same fluoride exposure in the field showed an approximate inverse relationship between the amount of injury to the blade tips and the fluoride concentration in the tips (Table 20). The smaller the amount of leaf injury, the higher the fluoride content of the tips. This inverse relationship has

Table 19. *Concentration of fluorine in leaf segments from the fourth leaf of blooming gladiolus, at various distances from an aluminum plant in Oregon* (COMPTON and REMMERT, 1960)

Date 1948	Distance-miles and direction	Segment distance from tip (cm)	Fluorine content (Dry Wt. basis) Beacon ppm	Picardy ppm	Snow princess ppm	Stoplight ppm
Aug 31	3 ESE	0—8	372	252	303	1009
		8—15	42	81	118	187
		15—23	31	21	38	15
		23—31	12	11	15	10
Aug 31	6 ESE	0—8	58	109	151	142
		8—15	11	12	7	3
		15—23	4	3	3	4
Sept 1	22 SW	0—8	11	9	7	5
		8—15	3	5	2	4
		15—23	2	3	2	2

Table 20. *Fluorine content and leaf scorch of four varieties of gladiolus near an aluminum factory in Oregon* (COMPTON and REMMERT, 1960)

Variety	Fluorine in 0—8 cm tip[1] ppm	Leaf scorch[1] cm
Beacon	134 ± 27[2]	9.1 ± 2.0[2]
Picardy	166 ± 21	5.3 ± 1.0
Snow princess . .	255 ± 19	5.3 ± 1.2
Stoplight	373 ± 63	1.5 ± 0.3

[1] Fourth leaf from base.
[2] Mean and standard error.

Table 21. *Relative susceptibility to injury and uptake of hydrogen flucride from the atmosphere by different varieties of gladiolus*

Variety	Scorch Index[1]	Scorch Tipburn cm[2]	Tipburn cm[3]	Tipburn cm[4]	Fluorine content of blade tips ppm[1]	ppm[2]	ppm[4]
Shirley Temple	54		20.8		138		
Ethyl Cave Cole.	32		13.5		180	191	
Beacon	34		12.7	9.1	246	111	134
Picardy	39	17.5	9.9	5.3	243		166
Snow Princess	36	18.0	10.7	5.3	—	142	255
Valeria.	—	19.0	9.9		—	160	
Surfside	24	18.0	11.9		422	194	
Yellow Emperor	—	13.0	9.9		—	278	
Rosa Van Luna	9	—	8.1		407	341	
Elizabeth the Queen. . .	—	11.5	6.6				
Spotlight.	—		4.6			310	
Stoplight.	—		3.6	1.5		309	373
Algonquin	7	7.0	3.0		611		

[1] JOHNSON et al. (1950). Comparable samples near two aluminum factories. Per cent of blade length scorched.
[2] HITCHCOCK et al. (1962). 0—10 pphm HF, 6—7 days.
[3] COMPTON and REMMERT (1960). Leaves not analyzed.
[4] Data from Table 20.

been confirmed for many varieties by JOHNSON et al. (1950) and HITCHCOCK et al. (1962) as indicated in Table 21.

ROMELL (1941) suggested that the absorption of hydrogen fluoride from the atmosphere by a leaf should be greater near the margins and tips than over the body of the leaf because of a "distortion of the diffusion field in the air around edges and protruding extremities." While this process may play a part, the principal factor in the large accumulation of fluoride in the blade tips has been shown conclusively by COMPTON and REMMERT to be translocation from the base or body of the leaf. Sodium fluoride, cryolite or hydrofluoric acid solutions were applied to the basal portions of attached and detached blades. Within 42 hours analysis of the leaves indicated a distribution like that shown in Table 19 (page 263).

b) Ponderosa pine blight at Mead

A study of fluoride damage to ponderosa pine trees due primarily to the operation of an aluminum plant at Mead, Spokana County, Washington, has been reported from Washington State University (ADAMS et al., 1952). An area of about 50 square miles was involved, including about three square miles immediately surrounding the industry in which the trees were all severely damaged or killed. Diagnosis of this so-called "pine blight" as fluoride injury was accomplished by pathological and meterological observations and by analysis of the atmosphere and vegetation for fluoride. The "blight" was characterized by a "reddening or browning" of the needles, progressing from the tip downward to the base. In severe cases the needles were shortened to one-fourth their normal length and the needle density on the twigs suffered a marked decline. The trees severely affected retained their needles for only one to two years instead of the usual five to six years. The damage pattern was quite consistent with the wind movements and fluorine concentrations in the area. High concentration of fluorine in the needles established the diagnosis conclusively.

Air analyses for gaseous fluorides were made from May to September, 1950, at 12 sampling stations located 0.5 to 7 miles in various directions from the Mead aluminum plant. The air was drawn at one cubic foot per minute through a dust filter, then through two absorption towers in series for 24-hour periods. Three stations nearest the source were sampled for 8-hour intervals. Fluoride was distilled by the Willard-Winter method and the distillates were titrated with thorium nitrate using alizarin sulfonate indicator. Ninety-five per cent of 1510 analyses ranged from 0 to 5 pptm and four per cent ranged from 5 to 20 pptm. The highest value was 351 pptm and the next highest, 73 pptm. The higher concentrations were all measured at low wind velocities.

c) Injury to gladiolus at Mead

For a two-week period in July, 1951, three varieties of gladiolus at the four-to-five leaf stage in gallon cans, and 5-year-old ponderosa pine trees in five-gallon cans, were exposed at three locations, 0.2, 0.5 and 0.8 miles from the Mead plant (ADAMS et al., 1956). These plants were grown at the Experiment Station at Pullman, Washington, both before and after the exposure period, and were transported to Mead for exposure.

Air analyses were made as before, except that the sample collection period was four hours. Injury indices were determined as the percentage of the blade or needle length that was necrotic.

Table 22 summarizes the results. If the injury index is plotted against the atmospheric fluoride concentration, straight lines are obtained indicating a linear relationship between these factors. The slope of the gladiolus line is over eight times as steep as that for pine.

Table 22. *Fluoride injury to potted gladiolus and pine trees due to a two-weeks exposure near the aluminium plant ad mead, Washington* (ADAMS et al. 1956)

Location miles from plant	Avg HF in air pptm	Injury index[1]	
		Gladiolus[2]	Pine
0.2 S	2.36	32.7	66.7
0.8 NNE	0.77	25.7	18.2
0.5 N	0.49	25.4	6.3

[1] Length necrotic tip/total length) × 100.
[2] Average of three varieties.

ADAMS et al. (1956) fumigated ponderosa pine and two varieties of gladiolus using different concentrations and exposure periods of hydrogen fluoride. Injury index data are presented in Table 23. Snow Princess appeared to be a little less sensitive than Ethyl Cave Cole. The pine needles were more sensitive when immature and about 50% elongated, but the mature needles absorbed more fluoride. The coefficient of correlation between injury index and exposure factor was 0.90 for the gladiolus and 0.96 for the pine needles.

Table 23. *Comparative injury indexes*[1] *of varieties of gladiolus and pine fumigated for different periods at three hydrogen fluoride levels* (ADAMS et al., 1956)

Hydrogen fluoride (ppb)	Time (hrs)	Factor (pphm × hrs)	Injury index: E. C. Cole	Injury index: Snow princess	Ponderosa pine needles: Immature	Ponderosa pine needles: Mature
	24	288	25.7	22.1	66.7	52.5
12	48	576	35.0	37.3	100.0	49.9
June 11—16, 1951	72	864	46.7	57.2	100.0	87.8
	96	1152	52.9	44.6	100.0	100.0
	120	1440	52.0	53.0	100.0	89.2
	24	28.8	1.9	0.0	0.5	0.0
	48	57.6	6.1	6.7	1.0	0.4
1.2	72	86.4	6.9	5.7	4.6	1.4
June 19—24	96	115.2	15.4	13.7	33.2	5.5
	120	144.0	20.7	15.3	34.0	5.0
	24	16.8	0.7	0.1	—	—
	48	33.6	2.0	1.2	—	—
0.7	72	50.4	3.1	1.4	—	—
June 26-July 1	96	67.4	2.9	2.3	—	—
	120	84.0	4.2	2.0	—	—

[1] (Length necrotic tip/total length) × 100.

3. Fumigation studies with higher plants

a) New techniques

COMPTON and REMMERT (1960) were the first investigators in the United States to carry out hydrogen fluoride fumigation studies using realistic concentrations and exposure periods. The selected range was originally calculated from emission data supplied by the Aluminum Company at Troutdale, Oregon. Most of the earlier work had been done with concentrations of the order of parts per million, whereas studies with parts per hundred million or thousand million (parts per billion) or even parts per ten thousand million, are required. Rapid replacement of the air in the fumigation chamber is also necessary because the gas is readily absorbed or adsorbed on all surfaces. COMPTON and REMMERT used large plastic-covered fumigation chambers (about 2.4 × 4.2 × 3.0 m) provided with an outlet blower that changed the air in the chamber about 1.5 times per minute. The hydrogen fluoride was added by oil displacement of pure gas in a large bottle and the analytical and calculated concentrations agreed rather closely. Many fumigations with this equipment established the time-concentration relations for fluoride injury to a number of plants but unfortunately, the studies were not published until 1960, although they were freely discussed earlier. These sound experimental techniques have enabled several other investigators to avoid some of the pitfalls of fluoride fumigations. Descriptions of satisfactory and effective fumigation equipment have been published by ADAMS et al. (1956, 1957), HILL et al. (1959a), MAVRODINEANU and COE (1957), and MAVRODINEANU et al. (1962). The dispensing of the hydrogen fluoride can be greatly facilitated by passing a measured stream of air through a bottle of dilute hydrofluoric acid of definite concentration and at a fixed temperature. The air stream charged with hydrogen fluoride is added to the large air volume passing through the fumigation chamber. By proper choice of aspiration rate, together with solution concentration and temperature, any desired fumigation condition can be readily established and maintained for long periods of time. It is particularly convenient to cool the fluoride solution in an ice bath to control the temperature and to avoid evaporating an appreciable amount of water into the system.

b) Uptake of fluoride and injury

Injury to the sensitive Picardy variety of gladiolus was noted as follows by COMPTON and REMMERT: 10 cm of tip necrosis at 10 pptm in 22 hours and 2.5 cm

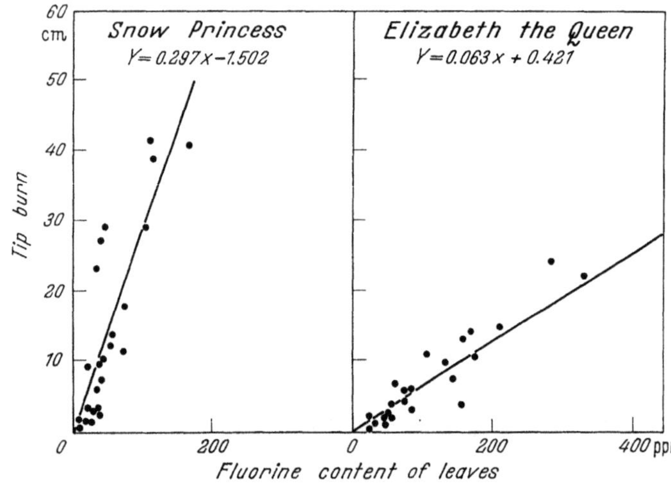

Fig. 7. Regression equations for "Snow Princess" and "Elizabeth the Queen" varieties of gladiolus (HITCHCOCK et al., 1962)

tip necrosis at 0.1 pptm in five weeks. The injured tissue accumulated 279 ppm fluorine in the first case and the tip 7.5 cm, 148 ppm, in the second. These concentrations are similar to those in Table 20 (p. 263).

HITCHCOCK et al. (1962) have summarized ten years' work at Boyce Thompson Institute on the effects of fluoride on gladiolus. Tip burn and accumulation of fluoride in the blades varied considerably with variety, culture and age of the plant and the leaf. Plants at the five-to-seven-leaf stage were more sensitive than plants at the three-leaf stage. Middle aged leaves exhibited maximum tipburn. The more resistant varieties accumulated the most fluorine with least injury, as found by COMPTON and REMMERT. A significant linear relationship was found between extent of tip burn and the fluoride content of the tissue of a given variety. Different varieties varied considerably. The slope of the regression equation for "Snow Princess" was nearly five times that for "Elizabeth the Queen," indicating a five-fold greater sensitivity of the former (Fig. 7).

c) Surface absorption

Hydrogen fluoride, like other gases, reaches the mesophyll of the leaf principally by way of the stomata. But an appreciable amount is also absorbed on the epidermis or cuticle. The latter can be partly removed by dipping the leaves in distilled water. In some plants, as much as 50–75 % of the total fluoride can be removed in this way, as shown by the Boyce Thompson studies using radioactive fluorine F^{18} (see page 254). However, the surface fluoride is evidently tenaciously held, because HITCHCOCK et al. (1962) found that fresh, fluoride-fumigated samples, without a lime treatment to fix the fluoride, could be dried at 80° for 12 hours without significant loss of fluorine as compared with lime-fixed aliquots similarly treated. Following a fumigation the fluoride content of the leaves tends to fall off due presumably to translocation, dilution by growth and slow loss to the atmosphere. For example, Snow Princess gladiolus leaves having 81 to 129 ppm fluorine after a protracted fumigation treatment lost 44 to 64 % of the element in one week, while Elizabeth the Queen gladiolus lost one-fifth as much. WEINSTEIN (1961) concluded that these decreases could not be explained by dilution due to growth or by root exudation but must represent mainly loss to the atmosphere.

d) Protection by lime sprays

ALLMENDINGER et al. (1950) found that repeated spraying of gladiolus with hydrated lime was quite effective in preventing damage to the leaves. The spray contained 450 g of hydrated lime, plus 40 g of a spreader, "Penetrol" and 30 g of casein in 19 l of water. It wetted the leaves uniformly. Treatment was begun shortly after the first injury due to fluoride from an aluminum plant was noticed. Dusts and sprays were applied at two- and four-week intervals for three months. Then the leaves were washed with water and leaves and washings analyzed separately.

Table 24. *Effect of lime dust and lime spray on injury to gladiolus by hydrogen fluoride* (ALLMENDINGER et al., 1950)

Treatment	Interval (weeks)	F Removed by washing ppm	F Remaining after washing ppm	Scorch %
		Snow Princess		
Untreated . . .	—	33	219	15.5
Lime dust . . .	2	95	197	6.1
Lime spray . .	4	155	152	2.5
Lime spray . .	2	327	91	1.9
		Ethyl Cave Cole		
Untreated . . .	—	35	275	19.3
Lime dust . . .	2	98	170	11.4
Lime spray . .	4	126	174	5.9
Lime spray . .	2	307	108	4.1

Table 24 gives typical data. Evidently part of the gas reacted with the lime coating before it could enter the leaf. The lime dust was considerably less effective than the lime spray and the four-week lime spray was less effective than the two-week lime spray schedule. The latter reduced the injury to the leaves of the two varieties to 1.9 to 4.1 %, which was 12 and 21 % of the injury on the untreated plant.

e) Color sensitivity of gladiolus

Hendrix and Hall (1958) grew 110 varieties of gladioli in replicated pots under comparable conditions. One set was fumigated with hydrogen fluoride at Pullman, Washington; another set was exposed near an aluminum factory. Foliar injury ranged from 10 to 60 % of the leaf area. The plants were arranged in six groups according to the extent of the injury. Leaf area measurements indicated that the most resistant varieties had leaves that were 22 % larger than the most sensitive varieties, but leaf thickness was about the same in both groups. The flower color of the different varieties was observed in relation to extent of injury. Plants with purple, lavender, red, pink, yellow, white and orange blossoms showed leaf area injury averaging 33.2, 35.2, 39.8, 44.6, 46.0, 47.5 and 53.3 %, respectively. Evidently, the plants with the darker colored blossoms were the most resistant to fluoride injury.

f) Time-concentration fumigations with hydrogen fluoride

Adams et al. (1956) carried out a fluoride fumigation program in August and September, 1953, involving 40 species and/or varieties of plants grown in potted soil. Dry hydrogen fluoride was diluted to one percent with dry nitrogen in compression cylinders. It was then fed into large air streams passing through four plastic-covered houses and a control house in which the air was changed once every two minutes. Fluoride concentrations of 1.5, 5 and 10 pptm, controlled by air analysis, were applied for 8 hours per day, 5 days a week, at the 1.5 pptm level and for 8 and 4 hours per day, respectively, twice a week at the two higher concentrations. Thus, the total nominal weekly exposure in the three treatments was 60, 80 and 80 "hours × pptm." As soon as a plant showed foliar injury due to the fluoride it was removed and analyzed for fluoride in the leaves. Some of the fumigation treatments were carried out in the dark by covering the houses with black cloth.

Results are summarized in Table 25, presenting only the data for treatments that caused incipient foliar injury, except with lilac. The plants are arranged in order of increasing fluoride content associated with injury, which indicates approximately a ten-fold range between the different species, in the amount of fluoride required to cause incipient lesions. Rate of gas uptake by the plants is indicated by the relative exposure and absorption volume. Again, the range is about ten-fold. Gladiolus was injured with one-third the exposure period and with one-tenth the absorbed fluoride required for carrots. It is interesting to note that injury to the sensitive species occurred with about the same, and to the resistant species, with about half, the foliar fluoride level in the dark as in the light.

For a majority of the plants, there is fairly good agreement in the exposure period and the amount of absorbed fluoride required to cause incipient injury at the three atmospheric concentrations. However, some anomalous variations are apparent. Possibly, special environmental factors affected the results at times. For example, one of the lilac fumigations caused no injury with double the exposure and absorption of a duplicate experiment that caused injury. The pines and corn

Table 25. *Exposures of various plants to hydrogen fluoride which caused incipient leaf damage in daylight and in the dark* (ADAMS et al., 1956)

Plant	Daylight								Dark	
	HF = 1.5 pptm		HF = 5 pptm		HF = 10 pptm		HF = Avg		HF = Avg	
	tc[1]	ppm[2]	tc[1]	ppm[2]	tc[1]	ppm[2]	tc[1]	ppm[2]	tc[1]	ppm[2]
Gladiolus . . .	97	37	119	46	137	57	118	47	102	52
Blueberry . . .	97	53	92	72	118	64	103	63	185	69
Pine, *etc*[3]. . . .	438	61	337	73	159	64	311	66	222	61
Apricot, *etc.*[4]. .	196	69	172	79	193	109	187	86	307	72
Rhododendron .	—		360	85	—	—	360	85	—	—
Larch.	107	53	119	147	118	106	115	102	83	68
Arbor vitae . .	318	138	286	104	—	—	302	121	—	—
Corn	—	—	747	178	496	47	622	113	—	—
Grape	—	—	252	138	344	122	298	130	442	68
Squash	—	—	631	134	421	179	526	157	—	—
Lilac[5].	138	123	248	216	—	—	193	170	—	—
Lilac[6].	381	267	381	230	506	123	—	—	—	—
Apple, *etc.*[7] . .	302	179	379	183	346	163	343	175	406	89
Pepper	218	149	274	203	188	244	227	199	188	136
Raspberry. . .	306	243	306	216	183	162	265	207	163	88
Sweet pea . . .	313	327	307	148	374	141	331	205	—	—
Elm, *etc.*[8] . . .	246	227	313	231	300	215	286	224	204	77
Tomato	—	—	327	278	302	207	315	243	—	—
Carrot	284	323	398	723	425	307	369	451	309	280

[1] Summation of hours of fumigation × pptm hydrogen fluoride.
[2] Fluoride in leaves (dry basis).
[3] Average ponderosa, lodgepole and white pine.
[4] Average apricot, cherry, peach and prune.
[5] Lilac—plants injured.
[6] Lilac—plants not injured.
[7] Apple, average of four varieties.
[8] Average elm, mulberry, willow and maple.

required much greater exposure at low concentrations than at high for the absorption of the same amount of fluoride. Correlation coefficients between 0.3 and 0.9 were found for the relationship between the exposure factor and absorbed fluoride in 20 out of 35 of the plants studied. Detailed statistical data for apples are given in Fig. 8.

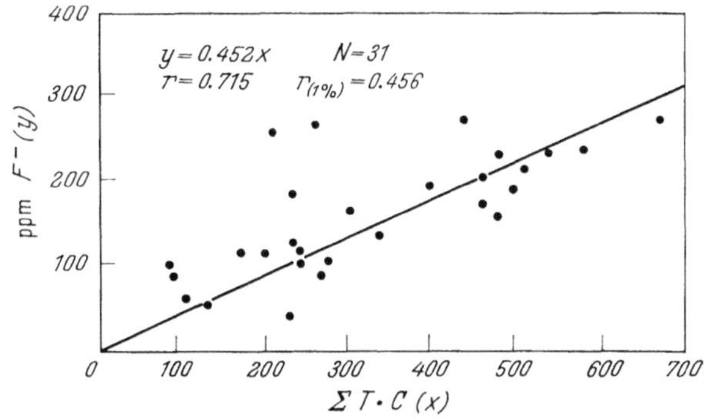

Fig 8. Correlation (r) of foliar fluoride content with exposure factor for apples (ADAMS et al., 1957)

g) Effects on polysaccharides

In a later report, ADAMS and EMERSON (1961) described the application to ponderosa pine trees growing in five-gallon cans of the three foregoing fumigation treatments and, in addition, a fourth treatment with 0.5 pptm hydrogen fluoride, 8 hours per day, 5 days per week, giving a nominal weekly exposure of 20 "hours × pptm." At weekly intervals in July and August, samples of the control and fumigated needles were analyzed for starch and total polysaccharides (Fig. 9). During the first five to six weeks of the experiment, total non-starch polysaccharides in the fumigated needles had an average concentration of about 2.4 % while the controls had 1.5 %. During the last week or two, these values were about 2.2

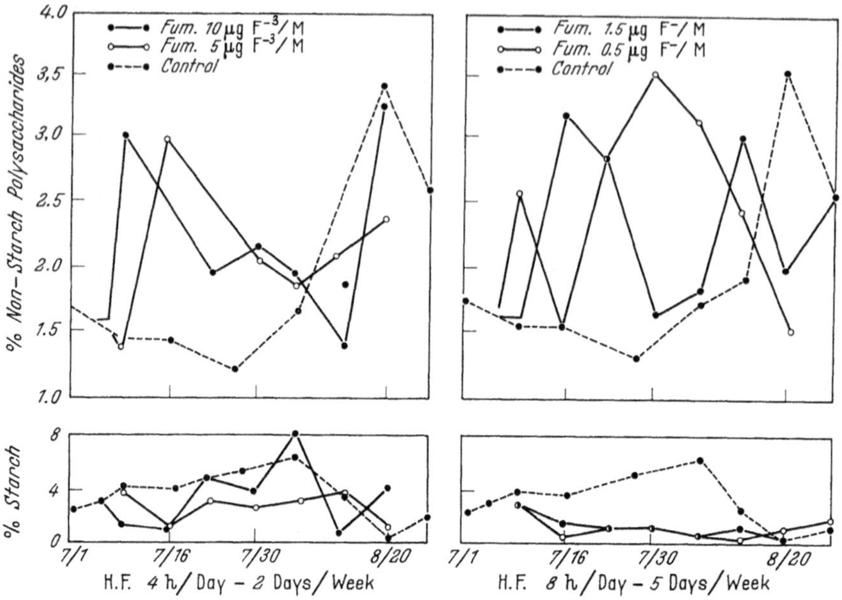

Fig. 9. Starch and non-starch polysaccharides in hydrogen fluoride fumigated and control pine needles (ADAMS and EMERSON, 1961)

and 2.9 %, respectively. The corresponding values for starch were: first five to six weeks – fumigated needles, 0.25 % and controls, 0.41 %; last one to two weeks – fumigated needles, 0.17 % and controls, 0.05 %. The four different fumigation treatments gave similar responses. They all increased the non-starch polysaccharides and decreased the starch by about the same amount. The concentration changes during the last two weeks of the experiments occurred in the control trees, primarily. The significance of the decreased starch and increased non-starch polysaccharides is not known in detail, but enzyme inhibition effects are probably involved.

h) *Effects on growth*

BENEDICT et al. (1964a) fumigated alfalfa, orchard grass, chard, endive, spinach and romaine lettuce growing in sand culture with a range of hydrogen fluoride concentrations from 1 to 100 $\mu g/m^3$ and with exposure periods up to four months. Two 3 × 5 m greenhouses were used in this study, supplied with carbon and lime filtered air and operated at 70–80° F. with a temperature difference of less than 1°.

In an early experiment with 100 $\mu g/m^3$ hydrogen fluoride for 20 days continuous fumigation, alfalfa, orchard grass and romaine lettuce were acutely marked (extent of leaf injury not quantitatively given) while spinach and endive were not marked. Table 26 gives dry weight data for ten plants, also fluoride uptake by the leaves. There was a significant reduction in dry weight of 25 to 41 % in the three plants that were marked as compared with the controls. The unmarked plants showed no significant difference from their controls. Fluoride in the tops of the different plants ranged from 1740 to 2542 ppm.

Table 26. *Fluoride content of tops and dry weight of plants fumigated for 20 days with 100 μg/M³ hydrogen fluoride* (BENEDICT et al., 1964a)

Plant	Dry weight, 10 plants grams		F/C	Fluoride in tops ppm — Dry basis	
	Control	Fumigated	%	Control	Fumigated
Alfalfa	4.00	2.86[1,2]	71	10	1943[1]
Orchard grass	2.24	1.68[1,2]	75	10	2423[1]
Romaine lettuce	1.24	0.73[1,2]	59	23	1740[1]
Endive	0.57	0.53[3]	92	51	2542[1]
Spinach	0.60	0.73[3]	122	35	2074[1]

[1] Difference between fumigated and control values significant at 1% level.
[2] Typical fluoride injury on leaves.
[3] Leaves uninjured.

A second experiment, Table 27, with 0.9 μg/m³ hydrogen fluoride for 120 days, produced no significant effect on the weight of the plants or plant parts although fluoride in the leaves ranged from 178 to 229 ppm in the different plants. The roots showed little or no increase in fluoride content above the controls.

Table 27. *Dry weight and fluoride content of plants fumigated 120 days with 0.9 μg/M³ hydrogen fluoride* (BENEDICT et al., 1964a)

Plants		Dry weight, 10 plants grams		Fluoride ppm — Dry basis	
		Control	Fumigated	Control	Fumigated
Alfalfa	Tops	13.3	13.2	6	178
	Roots	3.2	3.0	8	13
Orchard grass	Leaves	15.3	15.2	11	229
	Roots	3.2	3.1	30	28
Chard	Leaves	16.3	13.9	11	215
	Petioles	5.8	6.5	4	6
	Roots	10.3	9.0	23	22
Romaine[1]	Leaves	9.4	11.1	18	195
Lettuce	Stems	15.3	13.2	2	10
	Roots	3.0	2.0	17	24

[1] Plants bolted.

i) Histological studies of fluoride injury

SOLBERG and ADAMS (1956) carried out an histological study of ponderosa pine needles that were injured by hydrogen fluoride. They also observed the leaves of dicotyledonous plants injured by both hydrogen fluoride and sulfur dioxide. The histological responses to the two gases were indistinguishable, but the location of the injury on the leaves differed.

Acute hydrogen fluoride injury to pine needles started with browning at the apex and progressed gradually downward. It consisted of inward collapse of the interior needle surfaces. Immediately adjacent to the macroscopically browned areas, microscopic changes in the green tissue could be seen, representing a narrow transition zone between necrotic and healthy tissue. The mesophyll cells exhibited granulation, vacuolation, and finally, total collapse. The endodermal cells were

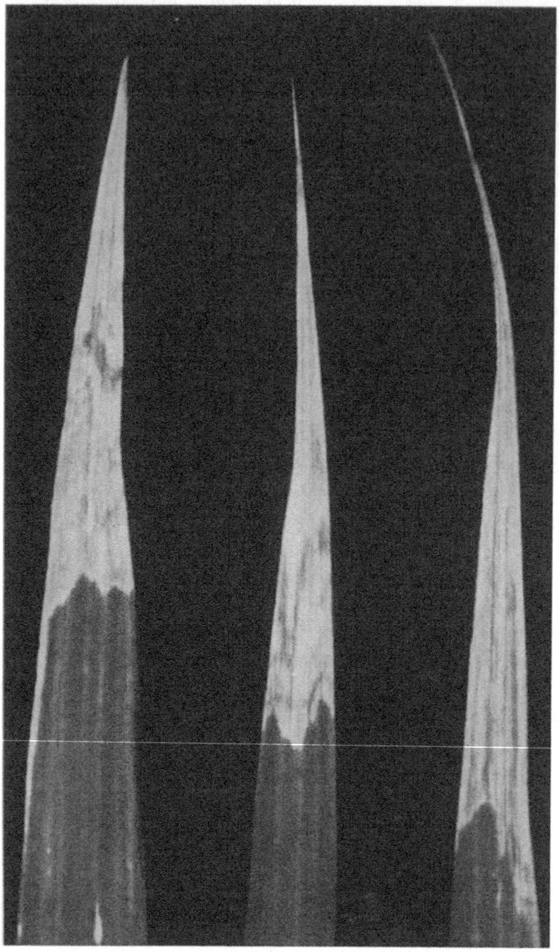

Plate 1. Gladiolus leaf damage by fluorides from the air

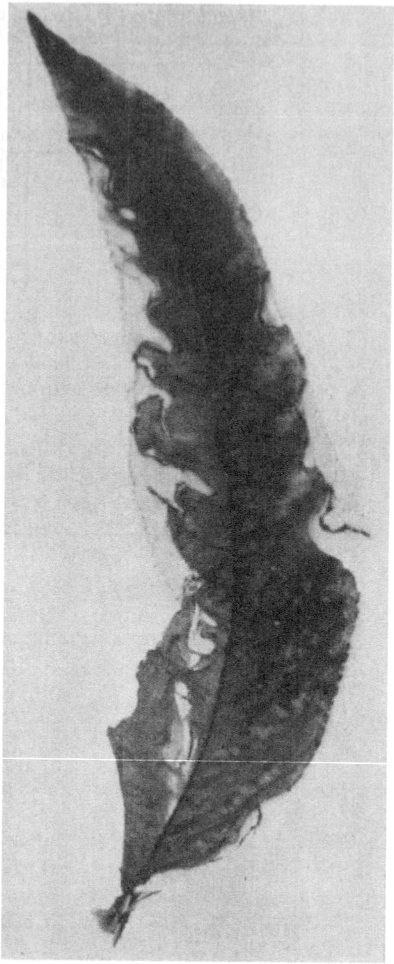

Plate 2. Acute hydrogen fluoride injury on peach

distorted, and there was extreme plasmolysis of cells in the epidermis and hypodermis. The transfusion parenchyma cells, the parenchyma cells of phloem and xylem and the epithelial cells in the resin ducts were all enlarged, even to the extent of distorting adjacent tracheidal cells, collapsing the phloem against the xylem and occluding the resin ducts. Only the xylem remained intact because of the thickness of their cell walls. The margins of the leaves of dicotyledonous plants were the site of initial response to fluoride intoxication characterized first by a collapse of the spongy mesophyll and lower epidermis, then distortion and disruption of the chloroplasts of the palisade cells, and finally, distortion and collapse of the upper epidermis. This area of the leaf dried to an ivory, brown or red color, depending on the species. This process proceeded inward until a substantial portion of the leaf surface was involved.

The foregoing histological observations were confirmed by TRESHOW (1956) who sought to determine the earliest observable anatomical effects prior to the

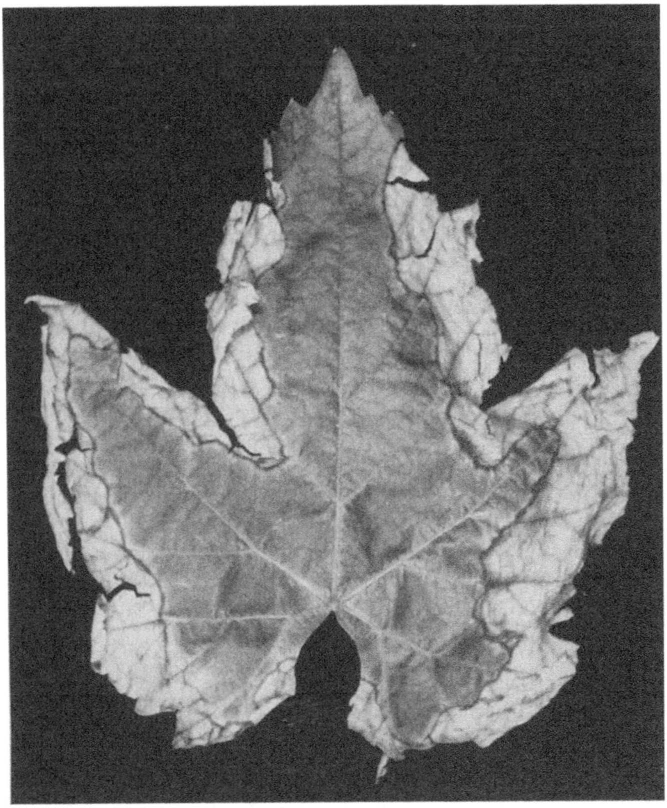

Plate 3. Acute hydrogen fluoride injury on grape

characteristic marginal necrosis on the leaves of Chinese apricots and prunes subjected to fumigation with hydrogen fluoride. Cell size, turgidity, starch content and suberization were observed on handcut sections. A narrow necrotic band spread from the tips of the leaf serrations after the appearance of macroscopically visible necrosis. This band was less than 2 mm wide and consisted of partly plasmolyzed spongy parenchyme and palisade cells adjacent to the necrotic areas. Epidermal cells looked normal, even those over the necrotic mesophyll. Cell size, starch content and suberization were normal in the areas immediately adjacent to the injured cells.

Plate 1 is a photograph of injured gladiolus leaves showing the characteristic sharp transition from the necrotic to the uninjured areas. Plates 2 and 3 depict grape and peach leaves injured by hydrogen fluoride. Excellent photographs in color of the leaves of a number of fluoride-injured plants have been published by MIDDLETON et al. (1956) and by THOMAS (1961).

4. Soft suture of peaches

a) *Occurrence*

A serious disorder in peach orchards near Wenatchee, Washington, involving a local premature ripening of the fruit, along the suture toward its stylar end, has been ascribed by Benson (1959) to fluoride emitted into the atmosphere by a neighboring aluminum factory. Surveys by Benson and others have indicated that this disorder can be found wherever peaches are grown near fluoride emitting industries. Fluoride sprays produce effects that are indistinguishable from the foregoing, while the hormone sprays, 2, 4 D and 2, 4, 5 T, cause similar but distinguishable lesions which have been described and illustrated with color photographs by Richards and Cochran (1956). Soft suture, closely resembling the fluoride type, may be caused by a number of other agencies, including viruses, also deficiencies of calcium and perhaps, of boron.

Dorsey and McMunn (1944) discussed "soft suture" as a disorder related to overloading of the tree with fruit. Recommended control consisted of cultural practices which maintained the trees in good vigor by pruning, nitrate applications and further thinning of the fruit after the June drop.

The disorder was also described by Hildebrand (1943). It occurred in an Elberta peach orchard on the shore of Lake Ontario, in Wayne county, New York. Similar or identical lesions were seen by the same observer in 1940 in the Niagara Peninsula of Ontario, Canada. The cause was not ascertained. No bacteria or fungi could be isolated and a virus origin was suggested. Anderson (1926, 1931) had previously noted that the use of sodium fluorosilicate sprays for the effective control of bacterial spot of peach had the disadvantage of causing a premature ripening of the fruit which "had a higher color, was somewhat smaller and had a peculiar mottled green area at the tip . . ." Later, in his book, *Diseases of Fruit Crops* (1956, pp. 306–307) Anderson wrote, ". . . the condition brought about by fluoride sprays was called 'soft suture' and resembles in many respects the virus disease of peach known as 'red suture.' The fruit matures several days ahead of normal ripening. The suture takes on a yellowish-red to deep-red color and softens even while the remainder of the fruit is quite firm. No decided difference is noted in the taste of the fruit but the soft suture is easily bruised in packing and the fruit becomes unsightly." Economic losses may be very large.

McCornack et al. (1952) described a rather recently-observed black spot condition at the tip of peaches growing in an area within 4 to 12 miles of the steel factory at Fontana, California. "The disorder is similar in appearance to blossom-end rot of tomatoes, suggesting that it may be caused by some factor which interferes with water uptake or translocation." Symptoms consisted of black, generally circular, sunken areas at the blossom end of the fruit with a gum pocket underneath the spot. These lesions are quite different from "soft suture." The cause was not ascertained. Both drought and chemical injury were suspected. Fluoride from the World War II steel plant was suggested as a possible cause. Further investigation was promised but nothing more has been published. The orchards were removed shortly after this study.

b) *Experimental studies*

Benson (1959) has studied the possibility of a fluoride etiology for the soft suture in orchards near Wenatchee, Washington. He sprayed control trees weekly with dilute solutions of various fluorine salts from April 30 to harvest. The 0.05% solution of ammonium fluoride caused soft suture on 68 to 100% of treated fruit of different varieties. Various amounts of soft suture were produced by the other salts. Benson also fumigated peach trees with fumes made by passing dry air through molten cryolite heated at 900° C. Subsequently, the cryolite fumes were washed with a water spray to remove hydrogen fluoride, then diluted with excess air. Three trees, each enclosed in an eight-foot-cube polyethylene-covered chamber, were fumigated in series, with additional dilution of the cryolite fumes in both the second and third chambers. Overnight (14-hour) fumigations were applied twice a week for three months.

Fluorine concentrations, found by drawing samples of the air through filter paper, were as follows: first tree, 14 to 58 pptm fluorine; second tree, 10 to 18 pptm; third tree, 3 to 19 pptm. The air which passed the filter paper was analyzed at first by impingers, but these analyses were discontinued when they "failed to show more than a few micrograms of fluoride." It is known that filter paper absorbs hydrogen fluoride readily. Presumably, some gaseous fluoride was present in the pptm or sub-pptm range which might account for the effects described. The leaves on the three trees accumulated maximum fluorine contents of 60, 29 and 25 ppm, respectively, in three months while the fruit peel absorbed 16, 11 and 13 ppm in two months, or 55, 7 and 11 ppm in three months. Soft suture developed on 91, 31 and 25% of the fruits, respectively. It may be noted that in the center of the polluted area where considerable soft suture was encountered, the leaves had absorbed 112 ppm on August 20, and the fruit peel, 34 ppm. Air analyses are not given but the concentrations are known to be of the order of 1 pptm or less.

In 1956, Benson sprayed trees of three varieties in the polluted area with lime sprays (10 pounds per 100 gallons) weekly, from post-full bloom to harvest. Zero to two percent of the fruit showed soft suture on the sprayed trees and 24 to 77% on the unsprayed trees.

Table 28. *The effect of date of application of lime sprays in preventing soft suture of peach in an area subjected to industrial fluoride fumigation* (Benson, 1957)

Sprays No.	Dates	Number Normal fruit Hale %	Elberta %
0	—	12	12
1	May 6	19	68
1	July 8	48	80
2	June 10 and 17	76	92
3	May 6, June 3, July 15	90	95
3[1]	May 13, June 3, July 8	100	94
3	Apr. 29 to May 13[2]	23	71
5	Apr. 29 to May 27	28	69
10	Apr. 29 to July 1[2]	99	88
13	Apr. 29 to July 22[2]	100	89
5	July 29 to Aug. 26[2]	30	54
8	July 8 to Aug. 26[2]	40	78
10	June 24 to Aug. 26[2]	97	95
13	June 3 to Aug. 26[2]	100	98

[1] Calcium chloride sprays; all others lime sprays.
[2] Applied weekly.

In 1957, the lime spraying program was designed to indicate the time when the sprays would be most effective in protecting the fruit from soft suture. Weekly sprays were applied according to 18 different schedules. Representative data are summarized in Table 28. It was noted that pit hardening began on June 19 and the period of retarded fruit enlargement extended from June 21 to July 20. The latter dates also covered the period when the sprays were most effective in preventing soft suture. A single spray as early as May 6 increased the yield of normal fruit appreciably above the "no spray" treatment and a single spray on July 8, or a spray at both June 10 and 17, increased the yield still more. Three sprays, spaced at about monthly intervals in May, June and July, gave nearly complete protection. The same was true of weekly sprays on the same tree extending through May and June, or starting June 24 and extending through July and

August. Evidently, in the latter treatments, the earlier spraying in May and the later spraying in August were unnecessary. Calcium chloride was at least as effective as lime as a spray material.

PILCHER (1958) reviewed the literature on soft suture and described experimental work by personnel of the Aluminum Company of America in the same Columbia River orchards which were studied by BENSON. Following are the principal results reported by PILCHER:

(1) Some entire orchards within the area were completely normal and some were apparently randomly affected with "suture red spot," with no obvious correlation between degree of affectation and location of fluoride levels.

(2) Samples of fruit from the area were tested for virus by the Dalzell-Reid hemaglutination test. "The results suggest that all the peaches were carrying a virus and that the concentration of the virus is much greater in the fruit showing suture trouble." However, the tests *per se* do not "establish the fact that a detected virus was responsible for symptoms observed."

(3) Ammonium fluoride sprays with 11 and 22 ppm fluoride gave fruit with 3 to 10 and 11 to 38% of "suture red spot," respectively. This tends to support BENSON's results with higher fluoride concentrations.

(4) BENSON's observations of the beneficial action of calcium sprays were confirmed. Boron sprays were also fairly effective in preventing soft suture. Potassium phosphate and magnesium salts were less effective.

Evidently, the problem is complex and it is difficult to make a decision as to the actual cause of a disorder that can involve several factors.

c) Calcium metabolism in peach

Soft suture in peaches, when due to fluorides, appears to be caused by interference with the calcium metabolism of the fruit and embryo, due probably to the precipitation of insoluble calcium fluoride. BIDDULPH (peronal communication, 1962) has carried out experiments on calcium transport in peaches which may be related to the soft suture problem, although he neither studied nor drew conclusions with regard to the action of fluorine compounds. He dipped fruit growing on the tree in a 0.22% solution of calcium chloride containing 57 microcuries per milliliter of Ca^{45} at the time the pit was commencing to harden (June 13). Cross-sections of the fruit were taken two weeks later (June 27), and cross, radial and tangental sections, five weeks later (July 18) for radioautographs and counting. Special attention was devoted to the suture area and also to the kernel and embryo.

The surface-deposited radiocalcium moved into the fruit to the embryo along with calcium supplied by the tree. Minimum transport occurred when the tree was not given extra calcium. Maximum transport occurred when the tree was given a calcium treatment the day before the fruit was dipped. The flesh of the fruit served as a calcium reservoir. A gradient was established from the flesh to the embryo with the major vascular connections passing through the apical suture area where "soft suture" develops. The autographs show these vascular tissues to be laden with Ca^{45} which must be in transit from the surface of the fruit to the embryo where it accumulates. Presumably, this region would be particularly vulnerable to a calcium deficiency, if the supply were reduced or cut off by precipitation of calcium fluoride, because of ready gradient transport to the embryo. Premature breakdown of the tissues might then be expected.

IX. Relative susceptibility of plant species to fluoride

In view of the wide range in the susceptibility of different species of plants, and even of different varieties in the species, to injury by hydrogen fluoride,

Table 29. *Relative sensitivity of cultivated and native plants to injury by hydrogen fluoride*

Sensitive		Intermediate		Resistant	
		Cultivated plants			
Class 1		*Class 3*		*Class 5*	
Gladiolus	ABC	Corn (Golden Cross Bantam)	B	Columbine and Canterbury bell	A
Pine (young needles)	B	Pepper (Calif. Wonder)	C	Dogwood and lilac	C
Apricot (Chinese)	BR	Raspberry (Washington)	C	Lobelia and petunia	A
Azalea	C	Aster and sweet William	A	Rose	B
Blueberry (Jersey)	C	Dahlia (immature leaves)	A	Apple (red Jonathon)	C
Prune (Italian PRH 1)	C	Dahlia	C	Live oak and pine	B
Tulip	B	Petunia petals	A	Tomato	ABC
Jerusalem cherry	B	Clover	B	*Class 6*	
Class 2		Barley, flax, oats, and rye (young plants)	A	Alfalfa (Ranger)	C
Milo maize	B	Apple (Delicious), cherry (Bing)	C	Corn (Golden Cross bantam)	C
Corn (Dixie 17, Funk 134 and 512)	B	Apple	B	Cotton	A
Corn (Spancross)	B	Birch, hawthorne, silver maple, mountain ash, mulberry, sycamore, and yellow willow	C	Tobacco	BC
Corn (bantam)	A	Peach	AB	Bean and celery	B
Sweet potato (Triumph)	B	Iris and begonia	B	Cucumber and squash	B
Apricot (Moorpark)	ABC	*Class 4*		Squash (Hubbard and zucchini)	AC
Prune (late Italian)	AB	Azalea	BC	Cabbage, cauliflower, eggplant, onion, pepper and soybean	A
Peach (some varieties under best conditions)	B	Begonia (some varieties)	B	Parsnips (hollow crown)	C
Peach (Elberta, Lovell stock)	C	Rose, geranium, coleus, lilac, spirea	B	Tomato (Marglobe)	C
Strawberry (Marshall)	C	Verbena	A	Chrysanthemum	AB
Grapes (some European varieties)	RW	Alfalfa	AB	Marigold, privet, and snapdragon	A
Iris	AB	Clover	B	Sweet pea (Spencer hybrid)	C
		Red clover	C	Rhododendron (Pink Pearl)	C
		Bean (Tendergreen bush)	C	Rose (Talisman)	C
		Carrot (Chantenay)	C	Zinnia	B
		Carrot	A	Citrus	A
		Grape (Concord)	CR	Laurel and locust	C
		Lettuce	C	Pine (old needles)	B
		Sweet potato (Nigger Killer)	B	Carrot	C
		Parsnip, peas, potato, rhubarb, spinach, sugar beet	A	Petunia	C
		Wheat	A		
		Barberry, bridal wreath, honeysuckle, and mock orange	A		
		Apple (Wealthy and Winesap)	C		
		Arbor vitae	C		

Table 29 (contd.)

Sensitive		Intermediate		Resistant	
		Native plants			
Class 1		*Class 3*		*Class 5*	
Pine (ponderosa, young needles	BC	Pokeweed, crabgrass	B	Pigweed dock	B
Larch	C	Smartweed Johnson grass	B	Carpet weed	B
Hypericum	B	Oxalis	B	Pine (lodgepole)	C
Class 2		Chickweed, barnyard grass	B	Pine (ponderosa, old needles)	C
Crabgrass	B	*Class 4*		*Class 6*	
Cattail	B	Pokeweed, pigweed lamb's quarters, dock, plantain	B	Dandelion, plantain, purslane, galinsoga, bidens, nightshade, and ragweed	B
Johnson grass, oxalis, smartweed	B			Douglas fir, grand fir, hemlock, white pine, Engelmann spruce	C
Buckwheat	B				
Pine (ponderosa, 3—4 month old needles)	C				

Source: Thomas and Hendricks (1956). By permission from "Air Pollution Handbook," by P. L. Magill, F. R. Holden and C. Ackley, editors. Copyright 1956. McGraw-Hill Book Co., Inc.

Concentrations required to cause slight injury in 7—9 days: classes 1 and 2 = 5 pptm or less; class 3 = 5—10 pptm; classes 4, 5 and 6 = more than 10 pptm.

A = American Smelting and Refining Company. — B = Boyce Thompson Institute. C = State College, Washington. — R = B. L. Richards. — W = F. W. Went.

Table 30. *Relative susceptibility to injury by hydrogen fluoride fumigation of different species and varieties of plants* (Zimmerman and Hitchcock, 1956)

Plant	Susceptibility[1]	Plant	Susceptibility[2]
Jerusalem cherry	4	Grape	S
Gladiolus sp	4	Hypernicum	S
Tulip	4	Regal lily	S
Milo maize	3	Peach	S
Ixora Sp.	3	Blueberry	S-I
Field corn	3	Azalea	I
Apricot (Moorpark)	3	Begonia	I
Prune (Italian)	3	Deutzia	I
Buckwheat	2	Honeysuckle	I
Smart weed, Grape (wild)	2	Lilac	I
Sweet corn, Iris	2	Peanut	I
Sweet potato, Apple	2	Plum	I
Lambsquarters	1	Pokeweed	I
Rose, Dock	1	Spirea	I
Stevia, Cotton	0	Chicory Sp	R
Turkish tobacco, Taxas Sp.	0	Cinquefoil	R
Bean, Chicory, Dandelion	0	Hibiscus	R
Spanish needles	0	Lettuce	R
Nightshade, Celery	0	Lilium speciosium	R
Tomato, Pumpkin	0	Philadelphius	R
Cucumber, Pigweed	0	Plantain	R
Alfalfa, Sweet clover	0	Purslane	R
Coleus, Geranium	0	Strawberry	R
Buttonbush, Eggplant	0	Weigelia	R
Galinsoga	0		

[1] Fumigation treatment: 50 pptm for 8 hours. 0 = no markings; 1 = slight markings; 2, 3, 4 = moderate to pronounced marking.

[2] Fumigation treatments: 1 to 100 pptm for 1 to 8 days. S = susceptible; I = intermediate; R = resistant.

THOMAS and HENDRICKS (1956) prepared Table 29 which summarized the experience of three laboratories and two independent investigators with regard to these relative responses. The attempt was made to classify the plants in six classes according to the concentration of the gas that would be required to cause "slight" injury in 7 to 9 days. This necessitated some calculations to allow for differences in the fumigation treatments. Cultivated and native plants are listed separately.

ZIMMERMAN and HITCHCOCK (1956) fumigated one group of 40 species and varieties of plants with 50 pptm hydrogen fluoride for 4 to 8 hours, and a second group of 28 other species and varieties with 1 to 100 pptm for 1 to 8 days. Susceptibility to injury on a scale of 0 to 4, with 0 representing no markings, and 4, pronounced markings, is given for the first group of plants in the first and second columns of Table 30. The second group is summarized in the third and fourth columns, with designations of "susceptible" (S), "intermediate" (I) and "resistant" (R) to characterize the fluoride effects.

The two tables are in fairly good agreement so far as they are comparable. It will be noted that different varieties of the same plant often vary considerably in their susceptibilities. Possibly some of the discrepancies in the tables are due to inaccurate identification of the varieties. However, there is no doubt as to resistant and sensitive plants. Small differences between species present considerable uncertainty.

X. Chemical and enzymatic effects of fluorides in plants

The mechanisms of the toxic properties of fluorides in plants are imperfectly understood at this time. It is known that fluoride exerts a strong inhibiting action on certain enzymes but it is not known why there is such a wide range of tolerance to fluoride in the leaves of different species, or even in the varieties within a single species. Some plants (*e.g.*, cotton) can tolerate 5000 ppm fluoride in the leaves; others are injured by less than 100 ppm. The role of both inorganic and organic fluorine compounds in plants is obscure, qualitatively and quantitatively.

LIPMAN (1929) assumed that enzyme inhibition by fluoride was due to an easily dissociable chemical combination between the enzyme and fluoride. The reaction obeys the requirements of the mass-action law. For example, methaemoglobin (M) + $F^- \rightleftharpoons MF$ is a monomolecular reaction which is displaced to the right by increasing acidity. Fluoride inhibition of lipase and fluoride inhibition of the decomposition of hydrogen peroxide by Fe^{+++} were cited as similar examples.

A. Inorganic fluorine compounds

The solubility of sodium fluoride is 4.8 g, and of potassium fluoride, 92 g per 100 g of water. Magnesium fluoride is only slightly soluble (130 ppm) while calcium fluoride is sufficiently insoluble (18 ppm) to interfere with calcium metabolism in the plant, as appears to be the case with soft suture of peaches, already described. The low solubility of magnesium fluoride may be a factor in the inactivation of magnesium bearing enzymes.

Fluoride has a strong tendency to form complex compounds of many kinds, some of which have biological significance (BOREI, 1945). For example, ferric salts complex readily with fluoride to form $(FeF_6)^{---}$, a reaction that can compete with the ferric reactions of many organic compounds such as dihydroxymaleic acid or catechol which form stable iron complexes also.

Fluoride reacts with the prosthetic groups of many haemoproteins, which always contain trivalent iron, including methaemoglobin, peroxidase, catalase and cytochrome C, usually causing more or less inhibition of the biological activity of the haemoprotein. The reaction is with the iron complex, not with the iron alone.

Fluoride forms fluoromanganates of the type $(MnF_5)^{--}$ and $(MnF_3)^{--}$ which inhibit the catalytic properties of manganic and manganous ions in permanganate oxidations of compounds like lactic, tartaric and oxalic acids.

B. Organic fluorine compounds

RECKENDORFER (1952, 1953) discussed invisible and visible fluoride injury to the leaves of plants. He postulated that when moderate amounts of hydrogen fluoride were absorbed into the leaf through the stomata, this fluoride was precipitated at first as insoluble calcium fluoride, rendering the gas more or less innocuous. If the supply of calcium was insufficient to precipitate all the fluoride, magnesium fluoride would be thrown down next, resulting in removal of magnesium from chlorophyll and magnesium-activated enzymes (such as enolase). This would cause premature aging of the leaves with the production of early autumnal coloring which the author has observed near fluoride-emitting industries.

Part of the absorbed fluoride may become organically bound, rendering it ether-soluble. The dark-brown necrotic areas of fluoride-injured cherry leaves were carefully cut away from the green areas and the two samples were analyzed separately. Total fluorine in the necrotic and green areas were 308 and 189 ppm respectively, and the corresponding ether-soluble values were $308 - 114 = 194$ ppm and $189 - 175 = 14$ ppm. Evidently, the necrotic areas had considerably more ether-soluble fluorine than the green areas. This suggests the possibility of the formation of organic fluorine compounds in the fumigated leaves due to the uptake of gaseous fluoride.

BENEDICT et al. (1964a) employed the soxhlet apparatus to extract with various solvents, alfalfa leaves and orchard grass tips which had been fumigated with hydrogen fluoride at 1 $\mu g/M^3$ for about 35 days without, however, causing any leaf lesions. The alfalfa contained 324 ppm fluorine and the orchard grass, 590 ppm. Four organic solvents in series extracted 14–17% of the fluorine in the leaves. Water extracted 65–75% from the alfalfa and 50–60% from the orchard grass; 19 and 32%, respectively, remained in the residue. Again, the presence of organic fluorine compounds in the fumigated leaves is suggested.

The South African plant, *Dichapetalum cymosum* (gifblaar) accumulates fluoroacetate which is toxic to animals. PETERS et al. (1953) have shown that the toxicity is due to an enzymatic reaction in the animal which changes the relatively non-toxic fluoroacetate to fluorocitrate. The latter "jams" the citric acid reactions in the tricarboxylic acid cycle and inhibits the disappearance of 300 times its weight of citric acid in 30 min. PETERS (1954) (Fig. 10) has discussed the unusual case of a relatively non-toxic compound being converted into a very toxic compound by enzymatic reactions in the animal.

PETERS and HALL (1960) isolated fluoroöleic acid from the seeds of *Dichapetalum toxicarium* (ratsbane). They also isolated in small amounts, a long chain fluoro-fatty acid with 16 to 18 carbon atoms, one fluorine and one double bond. Fluoroacetate was present only in traces. The plant causes a paralytic condition in man called "brokeback." The leaves of *D. toxicarium* had no detectable fluorine but the seeds had over 2000 μg fluorine per gram. Samples of *D. cymosum* had 70 to 270 μg fluorine per gram in the leaves while the seeds were fluorine-free. *D. cymosum* plants grown in England had 112 μg fluorine per gram while other grasses and alfalfa in the same location had 9 to 36 μg fluorine per gram. Six other species of *Dichapetalum* were examined and found to be less toxic to animals than toxicarium and cymosum.

It is interesting to note that a wide range in toxicity is exhibited by different organic fluorine compounds which are not greatly different from each other structurally. McCombie and Saunders (1946) have cited an extremely interesting example. Di-isopropylfluorophosphonate inhibits the enzyme choline esterase at a concentration of 10^{-10} M, whereas di-ammonium fluorophosphonate requires a concentration of 10^{-2} M to cause 50% inhibition.

Salisbury and Bonner (1960) completely inhibited flowering of cocklebur *(Xanthium pensylvanicus)* by applying the pyrimidine, 5-fluorouracil (5-FU) to the bud at the beginning of the dark period. They ascribed this inhibition to interference with processes in the bud which occur during the dark period and are essential to photoperiodic induction of flowering. Bonner and Zeevaart (1962) studied the synthesis of ribonucleic acid (RNA) and the multiplication of desoxyribonucleic acid (DNA) in the bud to explain this inhibition of flowering by 5-FU. When the latter is applied to the leaves, it is translocated to the bud but does not move in the opposite direction, indicating that the inhibition occurs entirely in the bud. Multiplication of DNA is inhibited by both 5-FU and another inhibitor, 5-fluorodeoxyuridine (5-FDU) which acts specifically on DNA and interferes only slightly with RNA synthesis. By using both inhibitors and two antidotes, orotic acid and thymidine, it was shown that DNA multiplication during the dark period is not essential to flowering, whereas RNA synthesis is essential in the *Xanthium* bud.

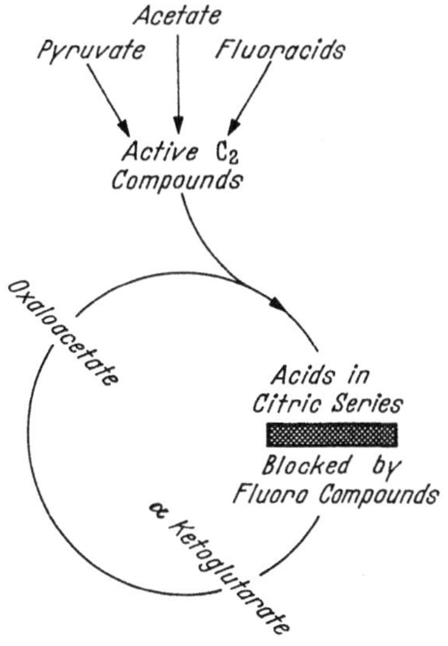

Fig. 10. Peters' "Jamming Theory." After activation to a C_2 fragment, fluoroacetate is condensed to form fluorocitrate (Peters, 1954)

Zeevaart (1962) found that 5-FU completely inhibits flowering in *Pharbitus nil* by suppressing DNA multiplication in the apex of the shoot. 5-FDU is 1000 times more effective than 5-FU as a flower inhibitor in this plant. Evidently, flowering in *Pharbitus nil* is controlled primarily by DNA multiplication in the plumule. Production of the floral stimulus in the cotyledons is not inhibited.

C. Enzyme inhibition by fluoride

1. Enolase

Lohmann and Meyerhoff (1934) studied the apparent hydrolysis of phosphoglyceric acid to form pyruvic and phosphoric acids as an essential step in glycolysis and fermentation. The reaction is not a simple hydrolysis but involves an enzyme-mediated, intramolecular transfer of oxygen in the presence of a coenzyme system, magnesium and adenylpyrophosphoric acid. This enzyme, which can be inhibited by fluoride, was identified by Warburg and Christian (1941a, b, 1942) as a magnesium phosphoprotein, enolase. Its inhibition by fluoride was found to be due to the formation of a magnesium fluorophosphate complex with the enzyme. With higher fluoride concentrations inactive magnesium fluoroenolase is also formed. Manganese or zinc can replace magnesium in enolase. Treatment with fluoride forms analogous inactive manganese or zinc fluoroenolase complexes. Other magnesium-protein enzymes can also be inactivated by fluoride, evidently by mechanisms analogous to those described for enolase. These include cocarboxylase and certain phosphatases from yeast, liver, kidney, *etc.* Some zinc phosphoproteins are not inactivated by fluoride. The rate equation for enolase as given by WARBURG and CHRISTIAN (1942) is

$$[Mg]\,[F^2]\,[PO_4] \times \frac{\%\ \text{Residual Activity}}{\%\ \text{Inhibited Activity}} = K = 3.2 \times 10^{-12}\,.$$

MILLER (1958) prepared pure enolase from pea seed, and found it similar to enolase from yeast. The relative activating capacities of Mg^{++}, Mn^{++}, Co^{++}, Zn^{++} and Ca^{++} were 1.0, 0.41, 0.30, 0.07, and 0.00, respectively. This compares with the activating capacity for Mg^{++}, Mn^{++} and Zn^{++} at 10^{-3} M by MALMSTROM (1953) using purified enzyme, of 1.00, 0.43, and 0.42. The discrepancy in the zinc value was not explained. Miller calculated the constant K in the foregoing equation from a range of values of the variables in the equation and found the average $K = 7 \times 10^{-12}$.

2. Cellular oxidation

BOREI (1945) has reviewed the literature to 1945 on inhibition by fluoride of cellular oxidation, with special reference to the work of RINNSTRÖM and coworkers

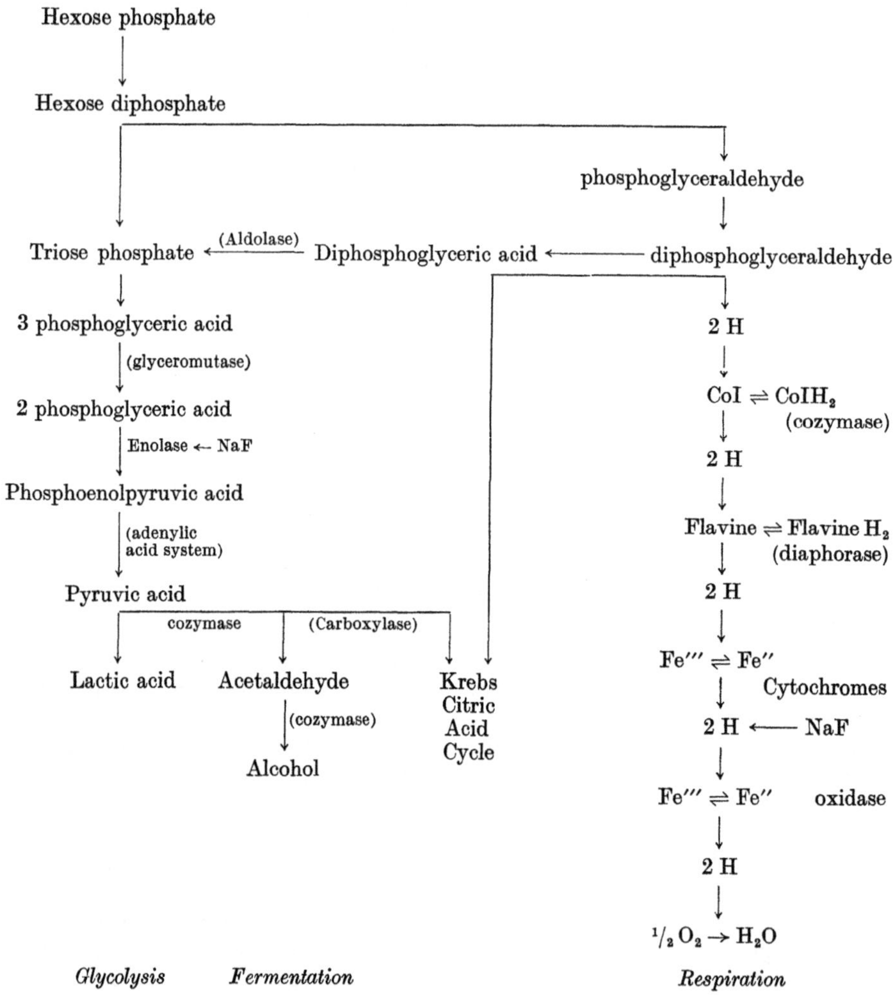

Fig. 11. Processe of glycolysis, fermentation and respiration including points of inhibition by fluoride (BOREI 1945)

at the Institute for Experimental Biology at the University of Stockholm. A scheme for the principal steps in glycolysis, fermentation, respiration and hydrogen transport in the oxidative processes in the cell is shown in Fig. 11. Fluoride inhibition of enolase and also of the cytochromes is indicated. Direct oxidation of primary triose phosphates seems to play a leading part in cell respiration.

The cytochrome system is coupled into the Krebs cycle at several points. An accumulation of phosphoglyceric acid due to fluoride inhibition of enolase will act indirectly on the cytochrome system. Fluoride and cytochrome oxidase compete for cytochrome C; two atoms of fluoride combine with one molecule of cytochrome C.

The transformation of glucose in intact bakers' yeast by respiration or fermentation is susceptible to the inhibiting action of fluoride. However, the degree of fluoride inhibition is smaller the more rapid the turnover of substrate in the cells. If the glucose is added to the yeast before the fluoride so that the respiration and fermentation processes are proceeding rapidly, inhibition by subsequently added fluoride is much less than if the additions are made in the reverse order. Pretreatment with fluoride thus enhances the inhibition, which is greater the longer the period of pretreatment. Fluoride inhibition is greatest under anaerobic conditions and when the yeast is starved, whereas under aerobic conditions the inhibiting power is greatly reduced. In fact, with low concentrations of fluoride there may be a stimulation of respiration and/or fermentation.

The greater sensitivity of starved yeast to fluoride inhibition and the protective action of added substrate cannot be explained by differences in the permeability of the cells to glucose or fluoride because the starved cells are more permeable than normal cells. It is suggested that the fluoride effects may be due to variations in the orthophosphate content of the cells which decreases when the substrate is respired or fermented, and increases when these processes are stopped. The phosphate level is higher under anaerobic than aerobic conditions; also, higher in starved than control cells. The extra phosphate could thus favor the formation of magnesium fluorophosphate enolase.

Chaix and Fromageot (1939) reported that 0.02 M fluoride inhibits the anaerobic degradation of glucose and lactic acid by the nonproliferating *Propionibacterium pentosaceum* and affects pyruvic acid similarly to a slight extent. Aerobic degradation is hardly affected at all. Iodoacetate at 0.0004 M inhibits like fluoride.

3. Metabolism of fructose diphosphate and glycerol

Stumpf (1948, 1950) and Tewfik and Stumpf (1949, 1951) studied carbohydrate metabolism in higher plants. The enzyme aldolase was prepared in concentrated form from pea seeds after an elaborate purification process. It catalyzes the decomposition of 1—6 fructose diphosphate (FDP) to dihydroxyacetone phosphate and 3-phosphoglyceraldehyde. Its central role in the transformation of sugars in plants is suggested by its presence in all forms of vegetation from fungi to the higher plants and in all plant parts from seeds and roots to leaves, flowers and fruits. Actively growing plant tissues carry the most aldolase.

Fluoride does not inhibit the aldolase reactions but stops subsequent glycolysis by inhibition of enolase. There was a marked difference between the enzymes in pea seed and pea leaves. The former oxidized FDP to carbon dioxide by the conventional glycolytic pathway. Daily extracts from the pea plant showed a steady decrease in glycolytic activity from the first to the eighth day after germination. On the sixth day, only the cotyledon had any activity. Stumpf showed that the pea leaf extract was lacking in triose phosphate dehydrogenase which was present in the pea seed extract. The leaf extract oxidizes FDP by a pathway that is not inhibited by fluoride, cyanide or iodo-acetamide which suggests that enolase, cytochrome oxidase, ascorbic acid oxidase and triosephosphate dehydrogenase are not involved.

STUMPF (1955, 1957) followed the oxidation of glycerol-1-C^{14} as a phase of fat metabolism. The glycerol, in the presence of enzymes and mitochondria from peanut cotyledons, was converted first to α-glycerol phosphate, then was dehydrogenated to dihydroxyacetone phosphate. The reactions proceeded via the glycolytic system to pyruvic acid and finally through the tricarboxylic cycle to produce carbon dioxide. Fluoride (0.01 N) inhibited the glycolytic system from glycerol as it did from FDP.

D. Fluoride effects on carotenoids and chlorophyll

VOGT-BEEKMANN (1954) determined the carotenoids in etiolated wheat sprouts by benzene extraction and chromatography. The carotenoid concentration increased continuously for the first 8 days of growth, remained constant for 4 days, then decreased rapidly. Glucose feeding maintained the rate of synthesis. Xanthophyll exceeded carotene in the mixture. Fluoroacetate at 10^{-3} M and a somewhat higher concentration of sodium fluoride inhibited the synthesis.

GROB et al. (1956) investigated the role of pyruvic acid in the biosynthesis of the carotenoids using cultures of the fungus *Mucor hiemalis*. When glucose was the sole source of carbon, sodium fluoride at 5×10^{-5} to 5×10^{-4} M reduced carotenoid synthesis to about ten percent of the control over a period of 4 to 14 days. The pyruvic acid concentrations fell off similarly. When sodium acetate was present in the medium instead of glucose, or along with glucose, there was no reduction in carotenoid synthesis by fluoride. Similarly, inhibition by fluoride did not occur with mixtures of glucose and pyruvate. It seems evident that glucose utilization for carotenoid synthesis requires pyruvate as an intermediate. Fluoride probably intervenes by blocking pyruvate formation at the enolase stage.

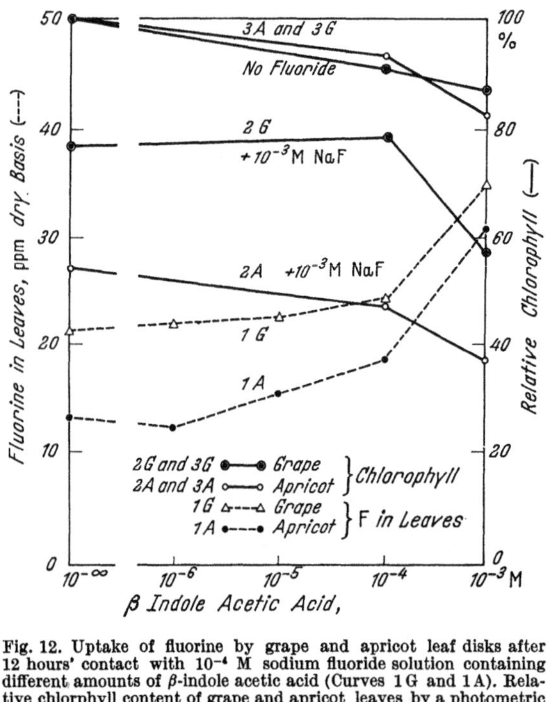

Fig. 12. Uptake of fluorine by grape and apricot leaf disks after 12 hours' contact with 10^{-4} M sodium fluoride solution containing different amounts of β-indole acetic acid (Curves 1 G and 1 A). Relative chlorphyll content of grape and apricot leaves by a photometric method, after 48 hours contact with 10^{-3} M NaF and 0, 10^{-4} or 10^{-3} M IAA (Curves 2 G and 2 A), and 48 hours contact with IAA alone (Curves 3 G and 3 A) (PILET, 1963)

PILET (1963) treated the leaves of apricot, cherry, apple and grape with several concentrations of sodium fluoride, then determined the chlorophyll content of leaf disks by a spectrophotometric method. Concentrations of 10^{-4} and 10^{-3} M sodium fluoride for 12 to 48 hours inhibited the synthesis of chlorophyll and also accelerated its decomposition. Lower concentrations and/or short-time treatments had little or no effect. β-indole acetic acid (IAA) also reduced the chlorophyll content of the leaves. Figure 12 shows that the uptake of fluoride by grape and apricot leaf disks from a 10^{-4} M sodium fluoride solution was about doubled by 10^{-3} IAA. The latter increased the destructive action of 10^{-3} M fluoride on the leaf chlorophyll, indicating a synergism between fluoride and IAA.

E. Growth and respiration of plants and plant parts

1. Growth

A major factor in the growth of a plant is the formation of polysaccharides for the construction of new cell walls. Observations by NICKERSON and CHUNG (1952) indicated that the inhibition of cell growth in yeasts due to fluoride could be overcome by the addition of glucose-1-phosphate but not by glucose-6-phosphate. Evidently, the fluoride inactivates the enzyme phosphoglucomutase which mediates the reactions:

(1) Glucose-6-phosphate $\overset{\text{NaF}}{\rightleftharpoons}$ glucose-1-phosphate $\rightarrow$ polysaccharides (growth)

(2) Hexose-6-phosphate $\overset{\text{NaF}}{\rightleftharpoons}$ mannose-1-phosphate $\rightarrow$ polysaccharides (growth)

CHUNG and NICKERSON (1954) presented a more general representation of these reactions, as shown in Fig. 13.

YANG and MILLER (1962, 1963) found that hydrogen fluoride-fumigated leaves of *Chenopodium murale* and *Glycine max.* (soybean) contained more reducing sugars and less sucrose than normal leaves, suggesting inhibition of sucrose synthesis.

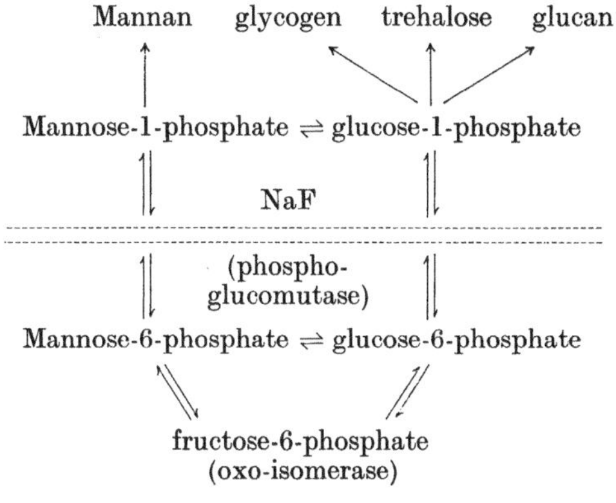

Fig. 13. Diagram of pathways leading to polysaccharide synthesis in growing yeasts, illustrating loci of fluoride-sensitive reaction (CHUNG and NICKERSON, 1954)

Necrotic leaves had higher concentrations of organic acids, particularly malic, malonic and citric acids; also higher concentrations of free amino acids and amides than unfumigated leaves.

These authors extracted phosphoglucomutase from bean meal and studied its activation *in vitro* by various metals and its inhibition by fluoride. The relative activations by 1 mM solutions of six divalent metals were as follows: None, 1.0; Mg^{++}, 3.2; Mn^{++}, 6.2; Co^{++}, 2.0; Ni^{++}, 0.65; Ca^{++}, 0.60; Zn^{++}, 0.50. Activation by manganese was twice as great as by magnesium but inhibition by fluoride of the magnesium enzyme was seven times greater than inhibition of the manganese enzyme. Inhibition was proportional to the fluoride content. Two other sucrose synthesizing enzymes, (uridine-diphosphate-glucose) fructose transglucosylase and UDPG pyrophosphorylase were similarly activated by these metals but the former was inhibited only slightly by fluoride while the latter was completely insensitive to fluoride.

NAJJAR (1948) proposed a rate equation for phosphoglucomutase that is similar to WARBURG's equation for enolase, except that glucose-1-phosphate replaces inorganic phosphate, and the value of K is about half the Warburg value for enolase:

$$[\mathrm{Mg}]\,[\mathrm{F}^2]\,[\text{glucose-1-phosphate}] = \mathrm{K} = 1.7 \times 10^{-12}\,.$$

Evidently, an inactive magnesium-fluoro-phosphate-enzyme complex is formed, analogous to the enolase complex.

NAJJAR and PULLMAN (1954) postulated a set of reactions somewhat different from the foregoing, involving group transfer from glucose-1-phosphate to glucose-6-phosphate

$$\text{glucose-1-phosphate} + \text{phosphoenzyme} \leftrightharpoons$$
$$\text{glucose-1,6-diphosphate} + \text{dephosphoenzyme} \leftrightharpoons$$
$$\text{glucose-6-phosphate} + \text{phosphoenzyme}$$

This mechanism assumes glucose-1,6-diphosphate is an actual reactant that is formed in the medium as a product of either phosphoenzyme reaction. It is not simply a part of a transient enzyme-substrate complex. Further, the enzyme exists in two independent states. Experiments were carried out which substantiated the mechanism.

BONNER and THIMAN (1950) observed that the growth of isolated sections of *Avena* coleoptiles and *Pisum* stems in solutions of 1 mg per liter auxin (indole acetic acid, IAA) was inhibited by sodium fluoride at concentrations greater than 10^{-3} M, also by fluoroacetate. A 2.5×10^{-3} M NaF or a 1.5×10^{-2} M solution of fluoroacetate inhibited growth 50% (Fig. 14). The inhibition was about the same on *Avena* sections breaking the surface of the liquid and on submerged *Pisum* sections. Submerged *Avena* sections exhibited over double the fluoride inhibition of sections on the surface. The enolase system was probably not involved in these

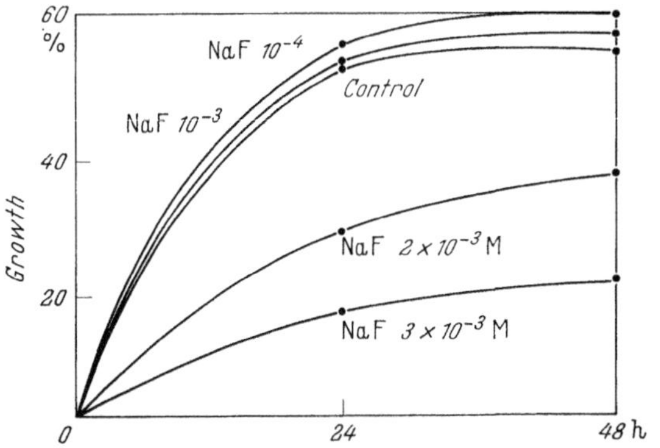

Fig. 14

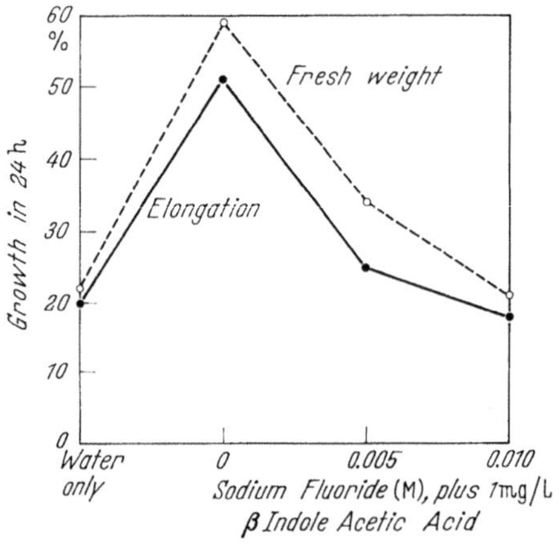

Fig. 15

Fig. 14. Time course of growth of coleoptile sections in various concentrations of fluoride, plus 1% sucrose and 1 mg per liter indole acetic acid (BONNER and THIMAN, 1950)

Fig. 15. Percentage elongation and increase of fresh weight of etiolated pea seedlings in water alone and in solutions containing 1 mg per liter β-indole acetic acid, with and without added sodium fluoride (CHRISTIANSEN et al., 1949) reactions since the inhibition was not affected by magnesium, phosphate, pyruvate or ATP. Fluoride concentrations that inhibited growth 50% had no effect on respiration but higher concentrations inhibited respiration also. Growth was promoted by 1-amino-2-naphthol-4-sulfonic acid, which is an inhibitor of carboxylase. Growth was also promoted in *Avena* by pyruvate and acetate. The latter is formed oxidatively from pyruvate and is an effective promoter of growth.

CHRISTIANSEN et al. (1949) and CHRISTIANSEN and THIMAN (1950) studied growth and inhibition of growth by fluoride of etiolated pea seedlings in the presence of 1 mg per liter auxin. Fluoride inhibited growth about 50% at 5×10^{-3} M and about 65% at 10^{-2} M (Table 31 and Fig. 15). Somewhat lower concentrations of iodoacetate or arsenite gave a similar inhibition. Growth in auxin plus 10^{-2} M fluoride was about the same as in water, above. Evidently, the fluoride counteracted the stimulation due to auxin. More reducing sugars were consumed during growth in the fluoride solution than in water or in auxin, in spite of the fact that there was less growth with fluoride. Only negligible amounts of sucrose, starch, dextrins and phosphorylated intermediates were present after growth inhibition, which was, therefore, not caused by the disappearance of reducing sugar *per se*, also there was no increase in growth in other experiments when various carbohydrates were added. The data in Table 31 also indicate that the reducing sugar which disappeared in the inhibited sections was not consumed by respiration. Probably it was changed to non-carbohydrate compounds.

Table 31. *Growth, reducing sugar and respiration of etiolated pea stems* (CHRISTIANSEN et al., 1949)

Treatment	Growth (24 hours)		Reducing sugar after 24 hours % of fresh wt.	Respiration O_2 Consumption Q_{O_2} after	
	Elongation %	Increase fresh weight %		2 hours	12 hours
Initial	—	—	1.12	—	—
In water	20	22	0.83	5.5	3.3
In auxin 1 mg/l	51	59	0.86	6.4	3.8
In auxin + $F^- = 5 \times 10^{-3}$ M	25	34	0.48	6.2	4.5
In auxin + $F^- = 1 \times 10^{-2}$ M	18	21	0.42	—	—

2. Growth and respiration

PILET (1964) found only a slight effect on growth of lentil root tips *(Lens culinaris)* by 10^{-6} M F^- per liter but greater concentrations reduced elongation substantially. A solution of 10^{-4} M F^- per liter inhibited growth by about 90%, as compared with the inhibition of about 50% in the case of pea seedlings treated with 5×10^{-3} M F^- (See Fig. 15). Indole acetic acid inhibited the elongation essentially like fluoride.

PILET (1964) found that respiration of the 18 mm end-sections of lentil roots was stimulated by 10^{-5} or 10^{-6} M fluoride or IAA (Fig. 16), but 10^{-4} M concentrations caused 18 and 9% inhibition, respectively. The 1 mm tip sections of the lentil roots were stimulated in respiration 11% by 10^{-4} M fluoride and 28% by 10^{-4} M IAA (Fig. 17). Presumably, higher concentrations would cause inhibition as with the 18 mm lentil roots or with pea seedlings. The inhibition of respiration by fluoride is reversible. For example, in one experiment, the addition for 50 min of 10^{-6} M sodium fluoride to root sections in one percent glucose caused oxygen evolution to remain constant while the control continued to show a steady increase. On removal of the fluoride the respiration rate soon reached that of the control.

Kandler (1953) studied the action of 2,4 D, α-naphthylacetic acid, thiamin, and indole acetic acid, along with sodium fluoride, on the metabolism of maize root tips which were prepared by germinating the seed under aseptic conditions, then transferring them to a sterile culture for five days' additional growth. The effects of the different compounds on the length, dry weight, assimilation of glucose, nitrogen content, oxygen uptake and respiration quotient were measured. In general, the metabolic functions were decreased if the concentrations of the growth substance exceeded certain levels. At lower concentrations, the metabolism was increased. Sodium fluoride inhibited all metabolic functions somewhat in proportion to the concentration.

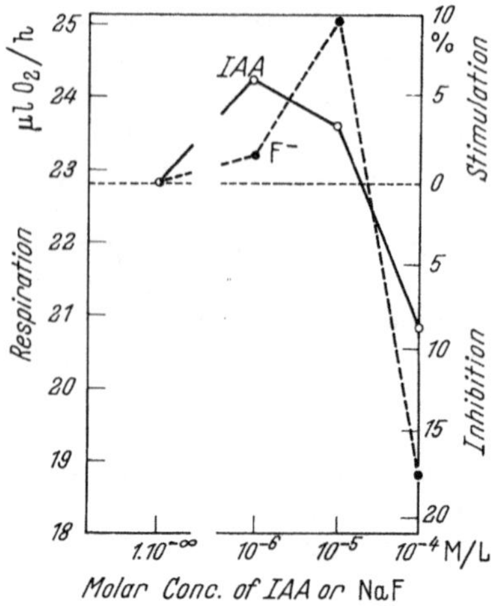

Fig. 16. Respiration of ten 18-mm end sections of lentil roots as affected by different concentrations of β-indole acetic acid or sodium fluoride (Pilet, 1964)

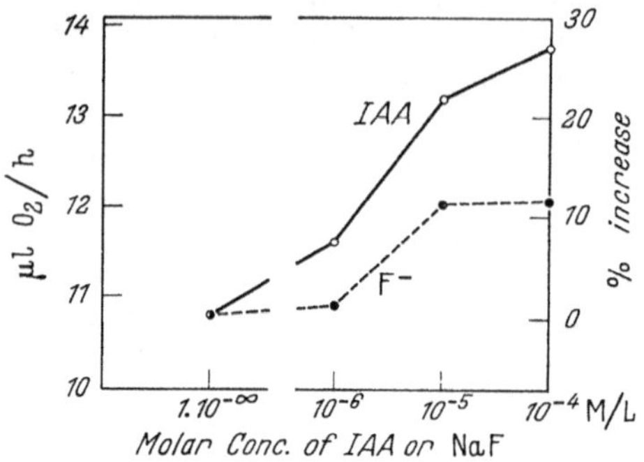

Fig. 17. Respiration of 10 mg (fresh weight) of 1-mm end sections of lentil root tips as affected by different concentrations of β-indole acetic acid and sodium fluoride (Pilet, 1964)

3. Respiration

Bonner and Wildman (1946) noted that excised spinach leaf tissue respired at a constant rate for about three hours, mediated by polyphenoloxidase, before depletion of the carbohydrate reserve in the tissue caused a reduction of respiration and the respiration quotient. Characteristic inhibition of this enzyme up to 90 to 100% was produced by p-nitrophenol. Fluoride also caused an inhibition of respiration that was reversed by pyruvate but not by glucose, as indicated in Table 32.

Laties (1949) found that the aerobic respiration of excised barley roots was comparable in the presence of either glucose or pyruvate. Respiration inhibited either by fluoride or iodoacetate could be restored by pyruvate.

Yamaguchi (1953) measured the respiration of hypocotyls of the kidney bean in the Warburg apparatus at 30° after soaking them in 0.67 M phosphate buffer. Ethyl alcohol was one product of the respiration and the respiration quotient (R. Q.) was 1.3–1.4. Sodium fluoride (0.01 M) or iodoacetate (0.001 M) inhibited oxygen consumption and carbon dioxide evolution progressively. Alcohol production declined to zero as the R. Q. fell to 1.0.

McNulty and Lords (1960) attempted to relate increased oxygen-uptake induced by low concentrations of fluoride in algae, yeasts, seedlings, and leaf tissue, with some phase of metabolism. They observed in algae that increased respiration with increased fluoride up to 10^{-3} M, was accompanied by increased nucleotide phosphates ADP and ATP. They, therefore, suggested that "fluoride probably

Table 32. *Inhibition of respiration of spinach leaf sections by sodium fluoride* (BONNER and WILDMAN, 1946)

Treatment	Gas measured	Gas exchange after 1 hour	2 hours	3 hours	Inhibition after 3 hrs
		mm³/200g leaf tissue/hr			%
Control	O_2	147	141	140	
+ 1 mg NaF/cc	O_2	54	22	16	89
Control	CO_2	133	139	141	
+ 1 mg NaF/cc	CO_2	67	28	19	87
Control	O_2	91	90	90	
+ 0.1 mg NaF/cc	O_2	45	23	19	79
+ 0.1 mg/cc NaF + 2.5 mg/cc Pyruvate	O_2	102	88	85	5
Control	O_2	78	72	76	
+ 0.1 mg NaF/cc	O_2	75	36	28	63
+ 0.1 mg/cc NaF + 10 mg/cc Glucose	O_2	64	34	29	62
+ 0.1 mg/cc NaF + 5 mg/cc Pyruvate	O_2	88	71	75	1

disrupts the basic energetics of the cell in some manner and increases oxygen consumption by increasing the phosphate acceptor or donor or at least by disturbing the relationship between PO_4, ADP and ATP."

KAUFMAN and ALIVISATOS (1955) have worked out the mechanism of the reactions mediated by the spinach phosphorylating enzyme in the presence of magnesium ions. The overall equation is:

$$ATP + CoA \cdot SH + Succinate \leftrightharpoons ADP + PO_4 + Succinyl\text{-}S\text{-}CoA$$

Inhibition by fluoride was not considered.

EICHENBERGER (1952) studied the respiration of tobacco leaves which are rich in organic acids and therefore, have a high respiratory quotient (1.15 to 1.35 during the daytime). Sodium fluoride (0.0025 M) inhibits respiration up to 90% in three hours, blocking the enolase. This inhibition can be reversed by pyroracemic acid, (suggesting that a tricarboxylic cycle functions in the leaves). Other enzymes detected in tobacco leaves include peroxidase, polyphenol oxidase, ascorbic acid oxidase, cytochrome oxidase and HCN-insensitive glycol and lactic acid oxidase.

Some enzymes are stimulated instead of inhibited by fluoride. ARRIGONI and MARRÉ (1955) found that the dehydrogenase activity of centrifuged extracts from the tips of small *Pisum sativum* plants in 0.015 M glucose-6-phosphate, increased 7 to 17% with the addition of 0.001 to 0.01 M sodium fluoride and 9 to 12% with 1 to 5×10^{-4} M ATP. The increase was 18% with 0.0004 M ATP plus 0.009 M sodium fluoride.

Using the Warburg apparatus, KIRALY and FARKAS (1955) measured the respiration of wheat seedlings infected with Erysiphe graminis or Puccinia graminas. Various respiration inhibitors dissolved in 0.05 M KH_2PO_4 were infiltrated into the leaves. The infection alone increased the respiration rate two and threefold, respectively. Infiltration of 0.01 M sodium fluoride (which inhibits glycolysis) reduced the respiration of the control plants 58% and of the infected plants, 64%. Iodoacetic acid behaved similarly but malonic acid (0.02 M) which inhibits succinic acid dehydrogenase, reduced the respiration of the healthy plants 31% and of the infected plants, 60 to 65%. Evidently, the parasite modifies the respiration mechanism.

Many other papers describe fluoride inhibition of various enzymes and enzymatic processes, including (1) anaerobic glycolysis in animal tissue, DICKENS and SIMER, 1929; (2) phosphatase in *Aspergillus oryzae*, BAMANN and SALZER, 1936; (3) catechol oxidase and succinic dehydrogenase in potato, BANGA and PORGES, 1938; (4) plant phosphatases, GIRI, 1937, 1938, 1941; (5) phosphatase in potatoes, HELFERICH and STETTER, 1947; (6) phosphatase in wheat bran, FLEURY and COURTOIS, 1947; (7) acid phosphatase, phytase and phosphomonoesterase in radish seed and in rye which hydrolyze glycerophosphate and inositol hexaphosphate, COURTOIS and PEREZ, 1949; and (8) polyphenolase and peroxidase in prunes, RAHMAN and JOSLYN, 1954.

By contrast, inactive amylase is activated by sodium fluoride and other salts, also by amino acids (DOBY, 1914 and SCHWEIGART, 1951).

4. Utilization of labelled glucose

Ross et al. (1962) used specifically labelled glucose to study the respiration pathways in normal and fluoride-injured leaves of *Chenopodium murale* and *Polygonum orientale.* The plants were grown under fluorescent lamps (1000 fc); then the leaves were treated with fluoride by two methods: (1) the third leaf below the tip of *P. orientale* was mounted with the petiole dipping in 5×10^{-3} M potassium fluoride solution for two days which caused extensive damage. The *C. murale* was treated with 10^{-3} M potassium fluoride. Control leaves were given potassium sulfate or chloride. (2) Other plants were fumigated with hydrogen fluoride at six pptm for 5 to 6 days which also caused extensive damage. Leaf disks, made with an 8 mm cork borer, were infiltrated under vacuum with glucose specifically labelled with C^{14} in the C_1, C_5 or C_6 position. Respiration measurements were made on the disks in Warburg apparatus. The carbon dioxide evolved was collected in potassium hydroxide, converted to barium carbonate and counted with a Geiger-Muller tube.

Table 33 and Fig. 18 summarize typical data. In all cases, the glucose C_6/C_1 ratio was reduced below 0.5 in the fluoride-treated leaves and ranged from 0.6 to 0.8 in the controls. The C_6/C_2 ratio ranged from 0.78 to 0.95. It was decreased slightly by hydrogen fluoride and increased by potassium fluoride. It is suggested that the respiration process tends to follow the pentose phosphate pathway with fluoride rather than the more usual glycolytic pathway, due possibly to inhibition

Table 33. *Effect of fluoride on the respiration of Chenopodium murale and Polygonum orientale as determined by uptake of specifically labelled glucose* (Ross et al., 1962)

Treatment	C_{14} Recovery (cpm)			Ratio		Respiration O_2 absorbed µl/hour/gram
	C_6	C_1	C_2	C_6/C_1	C_6/C_2	
Control[1]	173	310	—	0.63	—	4.2×10^3
HF Fum.	399	939	—	0.48	—	5.3×10^3
Control[1]	342	565	387	0.61	0.88	3.9×10^3
HF Fum.	338	691	435	0.49	0.78	5.0×10^3
KCl[1]	1297	2170	1430	0.62	0.87	3.5×10^3
KF	533	1081	555	0.49	0.95	3.1×10^3
KCl[1]	188	288	—	0.64	—	3.3×10^3
KF	312	778	—	0.40	—	3.0×10^3
K_2SO_4[2]	707	913	—	0.79	—	2.8×10^3
KF	2100	6040	—	0.35	—	4.1×10^3

[1] *C. murale.*
[2] *P. orientale.*

of enolase by fluoride. The hydrogen fluoride treatments increased respiration of *C. murale* above that of the unfumigated plants but potassium fluoride gave slightly lower respiration than did potassium chloride. In *P. orientale*, potassium fluoride increased respiration 50% above the sulfate.

Ordin and Skoe (1963) pretreated *Avena* coleoptile sections with 0.01 N sodium fluoride for two to eight hours at pH 6.0, which caused about 20 to 90% inhibition of growth rate, in 0.05 M glucose plus 2.9×10^{-5} M indole acetic acid and 0.0025 M potassium phosphate, as compared with sections similarly treated

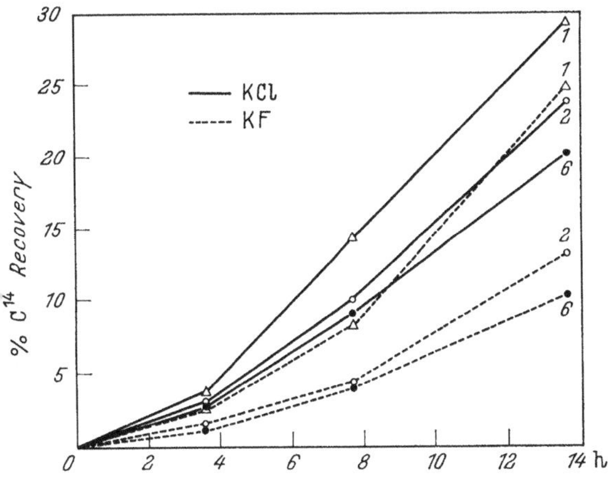

Fig. 18

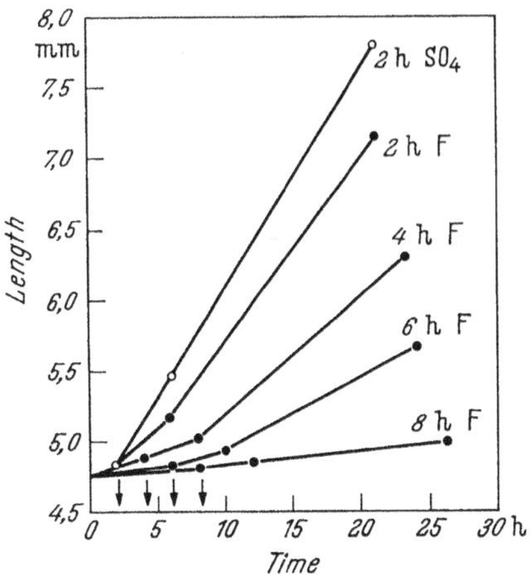

Fig. 19

Fig. 18. Respiration of $C^{14}O_2$ from glucose, specifically labelled in the C_1, C_2 or C_6 position, by excised leaves of *C. murale* pretreated for four days with 10^{-3} potassium chloride (solid lines) or fluoride (broken lines). Numbers on curves refer to the labelled carbon atom in glucose (Ross et al., 1962)

Fig. 19. Effect of duration of pretreatment with 0.01 N sodium fluoride or with 0.01 N sodium sulfate on the elongation of *Avena* coleoptile sections. Arrows indicate time of transfer to solutions of 0.05 M glucose plus 2.9×10^{-5} M IAA plus 0.0025 M potassium phosphate at pH 6.0 (Ordin and Skoe, 1963)

except that 0.01 N sodium sulfate was used for pretreatment. Fig. 19 shows the elongation of the *Avena* sections during 18 hours following fluoride pretreatment of 2, 4, 6 and 8 hours duration. The 2-hour sulfate curve has the same slope as those with 4, 6 and 8 hours pretreatment with sodium sulfate.

C^{14}-labelled glucose was used in the absence of auxin to study glucose utilization in the coleoptile. Absorption of the labelled sugar was normal but the fluoride treatment inhibited the incorporation of C^{14} into the cellulose and glucose components of the aqueous and acid-soluble fractions of the cell walls. There was little or no effect on the other sugar components or on $C^{14}O_2$ produced when potential growth was inhibited 50% or less, suggesting that phosphoglucomutase may have been the chief enzyme inhibited by fluoride. At higher levels of fluoride-induced inhibition the pattern of $C^{14}O_2$ production from glucose-1-C^{14}, glucose-2-C^{14} and glucose-6-C^{14} suggested that fluoride inhibited one or more of the following additional enzymes: uridine diphosphoglucose dehydrogenase, fructose diphosphatase and sedoheptulose diphosphatase. The data did not support the hypothesis that enolase had been inhibited.

5. Ion absorption and respiration

Ordin and Jacobson (1955) measured the uptake of potassium and bromide ions, and also respiration, by excised roots from six-day-old barley seedlings as influenced by pretreatment with potassium fluoride or fluoroacetate and a number of other glycolytic and Krebs Cycle inhibitors. Pretreatment with potassium sulfate served as control. Two-hour pretreatment with 0.02 N fluoride reduced uptake of potassium and bromide, both by 47%. Pretreatment with 0.04 N fluoride reduced uptake of potassium by 97% and of bromide by 60%. The corresponding values for 0.0025 N fluoroacetate were 49 and 52%, and for 0.01 N fluoroacetate, 83 and 59%. Reduction in respiration ranged from 24 to 60%, due to these treatments. Since fluoride inhibits both enolase and succinic dehydrogenase (SLATER and BONNER, 1952) intermediate treatments with 0.02 N potassium malate, glutamate and succinate, which are salts of Krebs Cycle acids, were applied after pretreatment with 0.02 N fluoride or 0.01 N fluoroacetate and before final treatment with 0.005 N potassium bromide. Some of the intermediate treatments removed the fluoride inhibition of potassium and bromide uptake, suggesting that absorption of these ions is mediated, at least in part, by enolase and succinic dehydrogenase.

F. Carbon dioxide exchange of intact higher plants

1. Respiration

The literature on the effects of fluorides in the atmosphere on plant respiration is limited and somewhat conflicting. MCNULTY and NEWMAN (1957) compared unsprayed and lime-sprayed prune and peach trees growing in an area where the presence of hydrogen fluoride was suspected. The sprayed trees that were protected against the fluoride had a somewhat lower respiration rate than did the unsprayed trees. However, the trees showed little or no fluoride injury, and their fumigation history was not known. Later, MCNULTY and NEWMAN (1961) fumigated 25-day-old bush bean plants with 30 pptm hydrogen fluoride, continuously for 18 days. Leaf samples were taken at 8, 12 and 18 days. Disks 16 mm in diameter were punched from these leaves (also from control leaves) and placed on moist filter paper in an upright position in Warburg reaction vessels for respiration measurements. The respiration rates of the fumigated leaves were increased 58% in 8 days, 74% in 12 days, and 7% in 18 days, as compared with the unfumigated control leaves. Slight intercostal chlorosis was present after 12 days. In another experiment, the bean plants were fumigated for 14 days which caused some chlorosis but no necrosis. When this treatment was started, the third-node leaves had reached full size and the sixth-node leaves were just starting to expand. After 14 days the fumigated leaves respired more rapidly than the controls, as follows: old leaves, 58%; middle-aged leaves, 66%; and young leaves, 8%.

Snow Princess gladiolus plants, some sprayed with calcium hydroxide plus spreader, and others unsprayed, were fumigated with 2.4 pptm hydrogen fluoride for 25 days. The unlimed plants had tip injury but no injury was found on the limed plants. Respiration measurements were made on the 3–5 mm chlorotic region between the brown collapsed tissue at the tip and the green, apparently healthy, tissue; also on the area 5 cm below the injured front. The corresponding areas on the lime-protected leaves were also measured as controls. The fumigation treatments increased respiration as follows; limed fumigated vs limed control, 7%; chlorotic tissue next to injured front, 61%, and tissue 5 cm below injured front, 20%.

HILL et al. (1959b) repeated the foregoing experiments with gladiolus and studied six other species also (Table 34). Fluoride fumigation treatments varied with the resistance of the plants. Gladiolus plants having 20 to 46% leaf necrosis showed a significant increase of 27 to 50% in respiration in the transitional area below the necrotic area, confirming the results of MCNULTY and NEWMAN.

Table 34. *Effect of hydrogen fluoride on the fluoride content and rate of oxygen uptake by plant leaves* (Hill et al., 1959b)

Plant	Variety	Fumigation		F in leaves		O_2 Uptake
		Days	$\mu g/M^3$	Control ppm	Fumigation ppm	$\frac{\text{Fum-Control}}{\text{Control}} \times 100$ %
Gladiolus	Snow Princess	40	0.97	9	58	40[1]
Gladiolus	Red charm	28	1.5	11	97	27[2]
Tomato	Moscow	26	5.7	24	500	—1.5
Tomato	Loran blood	21	47	18	2400	—6.0
Strawberry	Marshall	63	2.2	10	160	12
Strawberry	Marshall	49	6.9	14	670	—9.4
Celery	Utah 10 B	22	25	50	2500	4.3
Apricot	Chinese	44	1.1	8	58	—6.2
Prune	Italian	53	3.0	6	510	1.3
Barley	—	73	0.43	4	130	—5.9

[1] Statistically significant. 45% necrosis.
[2] Statistically significant. 20% necrosis.

The other six species were given fumigations ranging from 0.43 pptm for 73 days with barley to 47 pptm for 21 days with tomato. Fluorine uptake by the leaves ranged from 58 ppm in Chinese apricot treated with 1.1 pptm for 44 days, to 2400 ppm in the foregoing tomato and 2500 ppm in celery. Leaves with necrotic injury were avoided in making the respiration measurements. When this was done there was no statistically significant change in the respiration rate due to the fumigations, although differences between control and fumigated plants ranging from + 12 to − 14% were noted.

It is well known that plant tissue shows an increase in its respiration rate when it is injured mechanically (Richards, 1896). Attached leaves of Snow Princess gladiolus were injured for 20 cm from the tip by (1) crushing with a hammer, (2) heating with a hot iron, or (3) dipping in hot water. Three days later, respiration measurements were made on disks taken immediately below, 5 cm below and 15 cm below, the injured area. Data are given in Table 35. There was a significant increase in respiration adjacent to the mechanical injury, but at 5 or 15 cm distance, the increase was not statistically significant. The leaves injured by fluoride showed a greater increase in respiration than did the mechanically injured leaves.

Applegate and Adams (1960) treated bush bean seedlings with hydrogen fluoride at about 2 pptm, either continuously after germination, or for intermittent 24-hour periods. Oxygen uptake measurements were made in the Warburg respirometer at two-day intervals until the plants were 20 days old, using atmospheres containing 0 to 1% carbon dioxide. Whole plants minus the cotyledons

Table 35. *Increase of rate of respiration of Snow Princess gladiolus leaves due to mechanical and chemical injury* (Hill et al., 1959b)

Distance below injury, cm	Increased rate of O_2 uptake above control by			
	crushing %	dry heat %	scalding %	fluoride %
Adjacent	23	31	42	53
5	1	4	7	21
15	7	7	3	11
L.S.D. for P = 5%		14		13
L.S.D. for P = 1%		20		18

were measured on the second to sixth days; the plant parts above the cotyledons on the eighth and tenth days; and the first trifoliate leaf on the twelfth to twentieth days. All the fluoride-fumigated plants showed a consistently greater oxygen uptake, averaging about 15%, except during the initial days of the continuous fumigation. Infiltration treatments of 1.5 hours duration with 5.0 ppm solutions of several fluoride salts gave such small, complex relationships of respiration to light, temperature, carbon dioxide concentration and nature of the salt that no interpretation of the data was attempted (APPLEGATE and CARRIKER, 1960).

WEINSTEIN (1961) noted that the respiration of tomato and bean leaves was increased by 67 and 72%, respectively, by an eight-day fumigation with 1.6 pptm hydrogen fluoride.

Evidently, the fluoride effect on respiration is somewhat similar to mechanical injury. However, the fluoride concentration in the tissues can vary widely without causing more than a small effect on respiration if the leaf remains intact. The experiments of APPLEGATE and ADAMS indicate a small but definite increase in respiration due to hydrogen fluoride. Although, by definition, this can be called "invisible injury" it is too small to have a significant effect on the growth of the plant because it would represent only about one percent of the total carbon dioxide exchange.

2. Photosynthesis

Photosynthesis is a primary process in the growth and development of plants. Inhibition of photosynthesis implies interference with fundamental plant reactions essential for growth.

THOMAS and HENDRICKS (1956) and THOMAS (1958, 1961) measured the effects of hydrogen fluoride on the rate of photosynthesis of a number of different plants growing in the field or in large sand culture plots. A measured air stream was passed through a glass or plastic-covered chamber of four square meters area enclosing the plants. The air entering and leaving the chamber was analyzed continuously for carbon dioxide by means of an automatic recording analyzer. Hydrogen fluoride was metered into the air stream as required for the fumigation treatment and the air was sampled near the top of the plants for its fluoride content. Photosynthesis of the most sensitive plants, such as gladiolus and apricot, could be adversely affected by a few pptm hydrogen fluoride in a few hours, but more resistant plants, such as cotton and tomato, required several hundred pptm to give similar effects. In other experiments sodium fluoride was added to the nutrient to observe the effect of uptake through the roots.

In one experiment gladiolus was fumigated at 1 to 12 pptm for about seven hours per day, five days per week, for nearly two months. Tip injury developed continuously during this period until about 45% of the leaf area was necrotic. Photosynthesis, expressed as percentage of the photosynthesis of a comparable control plot, declined as the acute injury increased so that the curves for the percentage of green leaf tissue remaining and rate of photosynthesis were nearly coincident.

Another similar experiment is illustrated in Fig. 20 and gives the relative daily photosynthesis of two gladiolus plots from July through October. A series of fumigations on one plot, D 3, from September 20 to October 10, caused 20% reduction in photosynthesis along with 20% leaf destruction. A few light fumigations of plot D 1 in July raised the D 3/D 1 ratio slightly but did not cause an appreciable amount of leaf destruction.

It is apparent that the green areas remained fully functional while a large part of the leaf was killed. This must mean that the fluoride absorbed in the functional area of the leaf was translocated to the tip where it accumulated in sufficient concentration to kill those tissues while the green areas remained too low in fluoride to show any interference with photosynthesis.

Table 36 summarizes a number of experiments in which there were different amounts of acute injury to the plants but no "hidden injury" because reduction in photosynthesis corresponded closely with the acute leaf destruction. It may be

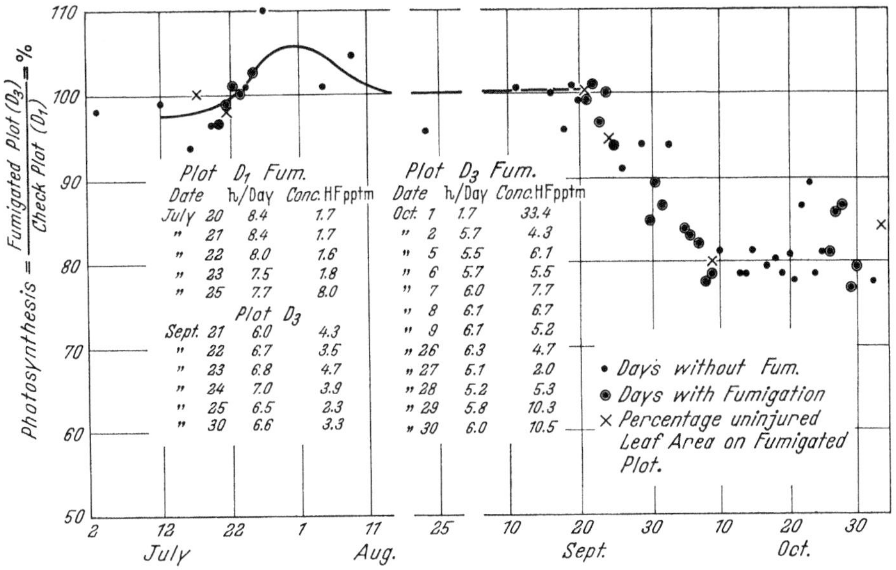

Fig. 20. Relative daily carbon assimilation of two similar gladiolus plots, one fumigated with hydrogen fluoride on certain days, compared with reduction of leaf area due to fumigation (THOMAS, 1958, 1961)

Table 36. *Effect of fumigation with relatively low concentrations of hydrogen fluoride on the photosynthesis of plants* (THOMAS, 1958)

Plant	HF Fumigation			Photosynthesis reduction[2]	Leaf area destroyed
	Duration[1]	Concentration			
		Max.	Avg.		
	hours	ppb	ppb	%	%
Fruit trees	183	9.0	2.6	14	10
	39	15.0	4.8	2	<5
	8	4.0	3.9	0	0
Gladiolus:					
Surfside	53	11.3	6.5	15	15
	44	9.8	6.4	28	30
	205	13.2	4.5	45	44
	128	33.4	5.7	20	22
Alladin	30	5.1	3.9	0	3
Algonquin	111	7.1	4.3	2	3
Commander Koehl	42	10.2	5.5	0	3
Mixed grain	10	200	145	0	Trace
Cotton	77	692	237	0	Trace
	138	33	17	0	0

[1] Fumigations 4 to 9 hours per day.
[2] Fumigated plot/check plot.

noted that the trees and gladioli were much more sensitive to absorbed fluorine than were grain or cotton.

In other experiments, higher concentrations of hydrogen fluoride were applied, usually causing only a small amount of leaf destruction. If the fumigation ex-

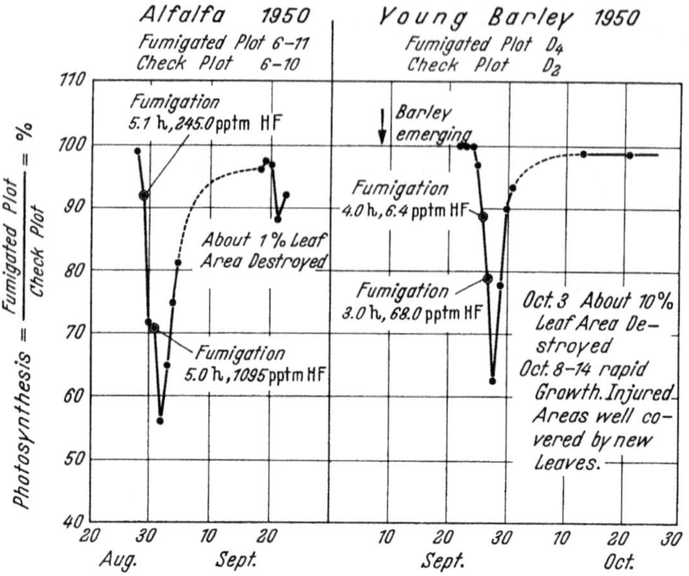

Fig. 21. Effect of relatively high concentrations of hydrogen fluoride on the total daily carbon assimilation of alfalfa and barley, expressed as percentage of control plots (THOMAS, 1958, 1961)

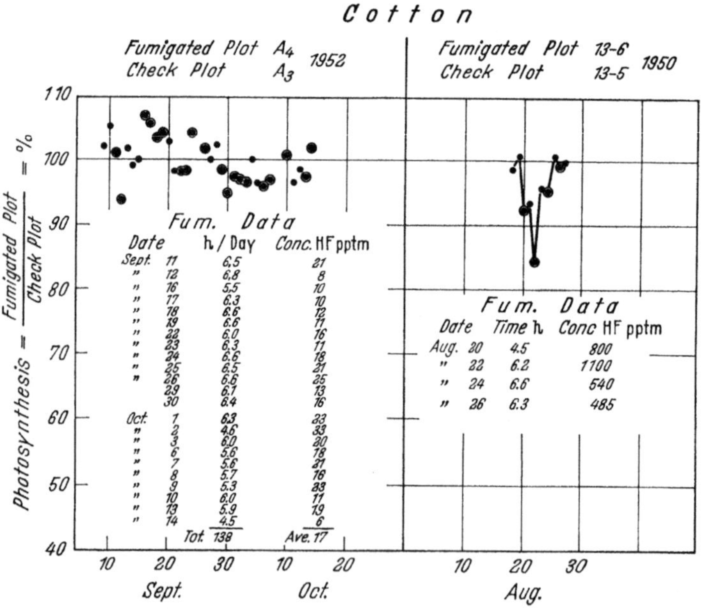

Fig. 22. Effect of hydrogen fluoride on carbon assimilation by cotton (THOMAS, 1958, 1961)

ceeded a threshold level of severity, photosynthesis fell to a low level, followed by a rapid partial recovery when the fumigation treatment was discontinued, then a slow recovery over a period of 4 to 25 days to the level expected from the amount of leaf area remaining intact. Fig. 21 shows the response of alfalfa and young barley to these super-threshold concentrations. Note that the fluoride levels for alfalfa are much higher than for young barley which resembles gladiolus in sensitivity. Cotton (Fig. 22) is more resistant than alfalfa.

This excessive reduction in photosynthesis below the level expected from the amount of leaf area destroyed represents "hidden" or "invisible" injury to the plant because the products of photosynthesis are correspondingly reduced in amount, without attendant visible injury.

Table 37 gives data for fumigation treatments that caused both visible and hidden injury. Visible injury caused permanent reduction of assimilation except as modified by growth of new leaves. The temporary reduction of photosynthesis was equivalent to total cessation of assimilation for 0.2 to 3.8 days in the different experiments. This represents only a few percent of the total photosynthesis of the crop. However, multiple severe fumigations, if applied at appropriately spaced intervals, could cause extensive interference with assimilation and growth without necessarily causing appreciable leaf damage.

Table 37. *Effect of fumigation with relatively high concentrations of hydrogen fluoride on the photosynthesis of plants* (THOMAS, 1958)

Plant	HF Fumigation			Decrease in photosynthesis (Fumigated plot/check plot)				Leaf area destroyed
	Duration[1]	Concentration		Temporary			Permanent	
		Max.	Avg.	Duration	Average[2]	Time lost		
	hours	ppb	ppb	days	%	days	%	%
Fruit trees	4	118	52	18	11	2.0	28[3]	50[4]
	13	22	18	25	15	3.8	35	22[5]
Gladiolus:								
Snow Princess	4	40	29	9	29	2.6	18	>10
Algonquin	46		12	21	12	2.5	17	15
Surfside	53	11	7	25	8	2.0	15	15
Young barley	7	68	37	7	15	1.1	1[6]	10
Alfalfa	10	1020	630	14	15	2.1	2	1
Cotton	20	1100	740	4	6	0.2	0	0

[1] All fumigations except on Algonquin gladiolus applied 4—7 hours per day.
[2] Temporary reduction below level of permanent injury.
[3] Some new growth of leaves reduced percentage loss.
[4] Approximate value 10 days after fumigation before new growth.
[5] Estimated before leaf fall.
[6] Rapid new growth restored activity.

Fluoride supplied through the roots permanently reduced photosynthesis, as shown in Fig. 23, for fruit trees. Ten to 50 ppm fluoride in the nutrient solution reduced assimilation by 30 to 50%. Evidently, the fluoride supply to the plant was continuous in this case, rather than intermittent as with many fumigation treatments.

HILL et al. (1958) carried out similar experiments with tomato plants fumigated continuously for three weeks with hydrogen fluoride concentrations ranging from 1 to 73 pptm (Table 38). Uptake of fluoride by the leaves ranged from 240 to 3000 ppm. Only very small amounts of fluoride accumulated in the fruit and peeling. There was no significant change in the rate of photosynthesis of the plants even with the most extreme of these treatments. Likewise, the chlorophyll content of the leaves and the rate of respiration were not significantly affected. Another experiment with a different variety of tomatoes but with lower hydrogen fluoride concentrations gave similar results.

It is evident that the threshold concentration required to cause invisible injury was not reached in these tomato experiments even though one of the fumigation treatments caused a rapid build-up of 3000 ppm fluorine in the leaves.

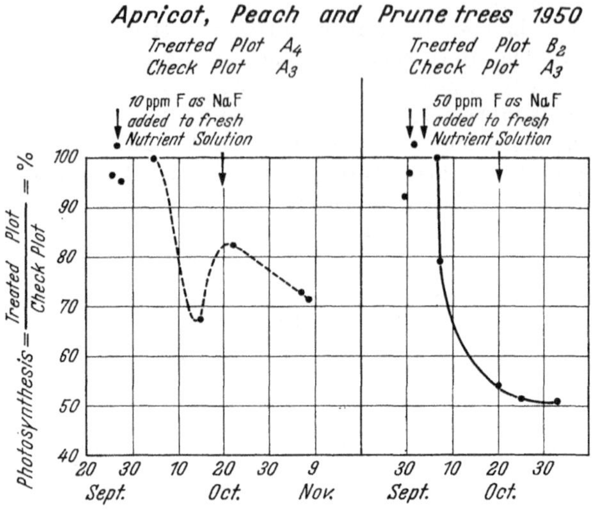

Fig. 23. Effect of sodium fluoride in the nutrient solution on carbon assimilation by fruit trees (THOMAS, 1958, 1961

Tomato is classified as a "resistant" plant to fluoride damage, along with alfalfa and cotton, for which the threshold concentration for injury appears to be several hundred pptm.

HILL et al. (1958) remark that invisible fluoride injury to most crop plants is improbable in the field because realistic fluoride concentrations near modern industries are presently only a small fraction of the threshold for such injury. This appears to be generally true, even for the most sensitive plants as well. However, the concept of the threshold fumigation treatment appears to be very important in view of the possibility of the occurrence of invisible injury in the

Table 38. *Rate of photosynthesis and fluoride content of washed tomato leaves in two fumigation experiments* (HILL et al., 1958)

Exposure	Experiment 1			Experiment 2		
	Fluoride in		Photosynthesis % of control	Fluoride in		Photosynthesis % of control
time (wks)	air μg/M³	leaves ppm		air μg/M³	leaves ppm	
1	0	—	98	0	—	98
2	0	(17)	97	0	(18)	100
3	0	—	104	0	—	103
4	1.0	240	103	3	440	106
5	14.0	840	103	73	1800	102
6	14.0	800	104	46	3000	100
6	fruit peel	11			42	
6	whole fruit	6			9	

field. A knowledge of the concentrations and durations of exposure, supplied preferably by automatic air analyzers, is needed to evaluate any area in which fluoride emissions are large and sensitive plants are grown. Unfortunately, the threshold exposures for different plants are very poorly defined at this time in terms of times and concentrations of fluoride treatment.

References

ADAMS, D. F.: Further applications of the limed filter paper technique in fluorine air pollution studies. J. Air Poll. Control Assoc. **7**, 88—91 (1957).
— An automatic hydrogen fluoride recorder proposed for industrial hygiene and stack monitoring. Anal. Chem. **32**, 1312—1316 (1960).
— A quantitative study of the limed filter paper technique for fluorine air pollution studies. Int. J. Air and Water Poll. **4**, 247—255 (1961).
— Diffusion method for microdetermination of foliar fluoride. Paper presented to Div. Water and Waste Chem. Am. Chem. Soc., New York, 1963.
—, and M. T. EMERSON: Variations of starch and total polysaccharide content of pinus ponderosa needles with fluoride fumigation. Plant Physiol. **36**, 261—265 (1961).
— J. W. HENDRIX, and H. G. APPLEGATE: Relationship among exposure period, foliar burn, and fluorine content of plants exposed to hydrogen fluoride. J. Agric. Food Chem. **5**, 108—116 (1957).
—, and R. K. KOPPE: Automatic atmospheric fluoride pollutant analyzer. Anal. Chem. **31**, 1249—1254 (1959).
— — Effect of pH on high-salt-thorium fluoride titration. Anal. Chem. **28**, 116—117 (1956).
— —, and N. E. MATZEK: Colorimetric method for continuous recording analysis of atmospheric fluoride. Anal. Chem. **33**, 117—119 (1961).
— D. J. MAYHEW, R. M. GNAGY, E. P. RICHEY, R. K. KOPPE, and I. W. ALLEN: Atmospheric pollution in a ponderosa pine blight area. Ind. Eng. Chem. **44**, 1356—1365 (1952).
— C. G. SHAW, R. M. GNAGY, R. K. KOPPE, D. J. MAYHEW, and W. D. YERKES, JR.: Relationship of atmospheric fluoride levels and injury indexes on gladiolus and ponderosa pine. J. Agric. Food Chem. **4**, 64—66 (1956).
AGATE, J. N.: Industrial Fluorosis. A study of the hazard to man and animals near Fort William, Scotland. A Report to the Fluorosis Committee, Med. Research Council Mem. No. 22, London, H. M. Stationery Office, 1949.
ALLMENDINGER, D. F., V. L. MILLER, and F. JOHNSON: Control of fluorine scorch on gladiolus with foliar dusts and sprays. Proc. Amer. Soc. Hort. Sci. **56**, 427—432 (1950).
ALTHER, E. W.: Chemisch-biologische Untersuchungen zur Fluorose des Rindes. (Diss.) Inst. für Tierernähr. der Landw. Hochschule, Hohenheim, 1961.
AMBERG, S., and A. S. LOEVANHART: Further observations on the inhibiting effect of fluorides on the action of lipase, together with a method for the detection of fluoride in food products. J. Biol. Chem. **4**, 149—164 (1908).
AMPOLA, G.: Esperienze culturali sull'azione del fluoruro di calcio nei vesuviani. Gazz. chim. ital. **34**, II, 156—165 (1904).
ANDERSON, H. W.: Spraying for control of bacterial spot of peach. Trans. Illinois State Hort. Soc. **60**, 147—154 (1926).
— Problems on spray to the peach. Trans. Illinois State Hort. Soc. **65**, 454—468 (1931).
— Diseases of Fruit Crops. New York: McGraw-Hill Book Co. 1956.
APPLEGATE, H. G., and D. F. ADAMS: Effect of atmospheric fluoride on respiration of bush bean. Botan. Gaz. **121**, 223—227 (1960).
— —, and R. C. CARRIKER: Effect of aqueous fluoride solutions on respiration of intact bush bean seedlings. I. Inhibition and stimulation of oxygen uptake. Am. J. Bot. **47**, 339—345 (1960).
ARRIGONI, O., and E. MARRÉ: Effect of adenosine phosphates on the direct oxidation of glucose-6-phosphate by plant extracts. Giorn. Biochim. **4**, 1—9 (1955).
ASO, K.: Stimulating influence of sodium fluoride on garden plants. Bull. Col. Agric., Tokyo Imperial Univ. **7**, 83—84 (1906).
—, and S. SUZIKI: Stimulating effect of iodine and fluorine compounds on agricultural plants. Bull. Col. Agric., Tokyo Imperial Univ. **6**, 159 (1904).
BALLCZO, H., u. O. KAUFMANN: Die Bestimmung des Fluorgehaltes von Heuproben aus rauchgasbeschädigtem Gebiet. Mikrochemie ver. Mikrochim. Acta **39**, 9—12 (1952).
BAMANN, E., u. W. SALZER: Die „Phosphatase“ aus Aspergillus oryzae, ein Gemisch isodynamer Phosphoesterasen: I. Abhandlung zur Kenntnis der pflanzlichen Phosphatasen. Biochem. Z. **287**, 380—399 (1936).

BANGA, I., u. E. PORGES: Über die dehydrierende Autoxydation und die biologischen Oxydationen. VII. Die Hemmung der Dehydrasen und der Polyphenoloxydase durch Cu-Komplex-Bildner. Hoppe-Seylers physiol. Chem. **254**, 200—204 (1938).
BARTHOLOMEW, R. P.: Fluorine: its effect on plant growth and its relation to the availability to plants of phosphorus in phosphate rocks. Soil Sci. **40**, 203—217 (1935).
BELCHER, R., M. A. LEONARD, and T. S. WEST: A new spot test for the detection of fluoride ion. Talanta **2**, 92—93 (1959).
BELLACK, E., and P. J. SCHOUBOE: Rapid photometric determination of fluoride in water. Anal. Chem. **30**, 2032—2034 (1958).
BENEDICT, H. M., J. M. ROSS, and R. H. WADE: The disposition of atmospheric fluorides by vegetation. Intl. J. Air and Water Poll. **8**, 279—289 (1964a).
— R. H. WADE, and J. M. ROSS: Some responses of vegetation to atmospheric fluorides. J. Air Poll. Control Ass. **15**, 253—255 (1965).
BENSON, N. R.: Fluoride injury of soft suture and splitting of peaches. Proc. Amer. Soc. Hort. Sci. **74**, 184—198 (1959).
BERGE, H.: Immissionsschäden an landwirtsch. und gärtnerischen Kulturen. Berlin: Paul Parey 1958.
BERTRAND, G.: Les engrais complémentaires. Ber. 5. Intern. Kongr. angew. Chem. III, 839. Berlin 1903.
BIRAGHI, A.: Determinazione della presenza di fluoro nei tessuti vegetali colpiti da emanazioni gassose. Boll. staz. patol. vegetale **18**, 360—366 (1938).
BOKORNY, T.: Über den Einfluß verschiedener Substanzen auf die Keimung der Pflanzensamen. Wachstumsförderung durch einige. II. Biochem. Z. **50**, 49—86 (1913).
BONNER, J., and S. G. WILDMAN: Enzymic mechanisms in the respiration of spinach leaves. Arch. Biochem. **19**, 497—518 (1946).
—, and J. A. D. ZEEVAART: Ribonucleic acid synthesis in the bud: an essential component of floral induction in Xanthium. Plant Physiol. **37**, 43—49 (1962).
BONNER, W. D., JR., and K. V. THIMAN: Studies on the growth and inhibition of isolated plant parts. III. The action of some inhibitors concerned with plant metabolism. Amer. J. Bot. **37**, 66—75 (1950).
BOREI, H.: Inhibition of cellular oxidation by fluorine. Arkiv. Kemi. Mineral, Geol. **20** A, No. 8, 215 (1945).
BOUYER, S., and L. COLLOT: (Trace elements and peanut growth). Ann. centre recherches agron. Bambey au Senegal, 1951. Bull. agron. (French) **7**, 77—88 (1952). [Chem. Abstracts **47**, 4537 (1953).]
BOVAY, E.: Les dépôts de chlore et de fluor sur la végétation dans le voisinage des usines de produits chimiques. Rev. romande agr. viticult. et arboricult. **10**, No. 9, 69—71 (1954).
— Dégâts occasionnés aux arbres fruitiers par les gaz fluorés. Landwirtsch. Jahrb. Schweiz **72**, 541—544 (1958).
BREDEMANN, G.: Biochemie und Physiologie des Fluors und der industriellen Fluorrauchschäden. Berlin: Akademie-Verlag 1951.
— Biochemie und Physiologie des Fluores, 2. Aufl. Berlin: Akademie-Verlag 1956.
—, u. H. RADELOFF: Zur Diagnose von Fluor-Rauchschäden. Phytopathol. Z. **5**, 195—206 (1933).
— — Über Fluor-Rauschchäden. Fluoraufnahme durch die Rinde der Sprosse und ihre Wirkung. Angew. Botan. **19**, 172—181 (1937).
BRENNAN, E. G., I. A. LEONE, and R. H. DAINES: Fluorine toxicity in tomato as modified by alterations in the nitrogen, calcium and phosphorus nutrition of the plant. Plant Physiol. **25**, 736—747 (1950).
BREWER, R. F., H. D. CHAPMAN, F. H. SUTHERLAND, and R. B. MCCOLLOCH: Effect of fluorine addition to substrate on navel orange trees grown in solution cultures. Soil Sci. **87**, 183—188 (1959).
— R. K. CREVELING, F. B. GUILLEMET, and F. H. SUTHERLAND: Effects of hydrogen fluoride gas on seven citrus varieties. Proc. Amer. Soc. Hort. Sci. **75**, 236—243 (1960a).
— R. C. MCCOLLOCH, and F. H. SUTHERLAND: Fluoride accumulation in foliage and fruit of wine grapes growing in the vicinity of heavy industry. Proc. Amer. Soc. Hort. Sci. **70**, 183—188 (1957).
— F. H. SUTHERLAND, F. B. GUILLEMET, and R. K. CREVELING: Some effects of hydrogen fluoride gas on bearing navel orange trees. Proc. Amer. Soc. Hort. Sci. **76**, 208—214 (1960b).
— — — Sorption of fluorine by citrus foliage from equivalent solutions of HF, NaF, NH_4F and H_2SiF_6. Proc. Amer. Soc. Hort. Sci. **76**, 215—219 (1960c).
BURGI, E.: Fluor, Chlor, Brom und Jod. Handbuch der experimentellen Pharmakologie, Bd. 3, S. 276—287. Berlin: Heffter-Heubner 1927.
CHAIX, P., and C. FROMAGEOT: Influence de fluorure de sodium et de l'acide monoidoacétique sur les dégradations anaérobie et aérobie de quelques substrats par Propioni bactérium pentosaceum. Enzymologia **7**, 353—361 (1939).

CHRISTIANSEN, G. S., L. J. KUNZ, W. D. BONNER, JR., and K. V. THIMAN: Action of growth inhibitors on carbohydrate metabolism in the pea. Plant Physiol. **24**, 178—181 (1949).

—, and K. V. THIMAN: Metabolism of stem tissue during growth and its inhibition. I. Carbohydrates; II. Respiration and ether soluble material. Arch. Biochem. **26**, 230—247, 248—259 (1950).

CHUNG, C. W., and W. J. NICKERSON: Polysaccharide syntheses in growing yeasts. J. biol. Chem. **208**, 295—407 (1954).

CLARK, F. W.: The Data of Geochemistry. U.S. Geol. Surv. Bull. 491 (1911).

COMPTON, O. C.: Effect of leaf clipping upon the size of gladiolus corms. Proc. Amer. Soc. Hort. Sci. **75**, 688—692 (1960).

—, and L. F. REMMERT: Effect of air borne fluorine on injury and fluorine content of gladiolus leaves. Proc. Amer. Soc. Hort. Sci. **75**, 663—675 (1960).

COURTOIS, J. E., and C. PEREZ: Recherches sur la phytase. XIV. Action de quelques effecteurs sur les phosphomonoesterases et phytophosphatases du radis et du seigle. Bull. Soc. Chem. Biol. **31**, 1234—1241 (1949).

DAINES, R. H., I. A. LEONE, and E. G. BRENNAN: Effects of fluorine on plants as determined by soil nutrition and fumigation studies. In: L. C. McCABE, editor, Air Pollution, pp. 97 to 105. New York: McGraw-Hill Book Co. 1952.

DICKENS, F., and F. SIMER: On tissue glycolysis: the effect of fluoride and some other substances. Biochem. J. **23**, 936—958 (1929).

DOBY, G.: Über Pflanzenenzyme. II. Die Amylase der Kartoffelknolle. Biochem. Z. **67**, 166—181 (1914).

DORSEY, M. J., and R. L. McMUNN: Tree-conditioning the peach crop. Bull. 507, 406—414, Agric. Exp. Station, Urbana, University of Illinois, 1944.

EICHENBERGER, E.: Über die Atmung lebender Tabakblätter. Ber. schweiz. botan. Ges. **62**, 123—163 (1952).

FABRE, R., R. TRUHAUT, and A. ROUQUETTE: Sur le microdosage du fluor dans les végétaux. Comp. Rend. **240**, 226—229 (1955).

FEIGL, F., u. P. KRUMHOLZ: Beiträge zur analytischen Auswertung komplex chemischer und induzierter Reaktionen. Ber. dtsch. Chem. Ges. **62**, I, 1138—1142 (1929).

FLEURY, P., and J. COURTOIS: Recherches sur la phytase. II. Cinétiques comparées de l'hydrolyse du glycerophosphate et de l'inositohexaphosphate par le son de blé. Biochim. biophys. Acta (Amst.) **1**, 256—269 (1947).

FRARY, F. C.: Aluminum in War. Chem. and Eng. News **21**, 2018—2019, 2042 (1943).

FRESENIUS, W.: Zum Nachweis des Fluors in Pflanzenteilen. Z. Untersuch. Nahr.- u. Genußm. **5**, 1035—1036 (1902).

GARBER, K.: Neuere Literatur über Rauch-, Staub- und Abgasschäden. Angew. Botan. **34**, 65—104 (1960); II, **36**, 127—184 (1962).

GARNER, W. W., J. E. McMURTREY, JR., J. D. BOWLING, and E. G. MOSS: Role of chlorine in nutrition and growth of the tobacco plant and its effect on the quality of the cured leaf. J. Agr. Research **40**, 627—648 (1930).

GAUTIER, A.: Influence du fluor sur la végétation. Comp. Rend. **160**, 194—195 (1915).

—, et P. CLAUSMANN: Influence des fluorures sur la végétation. A. Essais préliminaires en vases de jardin. Comp. Rend. **168**, 976—982 (1919).

GEMMELL, G. D.: Fluorine in New Zealand soils. New Zealand J. Sci. Technol. **27** B, 302—306 (1946).

GERICKE, S.: Fluor und Phosphorsäure. Z. Pflanzenernähr., Düngung u. Bodenk. **46**, 152—169 (1949).

—, u. B. KURMIES: Fluorgehalt und Fluoraufnahme von Kulturpflanzen. Phosphorsäure **15**, 50—63 (1955).

GIRI, K. V.: Über Pflanzenphosphatasen. I. Die Phosphatase gekeimter Sojabohnen (Glycine hispida). Z. physiol. Chem. **245**, 185—196 (1937); II. **254**, 126—138 (1938); III. Ann. Biochem. Exptl. Med. **1**, 297—306 (1941).

GISIGER, L.: Das Fluorion, microchemische Bestimmung und seine Wirkung auf Pflanzen. (Diss.) ETH, Zürich, 1931.

GREENHALGH, R., and J. P. RILEY: Determination of fluorides in natural water with particular reference to sea water. Anal. Chim. Acta **25**, 179—188 (1961).

GROB, E. C., R. BÜTLER u. V. GRUNDBACHER: Die Stellung der Brenztraubensäure in der Biosynthese der Carotinoide. Helv. Chim. Acta **39**, 168—173 (1956).

GWIRTSMAN, J., R. MAVRODINEANU, and R. R. COE: Determination of fluorides in plant tissues, air and water. Anal. Chem. **29**, 887—892 (1957).

HALL, R. J.: Determination of microgram amounts of fluoride by diffusion. Analyst **85**, 560—563 (1960).

— Spectrophotometric determination of submicrogram amounts of fluorine in biological specimens. Analyst 88, 76—83 (1963).

HAMMIG, H. W., C. SCHIFFNER u. H. WISLICENUS: Bericht über die zur Beseitigung von Ziegeleirauchschäden im Auftrage des Kgl. Sächs. Finanzministeriums vorgenommenen Versuche, 1911, 1912, 1913. Jahrb. Berg- u. Hüttenwesen (Saxony) A 47—86, 1913.

HASELHOFF, E.: Grundzüge der Rauchschadenkunde: Anleitung zur Prüfung und Beurteilung der Einwirkung von Rauchabgängen auf Boden und Pflanzen. Berlin: Gebrüder Bornträger 1932, 167 pp.

—, u. G. LINDAU: Die Beschädigung der Vegetation durch Rauch. Leipzig: Gebrüder Bornträger 1903.

— G. BREDEMANN u. W. HASELHOFF: Entstehung, Erkennen und Beurteilung von Rauchschäden. Chap. III. Fl. Comp. 174—186. Berlin: Gebrüder Bornträger 1932.

HELFERICH, B., u. H. STETTER: Zur Kenntnis der Kartoffelphosphatase. Liebigs Ann. Chem. 558, 234—241 (1947).

HENDRICKSON, E. R.: Dispersion and effects of air borne fluoride in Central Florida. J. Air Poll. Cont. Ass. 11, 220—232 (1961).

HENDRIX, J. W., and H. R. HALL: The relationship of certain leaf characteristics and flower color to atmospheric fluoride-sensitivity in gladiolus. Proc. Amer. Soc. Hort. Sci. **72**, 503—510 (1958).

HILDEBRAND, E. M.: Peach-suture spot. Phytopath. **33**, 167—168 (1943).

HILL, A. C., L. G. TRANSTRUM, M. R. PACK, and W. S. WINTERS: Air Pollution with relation to agronomic crops. VI. An investigation of the "Hidden Injury" theory of fluoride damage to plants. Agronomy J. **50**, 562—565 (1958).

— — —, and A. HOLLOMAN, JR.: Facilities and techniques for maintaining a controlled fluoride environment in vegetation studies. J. Air Poll. Cont. Ass. **9**, 22—27 (1959a).

— M. R. PACK, L. G. TRANSTRUM, and W. S. WINTERS: Effects of atmospheric fluorides and various types of injury on the respiration of leaf tissue. Plant Physiol. **34**, 11—16 (1959b).

HITCHCOCK, A. E., P. W. ZIMMERMAN, and R. R. COE: Results of ten years' work (1951—1960) on the effect of fluorides on gladiolus. Contrib. Boyce Thompson Inst. for Plant Research **21**, 303—344 (1962).

HOSKINS, W. M., and C. A. FERRIS: Method of analysis for fluoride. Application to determination of spray residue on food products. Ind. Eng. Chem., Anal. Ed. **8**, 6—9 (1936).

JOHNSON, F., D. F. ALLMENDINGER, V. L. MILLER, and C. J. GOULD: Leaf scorch of gladiolus caused by atmospheric fluoric effluents. Phytopath. **40**, 239—246 (1950).

—, V. L. MILLER, and D. F. ALLMENDINGER: Hydrogen fluorine injury to prune trees in Washington. Phytopath. **37**, 362 (Abstracts) (1947).

KANDLER, O.: Untersuchungen über die Wirkung von 2,4-Dichlorphenoxyessigsäure, α-Naphthylessigsäure, Natriumfluorid und Vitamin B_1 auf den Stoffwechsel in vitro kultivierter Maiswurzeln. Planta **42**, 304—348 (1953).

KAUDY, J. D., F. T. BINGHAM, R. C. MCCOLLOCH, F. G. LEIGIG, and A. P. VANSELOW: Contamination of citrus foliage by fluorine from air pollution in major California citrus areas. Proc. Amer. Soc. Hort. Sci. **65**, 121—127 (1955).

KAUFMAN, S.: Studies on the mechanism of the reaction catalyzed by the phosphorylating enzyme. J. biol. Chem. **216**, 153—164 (1955).

—, and S. G. ALIVISATOS: Purification and properties of the phosphorylating enzyme from spinach. J. biol. Chem. **216**, 141—152 (1955).

KIRALY, Z., u. G. L. FARKAS: Über die parasitogen induzierte Atmungssteigerung beim Weizen. Naturwissenschaften **42**, 213—214 (1955).

KOTTE, W.: Rauchschäden an Steinobst-Früchten. Nachrbl. dtsch. Pflanzenschutzdienstes **9**, 91—92 (1929).

KRÜGER, E.: Über den Nachweis von Fluor in rauchbeschädigten Pflanzen. Metall und Erz **38**, 265—266 (1941).

LATIES, G. G.: The role of pyruvate in the aerobic respiration of barley roots. Arch. Biochem. **20**, 284—299 (1949).

LEDBETTER, M. C., R. MAVRODINEANU, and A. G. WEISS: Distribution studies of radioactive fluorine-18 and stable fluorine-19 in tomato plants. Contrib. Boyce Thompson Inst. Plant Research **20**, 331—351 (1960).

LEONE, I. A., E. G. BRENNAN, R. H. DAINES, and W. R. ROBBINS: Some effects of fluorine on peach, tomato and buckwheat when absorbed through the roots. Soil Sci. **66**, 259—267 (1948).

— — — Atmospheric fluoride: its uptake and distribution in tomato and corn plants. Plant Physiol. **31**, 329—333 (1956).

LEROUX, D.: Influence de quelques oligo-éléments sur la fixation de l'azote atmosphérique au cours de la végétation d'une légumineuse. Comp. Rend. **212**, 506—507 (1941).

LINDBERG, Z. YA.: The amounts of fluorine in the soil and vegetables in the regions near superphosphate plants. Voprosy Pitaniya (Russian) **15**, No. 4, 41—45 (1956).

LIPMANN, F.: Mechanism of inhibition by fluoride and the dissociation curve of fluoromethaemoglobin. Biochem. Z. **206**, 171—185 (1929).

LOHMANN, K., and O. MEYERHOFF: Enzymic transformation of phosphoglyceric acid into pyruvic and phosphoric acid. Biochem. Z. **273**, 60—72 (1934).

MACINTIRE, W. H.: Fate of air borne fluorides and attendant effects on soil reaction and fertility. J. Ass. Off. Agric. Chem. **40**, 958—973 (1957).

— Resume of fluoride research of Tennessee Agricultural Experiment Station. J. Ass. Off. Agric. Chem. **38**, 913—931 (1955).

— Air versus soil as channels for fluoric contamination of vegetation in two Tennessee locales. In: L. C. MCCABE, editor, Air Pollution, pp. 53—58. New York: McGraw-Hill Book Co. 1952.

— et al.: Effects of fluorine in Tennessee soils and crops. Ind. Eng. Chem. **41**, 2466—2475 (1949).

— L. J. HARDIN, and M. HARDISON: Fluorine acquired by forage cultures in outdoor and washed atmosphere at Columbia, Tennessee. J. Agric. Food. Chem. **2**, 832—835 (1954).

— — F. D. OLDHAM, and J. W. HAMMOND: Development of P_2O_5 insolubility in phosphatic mixtures. Ind. Eng. Chem. **29**, 758—766 (1937).

— W. M. SHAW, and B. ROBINSON: A barium-fluoride study: the fate of added barium silico fluoride and its effect upon sulfates and other soil components as influenced by limestone and dolomite. Tenn. Agric. Exp. Sta. Bull. **155**, 31 pp. (1935).

— — —, and A. J. STERGES: Disparity in the leachability of fluorine from incorporations in phosphated and slagged soils. Soil Sci. **65**, 321—339 (1948).

—, S. H. WINTERBERG, L. B. CLEMENTS, L. S. JONES, and B. ROBINSON: Effect of fluorine carriers on crops and drainage waters. Ind. Eng. Chem. **43**, 1797—1799 (1951 a).

— — — L. J. HARDIN, and L. S. JONES: Crop and soil reactions to applications of hydrofluoric acid. Ind. Eng. Chem. **43**, 1800—1803 (1951 b).

MALMSTROM, B. A.: Interaction of pure enolase with its activating metal ions. Arch. Biochem. **46**, 345—363 (1953).

MAROTTA, D., D. VITA, and S. ANSELMI: Indagini sulle emanazioni di una fabbrica di alluminio in rapporto all'ambiente. Rend. Ist. Sanita pubbl. (Rome) **1**, 735—764 (1938).

MAVRODINEANU, R., and R. R. COE: Method of dispensing volatile fluoride in portable greenhouses. J. Agr. Food Chem. **5**, 852—854 (1957).

— and J. GWIRTSMAN: Use of sodium perotide fusion for the determination of fluorides in vegetation. Contrib Boyce Thompson Inst. 18, 419—420 (1956).

— J. GWIRTSMAN, D. C. MCCUNE, and C. A. PORTER: Summary of procedures used in the controlled fumigation of plants with volatile fluorides and in the determination of fluorides in air, water and plant tissues. Contrib. Boyce Thompson Inst. **21**, 453—464 (1962).

MAYRHOFER, J.: Über Pflanzenbeschädigungen, veranlaßt durch den Betrieb einer Superphosphatfabrik. Ber. 10. Versammlg. bayr. Vertreter, angew. Chem. Augsburg **1891**, p. 127.

MAZE, P.: Détermination des éléments minéraux rares nécessaires au développement du mais. Comp. Rend. **160**, 211—214 (1915).

MCCAUGHEY, W. J., and W. H. FRY: Microscopic determination of soil forming minerals. U.S. Dept. of Agric. Bur. of Soils Bull. **91**, 1—100 (1913).

MCCLENDON, J. F., and J. GERSHON-COHEN: Reduction of dental caries and goiter by crops fertilized with fluorine and iodine. J. Agr. Food Chem. **3**, 72—73 (1955).

MCCOMBIE, H., and B. C. SAUNDERS: Alkyl Fluorophosphonates. Nature (Lond.) **157**, 776—777 (1946).

MCCORNACK, A. A., L. C. COCHRAN, H. ENGLISH, and C. L. HEMSTREET: A black tip condition on peach fruits in California. Plant Disease Reporter **36**, 99—100 (1952).

MCNULTY, I. B., and J. L. LORDS: Possible explanation of fluoride-induced respiration in Chlorella pyrenoidosa. Science **132**, 1553—1554 (1960).

—, and D. W. NEWMAN: Effects of atmospheric fluoride on the respiration rate of bush bean and gladiolus leaves. Plant Physiol. **32**, 121—124 (1957).

— — Mechanism of fluoride-induced chlorosis. Plant Physiol. **36**, 385—388 (1961).

MELLOR, J. W.: Comprehensive Treatise on Inorganic and Theoretical Chemistry. Supplement II, Part I. New York: Longmans-Green and Co 1956.

MIDDLETON, J. T., A. S. CRAFTS, R. F. BREWER, and O. C. TAYLOR: Plant damage by air pollution. Calif. Agric. **10**, No. 6, 9—12 (1956).

MILLER, G. W.: Properties of enolase in extracts from pea seeds. Plant Physiol. **33**, 199—206 (1958).

MILLER, V. L., F. JOHNSON, and D. F. ALLMENDINGER: Fluorine analysis of Italian prune foliage affected by marginal scorch. Phytopath. **38**, 30—37 (1948).

MITCHELL, H. H., and M. EDMAN: Fluorine in soils, plants and animals. Soil Sci. **60**, 81—90 (1945).

MORSE, H. H.: The toxic influence of fluorine in phosphatic fertilizers on the germination of corn. Soil Sci. **39**, 177—193 (1935).

MÜHLSTEPH, W.: Notwendigkeit der Erforschung von Abgasschäden in der Natur. Chem.-Ztg. **66**, 436—437 (1942).
— Wege zum chemischen Nachweis von Abgas-(Rauch-)Schaden mit besonderer Rücksicht auf den Wald. Tharandt. forstl. Jahrb. **93**, 631—658 (1942).
MÜLLER, P. H., H. SCHMITT u. G. BISCHOFBERGER: Das Fluorproblem in der Aluminium-Industrie. Z. f. Erzbergbau u. Metallhüttenwesen **13**, 419 (1960); **12**, 400 (1959).
NAGELSMITH, G., and H. L. NIXON: Formation of apatite from superphosphate in the soil. Nature (Lond.) **154**, 428—429 (1944).
NAJJAR, V. A.: Isolation and properties of phosphoglucomutase. J. biol. Chem. **175**, 281—290 (1948).
—, and M. E. PULLMAN: Occurrence of group transfer involving enzyme (phosphoglucomutase) and substrate. Science **119**, 631—634 (1954).
NIELSEN, H. M.: Determination of microgram quantities of fluoride. Anal. Chem. **30**, 1009 to 1011 (1958).
NICHOL, A. A., H. M. BENEDICT, J. L. BYRNE, and C. P. MCCARTY: The determination of the fluoride content of natural vegetation. J. Air. Poll. Control Ass. **6**, 239—243 (1957).
NICKERSON, W. J., and C. W. CHUNG: Reversal of fluoride inhibition of yeast growth by glucose-1-phosphate. Amer. J. Bot. **39**, 669—679 (1952).
NOMMIK, H.: Fluorine in Swedish Agricultural Products, Soil and Drinking Water. Stockholm: Esselte Aktiebolag 1953.
OELSCHLÄGER, W., and M. KIRCHGESSNER: Die Fehlermöglichkeiten bei der Bestimmung des Fluorgehaltes von Futtermitteln. Landw. Forschung **13**, 64 (1960).
ONG, E. R. DE: Injury to apricot leaves from fluorine deposit. Phytopath. **36**, 469—471 (1946).
ORDIN, L., and L. JACOBSON: Inhibition of ion absorption and respiration in barley roots. Plant Physiol. **30**, 21—27 (1955).
—, and B. P. SKOE: Inhibition of metabolism in avena coleoptile tissue by fluoride. Plant Physiol. **38**, 416—421 (1963).
OST, H.: Der Kampf gegen schädliche Industriegase. Z. angew. Chem. **20**, 1689—1693 (1907).
— Untersuchung von Rauchschäden. Chem.-Ztg. **20**, 165—171 (1896).
PACK, M. R., A. C. HILL, M. D. THOMAS, and L. G. TRANSTRUM: Determination of gaseous and particulate inorganic fluorides in the atmosphere. Amer. Soc. Testing Materials Special Tech. Publ. **281**, 27—44 (1959).
PETERS, R. A.: Biochemical light on an ancient poison: a lethal synthesis. Endeavor **13**, 147—154 (1954).
—, and R. J. HALL: Fluorine compounds in nature; the distribution of carbon-fluorine compounds in some species of Dichapetalum. Nature (Lond.) **187**, 572—575 (1960).
— R. W. WAKELIN, and P. BUFFA: Fluoro-acetate poisoning—isolation and properties of the fluorotricarboxylic acid inhibitor of citrate metabolism. Proc. Royal Soc. B. **140**, 497—506 (1953).
PILCHER, L. S.: Peach suture red spot: a review. Unpublished manuscript, 1958.
PILET, P. E.: Sur la pénétration du fluor dans les feuilles; action de l'acide β-indolyl-acétique. Bull. Soc. Bot. Suisse **73**, 58—92 (1963).
— Influence of fluorine and β-indoleacetic acid on the respiration of root tissue. Rev. gen. Bot. **71**, 12—21 (1964).
POLHEIM, P. v., u. H. DIETRICH: Natürlicher Fluorgehalt wirtschaftseigener Futtermittel und Erfahrungen bei Anwendung der Destillationsmethode nach Gericke und Kermies. Landw. Forsch. **8**, 118—125 (1955).
PRINCE, A. L., F. E. BAER, E. G. BRENNAN, I. A. LEONE, and R. H. DAINES: Fluorine: its toxicity to plants and its control in soils. Soil Sci. **67**, 269—278 (1949).
QUANJER, H. M., and A. VÜRTHEIM: Een geval van beschadiging der vegetatie door rook. Pharm. Weekblad **43**, 181—187 (1906).
RAHMAN, B., u. M. A. JOSLYN: Die Phenolase und Peroxidase der Pflaumen. Mitt. Klosterneuberg Ser. B. Obst u. Garten **4**, 49—61 (1954).
RECKENDORFER, P.: Ein Beitrag zur Mikrochemie des Rauchschadens durch Fluor. Die Wanderung des Fluors im pflanzlichen Gewebe. I. Teil: Die unsichtbaren Schäden. Pflanzenschutz-Ber. **9**, 33—35 (1952); II. Teil: Die sichtbaren Schäden. Pflanzenschutz-Ber. **10**, 112—124 (1952).
REMMERT, L. F., T. D. PARKS, A. M. LAWRENCE, and E. H. MCBURNEY: Determination of fluorine in plant materials. Anal. Chem. **25**, 450—453 (1953).
REUSS, C.: Rauchbeschädigung in dem Gräflich v. Tiele-Winklerschen Forstreviere Myslowitz-Kattowitz. Goslar: J. Jäger u. Sohn 1893, and Goslar, Nachtrag, 1896.
RHODE, A.: Schädigung von Roggenfeldern, durch die einer Superphosphat-Fabrik entströmenden Gase. Z. Pflanzenkrankh. **5**, 135—136 (1895).
RICHARDS, B. L., and L. C. COCHRAN: Virus and viruslike diseases of stone fruits in Utah. Handbook for their identification and control. Utah State Agr. Exp. Sta. Bull. **384** (1956).

RICHARDS, H. M.: Respiration of wounded plants. Ann. Bot. **10**, 531—582 (1896).
RIEHM, E.: Über die Verwendung von Fluorpräparaten zur Schädlingsbekämpfung. Apotheker-Ztg. **42**, 136—137 (1927).
ROBINSON, W. O., and G. EDGINGTON: Fluorine in soils. Soil Sci. **61**, 341—353 (1946).
ROHOLM, K.: Fluor und Fluorverbindungen, Bd. 7, 1—62. Berlin: Heffter-Lorenz Ergänzungswerk 1938.
— Fluorschädigungen. Leipzig: Johann Ambrosius Barth 1937; English edition: Fluorine Intoxication. London: H. K. Lewis and Co. Ltd. 1937.
ROMELL, L. G.: Damage of plant organs by hydrofluoric acid and other acid gases. Svensk. Bot. Tidskr. **35**, 371—378 (1941).
ROSS, C. W., H. H. WIEBE, and G. W. MILLER: Effect of fluoride on glucose catabolism in plant leaves. Plant Physiol. **37**, 305—309 (1962).
ROSS, J. M., R. H. WADE, and H. M. BENEDICT: Rapid field method for determination of fluoride in plants. J. Ass. Off. Agr. Chem. **46**, 907—908 (1963).
ROWLEY, R. J., J. G. GRIER, and R. L. PARSONS: Determination of fluorine in vegetation. Anal. Chem. **25**, 1061—1065 (1953).
SALISBURY, F. B., and J. BONNER: Inhibition of photoperiodic induction by 5-fluorouracil. Plant Physiol. **35**, 173—177 (1960).
SALM-HORSTMAR: Über Lithium und Fluorkalium als Bedingungen zur Fruchtbildung der Gerste. J. Prakt. Chem. **84**, 140 (1861).
SCHARRER, K., u. W. SCHROPP: Die Wirkung des Fluorins auf Keimung und Jungwachstum einiger Kulturpflanzen. Landw. Vers. Stat. Berlin **114**, 203—214 (1932).
SCHMITZ-DUMONT, W.: Versuche über die Einwirkung von Fluorwasserstoff in der Atmosphäre auf Pflanzen. Tharandt. forstl. Jahrb. **46**, 50—57 (1896).
SCHÖNIGER, W.: Eine mikroanalytische Schnellbestimmung von Halogen in organischen Substanzen. Mikrochim. Acta, Feb.—Nov., 123—129 (1955).
SCHROEDER, J. V., u. O. REUSS: Die Beschädigung der Vegetation durch Rauch und die Oberharzer Hüttenrauchschäden. Berlin 1883.
SCHWEIGART, H. A.: Integrierende Spurenelemente in biologischen Systemen. Z. Pflanzenernähr. Düng.- u. Bodenk. **54**, 36—58 (1951).
SEMRAU, K. T.: Emission of fluorides from industrial processes — a review. J. Air Poll. Cont. Ass. **7**, 92—108 (1957).
SERTZ, H.: Über die Wirkung von Fluorwasserstoff und Fluorsilizium auf die lebende Pflanze. Tharandt. forstl. Jahrb. **72**, 1—13 (1921).
SINGER, L., and W. D. ARMSTRONG: Determination of fluoride (Procedure based upon diffusion of hydrogen fluoride). Anal. Chem. **26**, 904—906 (1954).
— — Determination of fluoride in blood serum. Anal. Chem. **31**, 105—109 (1959).
SLATER, E. C., and W. D. BONNER JR.: Effect of fluoride on the succinic oxidase system. Biochem. J. **52**, 185—196 (1952).
SOEP, H.: A combustion method for the quantitative estimation of chromatographic spots. Determination of organic compounds containing fluoride. J. Chromatography **6**, 122—130 (1961).
SOLBERG, R. A., and D. F. ADAMS: Histological responses of some plant leaves to hydrogen fluoride and sulfur dioxide. Amer. J. Botany **43**, 755—760 (1956).
STEINKOENIG, L. A.: Relation of fluorine in soils, plants and animals. Ind. Eng. Chem. **11**, 463—465 (1919).
STUMPF, P. K.: Carbohydrate metabolism in higher plants. I. Pea aldolase. J. biol. Chem. **176**, 233—241 (1948).
— Carbohydrate metabolism in higher plants. III. Breakdown of fructose diphosphate by pea extracts. J. biol. Chem. **182**, 261—272 (1950).
— Fat metabolism in higher plants. III. Enzymic oxidation of glycerol. Plant Physiol. **30**, 55—58 (1955).
— Biochemistry of fat formation. In: W. RUHLAND, editor, Handbuch der Pflanzenphysiologie, VIII, 201—208. Berlin-Göttingen-Heidelberg: Springer-Verlag 1957.
TEWFIK, S., and P. K. STUMPF: Carbohydrate metabolism in higher plants. II. Distribution of aldolase in plants. Amer. J. Bot. **36**, 613—623 (1949).
— — Carbohydrate metabolism in higher plants. IV. Observations on triosephosphate dehydrogenase. V. Enzymic oxidations of fructose diphosphate. J. biol. Chem. **192**, 519—533 (1951).
THOMAS, M. D.: The invisible injury theory of plant damage. J. Air Poll. Cont. Ass. **5**, 1—4 (1956).
— Unpublished data, 1933—1935.
— Air pollution with relation to agronomic crops: I. General status of research on the effects of air pollution on plants. Agronomy J. **50**, 545—550 (1958).

THOMAS, M. D.: Effects of air pollution on plants. In: Air Pollution. World Health Organization, Monograph Series, No. 46, Geneva, 233—278, 1961.
—, and R. H. HENDRICKS: Effects of air pollution on plants. In: P. Magill, F. R. Holden, and C. Ackley, editors, Air Pollution Handbook. Chap. 9. New York: McGraw-Hill Book Co. 1956.
— G. A. ST. JOHN, and S. W. CHAIKIN: An atmospheric fluoride recorder. Am. Soc. Testing Materials Special Tech. Publ. **25**, 29—57 (1958).
TRESHOW, M.: Effects of fluorine on the anatomy of Chinese apricot leaves. Phytopath. **46**, 640 (1956).
TRUHAUT, R.: Les Fluoroses. Paris 1948.
— Le Fluor dans les aliments: Aspects biologiques et analytiques du probleme. Ann. Fals. et fraudes **48**, 237—246, 290—312 (1955).
VOGT-BEEKMANN, H.: Untersuchungen über den Umsatz von Carotinoiden in höheren Pflanzen. Z. Botan. **42**, 387—435 (1954).
WADE, R. H., J. M. ROSS, and H. M. BENEDICT: Method for detection and isolation of traces of organic fluoride in plants. J. Chromatography **4**, 37—45 (1964).
WALLACE, D. H.: Market Control in the Aluminum Industry. Cambridge: Harvard University Press 1937.
WANDER, F. W., and J. J. MCBRIDE: A chlorosis produced by fluorine on citrus. Science **123**, 933—934 (1956).
WANG, T. H., C. S. LIN, C. WU, C. LIAO, and H. Y. LIN: The fluorine content of Fukien tea. Food Research **14**, 98—103 (1949).
WARBURG, O., u. W. CHRISTIAN: Isolierung und Kristallisation des Gärungsferments Enolase. Naturwissenschaften **29**, 589—590 (1941a).
— — Chemischer Mechanismus der Fluorid-Hemmung der Gärung. Naturwissenschaften **29**, 590 (1941b).
— — Isolierung und Kristallisation des Gärungsferments Enolase. Biochem. Z. **310**, 384—421 (1942).
WEINSTEIN, L. H.: Effects of atmospheric fluoride on metabolic constituents of tomato and bean leaves. Contrib. Boyce Thompson Inst. **21**, 215—231 (1961).
WHARTON, H. W.: Isolation and determination of microgram amounts of fluoride in materials containing calcium and orthophosphate. Anal. Chem. **34**, 1296—1298 (1962).
WILLARD, H. H., and O. B. WINTER: Volumetric methods for determination of fluorine. Ind. Eng. Chem. Anal. Ed. **5**, 7—10 (1933).
WILLE, F.: Die Rauchschadenfrage der Aluminiumfabriken mit besonderer Berücksichtigung der Aluminiumfabrik Chippis. pp. 66 Berlin: P. Parey
WILLIAMS, C. R.: Air pollution from fluorides. J. Air Pollut. Control. Ass. **6**, 199—202 (1956).
WILSON, L. B.: Effects of chlorine, bromine and fluorine on the tobacco plant. J. Agric. Res. **46**, 889—899 (1933).
WISLICENUS, H.: Resistenz der Fichte gegen saure Rauchgase bei ruhender und bei tätiger Assimilation. Tharandt. Forstl. Jahrb. **48**, 152—172 (1898).
— Zur Beurteilung und Abwehr von Rauchschäden. Z. angew. Chem. **14**, 689—712 (1901).
— Über experimentelle Rauchschäden in „Rauchversuchshaus" zu Tharandt. Ber. 57. Versamml. Sächs. Forstvereins, 78—93, 1913.
WOBER, A.: Über die Giftwirkungen von Arsen-, Antimon- und Fluorverbindungen auf einige Kulturpflanzen. Angew. Botan. **2**, 161—178 (1920).
YAMAGUCHI, S.: Respiratory metabolism of the hypocotyl in the kidney-bean seed. Misc. Rept., Research Inst. Nat. Resources, Japan **30**, 63—73 (1953).
YANG, S. F., and G. W. MILLER: Biochemical Studies on the effect of fluoride on higher plants. 2. The effect of fluoride on sucrose-synthesizing enzymes from higher plants. Biochem. J. 88, 509—516 (1963).
— — The effect of fluoride on phosphoglucomutase, U.D.P.G. pyrophosphorylase and U.D.P.G. transglucosylase from higher plants. Plant Physiol. **37**, Supp. lxix, (1962).
ZEEVAART, J. A. D.: DNA multiplication as a requirement for expression of floral stimulus in Pharbitus nil. Plant Physiol. **37**, 296—304 (1962).
ZIMMERMAN, P. W., A. E. HITCHCOCK, and J. GWIRTSMAN: Fluorine in food with special reference to tea. Contrib. Boyce Thompson Inst. **19**, 49—53 (1957).
— — Susceptibility of plants to hydrofluoric acid and sulfur dioxide gases. Contrib. Boyce Thompson Inst. 18, 263—279 (1956).

Chapter 6

The Effects of Fluorides on Livestock, with Particular Reference to Cattle

By

JAMES L. SHUPE[1] and ERNEST W. ALTHER[2]

With 46 Figures

I. Introduction

Fluorine occurs throughout the world in soil, vegetation, water, and animal tissues. Because of its chemical reactivity, it is found in nature in a combined (fluoride) form. The terms fluoride and fluorine will be used interchangeably in this chapter.

Under normal conditions, livestock consume variable low-level amounts of fluorine. No adverse effects are known to accompany this normal fluoride ingestion.

The total fluorine intake by an animal may be attributable to one or a number of sources. The most commonly encountered sources of potentially excessive fluorides are: (1) forages subjected to air-borne contamination in areas near industrial plants that heat fluorine-containing materials to high temperatures and expel fluorides, (2) drinking water high in fluoride content, (3) feed supplements and mineral mixtures high in fluoride content, and (4) vegetation growing on soils of high fluoride content.

When fluorides in amounts above the borderline or critical level (which varies with species and other factors detailed later) are ingested over long periods of time, chronic fluorine toxicosis may result. This is because fluorine is cumulative in the animal body as long as the animal continues to ingest a constant or increasing amount. Animals are also subject to acute fluorine toxicosis, but this condition is seldom encountered.

Fluorosis in livestock has been reviewed by AGATE et al. (1949), MITCHELL and EDMAN (1951/52), and SCHMIDT and RAND (1952) among others. In addition, the National Research Council (1960) has evaluated the research on fluorine and suggested tolerances. Early European literature has been reviewed by ROHOLM (1937) and more recently by ALTHER (1961). The literature citations in this chapter are not intended to be all-inclusive. The authors have cited only those references that seemed to them to be of maximum value to this discussion.

A. Relevant past European history

Apparently fluorosis was noted in sheep in Iceland 1000 years ago (1934a). According to the report the occurrence was correlated with volcanic eruptions.

[1] Research Veterinarian, Animal Disease and Parasite Research Division of the U.S. Agricultural Research Service, Logan, was formerly professor of veterinary medicine, Utah State University.

[2] Consulting Member, Fluorine Commission, Swiss Academy of Medical Sciences, Basle, Switzerland. Present address, Cantonal Agricultural College, Flawil, St. Gallen, Switzerland.

Stationery Office 1949.

In 1844 v. BIBRA found fluorine in all bones analyzed of herbivora and other species. HOPPE (1862) analyzed teeth of swine for their fluorine content in 1862. RABUTEAU, in 1867, tested the toxicity of fluorides on laboratory animals.

A sickness of cattle caused by pollutants from a nearby industrial plant was described by HAUBNER for the first time in 1878. Based on the circumstances and symptoms described by HAUBNER, the sickness was not the same as fluorine toxicosis as we know it today.

In their toxicity studies in 1891, BRANDL and TAPPEINER administered daily 0.1–0.9 g of pure sodium fluoride (NaF) to a dog. A total of 403 g was given during 21 months. After 3 weeks, fluorine was found in the urine. At the end of the experiment, post mortem analyses showed that much of the ingested fluorine (about 60 g) had been deposited in bones, cartilage, and teeth.

In 1902 JODLBAUER and STUBENRAUCH proved that excessive intake of NaF by dogs caused deposits of crystalline calcium fluoride (CaF_2) in the Haversian canals of bones. Exostosis and stiffness in the carpal joints of dogs were produced in 1908 by ROST who fed the animals up to 0.5 g NaF for 8–12 weeks.

The first poisoning of swine by a mineral mixture containing fluorine used as a feed supplement was reported in 1904 by DAMMANN and MANEGOLD (1904). Up to 4.42% of NaF was found in the feed.

BARTOLUCCI in 1912 reported some interesting cases of osteomalacia in cattle maintained near a fertilizer factory. Based on CHRISTIANI's results (1926), BARTOLUCCI in 1927 attributed his 1912 observations to fluorine effluents from the factory. CRISTIANI had fed hay contaminated by the effluent of a nearby aluminum factory to guinea pigs, and had caused cachexia or death of the animals. Since he did not find nitrates or nitrites in the forage (CRISTIANI, 1927), the cachexia of the experimental animals was attributed to fluorine compounds. The results of these experiments (CRISTIANI, 1926) have to be viewed with caution since no studies were made with cattle or other livestock.

In 1929, HUPKA and LUY frequently observed osteomalacia in cattle feeding in the neighborhood of a factory producing hydrofluoric acid. Cattle owners in the area had been reporting for several years that their animals became lame, lost weight, and decreased their milk production during grazing periods. The animals recovered during the winter when stabled and fed other forage. Vegetation in the path of prevailing winds had been damaged by the industrial effluents, and windows of homes and stables had become opaque. Bone changes in the cattle were observed.

Similar cases were reported in 1934 from the vicinity of aluminum plants in Norway (SLAGSVOLD, 1934a, b), and in 1935 from the neighborhood of an aluminum plant in Italy (BARDELLI and MENZANI, 1935). The descriptions of the affected animals were in general comparable to those given by BARTOLUCCI and by HUPKA. SLAGSVOLD (1934b) had found cases of chronic fluorine poisoning in livestock, especially sheep and cattle. He reported irregular molar and bone changes with white, porous exostoses on leg bones and skulls. BARDELLI (1937/38) had made similar observations on goats and cattle.

VELU (1931 b) established the relationship between the various soil and vegetative conditions found in the phosphate zones of Morocco, Algeria, and Tunisia and chronic fluorosis (darmous) in cattle and sheep. The author stressed (1931 a) the need to determine the fluorine content of the waters of these phosphatic zones (1932). In these areas one sheep may ingest daily 8.7 mg F from water and its sediments, 33.8 mg F from vegetation, and 113.6 mg F from dust. VELU and BALOZET (1931) later reproduced fluorine toxicosis in sheep experimentally by adding 3% natural phosphate to the diet.

B. Relevant past American history

Most of the endemic cases of fluorosis of livestock reported in America have occurred in cattle, thus most of the fluorine studies have been concerned with cattle.

HUFFMAN and REED in 1930 reported on the general symptoms and lesions associated with the feeding of raw rock phosphate to cattle. Then in 1934 PHILLIPS et al. (1934) reported observations made during a series of investigations in which the chronic toxicity patterns, tolerance levels, and physiological effects of fluorine in dairy cows were studied.

In 1936 DE EDS reported on fluorine in relation to bone and tooth development. This author also reported on factors related to the etiology of mottled enamel in 1941.

World War II caused a lapse in significant research relative to fluorosis, but in 1952 RAND and SCHMIDT reported the effect of Arizona waters of high fluoride content upon cattle. In 1954 HOBBS et al. discussed the physiological effects of various levels of fluorine fed to beef cattle and sheep.

SCHMIDT et al. (1954) issued a progress report in 1954 on controlled feedings of fluorine, as sodium fluoride to adult Holstein-Friesian cattle. Their 6-year study was made to determine the damaging and nondamaging levels of fluorine when fed under practical farm conditions. A more detailed presentation of their results was published in 1958.

In 1955, SHUPE et al. reported on the pathologic and physiologic aspects of chronic bovine fluorosis and evaluated the lesions useful in diagnosing fluorosis. A field survey to determine the possible presence and severity of fluorosis in cattle was published in 1956 (SPENCER et al.).

SUTTIE et al. (1957) have conducted fluoride feeding experiments with dairy cattle; these studies indicate that 50 ppm of fluoride in the ration of lactating cows will cause the development of fluorosis within $3-5^1/_2$ years.

HOBBS and MERRIMAN reported in 1962 on bovine fluorosis attributable to soil and water sources.

II. Experimental work with species other than cattle

Birds are more resistant than mammals to the toxic effects of fluoride ingestion. Rodents are more resistant than larger animals on a body weight basis, and omnivores and carnivores appear to be more resistant than herbivores.

A. Sheep

ROHOLM (1934b) fed 15 mg NaF per kg body weight daily to two sheep, producing exostoses on the mandibles of the animals within 30 days after the experiment began.

LILLEENGEN (1934) studied preparations of the bones of sheep that had been fed hay grown in the vicinity of a Norwegian aluminum reduction plant. Mandibles, leg bones, and skulls showed distinct exostoses. Microscopic examination demonstrated considerable bone atrophy around the extended marrow cavities and Haversian canals. Fibrous marrow and occasional osteoclasts were observed in the spongiosa of the mandible.

SHREWSBURY et al. (1944) reported that ingestion by sheep of 6 mg F/kg/day as phosphate rock was detrimental to feed consumption and growth.

HARRIS et al., in 1963, reported the physiological effects on lambs of ingesting various levels of fluorine. These workers concluded that lambs can safely ingest 100 parts per million (ppm) of fluorine (as NaF) for 84 days without any adverse effects. The tolerance level of fattening lambs for fluorine was determined to be between 100 and 200 ppm in their dry diet. Typical lesions of incisor and molar dental fluorosis in sheep are shown in Figs. 1 and 2.

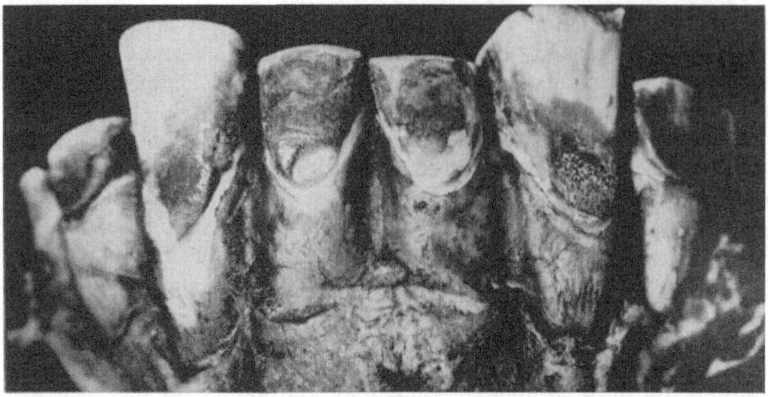

Fig. 1. Dental fluorosis in sheep as evidenced by abrasion, hypoplasia, and discoloration of the permanent incisors. From SHUPE et al., unpublished

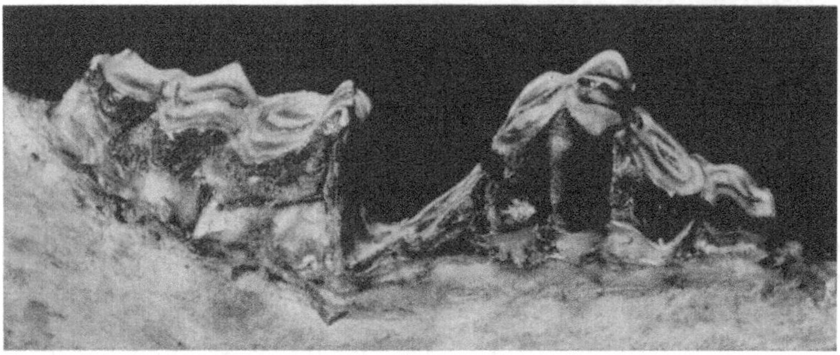

Fig. 2. Dental fluorosis in sheep as evidenced by severe molar abrasion. From SHUPE et al., unpublished

B. Swine

Bone and dental changes, and effects on growth and organs seen in pigs receiving fluoride in the ration as sodium fluoride or rock phosphate, were described by KICK et al. (1935).

Eight-week-old pigs, fed 15 mg of fluorine per kilogram of body weight daily for 171 days developed irregular calcification in teeth and jaw bones. The walls of the spongy framework of the periodontium showed osteoclastic destruction, and the bony tissue was hyperemic. The enamel of the teeth showed more hypoplasia than did the dentine itself (BRINCH, 1937).

Rock phosphate containing 2.4% F was used as a supplement to a commercial mixed feed and fed in equal parts with barley meal to a 6-months-old pig. Constipation and loss of appetite were attributed to the fluorine content of the phosphate. No control was maintained and no tests with other animals were made (PERO, 1945).

Based on experiments designed to establish the tolerated effective dose of NaF as a vermifuge against ascarids in swine, BENDIXEN et al. (1950) made the following recommendation. A dose of 1% NaF in 0.5 kg of the basic ration once when the pigs weighed 12.5–25.0 kg, again at the 25–37.5 kg weight, and once more at 37.5–50.0 kg would do no harm to the animal.

Comar et al. (1953) reported on the interrelated effects of dietary fluorine ingestion and feed intake on bone and body growth, Ca^{45} behavior and deposition patterns, bone pathology, and feed utilization in young pigs.

Wilder, in 1963, reported on the effects of fluorine compounds on swine.

C. Horses

Roholm (1934b) considers horses as being more tolerant to fluorine influence than other species of domestic animals. Dammann and Manegold (1904) produced acute fluorotic effects, including colic and diarrhea, in a horse that was fed increasing doses of NaF up to 100 g daily.

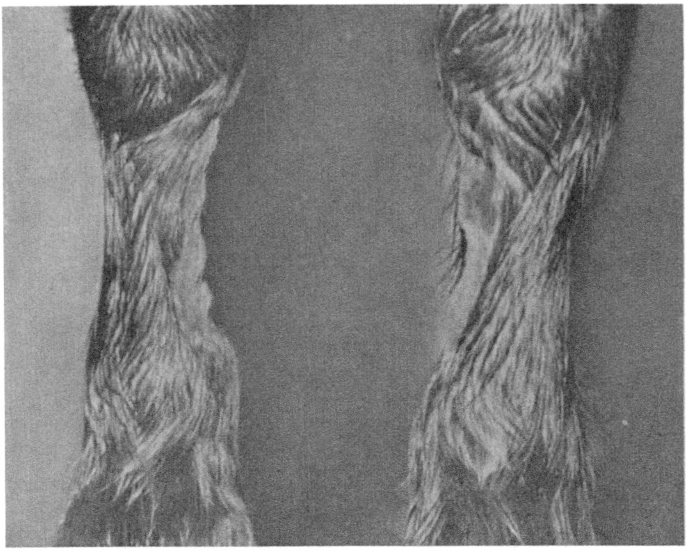

Fig. 3a. Bilateral periosteal hyperostosis on the medial aspects of the metacarpal bones of a horse. From Hupka, 1941

Velu (1931b) observed irregularities in the molars of a 5-year-old horse. The incisors were completely worn down. The horse lived in the same region where darmous was regularly found in sheep.

In 1941 Hupka published a picture of a horse $1^1/_2$ years of age, and another of two colts. During one entire summer the three animals had received the same fluorine-contaminated hay from the same pastures as had a herd of cows that were maintained in the vicinity of an industry producing fluoric acid. The cows had developed severe symptoms of fluorosis.

One of the horses showed distinct deformations of the leg bones with exostoses and thickening of the bones of the skull. The metacarpal regions of the fore-limbs are shown in Fig. 3a. Figure 3b depicts fluorine-induced periosteal hyperostosis on the medial aspects of the metacarpal bone of a 2 year old gelding that had ingested vegetation with a fluorine content of 280 ppm for ten months. The fluorine concentrations in the pastures varied according to the season between 70 and 1500 ppm F and averaged 280 ppm over the whole period of forage production.

Varying degrees of fluorosis in horses have been observed in some areas where fluorine poisoning of livestock was unequivocally diagnosed. The cattle in these areas evidenced marked to severe lesions of fluorosis. The permanent incisor teeth shown in Fig. 4 are from a horse that had grazed the same pasture where cattle with typical symptoms and lesions of fluorosis were grazing. The fluoride content of the vegetation in the pasture ranged from 89 ppm to 178 ppm and the drinking water contained 8 ppm.

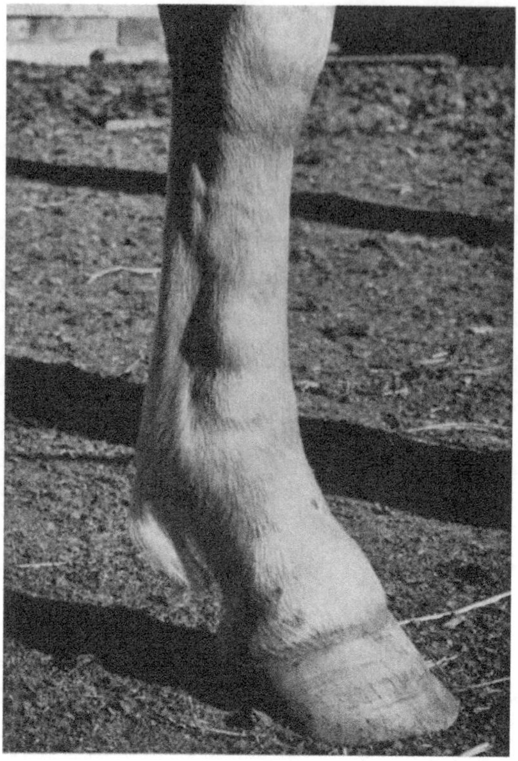

Fig. 3 b. Periosteal hyperostosis on the medial aspect of the metacarpal bone of a horse. The bone lesions were on the medial and lateral aspects of all four limbs. From SHUPE, unpublished

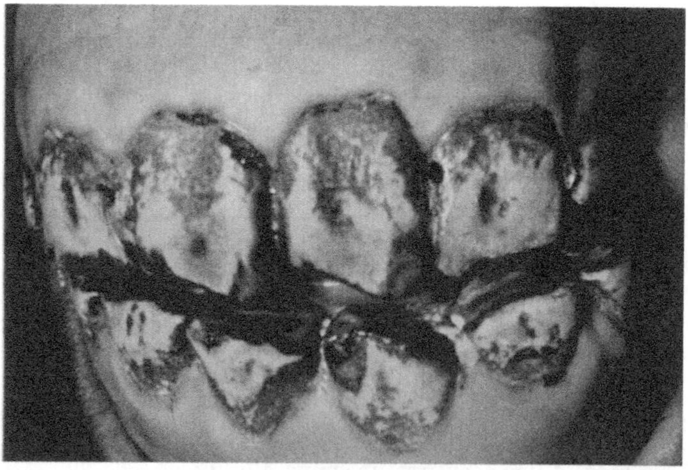

Fig. 4. Dental fluorosis in the permanent incisor teeth of a horse. Note abrasion, hypoplasia, and discoloration

D. Turkeys

ANDERSON et al. reported in 1955 on the effect of feeding various levels of sodium fluoride to growing turkeys. Performance of the turkeys was not affected by increasing the ration fluoride level to 10 ppm; however, weight gains were decreased when 200 ppm of fluoride were included in the ration.

III. The toxicity of fluorine compounds

Calcium fluoride, raw rock phosphate, and compounds of similar solubilities are less toxic than sodium fluoride (Fig. 5). Tolerances for such compounds would be higher, therefore, than the ones commonly quoted since these are usually based on NaF experiments. Fluorides emitted by some industrial plants may reach the toxicity range of sodium fluoride (Fig. 6).

SHUPE et al. (1962) have reported experimental findings on the relative effects of feeding hay atmospherically contaminated by fluoride residue, normal hay plus calcium fluoride, and normal hay plus sodium fluoride to dairy heifers. The results indicated that the calcium fluoride was less toxic than either the sodium fluoride or the hay containing fluoride emitted from an industrial plant (Fig. 7). The contaminated high F hay, containing fluoride emitted from an industrial plant, was as toxic as sodium fluoride.

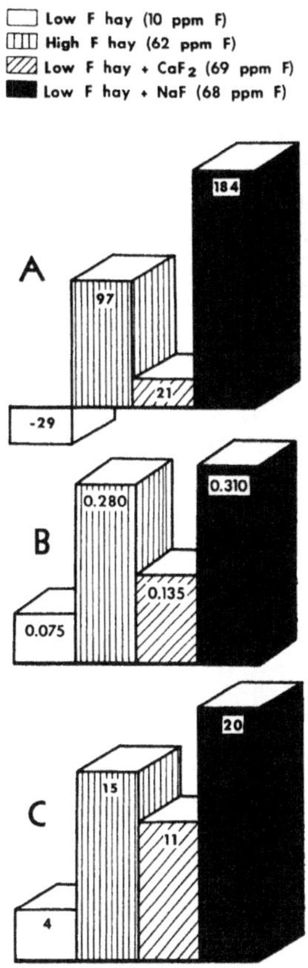

Fig. 5

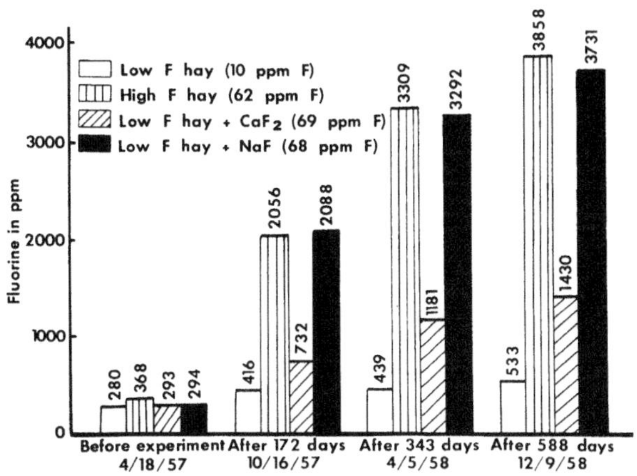

Fig. 6

Fig. 5. (A) Average daily fluorine balance (mg) of dairy heifers after 506 days on experiment. (B) Average fluorine (ppm) content of blood of dairy heifers after 543 days on experiment. (C) Average fluorine (ppm) content in urine of dairy heifers after 543 days on experiment. From SHUPE et al., 1962

Fig. 6. Average fluorine content of biopsied ribs from dairy heifers (dry fat-free basis). From SHUPE et al., 1962

The addition of aluminum chloride, aluminum sulfate, or calcium carbonate to the diet reduces the degree of toxicity that would otherwise result from the fluoride consumed. Controlled experiments on dairy cattle showed that as much as 42% less fluorine was stored in their osseous tissues when alleviators were included in their rations (GREENWOOD et al., 1964).

Although the toxic effects of various fluorides have been the subject of numerous investigations, few animal species have been studied thoroughly. The

FIRST INCISOR

Individual Classification	0	1	2	3	4	5
Treatment	No. Heifers					
Low F Hay	1	3				
High F Hay		2		2		
Low F Hay + CaF_2		3	1			
Low F Hay + NaF		2	1	1		

SECOND INCISOR

Individual Classification	0	1	2	3	4	5
Treatment	No. Heifers					
Low F Hay	2	2				
High F Hay				1	3	
Low F Hay + CaF_2		1	2	1		
Low F Hay + NaF				2	2	

THIRD INCISOR

Individual Classification	0	1	2	3	4	5	9
Treatment	No. Heifers						
Low F Hay	2	2					
High F Hay	1				3		
Low F Hay + CaF_2	2		2				
Low F Hay + NaF					3		1

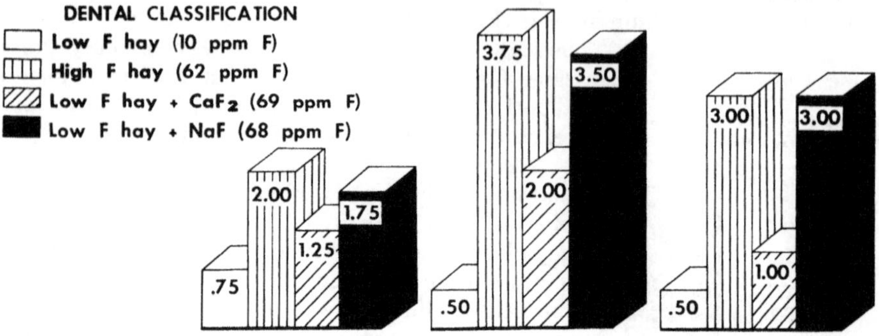

Fig. 7. Average classifications of incisor teeth of dairy heifers that received different sources of fluorine for 588 days on experiment (age 27 months). From SHUPE et al., 1962

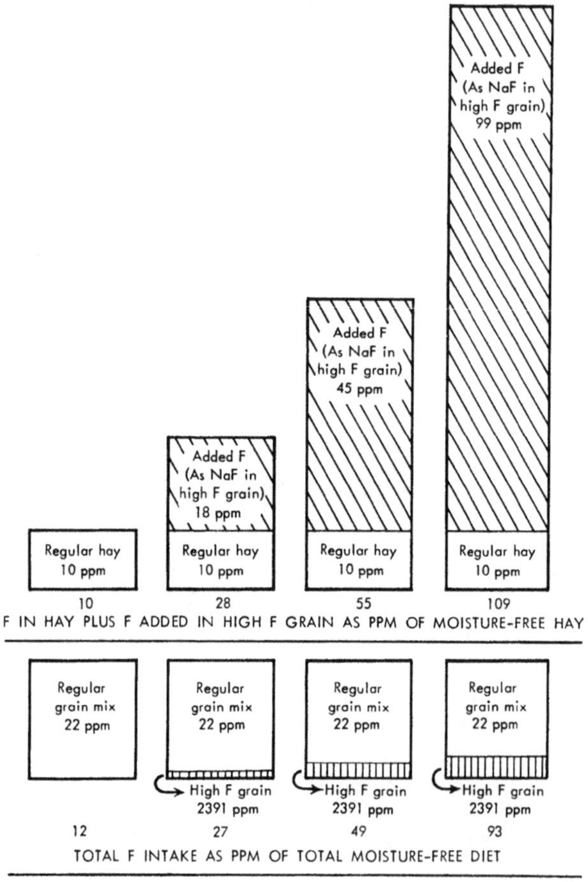

Fig. 8. Sources of fluorine in diets of Holstein cows in an 8-year experiment. (First appeared in J. Animal Sci. *23*, 537, 1964)

tolerance levels for various species cited later are based upon results of high-level short-term experiments, lower level long-term experiments, detailed necropsy studies, and clinical field studies. All of this work has been reported in various journals. The most comprehensive report can be found in a recently published monograph (GREENWOOD et al., 1964).

The remainder of this chapter is based largely upon one study that contributed extensive data to the monograph (Fig. 8). This recently completed, long-range (8-year) study involved dairy animals that were started on the controlled experiment when 3 to 4 months of age (SHUPE et al., 1963b). Information gathered over a 10-year period from examinations of more than 70,000 clinical field cases of fluorosis and detailed necropsy studies of 519 selected field cases involving animals of various ages and with varying degrees of fluorosis, has been correlated with the results from the controlled experiments to substantiate the conclusions drawn. Only especially pertinent literature citations are included.

IV. Response of cattle to ingested fluoride

A. General considerations

The various factors that govern the reactive processes of animals ingesting fluorides include the following: (a) level or amount of fluoride ingested, (b) duration of ingestion-time, (c) type and solubility of fluoride ingested, (d) age of animal during period of ingestion, (e) level of nutrition, (f) stress factors, and (g) individual biological response. All of these factors interact and affect the manifestation of the disease. In turn, the factors are influenced by the variable responses they elicit from reactive processes of the body, *e.g.*, elimination of fluorine in the urine, deposition of fluorine in the skeletal structures, and reduction of fluorine intake because of anorexia.

The clinical picture for all species is increased in complexity by the generally long time lapse or interval between ingestion of elevated levels of fluorine and manifestation of clinical symptoms. No single criterion should be used in diagnosing and evaluating fluorosis. All clinical, necropsy, and chemical findings must be carefully evaluated with reference to one another. Among the criteria usable at the clinical level are the following: (a) mottling and abrasion of the teeth, (b) intermittent lameness, (c) degree of osteofluorosis, (d) the amount of fluorine retained in the bone (can be obtained by biopsy), and (e) the amount of fluorine excreted in the urine.

In general, the following levels of sodium fluoride, calculated in ppm for the total dry ration, can be ingested over a normal life span without adverse effects on the normal animal: dairy heifer and cow, up to 30; beef heifer, up to 30; beef cow, up to 40; sheep, up to 50; swine, up to 70; horses, up to 90; turkeys, up to 100; and chickens, up to 150. Tolerances are higher over short time intervals such as normal fattening periods of 180 days for cattle and 70 days for sheep. Under such conditions cattle and sheep can safely ingest up to 110 ppm. The tolerance cited for horses is based primarily on field case studies and clinical observation correlated with lesions and chemical analysis of forage for fluorine.

B. Mineralizing matrix

The most consistent and reliable quantitative indication of fluorosis is achieved by measuring the amount of fluorine retained in the normal mineralizing matrixes of the body. In 1913 GAUTIER reported on determinations of fluorine made in various tissues of fluorosis-affected animals. He noted that the highest concentrations were in bones, enamel, and dentin, while lower concentrations occurred in tendons and cartilage. It has since been proved that about 96% of all fluorine retained in the body is found in the bone, enamel, cementum, and dentine. This retention pattern has made possible the establishment of certain criteria (defined later) that are useful in evaluating the degree of fluorosis. The primary effect of fluoride probably is on pre-enamel, pre-dentin, pre-cementum, and pre-skeletal matrices and the action probably is one of delaying and altering normal mineralization. The degree and extent of the reactive processes and the concentration of fluorine in the normal mineralizing tissues are governed by all of the factors itemized previously that potentially influence fluorosis.

1. Teeth

One of the most sensitive biological reactive processes of the body to fluorine intoxication occurs in the teeth. GARLICK (1954) reported on the gross anatomy, physiology, developmental anomalies, and general pathology of the teeth of the

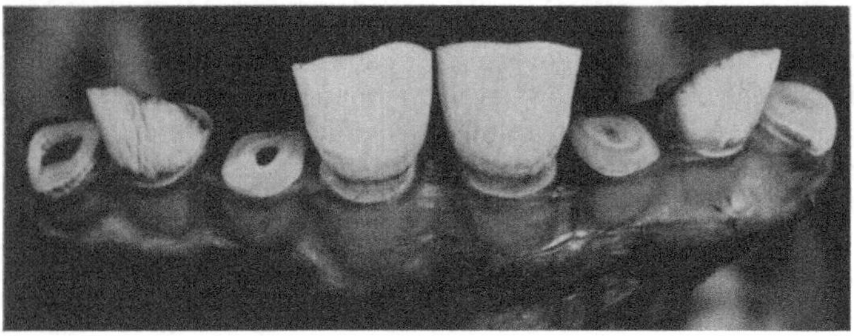

Fig. 9. Permanent incisor teeth of a cow that intermittently ingested various levels of fluorine at different stages of its life. Secondary dentine formation can be noted on second pair of incisor teeth. From GREENWOOD et al., 1964

ox in clinical diagnosis. In 1955 this same worker reported on dental fluorosis in the teeth of the ox in clinical diagnosis and stated that a knowledge of the lesions of dental fluorosis was essential when evaluating a clinical diagnosis of

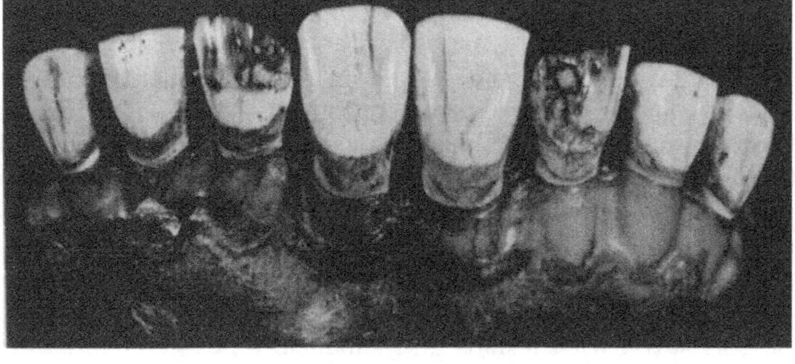

Fig. 10. Permanent bovine incisor teeth illustrating excessive fluoride effects of abrasion, discoloration, hypoplasia, and mottling. The bilateral nature and varying degrees of the lesions indicate intermittent ingestion of elevated levels of fluorine. From SHUPE, 1963

systemic fluorosis (GARLICK, 1955). HOBBS and MERRIMAN (1962) reported on experimental results and findings of fluorosis in beef cattle and correlated the dental fluorosis that was evident with the amount of fluoride ingested. BROWN et al., in 1960, reported on postnatal tooth development in cattle and described their studies relative to the development, eruption, and resorption of the teeth in cattle and the chronology of enamel and dentine development in the mandibular incisor and canine teeth. Dental fluorosis has not been observed in deciduous teeth of cattle, sheep, and horses.

The causative factor of dental fluorosis operates during the period of tooth development and indicates intake at that time. When elevated levels of fluorine are ingested during the formative stage of the teeth, both enamel and dentine are adversely affected. The teeth then erupt with characteristic changes such as: mottling (chalky white areas), staining, hypoplastic defects, and hypomineralization. The severity and combination of these dental changes vary depending upon the level of fluoride ingested while the teeth are forming.

Specific ameloblastic and odontoblastic damage will vary with the intake of varying levels of fluorine. A matrix laid down by damaged ameloblasts and odontoblasts does not accept minerals as does a normal matrix. This leads to poor and faulty mineralization. When a tooth has fully formed and erupted, the ameloblasts have lost their constructive ability and a fluoride-affected tooth has no reconstructive capacity to compensate for the fluorotic enamel lesions. Odontoblasts have the ability to form secondary dentine, however, and reconstructive secondary dentine can be noted in Fig. 9.

Oxidation of the organic material in the dental structures results in the characteristic brown or black discoloration which is observed in varying degrees in cases of dental fluorosis (Fig. 10).

After hypoplasia or a certain degree of mottling occurs in a tooth, it is subject to an increased rate of attrition regardless of type or quality of feed consumed. Abrasive feeds such as coarse and poor quality roughage, however, will hasten the rate of abrasion. Molar abrasion manifests itself later than incisor abrasion and exhibits greater variation in wear or erosion (Figs. 11a—c).

Dental fluorosis is usually diagnosed in cattle by clinical examination of the incisor teeth since these are more readily accesible for examination than are the molar teeth. Adequate diagnosis and evaluation of dental fluorosis, however, requires that the cheek teeth be evaluated along with the incisors. This is because of the following positive relations between the dental fluorosis of certain incisor teeth and the degree of abrasion of certain molar teeth in cattle:

First incisor and second molar
Second incisor and third molar
Third incisor and second premolar.

Field survey work in endemic areas has confirmed that dental lesions are useful in clinically diagnosing fluorosis. For the purpose of classifying clinically the various degrees of dental fluorosis, the following standards were adopted and have been used in classifying more than 70,000 cattle in endemic areas.

(0) Normal: smooth, translucent, glossy white appearance of enamel; tooth normal shovel shape.

(1) Questionable effect: slight change, unable to determine exact cause; may have enamel flecks; cavities, if present, may be unilateral or bilateral; absence of mottling.

(2) Slight effect: slight mottling of enamel; may have slight staining but no wear; teeth normal shovel shape.

(3) Mild effect: definite mottling and staining of enamel; coarse mottling (large patches of chalky poor quality enamel); teeth may show slight abrasion.

(4) Marked effect: definite mottling, staining, hypoplasia, and hypocalcification; may have pitting of enamel; definite abrasion of teeth; enamel may be a dirty cream color.

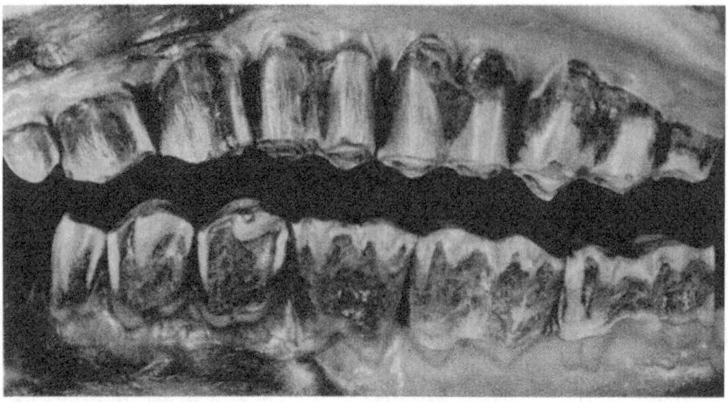

a

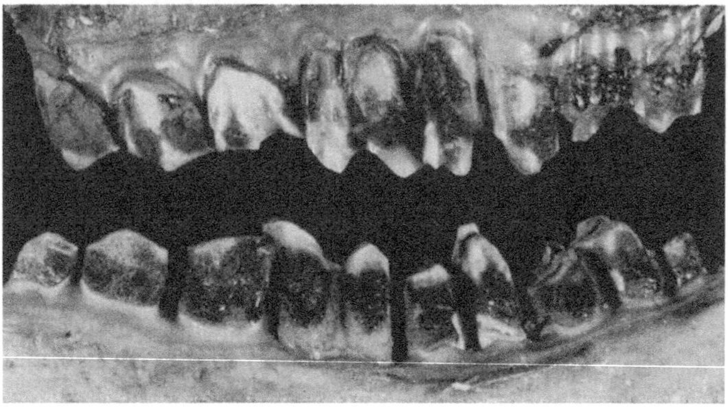

b

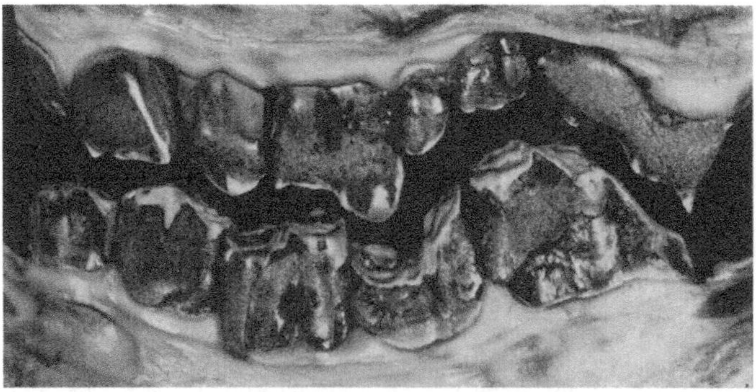

c

Fig. 11 a—c. a Molar teeth from cow ingesting 12 ppm F during the interval 3 to 4 months to 7.5 years of age. b Molar teeth from cow ingesting 93 ppm F for the same period. c Molar teeth from a severe field case of fluorosis. From SHUPE, 1963

(5) Excessive effect: definite erosion of enamel with excessive abrasion of teeth; staining and pitting of enamel may or may not be present.

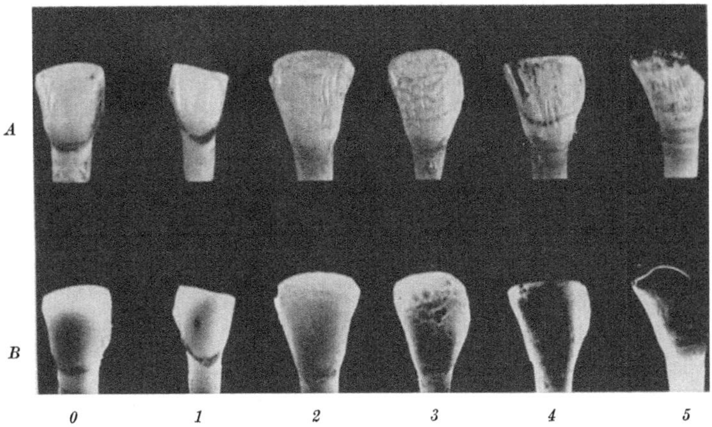

Fig. 12. Classification of representative incisor teeth from dairy cows is from 0 to 5 reading left to right in A and B. A is with direct lighting. B is with back lighting. From SHUPE et al., 1963b

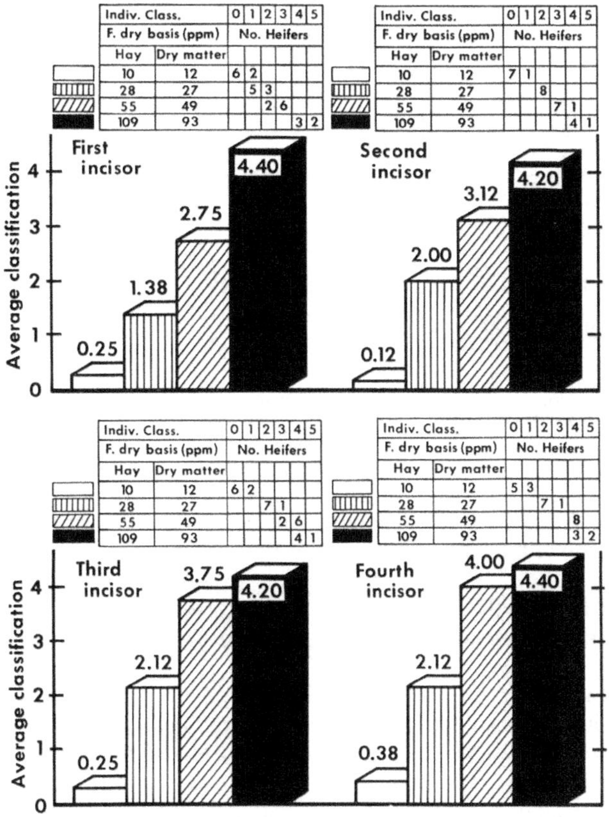

Fig. 13. Incisor tooth classification (0 to 5) of dairy cows receiving four levels of fluorine in the period from 3 to 4 months to 7.5 years of age. From SHUPE et al., 1963b

Typical incisor teeth are shown in Fig. 12.

Figure 13 depicts results of the dental examinations carried out on dairy animals during the 8-year Utah controlled experiment. The teeth were classified according to the code just described and illustrated in Fig. 14.

A

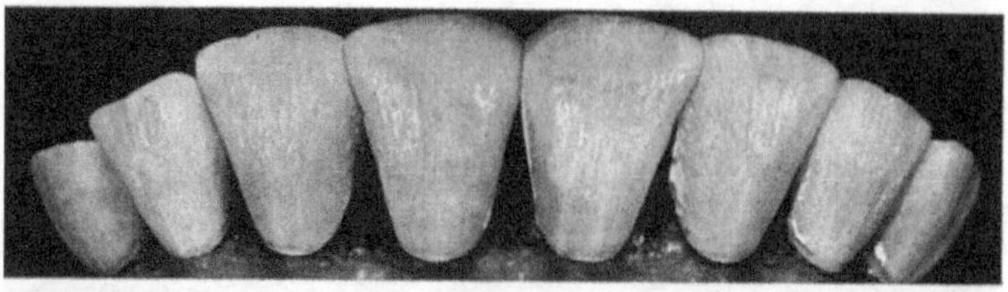

B

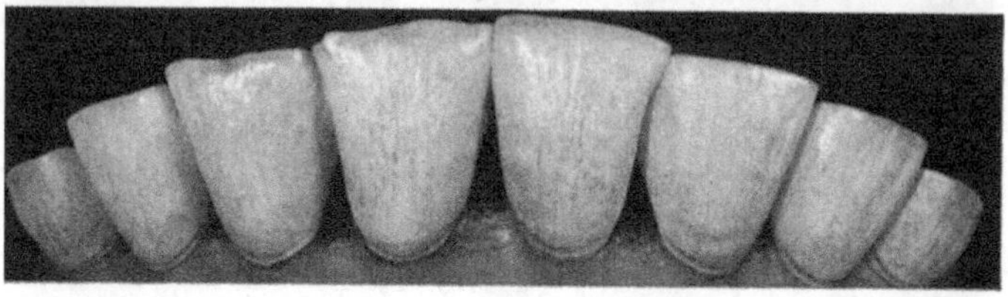

C

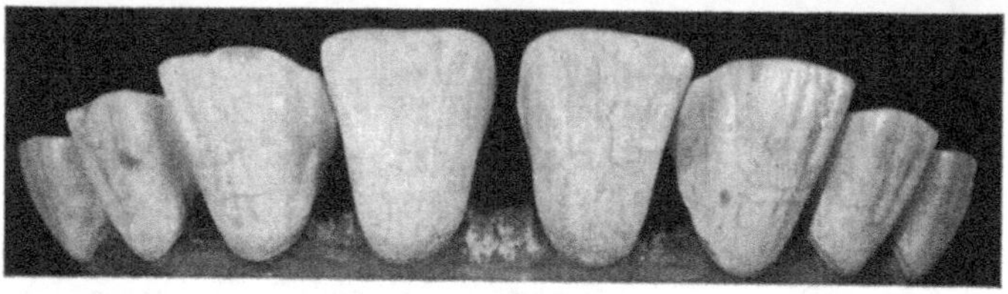

D

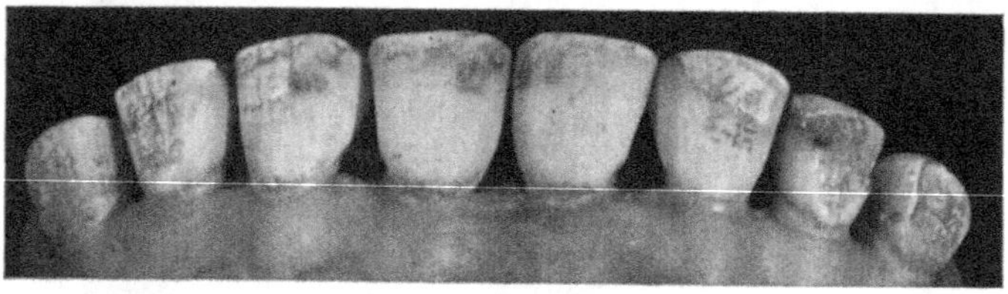

Fig. 14. Representative sets of incisor teeth from dairy cows fed four levels of fluorine from 3 to 4 months to 7.5 years of age; classifications read from left to right. Fluorine level: A - 12 ppm; B - 27 ppm; C - 49 ppm; D - 93 ppm; Tooth classification: 1-0-0-0; 1-2-2-2; 3-3-4-4; 5-5-5-5. From SHUPE et al., 1963b

2. Bones

Animals under normal conditions ingest small amounts of fluorine daily, and skeletal retention of fluorine usually is cumulative throughout the life of the animal (Fig. 15). Thus, the bones of young animals would be expected to contain less fluorine than those of old animals (Fig. 16). Aged animals on normal rations have been known to contain up to 1,200 ppm of fluorine calculated on a fat-free, dry bone basis.

Prolonged ingestion of low levels of fluorine has no discernibly adverse effects on normal bone structure and function. Unequivocal bone changes have been noted, however, in animals that ingest elevated levels of fluorine over long time periods (Figs. 17a, b).

Bone changes in cattle after fluorine consumption have been investigated microscopically by COHRS (1941). He compared the osteoporotic changes with the

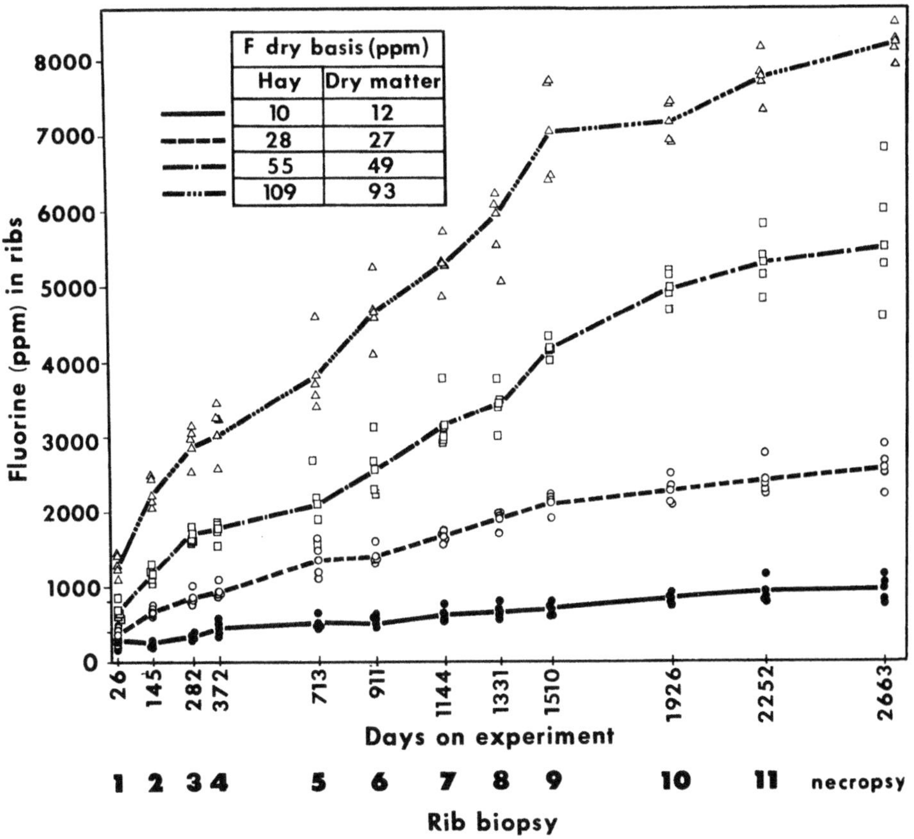

Fig. 15. Fluorine content of ribs of dairy cows receiving four levels of fluorine from 3 to 4 months to 7.5 years of age. From SHUPE et al., 1963b

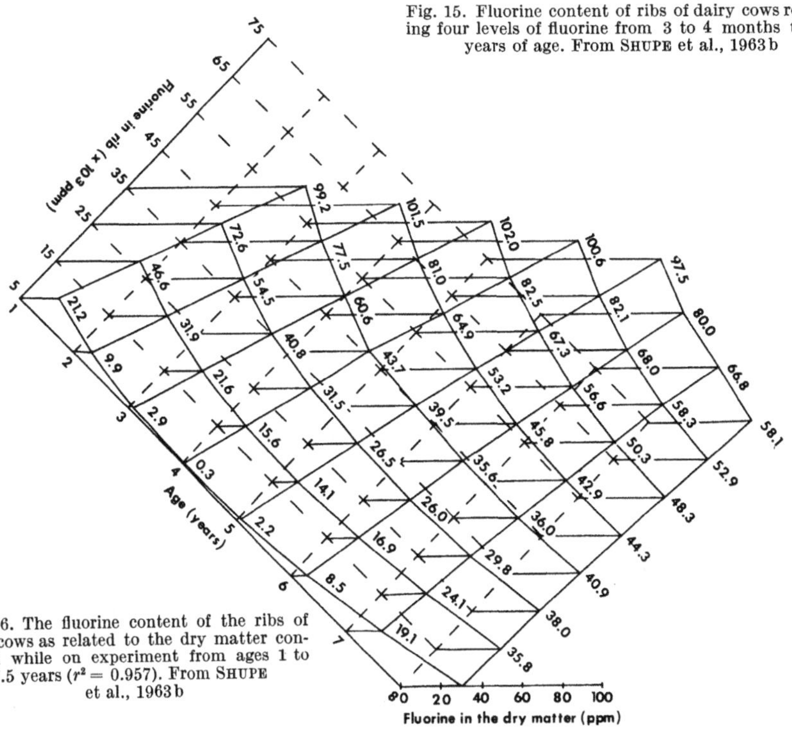

Fig. 16. The fluorine content of the ribs of dairy cows as related to the dry matter consumed while on experiment from ages 1 to 7.5 years ($r^2 = 0.957$). From SHUPE et al., 1963b

lesions of rickets and discussed sclerotic processes and osteomalacia. The chemistry, histology, and roentgenology of the teeth and bones of large animals, and changes following prolonged feeding of fluoride at various concentrations have been reported (SHUPE, 1960).

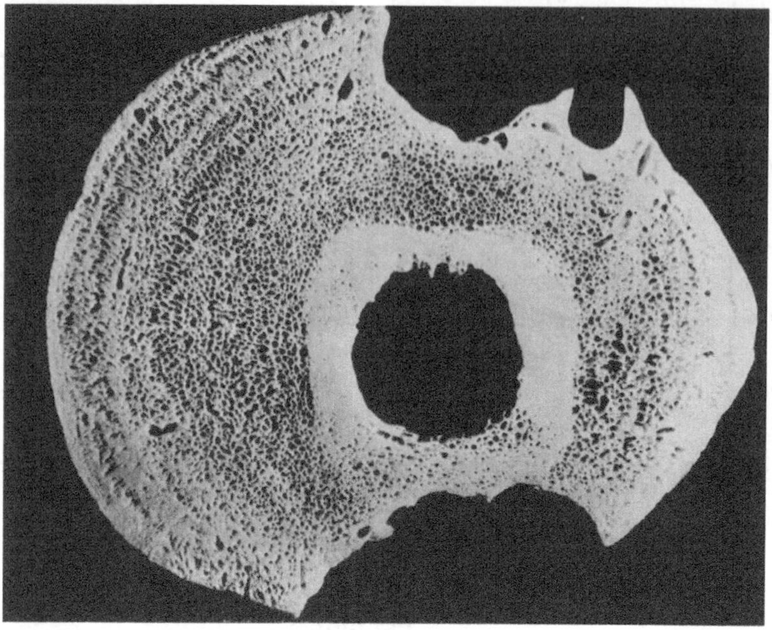

a

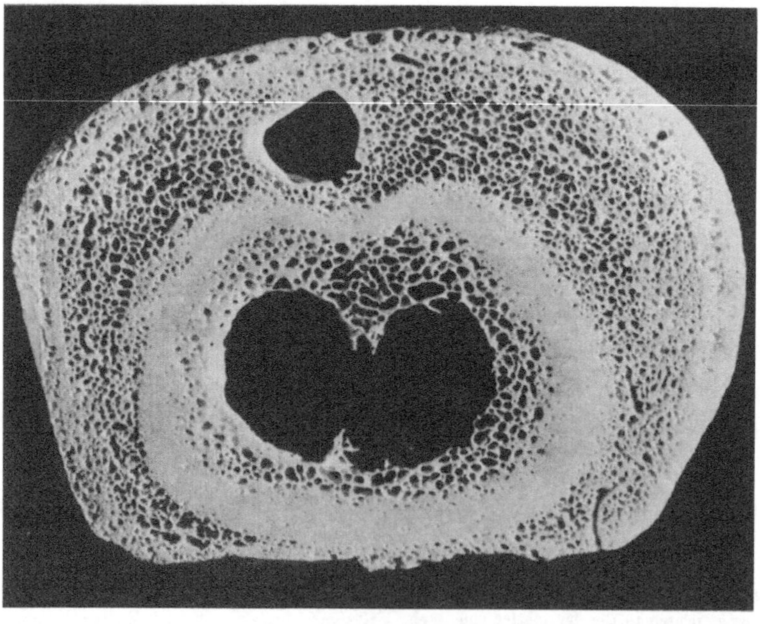

b

Fig. 17 a and b. Cross section of metatarsal bone. a Proximal aspect. b Distal aspect. Note excessive periosteal hyperostosis and endosteal resorption. From SHUPE, 1963

The bone pathogenesis and lesions that result from chronic fluorosis appear to be characteristic in nature. Fluoride deposition occurs most intensively in skeletal areas of high metabolic activity or greater vascularity. Thus, cancellous bone (*e.g.* rib, vertebrae, and sternum) accumulates more fluoride than does cortical bone. Also, in long bones, fluoride is incorporated most readily into the epiphyseal sections. This non-uniform distribution of fluoride must be considered in the evaluation of chemical analysis and long term effects.

SHUPE et al. (1963 b) reported on fluorine deposition in the bone and stated that the degree of abnormal reactive bone changes can be correlated among the various bones of the body and within certain anatomical and metabolic areas of specific bones. The more metabolically active proximal and distal areas of metacarpal and metatarsal bones proved uniformly and consistently higher than the diaphyseal areas in fluorine content (Fig. 18). Therefore, in taking bone samples for chemical analyses and other determinations, it is important to use bones for which standards have been established, and to compare like anatomical areas of given bones. Thus, both the age of the animal and the state of metabolic activity of its skeletal system influence the degree of fluoride retention in the skeleton and the actual bone changes that occur.

Grossly, bones that are adversely affected by fluorine appear enlarged and chalky white, and have an irregular, roughened periosteal surface (Figs. 19a-c). The lesions are diffuse and bilateral in nature. CORSICO (1955) observed cortical periostosis in some cases of fluorine intoxication; in other cases he described an osteoporotic and osteomalacic picture of the bone tissue.

Intra-articular structures are not primarily affected by fluorine toxicosis. Spurring and bridging of the joints may occur in advanced cases of fluorosis that also have marked periosteal hyperostosis (Fig. 20).

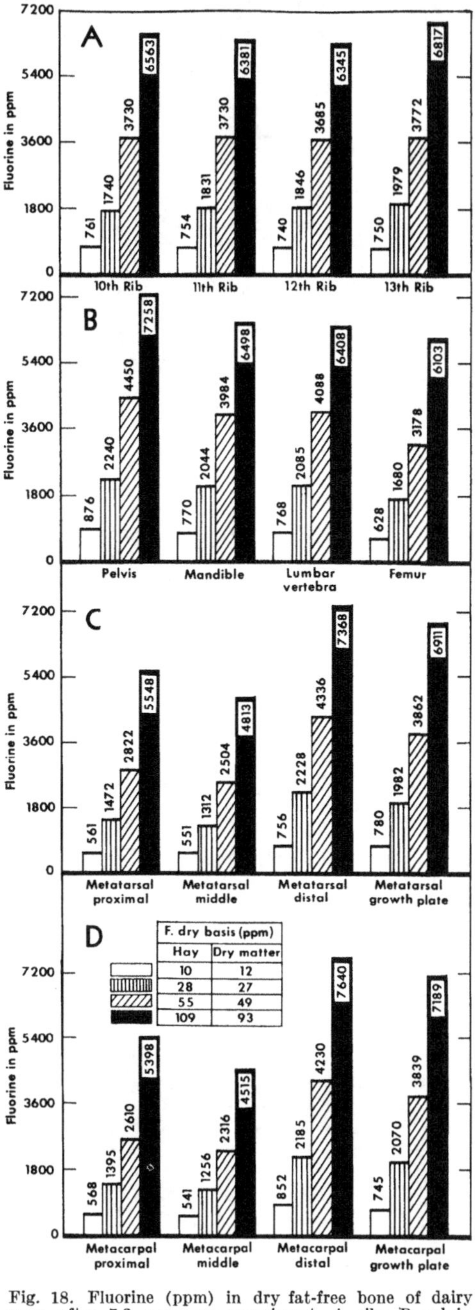

Fig. 18. Fluorine (ppm) in dry fat-free bone of dairy cows after 7.3 years on experiment. A rib; B pelvis, mandible, lumbar vertebra, and femur; C metatarsus; and D metacarpus. From SHUPE et al., 1963 b

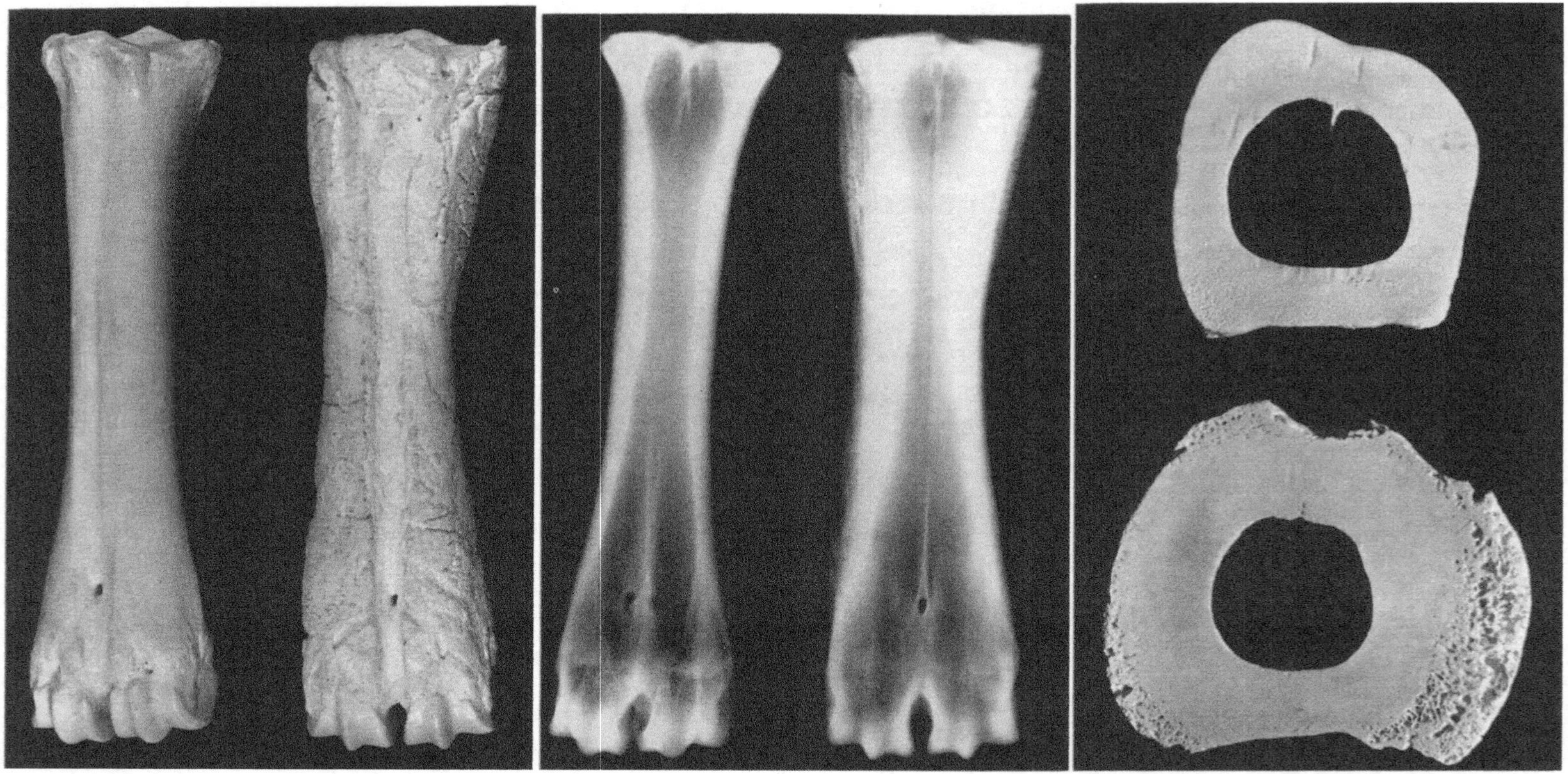

a b c

Fig. 19a—c. a Left: metatarsal bone from a dairy cow ingesting 12 ppm F in the period from 3 to 4 months to 7.5 years of age. The bone is normal. Right: metatarsal bone from a dairy cow ingesting 93 ppm F for the same period. The bone shows marked periosteal hyperostosis with a chalky white, roughened periosteal surface. b Radiographic comparison of bones in A. c Upper: cross section of a metatarsal bone from a dairy cow ingesting 12 ppm F from 3 to 4 months to 7.5 years of age. The bone is normal. Lower: cross section of a metatarsal bone from cow ingesting 93 ppm F for the same period. The bone evidences definite osteofluorosis. From SHUPE et al., 1963b

Some severe cases have shown a marked bridging that eventually led to complete rigidity of the involved joints.

In some advanced cases of bovine fluorosis that had developed marked skeletal lesions, the normal blood supply had been impaired. This situation obviously complicates efforts to understand the bone reactive processes. In differential dignoses it is important to remember that the initial stages of the bone lesions associated with degenerative arthrosis appear in the articular cartilage and are intra-articular in nature. By contrast, the first bone lesions clinically discernible

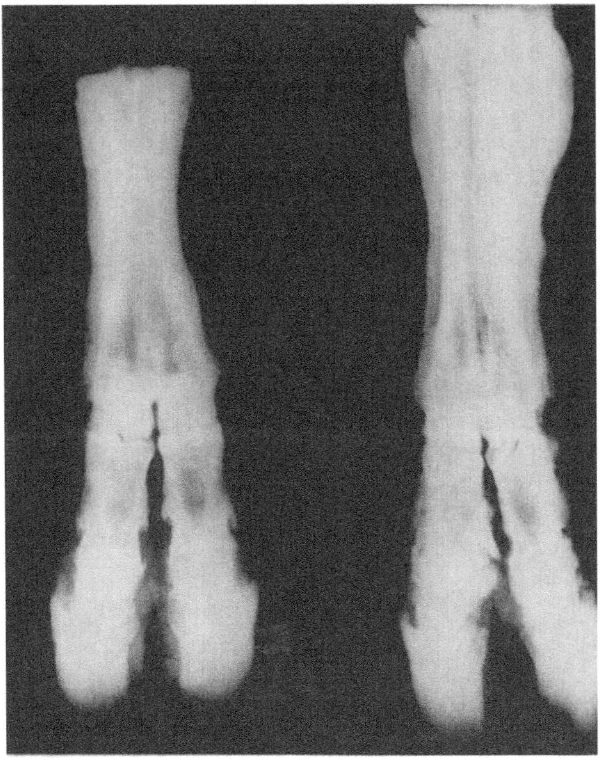

Fig. 20. Radiograph of the distal aspects of the fore and hind limb of a cow. Note the severe osteofluorosis with periosteal hyperostosis, spurring, and bridging of the joints. From SHUPE et al., unpublished

in early or mild cases of fluorosis are located on the medial surface of the proximal third of the metatarsal bones (Figs. 21 a - c). These lesions are bilateral in nature. They can be diagnosed by palpation and confirmed by radiographic studies.

The precise mechanisms of abnormal intracellular bone activity associated with bone formation, reconstruction, and remodeling that are associated with fluorine toxicosis are not fully understood at the present time. Abnormal osteoblastic activity is thought to cause the formation of an abnormal, inadequate matrix with resultant defective and irregular mineralization.

At present it is believed that fluoride ions replace the hydroxyl radical in the apatite-like crystal structure. Tests by KLEMENT and TRÖMEL (1932) have confirmed that the composition of bone substance is based principally on hydroxyapatite. In x-ray diffraction studies, Baud observed that as fluorine concentration in bone increases, the conversion of hydroxyapatite to fluorapatite causes a decrease in crystal lattice dimensions (BAUD, 1953).

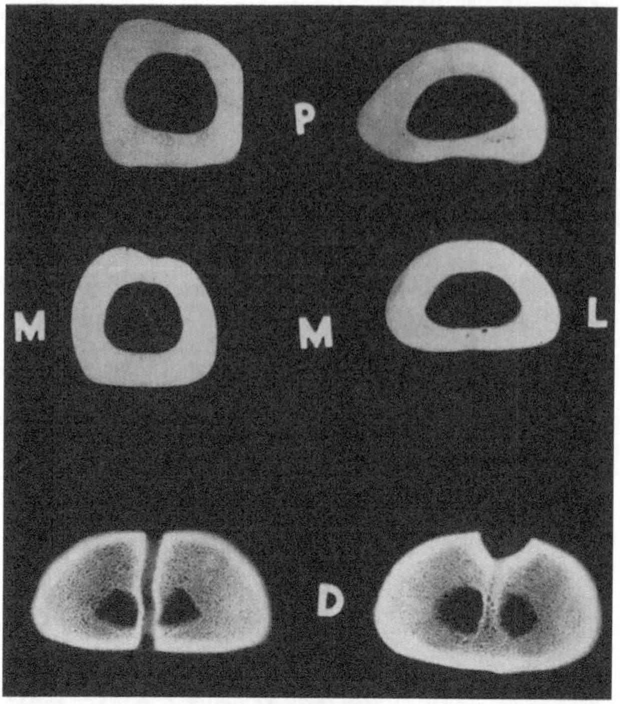

Fig. 21 a

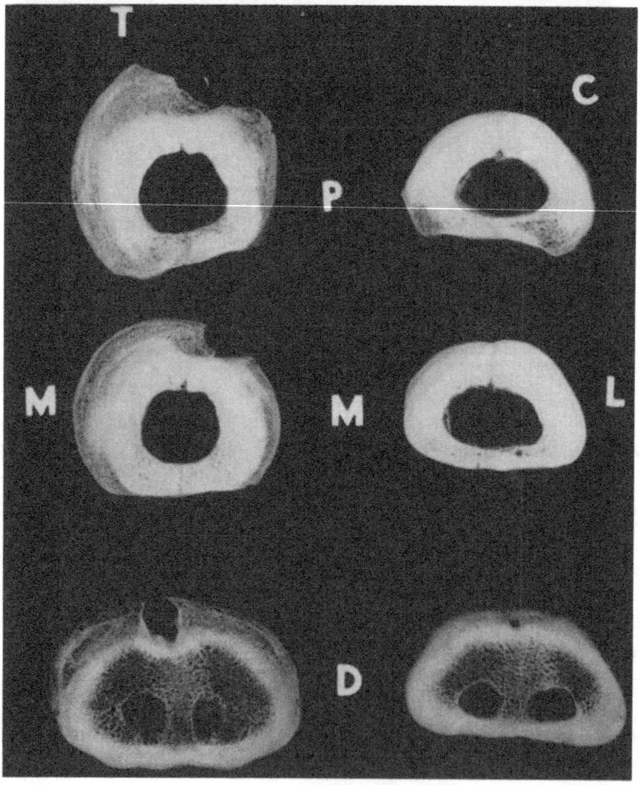

Fig. 21 b

In a recently completed study, the citrate concentration decreased from 1.2% to about 0.9% with a concomittant increase in "crystallinity". A 10-fold increase of fluoride concentration in the bovine metatarsal was accompanied by a 24% decrease in the citrate concentration and an approximate 21% increase in "crystallinity." Apparently over a 10-fold range of fluoride concentration in the bone ash of the bovine, human, and rat, there is a comparable reduction in citrate concentration and a comparable increase in "crystallinity" (ZIPKIN et al., 1964).

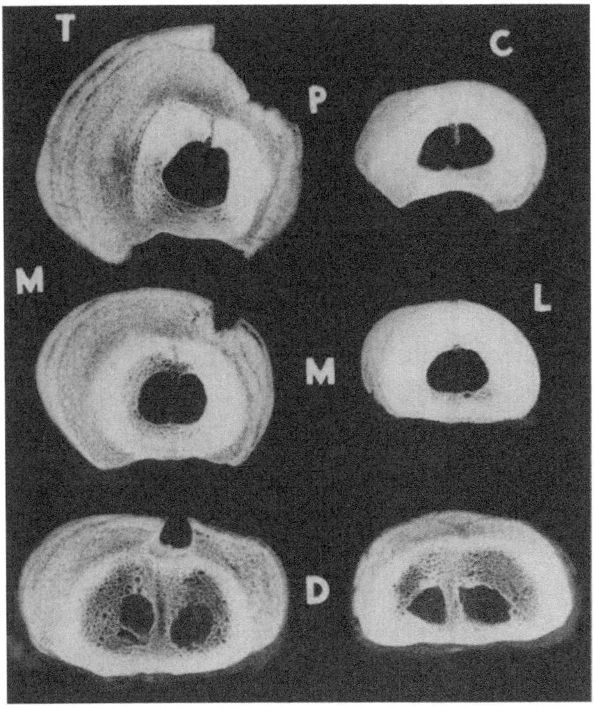

Fig. 21 c

Fig. 21 a—c. Radiograph of cross section of proximal (P), middle (M), and distal (D) aspects of metatarsal (left) and the metacarpal (right) bones from cows having varying degress of osteofluorosis. a slight, b marked, c severe. Left is the medial aspect, and right is lateral. From SHUPE et al., 1964

By giving tetracycline hydrochloride intravenously as a bone marker (20 mg per kilogram of body weight), it was established that resorption cavities may be formed in the bovine in 10 to 15 days, and that 2 to 3 months are required to refill such cavities with osteons.

Reabsorption of fluorine from bone following cessation of ingestion of fluorides appears to follow the same pattern as the deposition. A higher urinary excretion occurs during the first month after ingestion ceases because fluoride ions are being lost from the crystal surface and replaced by hydroxyl and carbonate ions. After the surface exchange and the relatively high fluoride losses that immediately follow cessation of fluoride ingestion, a slower rate of loss occurs during the process of remodeling.

a) Radiology

Pathological bone formations have been observed radiographically in animals that consumed elevated levels of fluorine over long periods of time. Ribs of cows showing clinical signs of fluorosis were examined roentgenologically by POMMER (1954). He concluded that an excessive intake of fluorine by cows induces a localized process of osteomalacic porosis and sclerosis. LEONE et al. (1955) reported

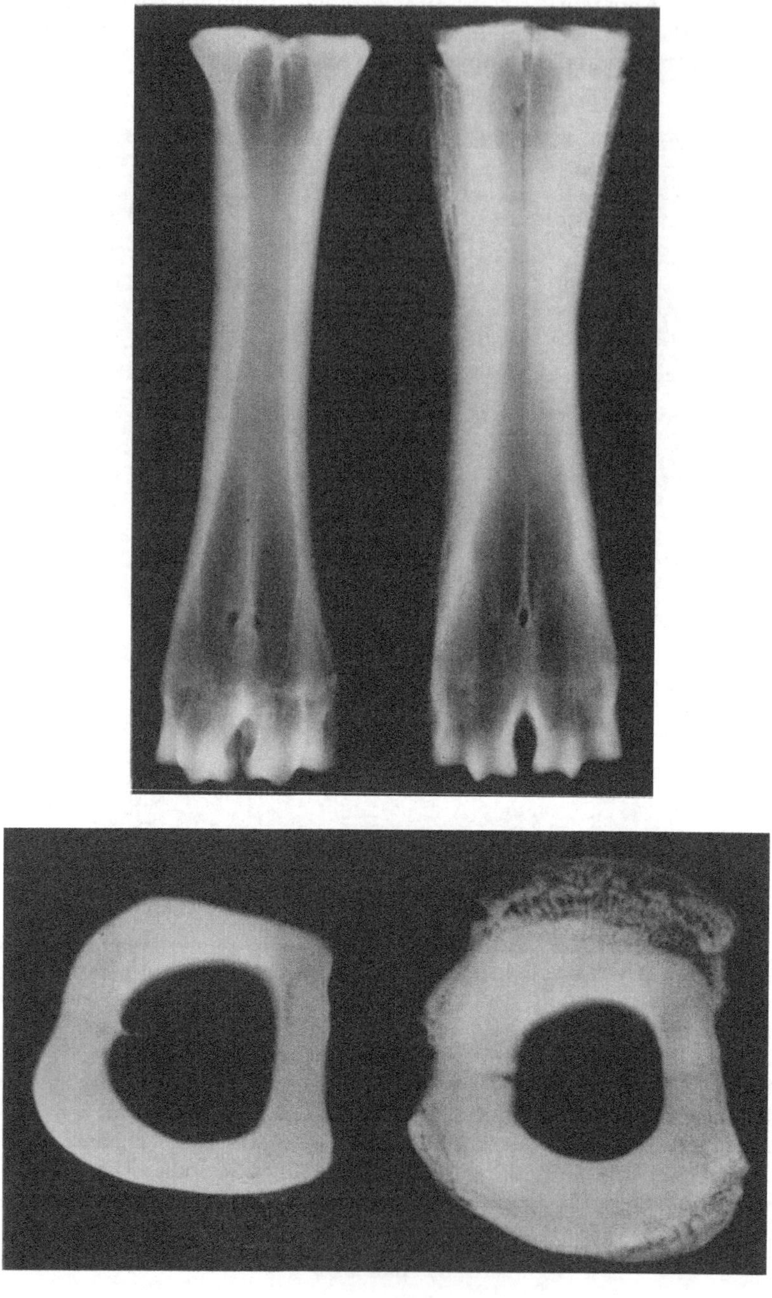

Fig. 22a. Left: normal. Right: osteofluorosis

Fig. 22a—c. Radiographs of bovine metatarsal bones illustrating normal and osteofluorotic bones. From SHUPE et al., 1963b on a roentgenologic study of a human population exposed to high fluoride domestic water and compared their findings in humans to roentgenographic bone conditions in cattle that had ingested prolonged toxic fluoride levels. Roentgenographic findings, however, vary greatly depending upon the interrelation and action of the multiple factors that govern the degree and duration of fluorosis (SHUPE et al., 1963 b).

Characteristic periosteal hyperostosis, increased subperiosteal density, endosteal porosity, narrowing of the marrow cavity, zones of increased density and porosity, and all possible combinations of these phenomena have been noted (Figs. 22 a-c). Increased coarsening and thickening of the trabecular pattern with a ground glass appearance have been noted in some cases. Bilateral fractures of the 8th, 9th, 10th, and 11th ribs with incomplete union and increased density and

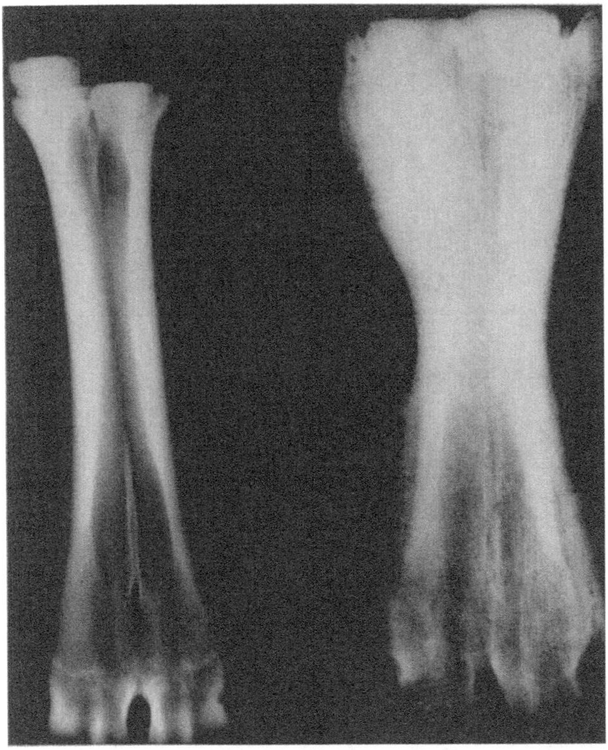

Fig. 22 b. Left: normal. Right: osteofluorosis

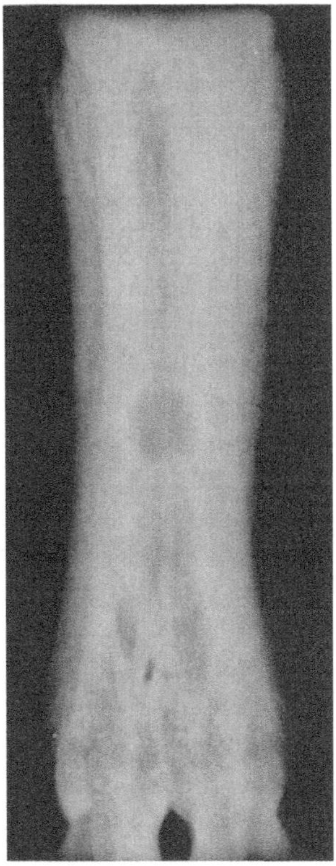

Fig. 22 c. Osteofluorosis

trabeculation of the bone have been noted occasionally. Mineralized spurs at the points of attachment of tendons to bones have been seen only in cases having marked periosteal hyperostosis.

b) *Histopathology*

Slight elevations of normal fluorine levels can occur in bone without causing detectable changes in bone structure or function. Slight or subtle microscopic changes in bone have been observed without any detectable alteration of function. In cases of fluorine toxicosis, however, a series of insidious progressive changes in bone structure and function results in altered bone properties and characteristic abnormal bone appearance (Figs. 23a—e).

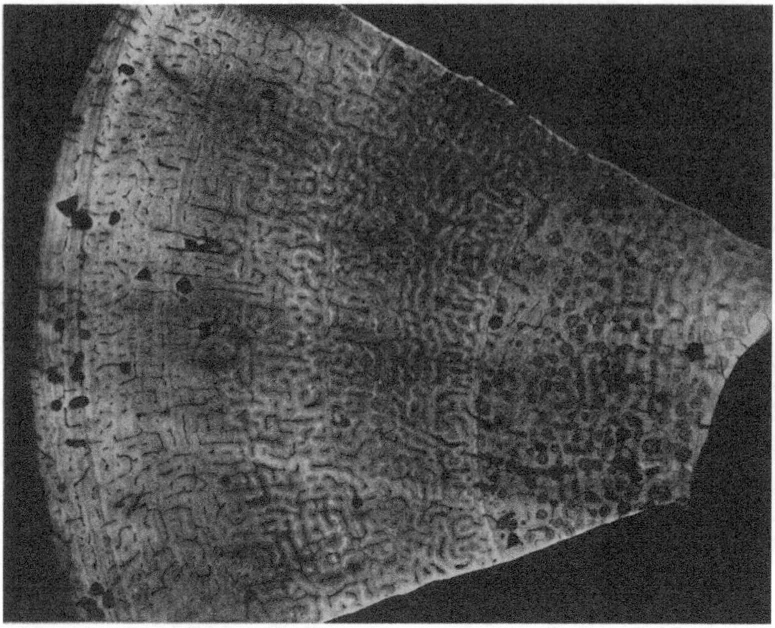

Fig. 23 b. 27 ppm, slight periosteal hyperostosis (× 6.6)

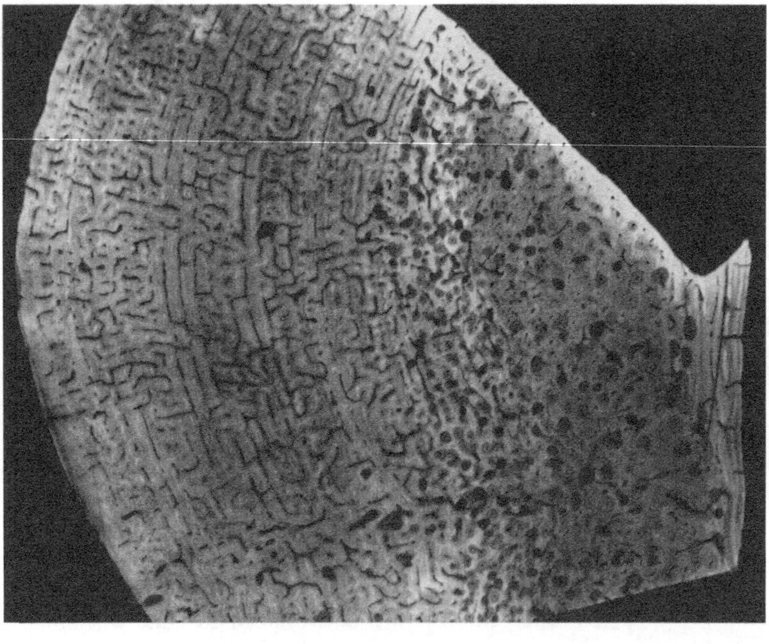

Fig. 23 a. 12 ppm normal (× 7.3)

Fig. 23 a—d. Microradiographs of metatarsal bones from dairy cows fed 4 levels of fluorine during the period from 3 to 4 months of age to 7.4 years of age
From SHUPE, 1963

Microscopic examinations of fluoride-affected bones have been completed using methods such as selective stains, ground macerated specimens (Fig. 24), infrared and ultra-violet light, polarization, and microradiographs (Shupe et al., 1963b). These studies have afforded better understanding of the changes in the bone that

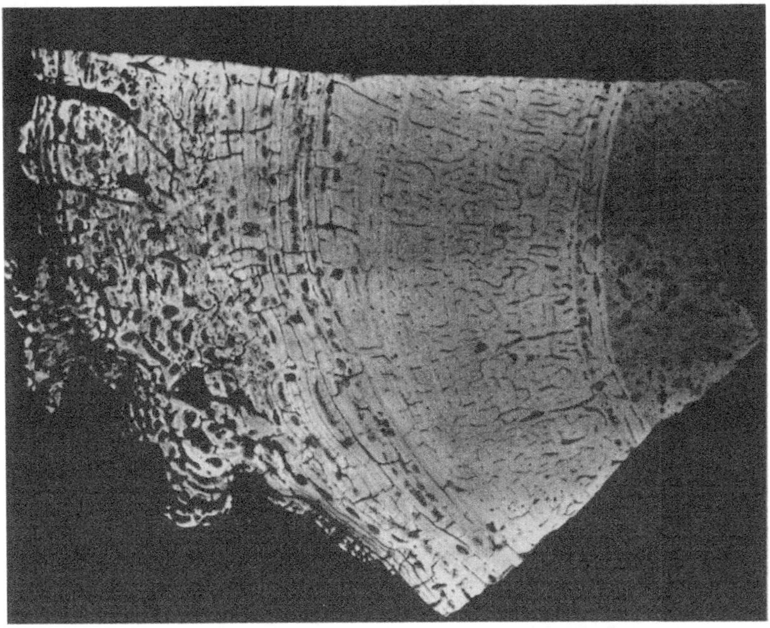

Fig. 23d. 93 ppm, marked periosteal hyperostosis (× 5)

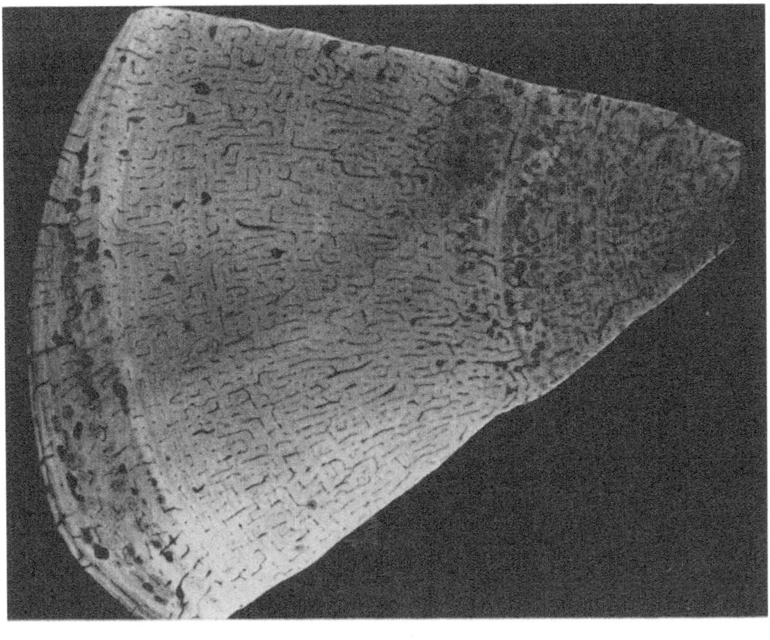

Fig. 23c. 49 ppm, moderate periosteal hyperostosis (× 5.5)

are caused by fluorine toxicosis. The amount of fluoride intake could be correlated with the degree of microscopic bone changes. The higher the fluoride intake the

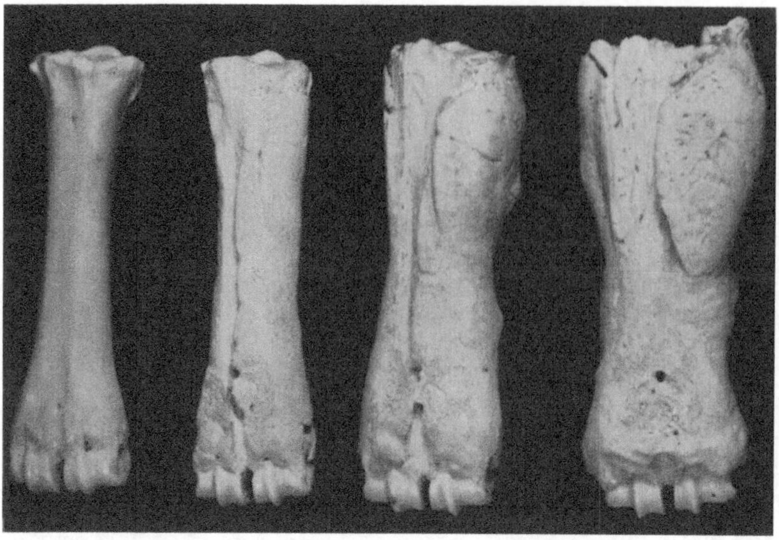

Fig. 23 e. Metatarsal bones from 4 cows of the same breed, size, and age illustrating varying degrees of osteofluorosis. Left to right: normal to severe periosteal hyperostosis

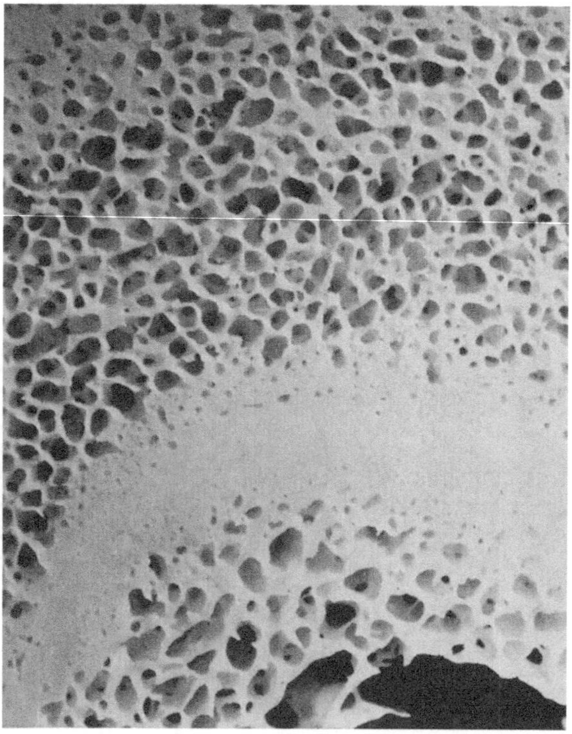

Fig. 24. Ground cross section of metatarsal bone illustrating severe periosteal hyperostosis and endosteal resorption (× 8.5). From SHUPE et al., unpublished

more abnormal the bone. It was demonstrated that the normal formation and structure of the organic matrix that normally precedes mineralization was altered, and that the osteoid did not calcify normally.

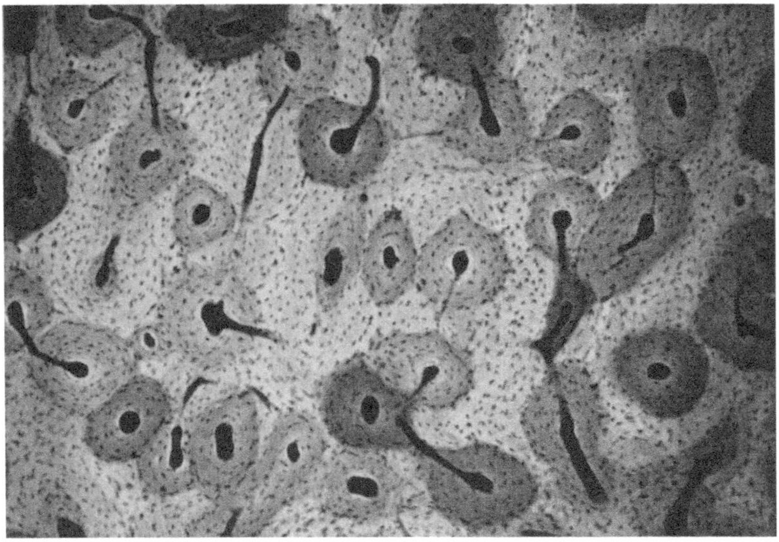

a

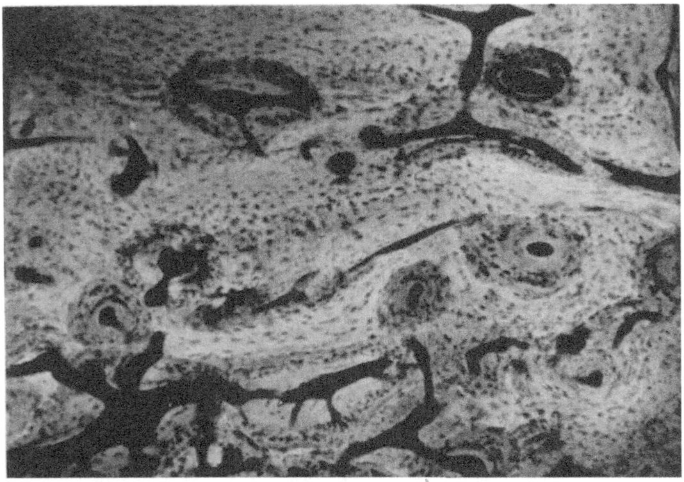

b

Fig. 25 a and b. a Enlargement of a section of Fig. 23 a, illustrating normal bone structure and various stages of remodeling activity. Note newly formed, slightly mineralized osteone, markedly mineralized osteone, moderately mineralized osteone, and interstitial bone (× 49). b Enlargement of a section of Fig. 23 d, illustrating abnormal bone structure with marked osteonal and interstitial changes. Note uneven distribution of large, irregular osteocytes and area devoid of osteocytes with marked clumping of osteocytes in peripheral zone of osteone (× 67). From SHUPE et al., 1963 b

An excellent and detailed discussion of the histogenesis and mechanisms in the development of osteofluorosis was reported by JOHNSON (1965).

Some of the more characteristic, definite, and meaningful histological changes associated with fluorosis are: (1) new bone formation on premorbid subperiosteal

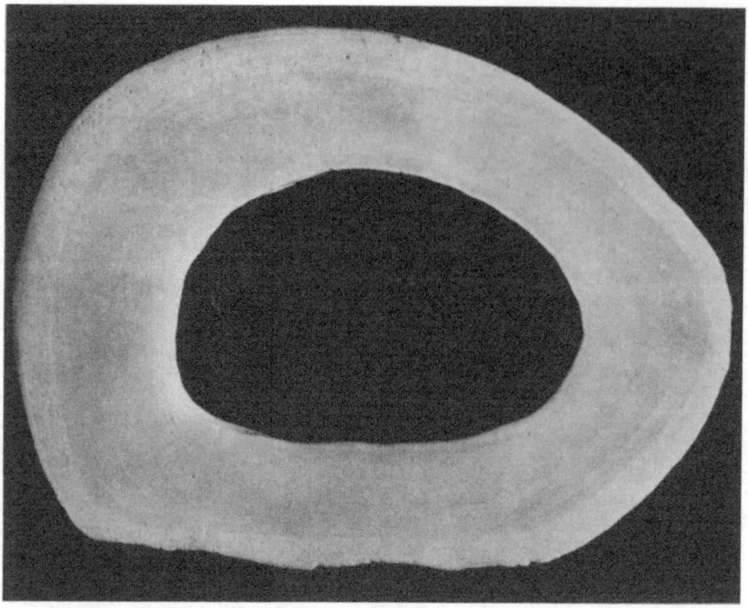

Fig. 26. Cross ground section of bovine metatarsal bone illustrating osteosclerosis. The animal received slightly elevated levels of fluorine over a long period of time. From SHUPE et al., unpublished

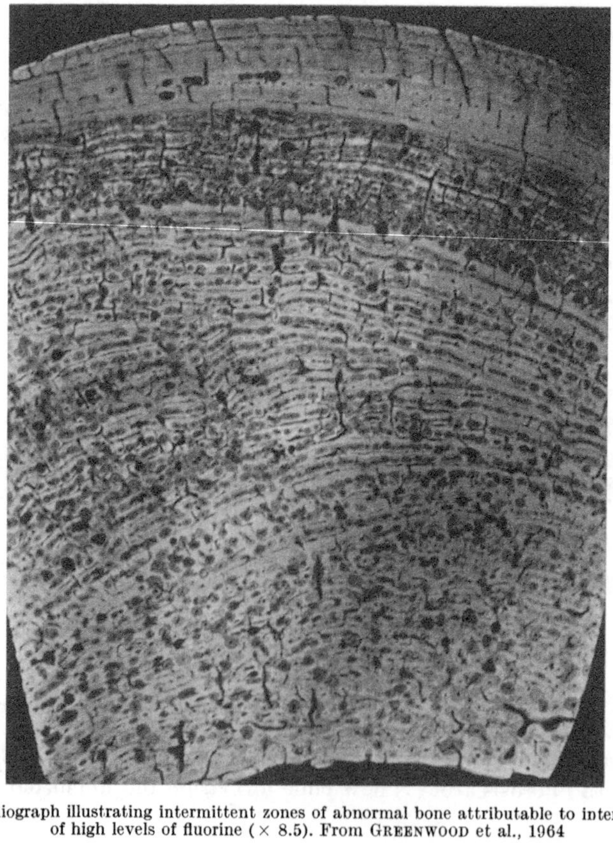

Fig. 27. Microradiograph illustrating intermittent zones of abnormal bone attributable to intermittent ingestion of high levels of fluorine (× 8.5). From GREENWOOD et al., 1964

surface, (2) thickened cortical substance due to periosteal hyperostosis, (3) irregular disorderly defective bone pattern, (4) uneven and irregular mineralization, (5) coarse, haphazardly arranged collagenous fibers, (6) loss of uniform osteonal pattern, (7) zones of immature bone, (8) islands of calcified cartilage in cortex, (9) excessive osteoid tissue, (10) immature coarse fibrillar bone, (11) deposits of mineral salts on surface of trabeculi, (12) increased osteoclastic reabsorption of the premorbid bone, (13) fibrous-like marrow in some advanced long-standing cases, (14) reabsorption on endosteal surface, (15) hypervascularization

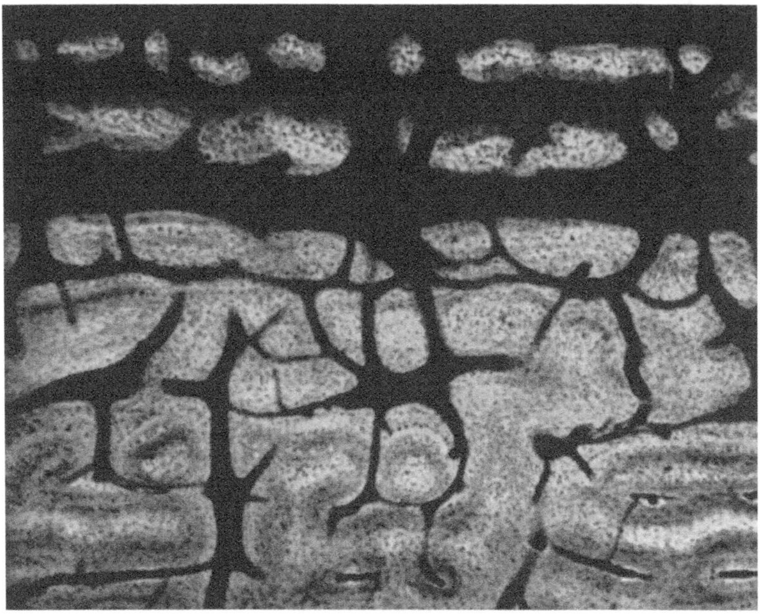

Fig. 28. Microradiograph of cross section of proximal aspect of bovine metatarsal bone. Note slight periosteal hyperostosis (× 67). From SHUPE et al., 1962

adjacent to resorptive cavities, (16) irregular shapes and sizes of osteons, (17) irregular and abnormal distribution of osteocytes in osteonal systems (Figs. 25 a and b), and (18) impairment and disturbance of normal blood supply in advanced cases.

The degree of these changes and their patterns of combination are governed by the same factors cited previously as influencing the degree and manifestation of fluorosis (Figs. 26 and 27). Early bone changes become discernible after four to five months when high levels of fluorine are being ingested (Fig. 28). The rapidity and degree with which the bone changes occurred were related to the amount of fluorine ingested. The amount of fluorine ingested also determined whether accelerated remodeling, porosis, sclerosis, hyperostosis, or osteomalacia was the predominant manifestation at any stage.

c) Joint appearance, lameness, stiffness

The general clinical appearance of joints has proved to be an inconclusive measure of fluorine effects. In the 8-year experiment with dairy animals (SHUPE et al., 1963 b), joint abnormalities did not become discernible until after periosteal hyperostosis was palpable [$1^1/_2$ to 2 years on experiment for 93 ppm F animals and $3^1/_2$ to 4 years for 49 ppm F animals (Fig. 29)]. Primary bone lesions were in evidence in all cases long before the joints started to evidence malalignment and malposition with marginal osteophytic formations.

When grass or hay polluted by effluent fluorine from a Dutch fertilizer plant was fed to cattle, LOURENS (1941) noted emaciation and lameness as principal

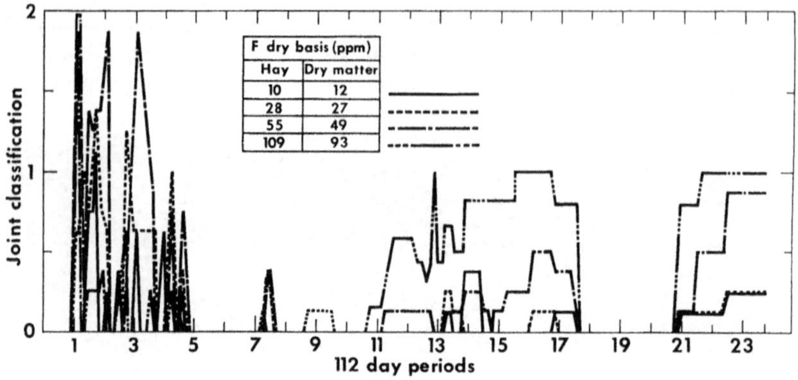

Fig. 29. Joint classification of dairy cows given 4 levels of fluorine for 7.3 years. Degree of severity rated from 0 to 2. From SHUPE et al., 1963b

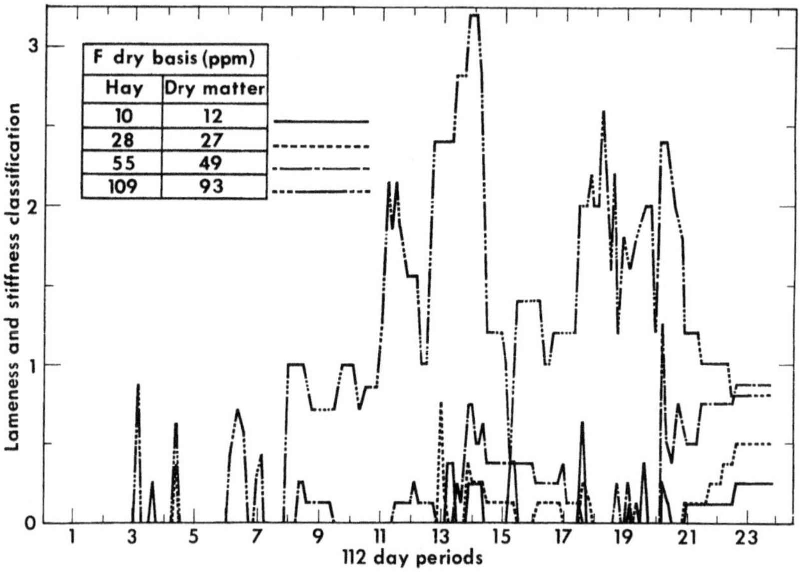

Fig. 30. Lameness and stiffness classifications of dairy cattle on experiment for 7.3 years. Degree of severity rated from 0 to 3. From SHUPE et al., 1963b

symptoms. These signs of chronic fluorosis correspond with those observed by MEYN and VIEHL (1941), who also described as symptoms the discoloration and abnormal wearing down of the incisor teeth. BLAKEMORE (1944), BURNS and ALLCROFT (1964), and ALLCROFT et al. (1965) studied fluorosis in cattle kept in the immediate neighborhood of fluorine-emitting industries in England. When severely affected, the animals showed lameness, exostoses, and mottled incisors.

Lameness and stiffness were inconclusive measures of fluorine toxicosis in the Utah work (Fig. 30). These symptoms were intermittent in nature, even in the animals receiving 93 ppm of fluorine. Animals on the 93 ppm F diet first showed definite signs of lameness at $2^1/_2$ years. Periosteal hyperostosis underlying the deep digital flexor tendons as shown in Fig. 31 may be one of the causes of lameness associated with progressive fluorosis. After $3^1/_2$ years on trial, two of the animals on the 93 ppm F diet went down on their knees. They moved around on their knees for 3 weeks. They then recovered and walked normally for 1 month. At that time they again went down and moved on their knees for a period of 3 weeks. After this they again recovered and remained so throughout the rest of the trial, although they showed intermittent lameness. Animals on the 49 ppm F evidenced lameness after $4^1/_2$ years.

By the time bone changes have progressed to the degree that they can be palpated (Fig. 32), the animal may show periods of intermittent lameness. Symptoms such as elevated body temperature, hot swollen joints, and suppressed ruminations, which are observed in most cases of acute inflammatory arthritis, were not associated with the characteristic intermittent lameness of advanced fluorine toxicosis. Crepitation was not noted in any of the fluorosis-affected animals.

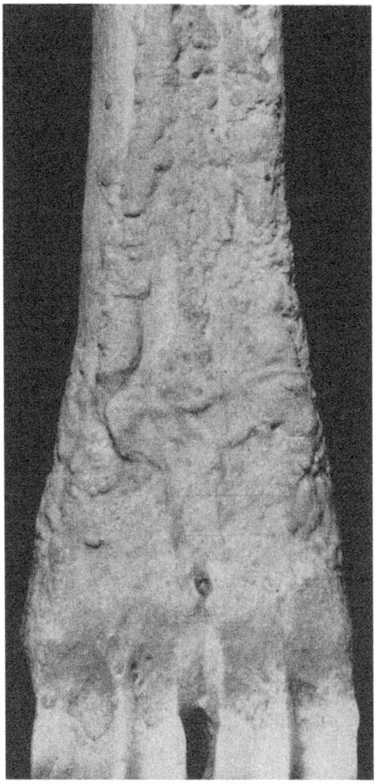

Fig. 31. Posterior distal aspect of metatarsal bone from a cow illustrating irregular rough periosteal hyperostosis

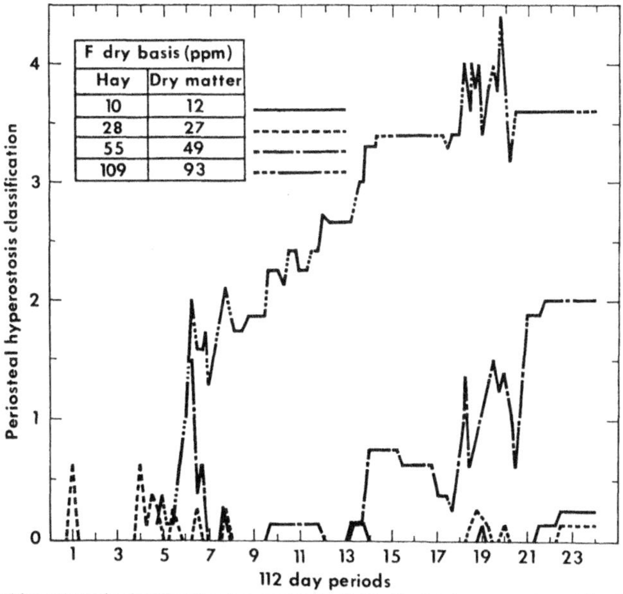

Fig. 32. Periosteal hyperostosis classification (see footnote, Table 2) of dairy cows given 4 levels of fluorine until 7.5 years of age. From SHUPE et al., 1963 b

d) Alkaline bone phosphatase

Data from controlled experiments indicate a close correlation between alkaline bone phosphatase activity and the amount of fluorine ingested, the fluoride content of the bone, and osseous abnormalities. The results suggest that fluorine accumulation in the bone and abnormal bone growth are accompanied by a marked increase in alkaline bone phosphatase activity. MILLER and SHUPE (1962) have reported that alkaline bone phosphatase activity in dairy cattle is related to the amount of fluoride ingested and the degree of abnormal bone formation.

C. Urine analysis

The amount of fluorine excreted in the urine can be used to estimate roughly what levels of fluorine are being ingested at a given time.

Boddie (1947) found fluorine tests of the urine a useful way to detect fluorine intoxication. He found 19–33 ppm F in the urine of cattle that had a continuous intake of pasture vegetation containing 776 ppm F. BLAKEMORE (1944) and KRUGER (1949) also found urinary analysis a valuable aid to early diagnosis of fluorosis.

A major limitation to using this particular analytical procedure as a basis for conclusion, however, is inherent in the individual variation that exists among animals in the ppm of fluorine that are excreted in the urine when a given level of fluorine is consumed in the ration. Thus, a single urine analysis for one animal

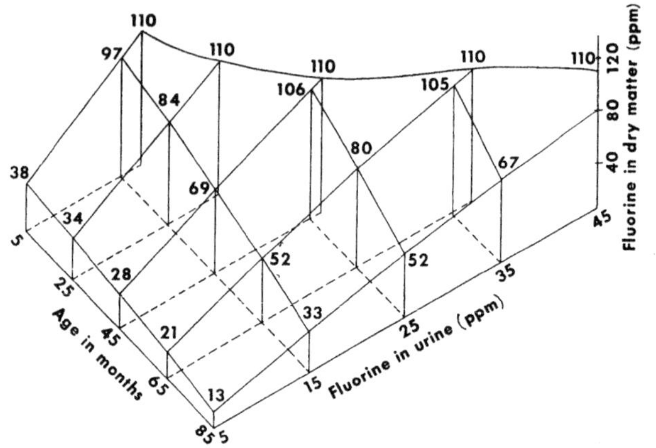

Fig. 33. The interrelation among age, fluorine in the urine, and fluorine in the dry matter as derived from data of an 8-year experiment. From SHUPE et al., 1963a.

should not be considered accurately indicative of current fluoride intake (SHUPE et al., 1963a). By sampling several animals, however, a more reliable value can be obtained. For best results, therefore, several animals should be sampled, and preferably in the morning. Fluorine and specific gravity determinations should be made and the results tabulated to arrive at a reasonably dependable index of fluorine consumed.

Factors such as age and urinary specific gravity must be kept in mind when using these procedures. Animals on different diets may excrete identical amounts of fluorine, but the urines may have different specific gravity values. This can happen because other extraneous material, which depends on the type of diet, is also excreted. Because urinary fluorine concentrations appear to vary with the specific gravity of the sample, conditions should be standardized for comparative purposes. Urinary values have been corrected to specific gravity 1.04 in several investigations. New findings, however, indicate that other bases may be more useful (SHUPE et al., 1963a).

Also, the older the animal, the more fluorine is voided in the urine relative to the amount of dry matter consumed (assuming a constant, continous fluorine intake) (SHUPE et al., 1963a). This is because older animals will retain proportionately less fluorine in their bones than will younger ones, because the bones of older animals are already relatively saturated with fluorine; therefore, additional storage is minimized and more fluorine is excreted in the urine (Fig. 33).

In addition, the normal urinary fluorine concentration from cattle is subject to considerable fluctuation. Urine of normal cattle generally contains less than 6 ppm of fluorine (Fig. 34).

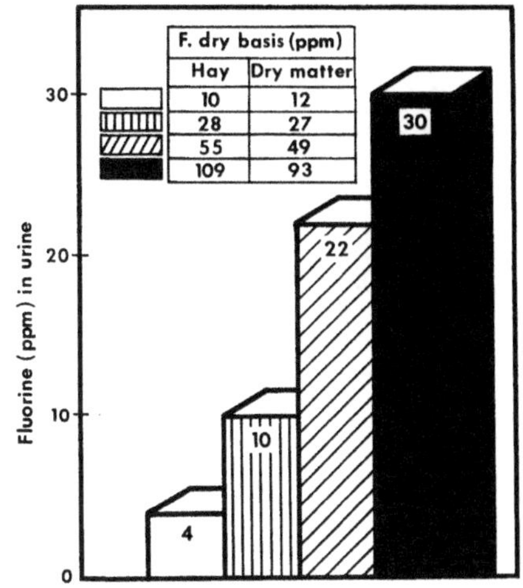

Fig. 34. Fluorine in urine of dairy cows on experiment 7.3 years. From SHUPE et al., 1963b

D. Other effects

The ingestion of various levels of fluorine may produce different combinations of miscellaneous effects. STODDARD et al. (1963b) reported effects of fluorine on the growth and feed consumption of dairy cattle on experiment for 8 years.

1. General condition

In the 8-year Utah experiment the 93 ppm and 49 ppm levels of fluorine intake affected the general condition of the animals (Fig. 35) primarily during lactation periods. In some cows on the 93 ppm F level, adverse effects were seen after

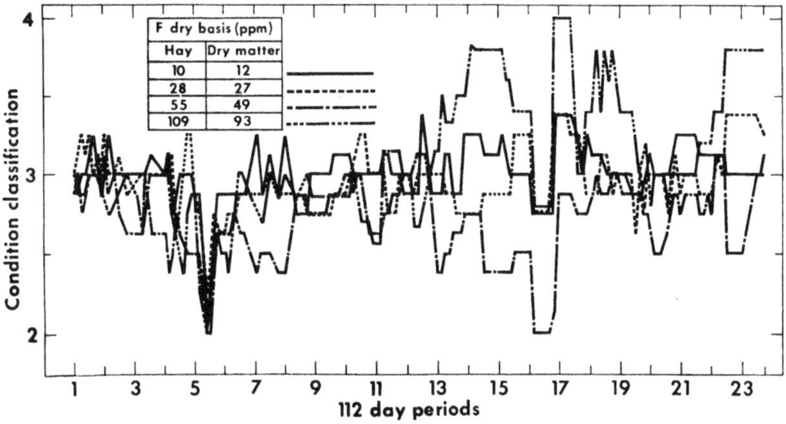

Fig. 35. Classification of general condition of animals on experiment for 7.5 years. The animals with fluorosis were primarily affected during lactation periods. From SHUPE et al., unpublished

$2^1/_2$ years on trial. Some animals receiving 49 ppm F showed adverse effects after $4^1/_2$ years. These general effects did not appear until after periosteal hyperostosis

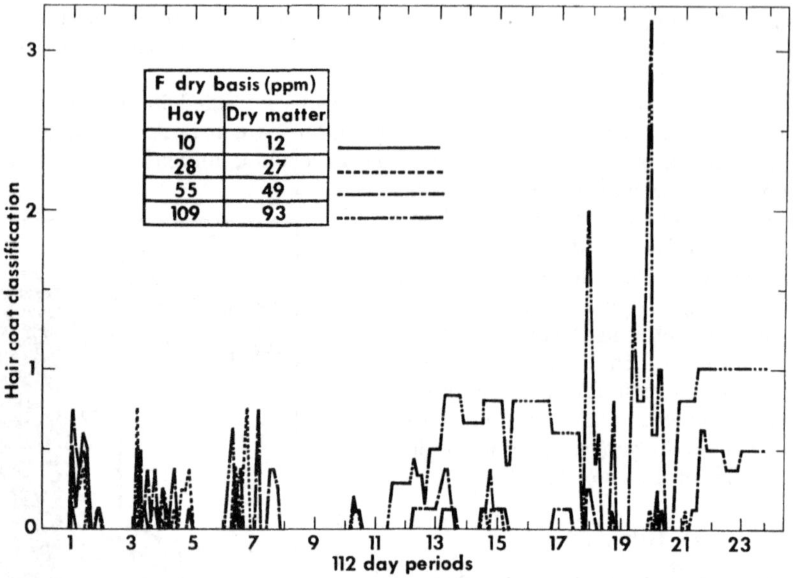

Fig. 36. Classification of hair coat of animals on experiment for 7.5 years. No effect was noted until toward the end of the trial after periosteal hyperostosis was clinically discernible. From SHUPE et al., unpublished

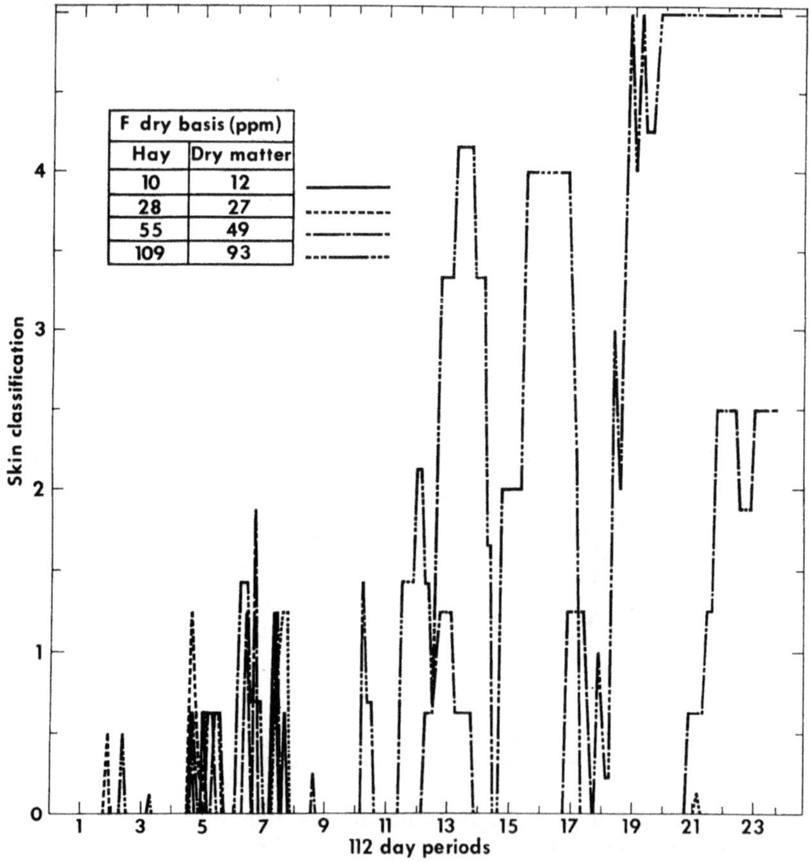

Fig. 37. Classification of skin condition of animals on experiment for 7.5 years. No effect was noted until the end of the trial after periosteal hyperostosis was clinically discernible. From SHUPE et al., unpublished

and lameness were discernible. Animals suffering from dietary deficiencies or metabolic malfunction may have increased susceptibility to elevated levels of fluoride ingestion.

2. Hair, coat and skin

No effect was noted until toward the end of the trial when some animals on the 93 ppm and 49 ppm fluorine intakes showed signs of dry hair coats and thick, non-pliable skin (Figs. 36 and 37). These conditions were manifested only after periosteal hyperostosis and intermittent lameness were apparent.

3. Hoofs

No adverse effects that could be associated with the fluorine treatments were noted throughout the 8-year trial on the growth and shape of the animals' hoofs. More variation occurred within a single treatment group than between groups (Fig. 38).

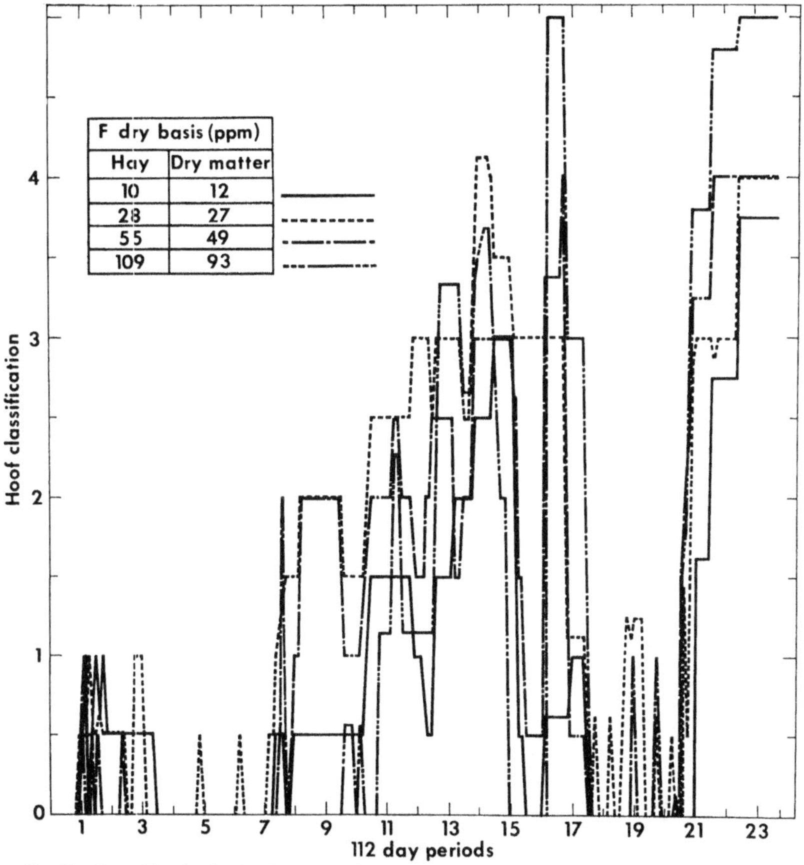

Fig. 38. Classification of hoofs of animals on experiment for 7.5 years. No adverse effect could be associated with fluorine treatments. From SHUPE et al., unpublished

4. Soft tissues

Only small, insignificant amounts of fluorine (less than 2.96 ppm) were retained in the soft tissues (Fig. 39). No gross or histologic changes in the brain, pituitary, liver, kidneys, adrenals, spleen, pancreas, thyroid, ovaries, mammary glands, uterus, rumen, reticulum, omasum, abomasum, or intestines could be correlated with fluorine consumption. Enzyme studies and the analyzed fluoride content of

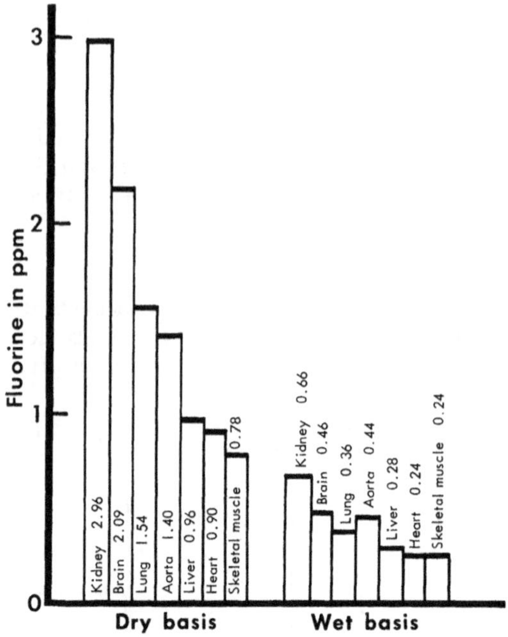

Fig. 39. Fluorine in the soft tissues of dairy cattle on experiments for 7.3 years. These data are an average of 4 treatments — 12, 27, 49, and 93 ppm of fluorine. From Shupe et al., 1962

selected soft tissues showed no significant effects related to fluoride ingestion.

5. Kidney and liver function

The kidneys were routinely higher in fluorine content than were any other soft tissues, probably because of their role in eliminating fluorides from the body. Measurements of the renal clearance of inulin and para-aminohippuric acid, however, did not indicate any kidney malfunction or damage.

BSP liver function tests revealed no correlation between the various fluoride treatments and fractional clearance, half-time clearance ($t^1/_2$), or percent of the dye dosage remaining in the blood at 30 min. A lower fractional clearance occurred during the last 20 min than during the first 10 min of a half-hour clearance test. Shupe et al. (1960), reported on the investigation of certain hepatic functions of dairy animals following prolonged ingestion of fluorides.

6. Reproduction

As measured by services per conception and calf size and viability, prolonged ingestion of fluorine had no adverse effect on reproduction. The conception rates

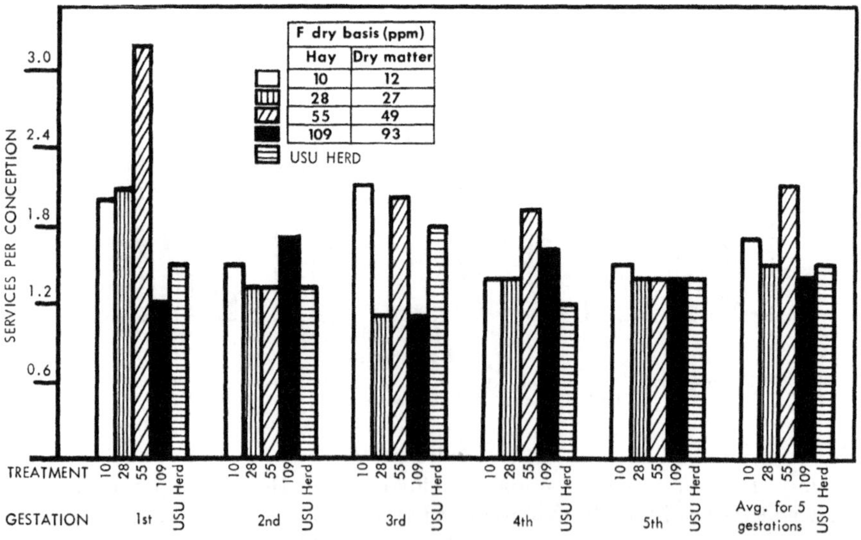

Fig. 40. Services per conception of dairy cows given 4 levels of fluorine during 5 lactations. From Shupe et al., 1963 b

of the experimental animals are shown and compared with those of the Utah State University dairy herd (Fig. 40). This herd is as good in this respect as other herds in the United States, in Europe, or elsewhere. SUTTIE et al. (1961) reported effects of fluorine ingestion by the dam on subsequent development of fluorosis in the offspring.

The factors known to influence reproduction include: plane of nutrition, condition of the animal, pathological conditions, climate, crowding, high milk production, metabolic disturbances, and general management of the herd. These may affect any herd of cows at any time. When they affect a herd that is also subject to fluorosis, their manifestations may be unjustifiably attributed to the fluorides.

7. Blood

None of the various fluoride diets had any harmful or detectable effects on the animals' blood morphology or the hemopoietic systems during the 8-year Utah experiment. No variations or differences were detected between or within the different fluoride treatment groups (HOOGSTRATEN et al., 1965). No correlation was found between the amount of fluoride in the diet and the concentration of calcium, inorganic phosphorus, or alkaline phosphatase in the blood serum. The amount of fluorine in the blood, however, was correlated with the amount of fluorine in the diet (Fig. 41).

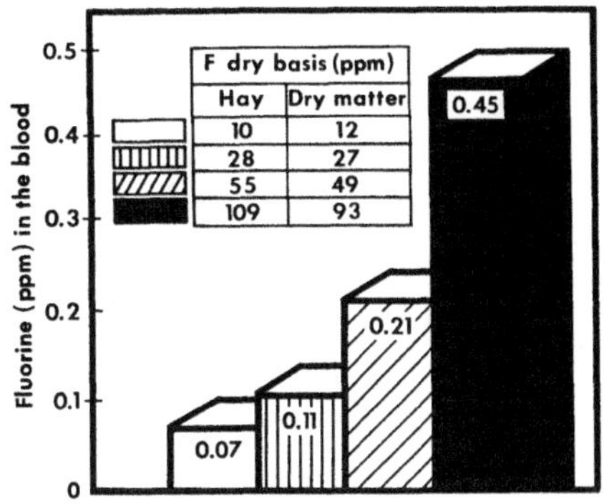

Fig. 41. Fluorine in blood of dairy cattle on experiment 7.3 years. From SHUPE et al., 1963b

THOMANN (1962) also investigated the influence of fluorine on the alkaline phosphatase of the blood serum of cattle. With concentrations of 6.8 and 15 mg fluorine per liter, no inhibition of phosphatase activity was found. Even with 20 mg F/l, the phosphatase level remained unchanged. These data are in agreement with those of ALTHER (1961). Alkaline phosphatase of blood serum remained normal throughout the 8-year Utah experiment for all animals on all levels of fluoride intake.

8. Placental transfer

Examinations of the calves from the animals on the long-term Utah experiment showed that fluorine passed the placental barrier. The amount of fluorine stored in the bones of the developing embryo and fetus could be correlated with the amount of fluorine ingested by the dam and with that in her blood (Fig. 42). In succeeding gestations, however, the amount of fluorine transmitted through the placental barrier did not increase above the levels noted in the calves from preceding gestations. BELL et al. (1961) have demonstrated an apparent barrier to the free passage of F^{18} from maternal placenta to fetal placenta.

9. Milk production

Milk production is not directly affected by ingestion of low levels of fluorine. In general, well-fed cows can consume 40 to 50 ppm of fluorine in their ration for two or three lactations and up to 90–100 ppm of F for at least one lactation without any measurable effect on milk production (STODDARD et al., 1963a). These tolerances are observed even when ingestion starts at 4 months of age. At these levels of fluoride ingestion, later lactations will be adversely affected in some animals. Amount and duration of intake that affected lactation varied among individual cows during the 8-year Utah study. In all observed cases, primary clinical manifestations of excessive fluoride intake preceded any alteration of milk

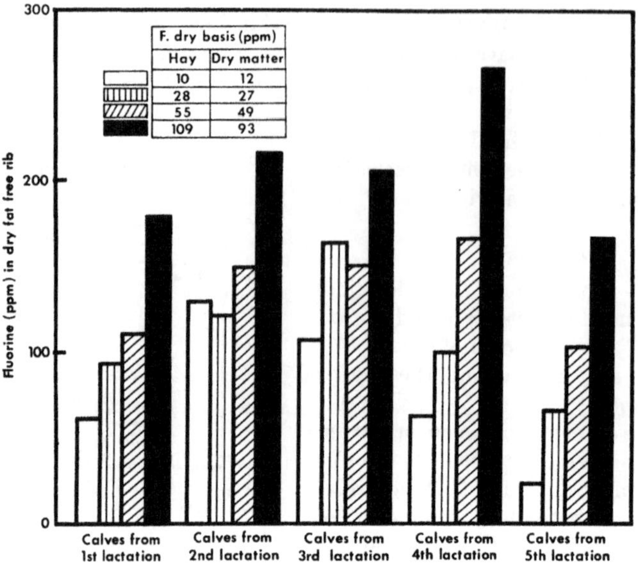

Fig. 42. Fluorine content of ribs of calves born to dairy cows fed various levels of fluorine, grain, and minerals for 7.3 years. From SHUPE et al., 1963b

production (Fig. 43). Even in cases of marked fluoride toxicity, any effects on milk production will probably be attributable to altered metabolic functions rather than to direct interference with lactogenesis.

In further substantiation of this hypothesis, MUSSIL (1954), for more than 10 years, observed lameness of seemingly obscure etiology in cattle in the vicinity of an aluminum plant. Other definite signs such as discoloration of incisor teeth with hypoplasia and enamel changes, and exostosis on ribs and long bones, supported his diagnosis of fluorosis. Mussil believed that the loss of body weight and decrease in milk production that were noted in these animals when they reached the more advanced stages of fluorosis were only secondarily due to fluorine ingestion.

Any of the primary effects of fluorosis which reduce feed intake or interfere with the cow's normal activity may secondarily reduce milk production. Such interferences include advanced periosteal hyperostosis with spurring and bridging of the joints and the concomitant intermittent lameness which in turn limits the animal's ability to graze or stand at the feed manger; advanced molar abrasion which makes mastication difficult; possible systemic or metabolic impairment; or a combination of these factors.

Genetic, disease, nutritional, management, and environmental influences all affect milk production. Fluorine toxicosis is only one of the many potentially influential factors, most of which are directly associated with milk production whereas fluorine has secondary effects. Even in clinical cases of fluorosis, these other factors may be the direct cause of any decreased milk production. In such instances, the added stress of fluorosis might indirectly enhance the more direct effects of the other factors.

10. Feed digestion and metabolism

Ingestion of 93 ppm fluorine by cattle for two years or more may reduce feed intake. Some animals on lower fluoride intakes may not evidence reduced feed intakes within a two-year period of ingestion. Fluoride-associated reductions in

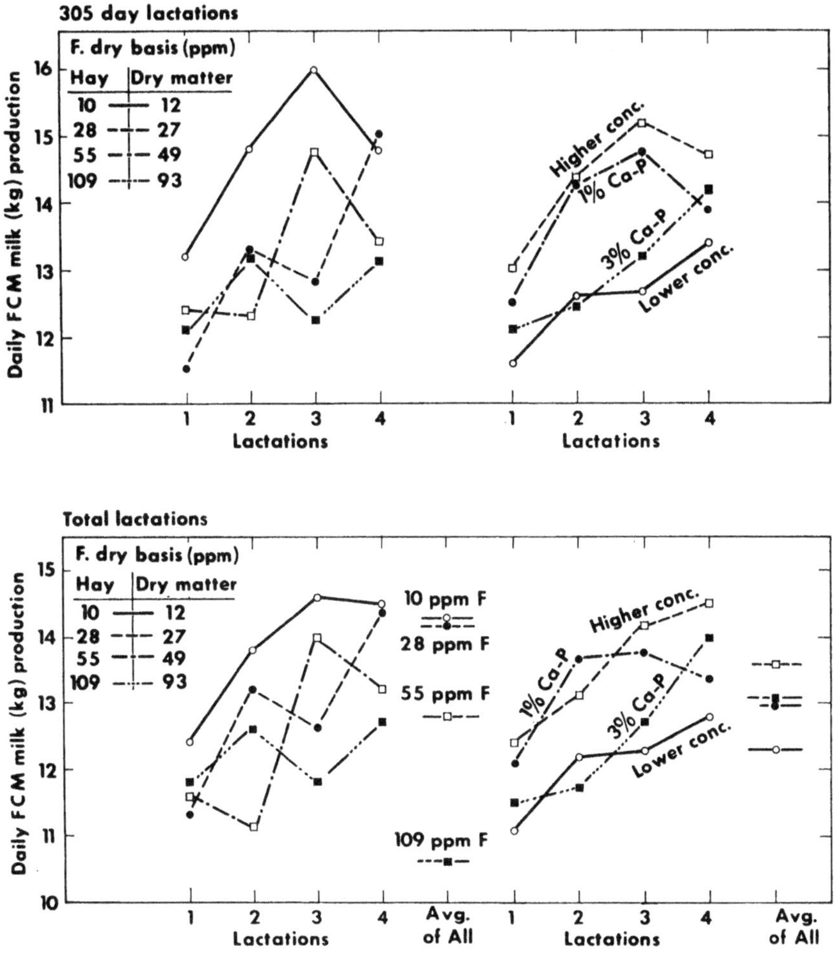

Fig. 43. Average daily milk (FCM) produced during the first four lactations (305-day and total) of Holstein females fed four levels of fluorine, two levels of concentrate mix, and two levels of a Ca-P mineral from three to four months to about 7.5 years of age. From STODDARD et al., 1963a

feed intake usually follow the primary effects of fluorosis on teeth and bones, and the secondary effects on joints which make it difficult for cows to stand at a feed manger or walk while grazing pasture forage.

Fluorine intakes up to 93 ppm appear to have little or no influence on nutrient digestibility. HARRIS et al. (1964) reported on digestion and metabolism trials on dairy animals fed various levels of sodium fluoride from 3 to 4 months of age to 8 years of age. Total nutrient absorption is decreased, but this is associated with a decrease in feed intake rather than in digestibility. The digestion coefficients of many nutrients are increased, but this also is more likely associated with variations in feed intake than with fluoride intake directly. Apparently the effects of fluorine on the digestion and absorption of nutrients are secondary.

11. Enzymes

The alkaline phosphatase in the blood serum remained normal throughout the 8-year Utah experiment for all animals on all levels of fluoride intake. Results indicated a correlation between bone alkaline phosphatase activity, the fluoride content of the bone, skeletal activity, and the degree of osteofluorosis. Bone phosphatase activity was highest in the animals fed the higher levels of fluorine. Soft tissue studies for succinic dehydrogenase in heart muscle, lipase and amylase in the pancreas, enolase and pyruvate kinase in skeletal muscle, and pepsin in the abomasal mucosa showed no treatment effects (GREENWOOD et al., 1964).

E. Data correlation

Correlation of the data accumulated during the 8-year Utah experiment with 32 Holstein-Friesian cows demonstrated that by taking into account the fluorine in the rib and the tooth classification, 95% ($r^2 = 0.950$) of the potential variability can be accounted for (Fig. 44). In other words, the tooth classification, the amount

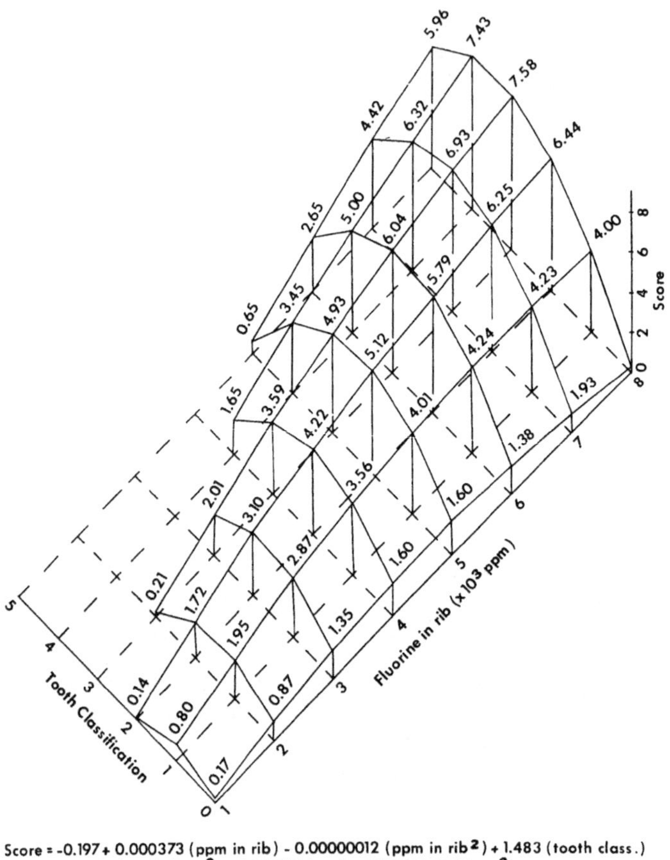

Score = -0.197 + 0.000373 (ppm in rib) - 0.00000012 (ppm in rib^2) + 1.483 (tooth class.) - 0.650 (tooth class.^{2}) + 0.00017 (days) - 0.00000015 (days^2) + 0.00044 (ppm in rib x tooth class.) + 0.00000027 (ppm in rib x days) - 0.00025 (tooth class. x days)

Fig. 44. The interrelations among tooth classification, fluorine in the rib, and score (degree of fluorosis) for 7.5-year-old dairy cows receiving four levels of fluorine from 3 to 4 months to 7.5 years of age ($r^2 = 0.950$). From SHUPE et al., 1963b of fluorine in the ribs, and the age of the animal can be used to predict the degree of fluorosis in an animal with a high degree of accuracy. Other examples of multiple correlation formulas are shown in Table 1.

Table 1. *The relationship of combined independent variables to their predicted expression of fluorosis in dairy cows*

Independent variable[1]	Dependent variable	Correlation R^2
$d, d^2, dm, dm^2, d \times dm$	Fluorine (ppm) in rib	0.957
$d, d^2, dm, dm^2, d \times dm$	Tooth classification	0.888
$d, d^2, dm, dm^2, d \times dm$	Fluorine (ppm) in urine	0.862
$d, d^2, r, r^2, d \times r$	Fluorine (ppm) in dry matter	0.900
$r, r^2, t, t^2, d, d^2, r \times t, r \times d, t \times d$	Fluorine (mg) consumption	0.971
$r, r^2, t, t^2, d, d^2, r \times t, r \times d, t \times d$	Score	0.950

[1] d = days; dm = fluorine (ppm) in dry matter; r = fluorine (ppm) in dry fat free rib; t = tooth classification (0, 1, 2, 3, 4, 5), depending on the degree of fluorosis. From SHUPE et al. 1963b.

F. Diagnosing fluorosis

1. Clinical

Fluorine has definite beneficial effects when ingested in small amounts but adverse or toxic effects when ingested in large amounts (Fig. 45). Criteria for large or small amounts vary with the species and the duration of time during which

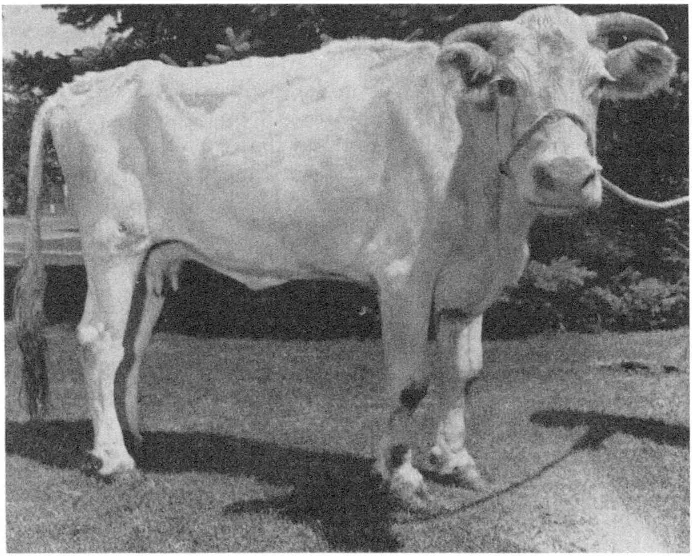

Fig. 45. Field case evidencing effects of severe chronic fluorosis. From SHUPE et al., 1955

ingestion takes place. Clinically, fluorine intoxication is usually seen in one of two typical forms, acute or chronic. SHUPE (1963) discussed the etiology, clinical aspects, pathogenesis, lesions, and diagnosis of fluorosis in cattle.

2. Acute

Acute fluorine intoxication most commonly results from accidental ingestion of high levels of fluorine compounds. The common sources of such poisonings in livestock are: (1) sodium fluoracetate "1080," used as a rodenticide, (2) sodium fluorosilicate used as a rodenticide, (3) sodium fluoride used as an ascaricide in swine, and (4) water, vegetation, and feeds containing excessively high levels of fluoride.

Depending upon a number of factors, such intoxication may simulate several different types of poisonings or toxicosis. The symptoms may appear in one-half hour after ingestion if the amount ingested is excessively high. The following symptoms are commonly characteristic: excitement, clonic convulsions, incontinence of urine and feces, high fluorine content of blood and urine, stiffness, weakness, loss of body weight, drop in milk production, necrosis of mucosa of digestive tract, excessive salivation, nausea, vomiting, severe depression in some cases, and cardiac failure.

In 1927 KRUG reported a severe case of intoxication of dairy cows from sodium fluosilicate. Eighteen cows died within 12–14 hours after ingesting the Na_2SiF_6, a pesticide, which was erroneously added to the ration instead of a mineral mixture. Convulsions, exaggerated chewing motions, and hyperemia were observed.

3. Chronic

Chronic fluorosis is the type of fluorine toxicosis most often observed in livestock. Its clinical manifestations relative to diagnosis will therefore be discussed in some detail here.

a) Sequential development of chronic fluorosis

Animals normally ingest low levels of fluorine throughout their lives. Clinically, the onset of chronic fluorosis is insidious and may be confused with chronic debilitating diseases such as degenerative arthritis or other debilitating diseases (SHUPE, 1961; 1963). In addition, every animal will evidence an individualized biological response. It is impossible, therefore, to define a precise point for all animals at which an instance of normal consumption will become a case of chronic fluorosis. The borderline or threshold point may tend to vary slightly in individual cases as the seven factors cited previously exert their influence. The time lapse or interval between ingestion of elevated levels of fluorides and any actual manifestation of the clinical symptoms of chronic fluorosis adds to the complexity of the clinical picture.

No single criterion should be relied upon in diagnosing fluorosis. All clinical, necropsy, and chemical findings must be carefully evaluated together before a definite diagnosis and evaluation of fluorosis is made. The following symptoms and lesions are of particular importance: (1) mottling and abrasion of teeth, (2) degree of osteofluorosis, (3) intermittent lameness, (4) the amount of fluorine retained in the bone, and (5) amount of fluorine in the urine.

Under field conditions the amounts of fluorine ingested and the lengths of time during which it is ingested are subject to wide variations. In some instances there may be intermittent periods during which no excessive fluorides are ingested. Different levels of nutrition and different management practices between farms can vitally affect manifestations of fluorotic lesions. The variability that can occur between individual animals within and between herds must also be taken into account. Whether an animal consumes elevated levels of fluorine throughout its life, or only after its teeth are formed will materially affect clinical manifestation of the disease.

b) Urine

When ingestion of elevated levels of fluorine is suspected, but clinical signs are lacking, urine analyses can be used as a diagnostic aid. Fluorine excretion in the urine, however, is affected by a variety of factors. Among these most important variables are the level and duration of ingestion, the resultant degree of fluorine saturation of the osseous tissue, and individual differences between animals. A definitive consideration of urine analysis as a tool in diagnosing fluorosis has been published (SHUPE et al., 1963a).

c) Teeth

If above normal fluorine ingestion takes place during the period of tooth formation, typical fluorotic dental lesions will be seen before any other clinical chronic symptoms become apparent. The extent and degree of such lesions will depend upon the seven factors cited previously. It also must be constantly borne in mind that dental lesions will not be seen if the animals are brought into endemic fluorosis areas after their permanent teeth have erupted.

The degree of dental fluorosis in an animal can be correlated with the amount of fluorine in the bones, the extent of osteofluorosis, the duration of exposure, the age of animal during exposure, the amount of fluoride ingested, and the reactive processes of the body. The dental lesions, therefore, are useful in diagnosing fluorosis clinically; however, to be most meaningful, the dental fluorotic changes must be correlated with other tissue changes and lesions indicative of fluorosis. In other words, dental lesions should not be used as the sole criterion when evaluating the degree of fluorosis.

d) Bone

The level of fluorine storage in the bone can increase within limits over a period of time without eliciting any demonstrable changes in structure and function. Eventually, if levels of fluorine ingestion are higher than normal for sufficient lengths of time, structural changes will become evident. Depending upon the operation of the seven factors influencing the degree of fluorosis, characteristic osteofluorotic lesions subsequently may develop and function may be adversely affected.

The first clinically palpable bone lesions occur on the medial surface of the proximate third of the metatarsal bones and are bilateral. Subsequently palpable and detectable bone lesions occur on the mandible, metacarpals, and ribs.

e) Lameness and stiffness

The intermittent lameness and stiffness that are seen in more advanced cases of fluorosis develop as a result of the osteofluorotic lesions and the mineralization of periarticular structures and tendon insertions. In turn, the intermittent lameness and stiffness deter the affected animals from standing at the manger or grazing pastures. The subsequently reduced feed intake then fosters reduced levels of performance of the animals.

f) Other diagnostic aids

The primary clinical lesions of chronic fluorosis-affected animals occur in their teeth and bones. The secondary, non-specific lesions and symptoms such as those involving reduced lactation, nonpliable skin, and dry, rough, hair coat will be discernible only after the primary dental and/or bone effects are evident.

Visible clinical lesions and signs sometimes are not definitive enough to warrant an unequivocal diagnosis of fluorosis. In such instances, or to substantiate a reasonably certain diagnosis, additional verification can be sought in several ways. When carefully interpreted, urine analysis is a useful diagnostic tool. Bone radiographs can supply valuable information. Biopsies or necropsies can be used to obtain tissues for chemical analysis of fluorine content and for gross and histopathological evaluations. Correlation of clinical observations with the ascertained fluorine contents of the animals' water and forage sources often can help substantiate suspected instances of fluorosis.

G. Methods of alleviating toxicity of fluorine

No substances are known to completely prevent the toxic effects of ingested elevated levels of fluorides (Allcroft et al. 1965). Some products, however, can counteract and lessen the damage that fluorides can cause (Fig. 46).

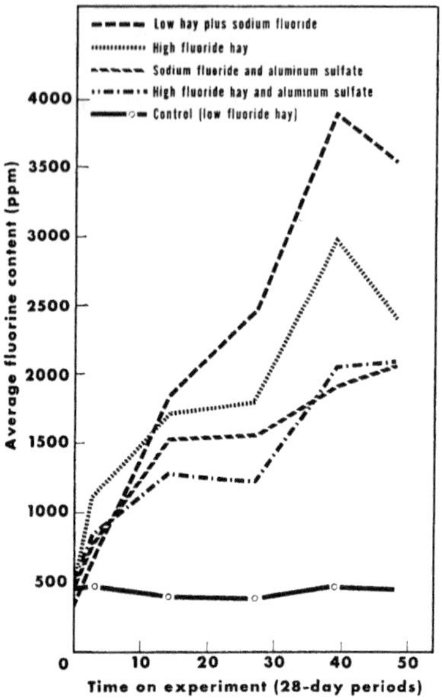

Fig. 46. Effect of varied fluorine and aluminum sulfate intake on deposition of fluorine in the ribs of dairy heifers on trial approximately 4 years. From Greenwood et al., 1964

Aluminum sulfate, aluminum chloride, calcium aluminate, calcium carbonate, and defluorinated phosphate have been successfully used to reduce the toxicity of fluorine. Heifers ingesting aluminum sulfate as a fluorosis inhibitor deposited 30 to 42% less fluorine in their ribs than did heifers ingesting comparable diets without aluminum sulfate (Greenwood et al., 1964). If the animals must be fed hay high in fluoride, it should at least be combined with hay of low fluoride content. If the drinking water available to the animals is unavoidably high in fluoride content, then it is advisable to feed roughage of low fluoride content. If the land commonly devoted to forage production is high in fluoride content, then it should be planted to cereal or nonroughage crops since grain does not accumulate fluoride from the soil the way forage crops do. In such cases, the necessary hay or roughage should be imported from nearby low fluoride areas. All mineral mixtures fed should use defluorinated phosphate.

H. Conclusions

Structural and physiological processes of animals that ingest fluorine are governed by a number of factors:

1. Level or amount of fluoride ingested,
2. Duration of ingestion – time,
3. Type and solubility of fluoride ingested,
4. Age of animal at time of ingestion,
5. Level of nutrition,
6. Stress factors, and
7. Individual biological response.

Prevention and control of fluorosis in livestock can be achieved, but only when the complexity of the disease is realized and the pathogenesis, symptomatology, and lesions are properly correlated, interpreted, and evaluated. A comprehensive guide that can be used in diagnosing and evaluating fluorosis is given in Table 2. The information in the Table is based on controlled experimental results and extensive necropsy findings.

Table 2. *Effects of ingested fluorine on dairy cattle fed various levels of sodium fluoride in the interval from 4 months to 7.5 years of age*

Average	Age (Years)	Normal conditions	Chronic fluorosis				Acute fluorosis
			No adverse effects	Borderline	Moderate	Severe	
Moisture-free diet F in ppm	2	up to 15	15—30	30—40	40—60	60—109	over 250
	4	up to 15	15—30	30—40	40—60	60—109	over 250
	6	up to 15	15—30	30—40	40—60	60—109	over 250
Teeth classification[1] (Incisors)	2	0—1	0—2	2—3	3—4	4—5	Characterized by: rapid onset — reduced food intake — high F content in urine — loss of body weight — reduced milk production — stiffness — weakness — even death
	4	0—1	0—2	2—3	3—4	4—5	
	6	0—1	0—2	2—3	3—4	4—5	
Teeth classification[1] (Molars)	2	0—1	0—1	0—1	0—1	0—3	
	4	0—1	0—1	0—1	1—2	1—4	
	6	0—1	0—1	1—2	1—3	1—5	
F in bone (ppm)	2	401— 714	714—1605	1605—2130	2130—3027	3027—4206	
	4	706—1138	1138—2379	2379—3138	3138—4504	4504—6620	
	6	653—1221	1221—2794	2794—3788	3788—5622	5622—8676	
F in urine (ppm)	2	2.27—3.78	3.78— 8.04	8.04—10.54	10.54—14.71	14.71—19.86	
	4	3.54—5.3	5.3 —10.32	10.32—13.31	13.31—18.49	18.49—25.63	
	6	3.51—6.03	3.03—11.29	11.29—14.78	14.78—20.96	20.96—30.09	
F in milk (ppm)	2	up to 0.12	up to 0.12	0.08—0.15	0.15—0.25	0.15 and above	
	4	up to 0.12	up to 0.12	0.08—0.15	0.15—0.25	0.15 and above	
	6	up to 0.12	up to 0.12	0.08—0.15	0.15—0.25	0.15 and above	
F in blood (ppm)	2	up to 0.30	up to 0.30	0.15—0.40	0.30—0.50	0.50 and above	
	4	up to 0.30	up to 0.30	0.15—0.40	0.30—0.50	0.50 and above	
	6	up to 0.30	up to 0.30	0.15—0.40	0.30—0.50	0.50 and above	
F in soft tissues (ppm)	2	up to 1.20	up to 1.20	up to 1.20	up to 1.20	up to 1.20	
	4	up to 1.20	up to 1.20	up to 1.20	up to 1.20	up to 1.20	
	6	up to 1.20	up to 1.20	up to 1.20	up to 1.20	up to 1.20	
Periosteal hyperostosis[2]	2	0	0—1	0—1	0—2	0—3	
	4	0	0—1	0—1	0—3	0—4	
	6	0	0—1	0—2	0—4	0—5	
Secondary changes may occur[3]	All	Absent	Absent	Occasionally noticed	Present	Present	

These data are based on controlled experiments, but can be correlated with numerous field cases that have been extensively studied and evaluated.

[1] Incisors and molars [average classification of erupted permanent teeth (degree of fluoride effects)]: 0-normal, 1-questionable, 2-slight, 3-moderate, 4-marked, 5-excessive.

[2] Periosteal hyperostosis: 0-normal, 1-questionable, 2-slight, 3-moderate, 4-marked, 5-excessive.

[3] Lameness and stiffness — loss of body weight — reduced feed intake — rough hair coat — unpliable skin — reduced milk production.

From Greenwood et al., 1964.

References

Agate, J. N., G. H. Bell, G. F. Boddie, R. G. Bowler, M. Buckell, E. A. Cheeseman, T. H. J. Douglas, H. A. Druett, J. Garrad, D. Hunter, K. M. A. Perry, J. D. Richardson, and J. B. de v. Weir: Industrial Fluorosis. A Study of the Hazard to Man and Animals Near Fort William, Scotland. A report to the Fluorosis Committee. Medical Research Council Mem. No. 22, 131 pp., 3 maps, 13 plates. London: H. M. Stationery Office 1949.

Allcroft, R., K. N. Burns, and C. N. Hebert: Fluorosis in cattle. 2. Development and alleviation: Experimental studies. London: Her Majesty's Stationery Office 1965.

Alther, E. W.: Chemisch-biologische Untersuchungen zur Fluorose des Rindes. Diss. Landw. Hochschule Hohenheim, Stuttgart, Februar 1961.

Anderson, J. O., J. S. Hurst, D. C. Strong, H. Nielsen, D. A. Greenwood, W. Robinson, J. L. Shupe, W. Binns, R. A. Bagley, and C. I. Draper: Effect of feeding various levels of sodium fluoride to growing turkeys. Poultry Sci. **34**, 1147—1153 (1955).

BARDELLI, P., e C. MENZANI: Richerche sulla fluorosi spontanea dei ruminanti. Nota preventiva. Ann. igiene **45**, 399—404 (1935).
— — La fluorosi. Atti ist. veneto sci. Pt. II **97**, 623—674 (1937/38).
BARTOLUCCI, A.: Casi interessanti di osteite malacia nei bovini. Mod. zooiat. **23**, Parte sci. 194 (1912).
— Della fluorosi o cachessi afluorica nei bovini. Nuova vet. **5**, No. 1: 18—20; No. 2: 20—40 (1927).
BAUD, C. A.: Etude biocristallographique des remaniements de la substance minerale osseuse en rapport avec son enrichissement en fluor. Compt. rend. soc. biol. **150**, 103—104 (1956).
BELL, M. C., G. M. MERRIMAN, and D. A. GREENWOOD: Distribution and excretion of F^{18} fluoride in beef cattle. J. Nutrition **73**, 379—385 (1961).
BENDIXEN, H. C., H. ROTH, and A. THORDAL-CHRISTENSEN: Natriumfluorid som middel mod spolorm hos svin. Nord. Vet.-med. **2**, 385—404 (1950).
BIBRA, E. v.: Chemische Untersuchungen über die Knochen und Zähne des Menschens und der Wirbelthiere, 435 pp. Schweinfurt 1844.
BLAKEMORE, F.: Industrial fluorosis of animals in England. Proc. Nutr. Soc. (Engl. and Scot.) **1**, 211—212; discussion 212—215 (1944).
BODDIE, G. F.: Fluorosis in domestic animals. Vet. Rec. **59**, 301—303 (1947).
BRANDL, J., u. H. TAPPEINER: Über die Ablagerung von Fluorverbindungen im Organismus nach Fütterung mit Fluornatrium. Z. Biol. **28**, 518—539 (1891/92).
BRINCH, O.: Pathologische Veränderungen in Zähnen und Kieferknochen von experimentell fluorvergifteten Versuchstieren. Z. Stomatol. **35**, 890—896 (1937).
BROWN, W. A. BARRY, P. V. CHRISTOFFERSON, M. MASSLER, and M. B. WEISS: Postnatal tooth development in cattle. Amer. J. vet. Res. **21**, 7—34 (1960).
BURNS, K. N.. and R. ALLCROFT: Fluorosis in cattle. 1. Occurence and effects in industrial areas of England and Wales 1954—1957. London: Her Majesty's Stationery Office 1964.
COHRS, P.: Zur pathologischen Anatomie und Pathogenese der chronischen Fluorvergiftung des Rindes. Dtsch. tierärztl. Wschr. **49**, 352—357 (1941); Berlin u. Münch. tierärztl. Wschr. **1941**, 366 (Proceedings).
COMAR, C. L., W. J. VISEK, W. E. LOTZ, and J. H. RUST: Effects of fluorine on calcium metabolism and bone growth in pigs. Amer. J. Anat. **92**, 361—389 (1953).
CORSICO, G.: Sui reperti istomorfologici sulla istogenesi della osteopatia da fluorosi nel bovino. Clin. vet. Milano **78**, 385—392 (1955).
CRISTIANI, H.: Une nouvelle maladie. La fluorose ou cachexie fluorique. Presse méd. **34**, 469—470 (1926).
— La fluorose du bétail et les gaz nitreux. C. R. Soc. Biol. (Paris) **96**, 388—389 (1927)
DAMMANN, C., u. O. MANEGOLD: Vergiftungen durch fluorhaltigen phosphorsauren Futterkalk. Dtsch. tierärztl. Wschr. **12**, 129—131, 141—143 (1904).
DEEDS, F.: Fluorine in relation to bone and tooth development. J. Amer. dent. Assoc. **23**, 568—574 (1936).
— Factors in the etiology of mottled enamel. J. Amer. dent. Assoc. **28**, 1804—1814 (1941).
GARLICK, N. L.: The teeth of the ox in clinical diagnosis. II. Gross anatomy and physiology. Amer. J. vet. Res. **15**, 385—394 (1954); and III. Developmental anomalies and general pathology. Amer. J. vet. Res. **15**, 500—508 (1954).
— The teeth of the ox in clinical diagnosis. IV. Dental Fluorosis. Amer. J. vet. Res. **16**, 38—44 (1955).
GAUTIER, A., et P. CLAUSMANN: La fluor dans l'organisme animal. B. Squelette, cartilages, tendons. Compt. rend. **156**, 1425—1430 (1913).
GREENWOOD, D. A., J. L. SHUPE, G. E. STODDARD, L. E. HARRIS, H. M. NIELSEN, and L. E. OLSON: Fluorosis in Cattle. Special Report No. 17, Utah Agricultural Experiment Station, 1964.
HARRIS, L. E., R. J. RALEIGH, M. A. MADSEN, J. L. SHUPE, J. E. BUTCHER, and D. A. GREENWOOD: Effect of various levels of fluorine, stilbestrol, and oxytetracycline, in the fattening ration of lambs. J. Animal Sci. **22**, 51—55 (1963).
— Digestion and metabolism trials on dairy animals fed various levels of sodium fluoride from 3 to 4 months of age to 7.5 years of age (In preparation).
— R. J. RALEIGH, G. E. STODDARD, D. A. GREENWOOD, J. L. SHUPE, and H. M. NIELSEN: Effects of fluoride on dairy cattle. III. Digestion and metabolism trials. J. Animal Sci. **23**, 537—546 (1964).
HAUBNER: Die durch den Hüttenrauch veranlaßten Krankheiten des Rindviehs im Hüttenrauchbezirk der Freiburger Hütten. Arch. wiss. u. prakt. Tierheilk. **4**, 97 und 241 (1878).
HOBBS, C. S., R. P. MOORMAN JR., J. M. GRIFFITH, J. L. WEST, G. M. MERRIMAN, S. L. HANSARD, and C. C. CHAMBERLAIN: Fluorosis in cattle and sheep. Bull. No. 235, Univ. of Tennessee. Agr. Expt. Sta. pp. 1—163, November 1954.

HOBBS, C. S.. and G. M. MERRIMAN: Fluorosis in beef cattle. Univ. of Tennessee, Bull. No. 351, pp.1—183, October 1962.
HOOGSTRATEN, B., N. C. LEONE, J. L. SHUPE, D. A. GREENWOOD, and J. LIEBERMAN: The effect of fluorides on hemopoietic system, liver, and thyroid gland in cattle. J. Amer. Med. Ass. **192**, 26—32 (1965).
HOPPE, F.: Untersuchungen über die Constitution des Zahnschmelzes. Virchow's Arch. path. Anat. **24**, 13—32 (1862).
HUPKA, E., u. P. LUY: Gehäuftes Auftreten von Osteomalacie unter Weiderindern, verursacht durch Fluorwasserstoffsäure enthaltenden Fabrikrauch. Arch. wiss. prakt. Tierheilk. **60**, 21—39 (1929).
— Klinische Beobachtungen über Vergiftungen durch Flußsäureabgase bei Weidetieren. Dtsch. tierärztl. Wschr. **49**, 349—352 (1941).
JODLBAUER, A., u. v. STUBENRAUCH: Über den normalen Fluorgehalt der Knochen und dessen Beeinflussung durch Fluornatriumfütterung. Sitz.-Ber. Ges. Morph. Physiol. München **1902**, 18.
JOHNSON, L. C., C. S. HOBBS, G. M. MERRIMAN, J. L. SHUPE, D. A. GREENWOOD, and E. L. LARGENT: Histogenesis and mechanisms in the development of osteofluorosis. Fluorine Chemistry, IV, edited by J. H. Simons, Academic Press Inc., New York and London 1965.
KICK, C. H., R. M. BETHKE, B. H. EDGINGTON, O. H. M. WILDER, P. R. REARD, W. WILDER, T. J. HILL, and S. W. CHASE: Fluorine in animal nutrition. Ohio Agr. Expt. Sta. Bull. No. 558, 1935, 77 pp.
KLEMENT, R., u. G. TRÖMEL: Hydroxylapatit, der Hauptbestandteil der anorganischen Knochen- und Zahnsubstanz. Hoppe-Seyler's Z. physiol. Chem. **213**, 263—269 (1932).
KRUG, O.: Eine Vergiftung von Milchkühen durch Kieselfluornatrium. Z. Fleisch- u. Milchhyg. **37**, 38—39 (1927).
KRÜGER, E.: Nachweis fluorhaltiger Industrieexhalationen durch Analyse von Rinderharn. Dtsch. tierärztl. Wschr. **56**, 325 (1949).
LEONE, N. C., C. A. STEVENSON, TH. F. HILBISH, and M. C. SOSMAN: A roentgenologic study of a human population exposed to high-fluoride domestic water. Amer. J. Roentgenol., Radium Therapy Nuclear Med. **74**, 874—885 (1955).
LILLEENGEN, K.: Mikroskopisk undersökelse av benpreparater fra sauer lidende av kronisk fluorforgiftning. Norsk. Vet. **46**, 68 (1934).
LOURENS, L. F. D. E.: Fluorose bij het rund. Tijdschr. Diergeneesk. **68**, 229—243 (1941).
MEYN, A., u. K. VIEHL: Über chronische Fluorvergiftungen bei Rindern. Arch. wiss. prakt. Tierheilk. **76**, 329—339 (1941).
MILLER, G. W., and J. L. SHUPE: Alkaline bone phosphatase activity as related to fluoride ingestion by dairy cattle. Amer. J. vet. Res. **23**, 24—31 (1962).
MITCHELL, H. H., and M. EDMAN: The fluorine problem in livestock feeding. Nutr. Abstr. Rev. **21**, 787—804 (1951/52).
MUSSILL, J.: Beobachtungen bei Fabriksrauchschäden an Rindern. Wien, tierärztl. Mschr. **41**, 569—583 (1954).
National Research Council. The fluorosis problem in livestock produktion. Pub. 824, National Academy of Sciences — National Research Council, Washington, D.C. 1960, pp. 1—29.
PERO, R.: Expériences portant sur l'assimilation des phosphates tricalciques naturels finement moulus par l'organisme du porc.Ann. agron. **15**, 288—300 (1945).
PHILLIPS, P. H., E. B. HART, and G. BOHSTEDT: Chronic toxicosis in dairy cows due to the ingestion of fluorine. Research Bull. 123, Agr. Expt. Sta., Univ. of Wisconsin, pp. 1—29, 1934.
POMMER, A.: Röntgenbefunde an den Rippen fluorosekranker Rinder. Wien. tierärztl. Mschr. **41**, 583—589 (1954).
RABUTEAU, A. P. A.: Étude expérimentale sur les effects physiologiques des fluorures et des composés métalliques en général. Thêses, Paris, 1867, 151 pp.
ROHOLM, K.: Fluorosis in sheep in Iceland after volcanic eruptions. Nord. med. Tidskr. 8, 1093—1102 (1934a).
— Fluorose der Schafe auf Island nach Vulkanausbrüchen? Arch. wiss. prakt. Tierheilk. **67**, 420—435 (1934b).
— Fluorine intoxication; a clinical-hygienic study with a review of the literature and some experimental investigations, 364 pp., H. K. Lewis and Co., London (1937).
ROST, E.: Ber. 14, intern. Kongr. Hygiene u. Demographie, Berlin, 1907, 4: 166, 1908.
SCHMIDT, H. J., and W. E. RAND: A critical study of the literature on fluoride toxicology with respect to cattle damage. Amer. J. vet. Res. **13**, 38—49 (1952).
— G. W. NEWELL, and W. E. RAND: The controlled feeding of fluorine, as sodium fluoride to dairy cattle. Amer. J. vet. Res. **15**, 232—239 (1954).
SHREWSBURY, C. L., J. D. HATFIELD, L. P. DOYLE, and F. N. ANDREWS: Some effects of fluorine in the nutrition of sheep. Indiana Agr. Expt. Sta. Bull. No. 499, 1944. 20 pp.

SHUPE, J. L., M. L. MINER, W. BINNS, D. A. GREENWOOD, H. M. NIELSEN, G. E. STODDARD, G. Q. BATEMAN, and L. E. HARRIS: Pathology of chronic bovine fluorosis. "Proceedings Book," Amer. Vet. Med. Assoc. 92nd Annual Meeting, Minneapolis, Aug. 15—18, 1955, pp. 195—201.
— The chemistry, histology, and roentgenology of the teeth and bones of large animals. Arch. Industr. Health **21**, 346—347 (1960).
— N. C. LEONE, E. G. FRAME, D. A. GREENWOOD, and M. L. MINER: Investigation of certainhepatic functions of dairy animals. Arch. Industr. Health **21**, 348—349 (1960).
— Arthritis in cattle. Can. Vet. J. **2**, 369—376 (1961).
— M. L. MINER, L. E. HARRIS, and D. A. GREENWOOD: Relative effects of feeding hay atmospherically contaminated by fluoride residue, normal hay plus calcium fluoride, and normal hay plus sodium fluoride to dairy heifers. Amer. J. vet. Res. **23**, 777—787 (1962).
— Diseases of Cattle, edited by Walter J. Gibbons, Revised Second Edition, American Veterinary Publications, Inc. Santa Barbara, Calif., (1963), pp. 735—746.
— L. E. HARRIS, D. A. GREENWOOD, J. E. BUTCHER, and H. M. NIELSEN: The effect of fluorine on dairy cattle. V. Fluorine in the urine as an estimator of fluorine intake. Amer. J. vet. Res. **24**, 300—306 (1963a).
— M. L. MINER, D. A. GREENWOOD, L. E. HARRIS, and G. E. STODDARD: The effect of fluorine on dairy cattle. II. Clinical and pathologic effects. Amer. J. vet. Res. **24**, 964—979 (1963b).
— — .— Clinical and pathological aspects of fluorine toxicosis in cattle. Ann. N. Y. Acad. Sci. v. 111, Art 2, 618—637 (1964a).
— International Encyclopedia of Veterinary Medicine, London, England, 1964.
SLAGSVOLD, L.: Fluor poisoning in animals. Vet. Med. **30**, 375 (1934a).
— Fluorforgiftning. Norsk Vet. Tidsskr. **46**, 2—16, 61—68 (1934b).
SPENCER, G. R., G. K. GARLICK, E. C. STONE R., L. ALBROOK, and D. F. ADAMS: A field survey for the detection of bovine fluorosis. Northwest Sci. **30**, 24—32 (1956).
STODDARD, G. E., G. Q. BATEMAN, L. E. HARRIS, J. L. SHUPE, and D. A. GREENWOOD: Effects of fluorine on dairy cattle. IV. Milk production. J. Dairy Sci. **46**, 720—726 (1963a).
— L. E. HARRIS, G. Q. BATEMAN, J. L. SHUPE, and D. A. GREENWOOD: Effects of fluorine on dairy cattle. I. Growth and feed consumption. J. Dairy Sci. **46**, 1094—1102 (1963b).
SUTTIE, J. W., R. F. MILLER, and R. H. PHILLIPS: Studies of the effects of dietary NaF on dairy cows. I. The physiological effects and the developmental symptoms of fluorosis. J. Nutr. **63**, 211—224 (1957).
R. GESTELAND, and P. H. PHILLIPS: Effects of dietary sodium fluoride on dairy cows. VI. In young heifers. J. Dairy Sci. **44**, 2250—2258 (1961).
THOMANN, P. E.: Die Beeinflussung verschiedener Stoffwechselabläufe durch Fluor. Inaugural-Dissertation, Vet.-Med. Klinik der Univ. Zürich, 1962.
VELU, H.: Dystrophie dentaire des mammiféres des zones phosphatées (darmous) et fluorose chronique. C. r. soc. Biol. (Paris) **108**, 750—752 (1931a).
— Relations du darmous et de la nappe phréatique des zones phosphatées. Bull. acad. vét. France **4** (n.s.), 392—394 (1931b).
—, et L. BALOZET: Reproduction expérimentale chez le mouton de la dystrophie dentaire des animaux des zones phosphates. Bull. acad. vét. France **4** (n.s.), 373—376 (1931).
— Le darmous (ou dermes); fluorose spontanée des zones phosphatées. Arch. Inst. Pasteur d'Algérie **10**, 41—118 (1932).
WILDER, O. H. M.: Effects of fluorine compounds on swine. Presented at the Seminar, "Biological Effects of Fluorine Compounds on Plants, Animals, and Man," Utah State University, August 1—2, 1963.
ZIPKIN, I., E. D. EANES, and J. L. SHUPE: Effect of prolonged exposure to fluoride on the ash fluoride, citrate and crystallinity of bovine bone. Amer. J. vet. Res. **25**, 1595—1597 (1964).

Chapter 7

Fluorine-Containing Insecticides

By

R. L. METCALF

I. Introduction

Fluorine has played a significant role in insect control since about 1896 when sodium fluoride and various iron fluorides were patented in England as insecticides. Sodium fluoride was used in the United States for cockroach control before 1900 and was introduced in 1915 for the control of poultry lice. However, the use of fluorine insecticides did not become general until the 1930's when the disadvantages of arsenical residues on food crops became apparent and the inorganic fluorine compounds were introduced as safer substitutes.

Systematic investigation of organofluorine insecticides began about 1935 in the I.G. Farbenindustrie and the fluoroalcohols and fluorophosphates (phosphorofluoridates) were intensively investigated largely through the research of SCHRADER (1952). During World War II fluoro-DDT or "Gix" was used for the control of insects of medical importance. More recently, fluoroacetamide and analogues have been used as systemic insecticides and a large variety of other fluorinated organic compounds have shown insecticidal activity. Sulfuryl fluoride has recently been marketed as a fumigant for household and structural pests. These and related developments will be discussed in detail in this chapter.

II. Elemental fluorine

Elemental fluorine F_2, b. $-187°$, is a pale yellow gas at ordinary temperatures and is exceedingly reactive. METCALF and LINDGREN (1948) have evaluated the fumigant action of elemental fluorine to 8 species of insects and mites and found that the effective insecticidal concentration for a one hour exposure at 20° was between 1 g per 100 cu. ft. (227 p.p.m.) and 5.75 g per 100 cu. ft. (1305 p.p.m.). The lower concentration did not cause any injury to citrus seedlings but the upper burned them severely. The dosage of 1305 p.p.m. killed 96% of the adults of California red scale *Aonidiella aurantii* while hydrogen cyanide at 1000 p.p.m. under the same conditions produced a mortality of 97%. It is evident that elemental fluorine is highly toxic to insects but because of its hazardous nature and corrosive action it seems exceedingly doubtful that it will ever play a practical role in insect control.

III. Inorganic fluorine insecticides

A. Fluorides

As has been mentioned, sodium fluoride, NaF, was the first widely used fluorine containing insecticide. Sodium fluoride has had extensive use as an undiluted dust for the control of cockroaches and chewing lice of poultry and cattle. It has also been used as a stomach poison in poison baits for the control of grasshoppers, cutworms, and earwigs. A bait suggested for the control of the silverfish, *Lepisma saccharina*, contains sodium fluoride 16 parts by weight, oatmeal 200 parts, powdered sugar 10 parts, and powdered salt 5 parts (METCALF et al. 1962). Sodium fluoride has an oral LD_{50} to the rat and rabbit of ca. 200 mg per kg and to the dog of 50 to 100 mg per kg (NEGHERBON 1959).

Sodium fluoride is a white powder containing 45% fluorine and soluble in water at 18° to 4.22 g per 100 cc. Sodium fluoride is commonly produced by the following reactions:

1) $2\,HF + Na_2CO_3 \rightarrow 2\,NaF + H_2O + CO_2$

2) $Na_2SiF_6 + 2\,Na_2CO_3 + H_2O \rightarrow 6\,NaF + H_2SiO_3 + 2\,CO_2$

In the latter process (U.S. Pat. 1,382,165) caustic soda is added to dissolve the colloidal silicic acid leaving the sodium fluoride as a precipitated solid. The regulations of the U.S. Federal Insecticide, Fungicide, and Rodenticide Act require that sodium fluoride be colored green or blue to prevent its mistaken use as flour.

Other fluorides which have been evaluated for insecticidal use are those of ammonium, barium, calcium, chromium, copper, iron, lead, lithium, magnesium, manganese, potassium, strontium, and zinc (MARCOVITCH 1928). Pertinent insect toxicity data are given in Table 1. It appears that the insecticidal properties largely depend upon the fluorine content. These compounds generally produced severe plant damage because of their relatively high water solubility and have had little or no practical use.

Table 1. *Solubility and toxicity of inorganic fluorine compounds to insects*[1]

Compound	Water solubility g per 100 ml 25°	Oral LD_{50} γ per g	
		Bombyx mori 4th Instar	Apis mellifera as fluorine
NaF	4.054	110—150	60—70
CaF_2			>540
MgF_2	0.013	>570	
MnF_2	0.186	200—400	
PbF_2	0.066	250—400	
Na_2SiF_6	0.762	100—130	240
K_2SiF_6	0.177	70—100	50
$BaSiF_6$	0.025	90—120	60—70
Na_3AlF_6	0.061	50—70	60—70
K_3AlF_6	0.158	80—100	
$(NH_4)_3AlF_6$	1.031	110—140	

[1] Data from SHEPARD and CARTER (1933), KÖRTING (1933) corrected for approximate body weight and fluorine content.

B. Fluoroaluminates

Cryolite or sodium fluoroaluminate which occurs naturally as a mineral of Greenland, Na_3AlF_6 or $AlF_3 \cdot 3\,NaF$, was first used as an insecticide by MARCOVICH in 1929. Cryolite is commonly used as a spray at 0.35 to 1%, and as a 20 to 80% dust diluted with inert diluents such as clays, talcs, *etc.* for the control of chewing insects such as the codling moth, *Carpocapsa pomonella*, Mexican bean beetle, *Epilachna varivestis*, flea beetles, tomato worms and many others. Its greatest advantages are its safety on foliage and its low toxicity to mammals. The oral LD_{50} to the rat is greater than 13,500 mg per kg (MARKOVITCH and STANLEY 1942).

This compound contains 54.2% fluorine and is soluble in water to 0.035 g per 100 cc. The naturally occurring material when ground forms a rather heavy powder not entirely suited for insecticidal purposes and synthetic cryolite which is lighter and fluffier is often preferred. It may be produced by the following reaction (HOWARD 1924):

$$AlF_3 + 3\,NH_4F + 3\,NaCl \rightarrow Na_3AlF_6 + 3\,NH_4Cl$$

Synthetic cryolite is also recovered from the discarded pot linings of electrolytic cells used in the production of aluminum by the Hall processes. The fused cryolite is dissolved in sodium hydroxide or sodium aluminate and sodium fluoride and precipitated at about 60° F by acid, such as carbonic acid, to give a light fluffy product that suspends well in water and adheres well to foliage (MORROW 1941). The synthetic cryolites contain about 86 to 98% sodium fluoroaluminate and are soluble in water to about 0.061 g per 100 cc.

Sodium fluoroaluminate although relatively insoluble in water is soluble in dilute acids and alkalies. Spray residues have been removed from apples by washing in dilute hydrochloric acid. With lime, cryolite reacts to form calcium fluoride and sodium aluminate. These may cause foliage injury and sodium fluoroaluminate should therefore not be used in combination with lime in spraying plants (MARCOVITCH and STANLEY 1942). The reaction with lime is:

$$2\,Na_3AlF_6 + 6\,Ca(OH)_2 \rightarrow 2\,Na_3AlO_3 + 6\,CaF_2 + 6\,H_2O$$

C. Fluorosilicates

A number of fluorosilicates of various metals have been investigated as insecticides. The water solubility of the various fluorosilicate salts at 17.5° has been given by MARCOVITCH (1928) as: Cu — 41.6%, Ca — 34.5%, Mg — 26.3%, Pb — 23.3%, NH_4 — 20%, Al — 0.85%, Na — 0.65%, K — 0.118% and Ba — 0.0266%. Of these only the sodium and barium salts have been used commercially as insecticides.

Sodium fluorosilicate Na_2SiF_6 is a white granular material containing 60.6% fluorine. It is used as a toxicant for baits for grasshoppers, crickets, cutworms, and weevils at about 4 to 6 parts to 100 parts of bran and 60—100 parts of water. Its other principal use is as a home mothproofing agent using 0.5 to 0.7% in water solution together with 0.25 to 0.5% wetting agent. The sodium fluorosilicate which has a decided affinity for wool is applied by spraying or dipping and is not removed by dry cleaning. Sodium fluorosilicate has an oral LD_{50} to the rat and rabbit of about 125 mg per kg (NEGHERBON 1959).

Sodium fluorosilicate is prepared by reacting fluorosilicic acid obtained as a by-product of the production of superphosphate fertilizer with salt (MARCOVITCH and STANLEY 1942).

$$H_2SiF_6 + 2\,NaCl \rightarrow Na_2SiF_6 + 2\,HCl$$

An especially light and fluffy product has been produced by passing sodium tetrafluoride into sodium carbamate solution to form a gel which when dried contains 79.5% sodium fluorosilicate and has a specific gravity of 0.25.

The commercial product has been stated to be more than 98% pure. In water, hydrolysis occurs and a saturated solution has a pH of 3.6 due to the formation of HF:

$$Na_2SiF_6 + 2\,H_2O \rightarrow 2\,NaF + 4\,HF + SiO_2$$

With lime the following reaction occurs:

$$Na_2SiF_6 + 2\,Ca(OH)_2 \rightarrow 2\,CaF_2 + 2\,NaF + SiO_2 + 2\,H_2O$$

These two reactions which result in the formation of soluble fluorides may cause plant damage and therefore the compound is not used for foliage applications.

Barium fluorosilicate $BaSiF_6$ which contains 40.8% fluorine has the lowest water solubility of the common fluorosilicates and was at one time favored for use on plants to control chewing insects as a spray at 3–8 lb. per 100 gallon or as a 25% dust. Like sodium fluorosilicate it gives an acid reaction in water, a saturated solution having a pH of 3.4 (MARCOVITCH and STANLEY 1942). The commercial product contains about 72% barium fluorosilicate, 8% cryolite, and 20% inert materials. Barium fluorosilicate has an oral LD_{50} to the rat and rabbit of about 175 mg per kg (NEGHERBON 1959).

1. Mode of action of fluorides, fluoroaluminates, and fluorosilicates

SHAFER (1915) made a comprehensive investigation of the action of sodium fluoride upon the American cockroach *Periplaneta americana*. When this insect ran about through deposits of the insecticide, this adhered and partially dissolved in exudations of the bases of the legs and thinner areas of the cuticle. The presence of the material produced (a) symptoms of irritability; (b) torpor with occasional nervous starts; and (c) paralysis and death. It was concluded that this insect ingested considerable quantities of sodium fluoride by cleaning off the irritating material with its mouthparts. HOCKENYOS (1933) investigated the mechanism of absorption of sodium fluoride by *P. americana* and *Blatta orientalis* and concluded that the compound was absorbed directly through the membranous areas of cuticle at the junction of the head and thorax and of the coxa. SWEETMAN (1941) and GRIFFITHS and TAUBER (1943) showed by sealing the mouthparts of *P. americana* that sodium fluoride could act both as a stomach and a contact poison. The latter authors found no significant differences in the mortalities of normal roaches or those with sealed mouthparts after walking in sodium fluoride powder, and concluded when the roach walked in NaF, death resulted from contact action rather than as a result of cleaning of the appendages. This, however, is not in agreement with the LD_{50} values for NaF to male *Periplaneta* obtained by HEAL and MENUSAN (1948): injection 125, oral 100–200, and contact 1200 γ per g.

In most chewing insects, the inorganic fluorine insecticides act largely if not entirely as stomach poisons. WOKE (1940) describes the following sequence of symptoms as occurring in the southern armyworm *Prodenia eridania* larvae fed leaf sandwiches containing 2 to 5 mg of sodium fluoride: (a) rearing of the head and thorax, (b) turning onto the back, (c) twisting from side to side, and (d) regurgitation. When fed 1 mg of cryolite or 0.2 to 1 mg barium fluorosilicate the larvae (a) became sluggish, (b) showed occasional spasms, and (c) died after flaccid paralysis. Histological investigation of larvae poisoned by sodium fluoride or cryolite revealed pronounced disintegration of the nuclei and cytoplasm of the epithelial cells of the mid-gut. Similar effects were observed in the larvae of *Aglais urticae* and in *Locusta migratoria* poisoned by sodium fluoride and sodium fluorosilicate (PILAT 1935). However, sodium fluorosilicate did not produce these histological effects in larvae of *Porthetria dispar* or *Pieris rapae* and barium fluorosilicate did not produce histological changes in the mid-gut epithelium of *Prodenia* (WOKE 1940). These variable results suggest that fluoride poisoning is the result of a much more subtle biochemical lesion whose grossest manifestation may be the disintegration of the epithelial tissues.

The poisoning of *Tribolium confusum* by sodium fluoride results in slow and progressive decline in respiratory rate (LORD 1950).

Sodium fluoride at concentrations as low as 0.005 M was found to decrease the *in vitro* oxidative and glycolytic activity of muscle and fat of *Carpocapsa pomonella* (GRAHAM 1946). It was concluded that the inhibition of muscle glycolysis was the more probable site of activity for inorganic fluoride and that this process could account for the flaccid paralysis commonly observed after poisoning.

From the studies of WARBURG and CHRISTIAN (1942), fluoride ion has been shown to inhibit the enzyme enolase which catalyzes the interconversion of:

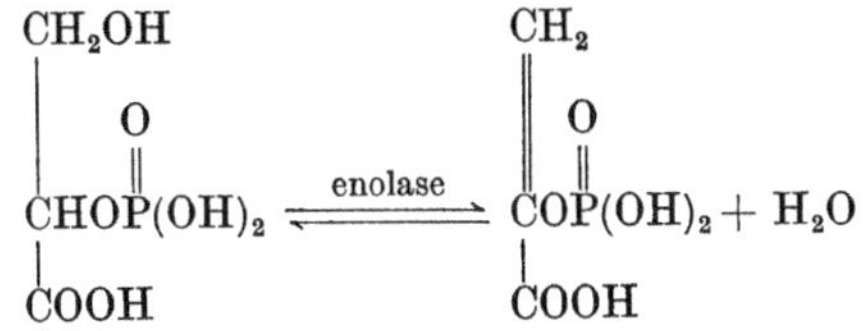

D-2-phosphoglyceric acid *enol*-2-phosphopyruvic acid

and is of great importance in oxidative metabolism as the enol-phosphate liberates a large amount of energy upon hydrolysis and can phosphorylate the adenylic system.

Enolase is believed to be a magnesium complex and is inhibited by fluoride ion as a result of the formation of a complex magnesium fluorophosphate which removes the Mg^{++} from the prosthetic group of the enzyme. In the house fly, enolase is inhibited by fluoride ion at 10^{-4} M (CHEFURKA 1954).

Fluoride also inhibits other insect enzymes which require Mg^{++} as a prosthetic group. SACKTOR (1953) found that although fluoride did not affect the specific ATPase of house fly mitochondria, fluoride at 1×10^{-2} M completely inhibited the soluble pyrophosphatase activity. Fluoride at 2×10^{-3} M produced about 50% inhibition of hexose-1-phosphatase activity in silkworm blood (FAULKNER 1955).

D. Sulfuryl fluoride

SCHRADER (1947a) states that *thionyl fluoride* SOF_2 b. −30°, d. 2.93 g per l has the same order of effectiveness as a fumigant to grain weevils as ethylene oxide. Sulfuryl fluoride SO_2F_2 was stated to have no insecticidal action. However, more recent investigation has disclosed the valuable fumigant properties of sulfuryl fluoride for structural and commodity fumigation (STEWART 1957).

Sulfuryl fluoride, SO_2F_2, is a colorless, non-inflammable, odorless substance which boils at −55.2° at 760 mm. The compound has a melting point of −136.67° and a liquid density of 1.34 g per cc. at 25°. The gas has a density of 3.52 compared to air and has the following solubilities in g per 100 g at 22 to 25°: water 0.075, propylene glycol 0.2, peanut oil 0.62, acetone 1.74, chloroform 2.12, ethylene dibromide 0.5, petroleum ether (hexane fraction) 0.77, isopropyl formate 1.4, and propylene oxide 0.62. The compound is highly stable and showed no corrosive action to metals, plastic, paper, rubber, cloth, and other household items.

Sulfuryl fluoride has a boiling point much lower than any other commercial fumigant and a consequently higher vapor pressure as shown in Table 2. This

Table 2. *Properties of sulfuryl fluoride compared to other common fumigants* (KENAGA 1957)

Fumigant	d. 25° H_2O = 1.00	Vapor density air = 1.00	b.p. 760 mm °C	Vapor pressure mm Hg 25° C	Latent heat of vaporization at B.P. Cal. per mole
SO_2F_2	1.342	3.52	−55.2	13,442.0	4,600
CH_3Br	1.732 (%°)	3.28	4.5	1,580.0	5,750
CS_2	1.256	2.62	46.2	361.6	6,399
CCl_4	1.584	5.31	76.5	114.5	7,110
CH_2ClCH_2Cl	1.246	3.41	83.0	79.9	7,652
CH_2BrCH_2Br	2.17	6.48	131.6	11.6	7,688

Table 3. *Comparison of toxicity of sulfuryl fluoride and methyl bromide* (KENAGA 1957)

	Hours exposure	Oz. per 1000 cu. ft. at 80° F			
		Tribolium confusum		Attagenus piceus	
		LD_{50}	LD_{95}	LD_{50}	LD_{95}
Sulfuryl fluoride	0.5	36.16	43.84	27.84	42.08
	1	19.36	22.56	18.40	26.32
	2	12.77	14.32	11.71	14.45
	5	6.86	8.06	5.19	6.75
	16	3.14	3.45	2.08	2.39
Methyl bromide	0.5	46.08	55.20	48.58	53.90
	1	29.92	36.00	29.92	36.16
	2	20.03	22.75	18.72	24.48
	5	8.34	9.49	8.64	9.60
	16	3.29	3.71	3.60	4.02

favors the dispersion and penetration of the fumigant through commodities and structures. Sulfuryl fluoride has proved to be a highly toxic fumigant to many species of insects as is shown by the comparative toxicity to methyl bromide given in Table 3. Sulfuryl fluoride is effective against all stages of insects as shown by the following LD_{50} values in oz. per 1000 cu. ft. at 80° F: granary weevil, *Sitophilus granarius* – adult 0.63, pupa 0.76, larva 0.36, and egg 24.9; angoumois grain moth, *Sitotroga cerealella* – adult 0.74, larva 0.82, and egg 4.81 (KENAGA 1957). Its principal field of usefulness is in the fumigation of dwellings for the drywood termite *Kalotermes minor*. It is applied under polyethylene sheeting at a dosage of 2 to 4 lb. per 1000 cu. ft. Sulfuryl fluoride is highly toxic to green plants, vegetables, fruits and tubers at 1 to 3 lb. per 1000 cu. ft. but showed little effect on the germination of seeds at 1 to 5 lb. per 1000 cu. ft. over a 16 hour period at 80° F. It is about one-third as toxic as methyl bromide to mammals based on the inhalation of a single acute exposure and the safe limit for prolonged human exposure is 100 p.p.m.

1. Mode of action of sulfuryl fluoride

MEIKLE et al. (1963) have investigated the mode of action of sulfuryl fluoride to the drywood termite *Kalotermes minor* exposed to a concentration of 1 mg per liter for 24 hours at 20° (or 40% LD_{100}). Experiments with S^{35}-labeled SO_2F_2 showed that the fumigant was excreted as inorganic $SO_4^=$ indicating the *in vivo* release of F^-. By using labeled metabolic pools of sodium acetate (1-C^{14}) and of $P^{32}O_4^{\equiv}$, the following metabolic intermediates were shown to be affected:

	Per cent total radioactivity	
	untreated	treated
Hexose monophosphate	27.0 ± 0.9	29.5 ± 0.6
Hexose diphosphate	18.8 ± 0.2	20.5 ± 0.4
Pentose diphosphate	9.6 ± 0.5	10.3 ± 0.6
Adenosine triphosphate	15.1 ± 1.7	10.0 ± 1.3
Phosphoenol pyruvate	0	0.9 ± 0.3
Argenine	0.1 ± 0.1	2.3 ± 0.6

The authors suggest that the variations found are the result of F^- inhibition of Mg^{++} containing enzymes. For example, the increase in phosphoenol pyruvate may occur as a result of blocking of glycolysis through inhibition of phosphopyruvate carboxylase, pyruvate kinase, and enolase. The decreased amount of adenosine triphosphate in the treated termites is the result of inhibition of oxidative phosphorylation.

IV. Organic fluorine insecticides

A. Fluoroalcohols and derivatives

1. Fluoroethanol, its esters, and acetals

UFER of I.G. Farben found in 1935 that fluoroethyl alcohol and 2′-fluoroethyl-2-hydroxyethyl ether $FCH_2CH_2OCH_2CH_2OH$ were highly toxic to mammals (the subcutaneous lethal dosage to the dog is about 1 mg per kg) and these substances were patented as rodenticides. However, neither of these substances has contact insecticidal action although fluoroethyl acetate $FCH_2CH_2O\overset{\overset{O}{\|}}{C}CH_3$ was found to be insecticidal at 0.1% in water (SCHRADER 1947a). This was apparently the result of enhanced penetration of the cuticle by the more lipid soluble ester. SCHRADER investigated a number of other esters of fluoroethyl alcohol. Bis-(2-fluoroethyl) sulfite $(FCH_2CH_2O)_2S{=}O$ b.$_{17}$ 108° and bis-(2-fluoroethyl) carbonate $(FCH_2CH_2O)_2C{=}O$ b.$_{14}$ 89° had a toxicity to aphids approaching that of nicotine, although they killed much more slowly. Bis-(2-fluoroethyl) sulfate $(FCH_2CH_2O)_2S\genfrac{}{}{0pt}{}{\diagup O}{\diagdown O}$ was somewhat less active. Two acetals, bis-(2-fluoroethyl)-acetal $FCH_2CH_2OCH_2OCH_2CH_2F$ b.$_{11}$ 43° and bis-(2-fluoroethoxyethyl)-acetal $FCH_2CH_2OCH_2CH_2OCH_2OCH_2CH_2$-$OCH_2CH_2F$ b.$_3$ 120° were found to be toxic to aphids as contact sprays at 0.05 to 0.1% in water. KÜKENTHAL then demonstrated that when watered about the roots of maize at 0.1% they were translocated to the leaves in amounts toxic to aphids. When sprayed on grape vines at 0.1% bis-(2-fluoroethyl)-acetal killed the grape phylloxera *Phylloxera vitifoliae* feeding on the roots. Thus these fluoroacetals were the first organic insecticides for which pronounced systemic action was demonstrated. The fluoroacetals are, however, very toxic to mammals and this has prevented their practical use as insecticides.

2. Carbamates of fluoroethanol

SCHRADER (1947a) also studied the carbamates or urethanes of fluoroethyl alcohol. The following compounds had no contact insecticidal activity: 2-fluoroethyl carbamate, b.$_{12}$ 105°; 2-fluoroethyl *N*-methylcarbamate ,b.$_{13}$ 92°; 2-fluoroethyl *N*,*N*-dimethylcarbamate b.$_{13}$ 65°; 2-fluoroethyl *N*,*N*-diethylcarbamate b.$_{14}$ 75°; 2-fluoroethyl *N*,*N*-dipropylcarbamate b.$_{13}$ 126°; 2-fluoroethyl *N*-ethyl, *N*-phenylcarbamate b.$_{12}$ 130°; and 2-fluoroethyl *N*-morpholinocarbamate b.$_{12}$ 120°. However, they were highly toxic to rodents and 2-fluoroethyl *N*,*N*-dimethylcarbamate was an outstanding rodenticide with toxicity values to mice, upon injection, of 0.3 to 0.4 mg per kg (SCHRADER 1947b).

In contrast to the carbamates of fluoroethyl alcohol, the carbamates of 2-hydroxyethyl-2′fluoroethyl ether were strong contact insecticides but with only slight action as stomach poisons. 2-Fluoroethoxyethyl *N*-methylcarbamate b.$_{11}$ 140°; 2-fluoroethoxyethyl *N*,*N*-dimethylcarbamate b.$_{12}$ 118°; and 2-fluoroethoxyethyl *N*-morpholinocarbamate b.$_{12}$ 164° gave 100% mortality of aphids when sprayed at 0.1% and were thus of the same toxicity as the esters of fluoroethylalcohol.

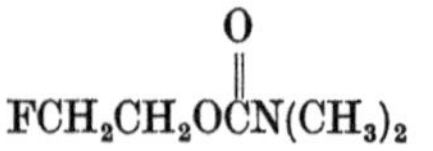

2-fluoroethyl *N,N*-dimethylcarbamate

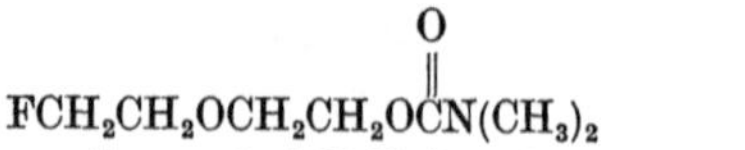

2-fluoroethoxyethyl *N,N*-dimethylcarbamate

3. Mode of action of fluoroalcohols and derivatives

The 2-fluoroethylacetals are readily converted to 2-fluoroethylalcohol by hydrolysis, and this alcohol by the successive action of alcohol dehydrogenase and aldehyde dehydrogenase forms fluoroacetic acid (Bartlett 1952).

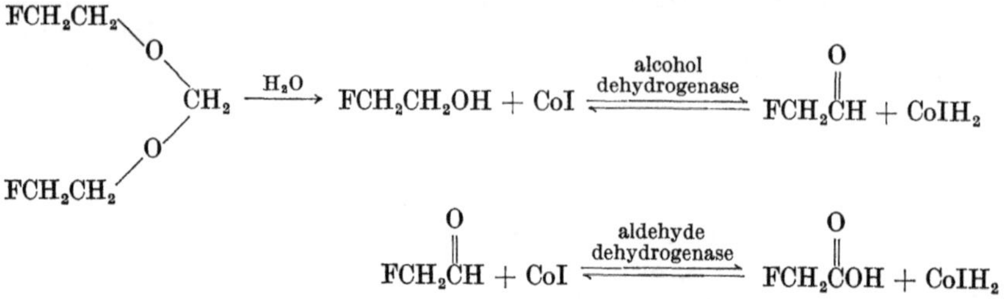

The various esters of fluoroethanol are readily hydrolyzable *in vivo* to fluoroethanol. Thus it appears that all of the toxicants discussed in this section share a common mode of action with fluoroacetic acid as described in the following section.

B. Fluoroacetic acid, fluoroacetamide, and derivatives

Fluoroacetic acid, $FCH_2\overset{O}{\overset{\|}{C}}OH$, is the subject of Chapter 8 of this volume and as the sodium salt has been shown to be highly toxic to insects (David and Gardiner 1951). However, it is also extremely toxic to warmblooded animals with an oral LD_{50} to the rat of about 1 to 2 mg per kg. Many other species including man have equivalent susceptibility (Negherbon 1959). Thus the compound is entirely too toxic to be considered for general insecticidal usage although it is employed as a rodenticide for use under careful supervision.

Fluoroacetamide also has useful insecticidal properties (David and Gardiner 1958, 1959) and is considered to be much safer to warm-blooded animals with an oral LD_{50} to the rat of about 15 mg per kg. This compound $FCH_2\overset{O}{\overset{\|}{C}}NH_2$ is a white crystalline salt, m. 108°, soluble in water and slightly soluble in some organic solvents. It is employed commercially as a systemic insecticide especially in Japan where 75 tons were used in 1960 as a 10% liquid or a 30% wettable powder. The closely related fluoroacetanilide, $FCH_2\overset{O}{\overset{\|}{C}}NHC_6H_5$, m. 75°, is a white solid soluble in water to 0.1% and in some organic solvents. It has been suggested for use as a systemic and contact insecticide with some fumigant action (Phillips 1955, Harrison 1956). The acute oral LD_{50} to the rat is 10 to 12 mg per kg.

N-substituted derivatives of fluoroacetamide such as the phenyl, *p*-methoxyphenyl, *p*-fluorophenyl, *p*-chlorophenyl, and *N,N*-diisoamyl had a weak contact toxicity to the house fly when applied as residues at 1 g per sq. meter (Ascher

1958a). Esters of fluoroacetic acid such as 2-fluoroethyl fluoroacetate are also insecticidal (RIPPER 1957).

Fluoroacetylphenyl urea, $FCH_2\overset{O}{\overset{\|}{C}}NH\overset{O}{\overset{\|}{C}}NHC_6H_5$, m. 159°, is a white solid soluble in water to 0.014% and in most organic solvents. It is a powerful contact and systemic insecticide which penetrates slowly into plant tissues and has given control of sucking insects for several weeks without plant damage. As a spray it is active against aphids, spider mites, and scale insects at 0.001 to 0.025%. It is fully effective against aphids and mites resistant to organophosphorus insecticides. Fluoroacetylphenyl urea has an oral LD_{50} to the rat of between 25 and 62.5 mg per kg (HOECHST 1963).

1. Insecticidal activity of fluoroacetic acid and derivatives

DAVID and GARDINER (1959) have conducted careful comparisons of the systemic activity of fluoroacetamide, fluoroacetate, and the well known systemic insecticide, octamethyl pyrophosphoramide or schradan and have found the quantitative values for the systemic toxicity of the compounds as shown in Table 4. Fluoroacetamide and sodium fluoroacetate were about equally effective as systemic insecticides to *Aphis fabae*, *Brevicoryne brassicae*, *Myzus persicae* and the eggs and larvae of *Pieris brassicae*. Both fluorine compounds were absorbed and translocated in toxic amounts from solutions applied to bean and cabbage plants and were approximately 100 times as effective as schradan. Fluoroacetamide and sodium fluoroacetate applied to the lower leaves of the broad bean were rapidly translocated upward in amounts toxic to aphids. Both fluorine compounds were also translocated downward from younger to older broad bean leaves in amounts toxic to aphids but schradan was not. Translocation of the fluoro-compounds was also demonstrated from the older outer leaves of cabbage to the younger inner leaves. At equal dosages, plants treated with fluoroacetate remained toxic to aphids for 5 days or so longer than those treated with fluoroacetamide. In ovicidal experiments where eggs of *Pieris brassicae* were dipped in solutions of the insecticides at 20° C, fluoroacetamide gave 100% prevention of hatching at 0.2% w/v while fluoroacetate gave only 2%.

Table 4. *Comparative systemic toxicity of fluoroacetamide, fluoracetate, and other insecticides*[1]

Compound	LD_{100} to Aphis fabae feeding on broad beans mg per kg of leaf	Dosage preventing growth of Pieris brassicae on cabbage leaves mg per kg of leaf
Fluoroacetamide	0.09—0.9	20
Sodium fluoroacetate	0.7	20
Schradan	50	>2,900
Demeton	1	140—310
Para-oxon	—	6

[1] DAVID and GARDINER (1951, 1959).

TAHORI (1963) selected the house fly *Musca domestica* for 33 generations by feeding the adults on a sugar-water solution of sodium fluoroacetate of such a concentration that 80 to 90% mortality was obtained. The degree of resistance developed was measured by oral feeding upon 1.0 microliter droplets of the toxicant. The LD_{50} of fluoroacetate was 0.6 γ per female fly before selection and after 25 generations of selection this had increased to 4.2 γ per female fly. The fluoroacetate-selected, resistant flies had also developed the following degrees of resistance, measured by topical application, to various contact insecticides: DDT 66 ×, methoxychlor 12 ×, lindane 26 ×, and dieldrin 400 ×. No resistance had developed to the organophosphorus insecticides parathion, malathion, or Dipterex, or to the carbamate Sevin as synergized with piperonyl butoxide. No suggestion was advanced to account for these interesting findings.

In connection with insecticide resistance, ASCHER (1960) found that larvae of DDT-resistant house flies were more susceptible to cetyl fluoride $C_{16}H_{33}F$ and to cetyl fluoroacetate $FCH_2\overset{O}{\overset{\|}{C}}OC_{16}H_{33}$ than the larvae of a susceptible strain.

2. Mode of action of fluoroacetic acid and derivatives

Fluoroacetate has been shown by the classical work of PETERS (Chapter 8) to be incorporated into the tricarboxylic acid cycle where it is activated with coenzyme A and then condensed with oxaloacetic acid to form optically active fluorocitric acid. This substance is a competitive inhibitor of the enzyme *cis*-aconitase which catalyzes the conversion of citric acid to isocitric acid prior to its oxidative decarboxylation. This action of fluoroacetic acid appears to represent the fundamental biochemical lesion resulting from the toxic action of the fluoroacetates, fluoroacetamides, and fluoroacetals.

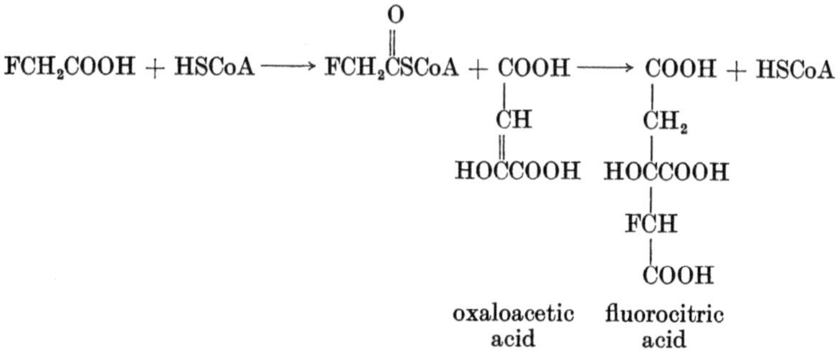

The enzyme aconitase has been demonstrated in the fat body of the grasshopper *Schistocerca* and there is evidence that it is present in other insects (GILMOUR 1961). The high toxicity of fluoroacetate to insects is, in fact, presumptive evidence of the existence of these metabolic pathways.

Fluoroacetamide is hydrolyzed in animal tissues to fluoroacetic acid (PETERS et al. 1953), (BUCKLE et al. 1949).

$$FCH_2\overset{O}{\overset{\|}{C}}NH_2 \xrightarrow{H_2O} FCH_2\overset{O}{\overset{\|}{C}}OH + NH_3$$

Therefore fluoroacetamide may be expected to exert approximately the same ultimate degree of toxicity as fluoroacetate to both insects and mammals. SAUNDERS (1957) records that the intravenous toxicity to rabbits for fluoroacetamide, fluoroacetate and methyl fluoroacetate was almost identical (LD_{50} 0.25 mg per kg) and that the symptoms of intoxication were the same. However, the fact that fluoroacetamide is a solid obviously changes its absorption characteristics. A similar *in vivo* conversion to fluoroacetate may be expected for fluoroacetanilide and fluoroacetylphenyl urea. The rate of conversion is undoubtedly different for the various compounds and influenced by enzymes in the insect and, in the case of systemic use, by those in the plant. Thus the speed and duration of toxic action are functions of the overall effects of these factors and in the systemic use of these compounds, of the rate of absorption by the plant roots or leaves.

C. Phosphorofluoridates

The discovery of the physiological activity of the organophosphorus anticholinesterases began with the observation of LANGE and VON KREUGER (1932) that the vapors of *diethyl phosphorofluoridate* when breathed in small amounts produced symptoms of breathlessness and constriction of the pupil of the eye. This chance observation has led to the development of a vast number of organophosphorus esters which have been utilized as insecticides, nematocides, war gases, and pharmaceuticals. The phosphorofluoridates form only a very small proportion of the compounds of insecticidal interest and are dealt with in a succeeding volume. However, a few of these phosphorofluoridates have interesting and unique insecticidal action and are discussed in some detail here.

GERHARD SCHRADER of I.G. Farbenindustrie began his extensive investigations of organophosphorus compounds as insecticides in 1936. By analogy with methane sulfonyl fluoride (Section I), *N*,*N*-dimethyl phosphoramidodifluoridate $b._{22}$ 38° was produced and was found to have similar fumigant action but no contact insecticidal action (DRP 664,438). In December of 1936 SCHRADER patented *O*-ethyl *N*,*N*-dimethyl phosphoramidofluoridate as an insecticide with strong miotic properties and lethal to aphids when sprayed at 0.005%. This compound was too volatile and much too toxic to mammals (LD_{100} to the dog is about 0.1 mg per kg) to have practical use as an insecticide but has an obviously close resemblance to the war gases tabun and sarin. The related *O*-2-chloroethyl *N*,*N*-dimethyl phosphoramidofluoridate $b._3$ 63° was found to be a contact insecticide, water stable and of lower toxicity to higher animals (SCHRADER 1947a).

SCHRADER patented the dialkyl phosphorofluoridates as insecticides in 1939 (German Patent 645/39 Secret D.P. 767,153) and his continuing researches led to the discovery of tetramethyl phosphorodiamidofluoridate or dimefox in 1940.

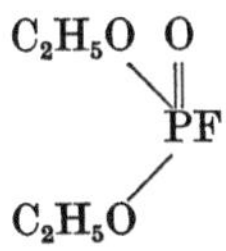

diethyl phosphorofluoridate

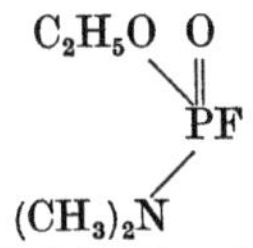

O-ethyl *N*,*N*-dimethyl phosphoramidofluoridate

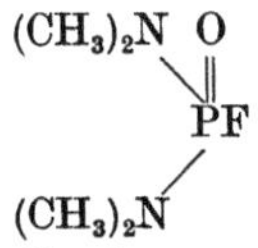

dimefox

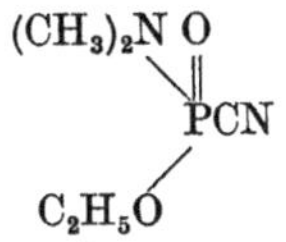

tabun

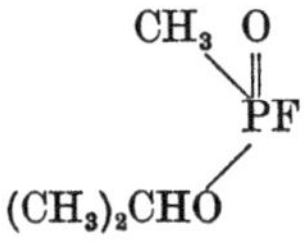

sarin

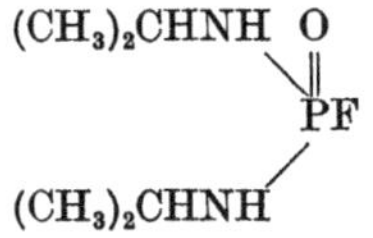

mipafox

Dimefox. This compound in the pure state is a colorless, mobile liquid $b._4$ 67°, d. 1.12, with a faint odor and a v.p. of 0.4 mm Hg at 30°. Dimefox is water miscible and has a half life of 8.6 days at pH 4, 2 years at pH 6, and 710 years at pH 8 (METCALF 1955).

Dimefox has systemic insecticidal properties and has been used commercially in England as a soil drench for hops to control the two-spotted spider mite *Tetranychus telarius* and the hop aphid *Phorodon humuli*. A dosage of 1 quart of 50% material to 25 gallons of water is applied at 4 fluid oz. to the crown of the plant by dipper or low pressure lance. A single application has given seasonal protection and should not be made closer than 8 weeks of harvest. Such treatments have resulted in increased yields of 6 to 40% and in 1955 were applied to about 20% of the acreage in England and 66% in Belgium (METCALF 1957).

Perhaps the most interesting use of dimefox has been for the control of the mealybug vectors *Pseudococcus njalensis*, *P. citri*, and *Ferrisia virgata* of the swollen-shoot virus of cacao in Ghana (HANNA et al. 1955). The most effective control has been obtained by watering the compound as a 5% solution directly about the trunk of the tree at a dosage proportioned to the weight of the aerial portion of the tree (estimated by a girth vs. weight correlation). Treatment rates range from about 20 g of active ingredient for a 10-inch tree to 230 g for a 30-inch tree. The treatment was effective for about seven weeks and resulted in reduction of the mealybug populations to as low as 0.08% of pretreatment values. Trunk implantations of dimefox using aqueous solutions poured into holes bored at intervals about the base at 160—250 p.p.m. of tree weight gave satisfactory control of the mealybugs at about one-tenth the dosage required with the root application.

A number of related bis-(*N*,*N*-dialkyl) phosphorodiamidofluoridates have been synthesized (HEAP and SAUNDERS 1948) and these together with their subcutaneous LD_{50} values (in mg/kg) to the mouse are: bis-(*N*,*N*-dimethyl), 1; bis-(*N*,*N*-diethyl), 160; bis-(*N*,*N*-dibutyl), 16; bis-(*N*,*N*-cyclohexyl), 9; and bis-(*N*,*N*-dibenzyl), 10. SAUNDERS (1957) lists in addition the bis-(*N*-methyl-*N*-phenyl), 160; bis-piperidino, 320; and bis-morpholino, 400.

Mipafox — or bis-(*N*-mono-isopropyl) phosphorodiamidofluoridate, m. 60°, $b._2$ 125°, $d._{25}$ 1.2, and v.p. 0.001 mm at 15°, is a white crystalline solid, soluble in water to about 8% and in polar organic solvents. In water solution it has a half life of 14 days at pH 4, 200 days at pH 6, and 6 days at pH 8. Its oral LD_{50} to laboratory mammals, 25 to 50 mg per kg, is notably lower than that of dimefox, 7.5 mg per kg (RIPPER 1952). Mipafox was found to be an effective systemic insecticide for leaf or soil application to control aphids, spider mites, thrips, white flies, scale insects, and mealy bugs (RIPPER et al. 1951), but is less persistent than schradan. However, it was withdrawn from practical use after it was found that chronic exposure in birds, rats, and humans could result in severe neurotoxic symptoms. These may be caused by the ability of this compound along with diisopropyl phosphorofluoridate to cause demyelination of the nerve, possibly because of strong inhibition of pseudocholinesterase. In three humans exposed during the manufacture of mipafox, symptoms of severe muscular weakness developed together with gastrointestinal disturbances, bronchospasms, and miosis or pupillary contraction. About three weeks after the acute symptoms, the victims developed flaccid paralysis of all limbs resembling that of "ginger paralysis" produced by tri-*o*-cresyl phosphate (BIDSTRUP et al. 1953; DAVIES 1954). The specific and pseudocholinesterase levels of the blood were lowered in all the subjects.

Dialkylphosphorofluoridates — SCHRADER (1952, 1963) lists the following dialkylphosphorofluoridates as toxic to aphids[1] when sprayed at concentrations of 0.05 to 0.2%:

dimethyl- $b._{10}$ 50°; diethyl- $b._{11}$ 62°; di-*n*-propyl- $b._2$ 62°; di-isopropyl- $b._{10}$ 71°; di-*n*-butyl- $b._5$ 80°; di-isobutyl- $b._6$ 79°; di-*n*-pentyl- $b._4$ 102°; di-*n*-hexyl- $b._4$ 132°; di-isohexyl- $b._6$ 120°; di-isoheptyl- $b._{10}$ 145°; di-isooctyl- $b._4$ 158°; di-dodecyl- $b._5$ 195°; di-cyclohexyl- $b._3$ 120°; di-2-chloroethyl- $b._5$ 123°; di-2,2,2-trichloroethyl- $b._3$ 160°; di-1,3-dichloroisopropoxy- $b._3$ 155°; di-isoheptoxy- $b._2$ 87°; diphenyl- $b._3$ 142°; di-*p*-tolyl- $b._3$ 175°; di-*o*-tolyl- $b._3$ 174°; di-*p*-chlorophenyl- $b._7$ 195°; methyl,ethyl- $b._{13}$ 55°; methyl,*n*-propyl- $b._{15}$ 63°; methyl,isopropyl- $b._3$ 41°; methyl-*n*-butyl- $b._{14}$ 90°; ethyl,*n*-propyl- $b._{14}$ 79°; ethyl,*n*-butyl- $b._{17}$ 93°; ethyl,isopropyl- $b._{17}$ 75°; ethyl,isobutyl- $b._{15}$ 83°; ethyl,pentyl- $b._{16}$ 110°; ethyl,hexyl- $b._{11}$ 120°; ethyl,heptyl- $b._{24}$ 145°; ethyl,octyl- $b._{24}$ 152°; ethyl,isohexyl- $b._{23}$ 135°; ethyl,

[1] Species not identified.

2-chloroethyl- b.$_{12}$ 105°; ethyl,2,2,2-trichloroethyl- b.$_4$ 98°; ethyl,1,3-dichloroiso-propyl- b.$_1$ 100°; ethyl,2-fluoroethyl- b.$_{14}$ 80°; ethyl,2,2,2-trifluoroethyl- b.$_{13}$ 56°.

None of these compounds appear to have had serious consideration as insecticides.

SCHRADER (1952) lists the following *N*-substituted phosphoramidofluoridates as toxic to aphids when sprayed at concentrations of 0.002 to 0.05%:

O-ethyl *N*,*N*-dimethylphosphoramidofluoridate, b.$_2$ 50°;
O-ethyl *N*,*N*-dimethylthiophosphoramidofluoridate, b.$_{14}$ 70°;
O-ethyl *N*-methylphosphoramidofluoridate, b.$_{15}$ 87°;
O-ethyl *N*-methylthiophosphoramidofluoridate, b.$_5$ 74°;
S-methyl *N*-methylphosphoramidofluoridate, b.$_8$ 110°;
S-methyl *N*,*N*-dimethylphosphoramidofluoridate, b.$_8$ 79°;
S-ethyl *N*,*N*-dimethylphosphoramidofluoridate, b.$_{10}$ 83°.

Similarly the following *N*,*N*-substituted phosphorodiamidofluoridates were toxic to aphids when sprayed at 0.005% to 0.02%:

N,*N*,*N'*,*N'*-tetramethylphosphorodiamidofluoridate, b.$_4$ 67°;
N,*N*,*N'*,*N'*-tetramethylthiophosphorodiamidofluoridate, b.$_{15}$ 58°;
N,*N*-dimethyl, *N'*-methyl, *N'*-ethyl phosphorodiamidofluoridate, b.$_{11}$ 90°;
N,*N*,*N'*,*N'*-tetraethylphosphorodiamidofluoridate, b.$_8$ 113°;
N,*N*,*N'*-trimethylphosphorodiamidofluoridate, b.$_3$ 110°;
N,*N*,*N'*-trimethylthiophosphorodiamidofluoridate, b.$_6$ 93°;
N,*N'*-dimethylthiophosphorodiamidofluoridate, b.$_2$ 165°.

1. Mode of action of phosphorofluoridates

The phosphorofluoridates, like the other organophosphorus insecticides owe their insecticidal properties to the fundamental biochemical lesion produced by the inhibition of the enzyme cholinesterase. This specific action is discussed at length in a succeeding volume and only the aspects pertinent to the mode of action in insects will be reviewed here (see O'BRIEN 1960 for a comprehensive review of organophosphorus cholinesterase inhibitors).

The insect central nervous system contains very high levels (10 to 20 times those in vertebrates) of the neurohormone acetyl choline and its hydrolyzing enzyme cholinesterase. Acetyl choline occurs in concentrations ranging from about 60 γ per g in the nerve cord of the cockroach *Periplaneta* to 500 γ per g in the brain of the blow fly *Calliphora*, with the house fly brain having a value of about 170 γ per g (LEWIS and SMALLMAN 1956). The brain of the house fly contains cholinesterase at a level which will split about 2 g of acetyl choline per g of tissue per hour, a level about 10 to 50 times that of vertebrate tissue. Insect cholinesterase has properties virtually identical with that from the electric organ of the eel *Electrophorus electricus* or the mammalian brain (METCALF et al. 1955).

The phosphorofluoridates react with cholinesterase by the well known bimolecular displacement reaction of the SN_2-type, in which the esteratic site of the cholinesterase enzyme makes a nucleophilic attack on the electrophilic phosphorus atom, displacing fluoride and irreversibly phosphorylating the esteratic site. The overall reaction is:

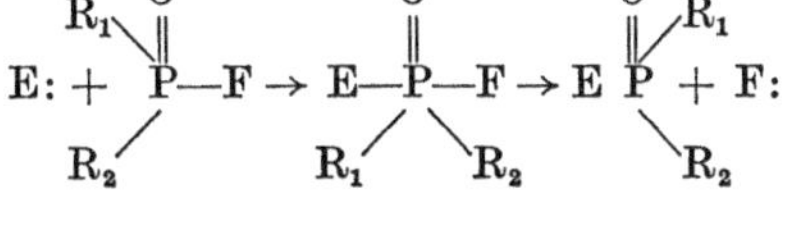

The reactivity of the individual phosphorofluoridate is determined by (a) the magnitude of the electrophilic character of the phosphorus atom, and (b) the steric effects of the substituents R_1 and R_2 (FUKUTO 1957).

Thus CHADWICK and HILL (1947) have shown that the injection of various amounts of diisopropyl phosphorofluoridate (DFP) into *Periplaneta americana* produced the indicated inhibition of cholinesterase in the nerve cord.

DFP γ	inhibition ChE %
0.9	3
2.25	41
4.5	53
9.0	95
18.0	100

The mortality after injection closely paralleled the cholinesterase inhibition and the dosage of 10.8 γ per roach which produces over 90% mortality, would if distributed throughout the insect be of the order of 1×10^{-4} M.

Two independent studies with the house fly (LEWIS and FOWLER 1956) and the blow fly (SMALLMAN and FISHER 1958) have demonstrated that in insects poisoned with DFP there is an increase in the amount of acetyl choline, which in the house fly body reached about 250% of normal within six hours after poisoning. DFP produced only about one-half as much increase in acetyl choline as the organophosphorus insecticides parathion (*O,O*-diethyl *O*-*p*-nitrophenyl phosphorothionate) and tetraethyl pyrophosphate, and it was suggested that DFP differs from the other O-P-toxicants in interfering with the synthesis of acetyl choline (see WINTERINGHAM et al. 1957).

Sarin – or isopropyl methylphosphonofluoridate – is one of the most toxic of all known organophosphorus compounds to both mammals and to the house fly. MENGLE and CASIDA (1958) determined the topical LD_{50} to the latter to be about 0.8 γ per g. Survivors from this dosage had about 70% depression of brain cholinesterase in 20 min with recovery to normal in about 320 min. Hyperactive symptoms appeared just prior to and during the period of maximum inactivity and paralytic symptoms appeared when the enzyme activity had recovered to 55% of normal and continued until brain cholinesterase had reached 93% of normal activity. A large proportion of deaths occurred during the interval following the time of minimum enzyme activity.

ROEDER and KENNEDY (1955) have studied in detail the action of sarin, soman or 1-methyl-2,2-dimethylpropyl methylphosphonofluoridate and related compounds upon synaptic and axonal transmission in the central nervous system of *Periplaneta americana*. These compounds when applied as perfusates to the sixth abdominal ganglion, which contains the synapses between the cercal nerves and giant fibers, produced the following sequence of events:

1) after discharge – a brief burst of stimulation from the cercal nerve causes an after discharge in the giant fibers appearing 5 to 20 min after exposure to the compound. This effect is completely irreversible;

2) synchronized synaptic responses – each stimulus of the cercal nerve produces a normal-appearing synchronized spike from the giant fibers;

3) synaptic block – associated with after discharge;

4) axonic block.

The authors suggest that the irreversible synaptic instability and after discharge result from cholinesterase inhibition while the reversible effects, observed after washing, upon synaptic conduction, may result from competition of the mediator with the acetyl choline receptor. The concentrations of the various compounds which produced these effects are shown in Table 5.

In summary, the mode of action of the phosphoro- and phosphonofluoridates upon insects may be summed up as (1) the inhibition of cholinesterase, (2) the

Table 5. *Effects of phosphonofluoridates upon synaptic and axonal transmission in Periplaneta americana* (ROEDER et al. 1947, 1955)

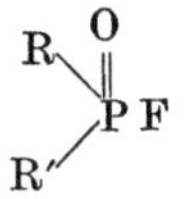

R	R′	Approximate M conc. for			
		After discharge	Synchronized response	Synaptic block	Axonal block
so-C_3H_7O	iso-C_3H_7O (DFP)	5×10^{-5} —1×10^{-4}	—	1×10^{-4} —5×10^{-3}	6×10^{-2}
so-C_3H_7O	CH_3 (sarin)	6.5×10^{-8} —6.5×10^{-7}	6.5×10^{-6} —6.5×10^{-4}	6.5×10^{-6} —6.5×10^{-5}	6.5×10^{-3}
$CH_3C(CH_3)_2CH(CH_3)O$	CH_3 (soman)	5.7×10^{-11} —5.7×10^{-10}	5.7×10^{-10} —5.7×10^{-9}	5.7×10^{-10} —5.7×10^{-9}	none at 5.7×10^{-3}

accumulation of excess acetyl choline, and (3) the disruption of synaptic transmission. These biochemical phenomena lead to the sequence of toxic symptoms observed in DFP poisoning of: hyperexcitability, hyperactivity, exaggerated tonus, muscular incoordination, clonic and tonic convulsions, incoordination and death (CHADWICK and HILL 1947). Such gross physiological abnormalities also give rise to other biochemical disturbances and WINTERINGHAM et al. (1957) have shown that DFP injected into the house fly increased the production of glutamine from acetate by about three fold, and caused a 10% decrease in the glutamate and proline level. The DFP also reduced the rate of acetyl choline synthesis from acetate.

Unlike the phosphoro- and phosphonofluoridates the phosphoramidofluoridates are not direct inhibitors of cholinesterase. Dimefox or tetramethylphosphorodiamidofluoridate (I_{50} 1.1×10^{-2} M) is less than one-thousandth as reactive with red cell cholinesterase as DFP (I_{50} 1.8×10^{-6} M) (ALDRIDGE 1953). However, oxidation with peracetic acid was found to convert dimefox to an active anticholinesterase (I_{50} 1×10^{-6} M) and oxidation *in vivo* in *Periplaneta americana* and in the rat, and *in vitro* by rat liver slices or in pea plants resulted in a similar activation leading to products with I_{50} values for cholinesterase of 1.3×10^{-5} to 6.7×10^{-6} M (ARTHUR and CASIDA 1958). The active oxidative metabolite from *Periplaneta americana* yielded formaldehyde upon acidification and from this and from infrared absorption studies especially in analogy with schradan or octamethyl pyrophosphoramide it appears that the activation of dimefox occurs through oxidation of one of the methyl groups to form a much more electrophilic phosphorus atom which then readily reacts with cholinesterase:

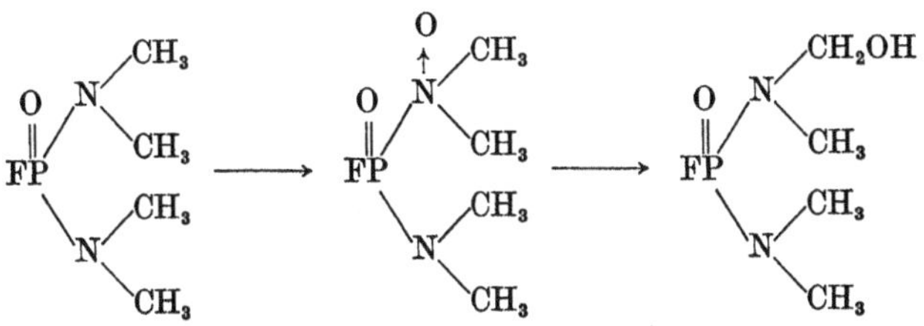

Tissue distribution studies with P^{32} dimefox in *Periplaneta americana* showed that following topical application, the highest radioactivity was found in the malpighian tubes and hind-gut with relatively large amounts also present in the fat body, gastric caeca, nerve cord, and salivary glands.

D. Fluorinated diphenylethanes

1. DFDT or fluoro-DDT

The *p,p'*-difluoro- analogue of DDT 2,2-bis-(*p*-fluorophenyl)-1,1,1-trichloroethane or DFDT was developed as a general purpose insecticide "Gix" by Farbwerke Hoechst of Germany during World War II and according to KILGORE (1945) was manufactured at about 40 tons per month in 1944. The crude material was compounded as an insecticide concentrate which consisted of 60% DFDT, 20% high boiling petroleum oil, (b. 240—360°), and 20% emulsifier (polydioxyethylated iso-octyl phenol type).

According to PERKOW (1956) DFDT was employed largely for special purposes where its much greater cost than DDT was not a factor. Because of its more rapid "knockdown" properties, it was favored over DDT for the control of flies and mosquitoes and was used by the German Army in North Africa. It was also very effective against flies and lice attacking animals and bedbugs and human lice.

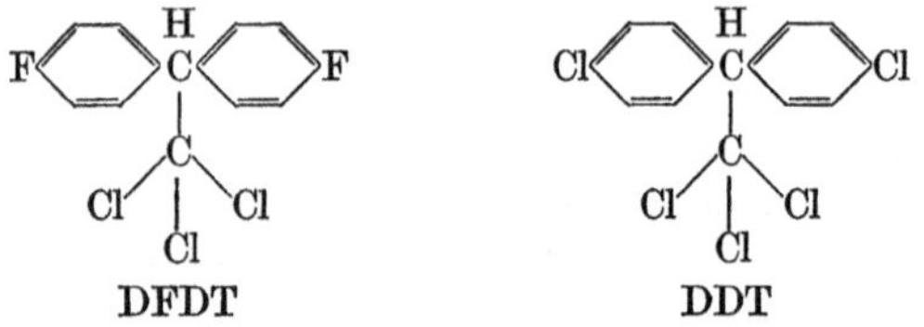

DFDT is prepared in yields up to 81% by reacting 2 moles of fluorobenzene with one mole of chloral in the presence of 98% sulfuric acid. The technical product is a viscous, colorless oil containing as much as 90% *p,p'*-isomer and from 1 to 10% *o,p'*-isomer b. 135° but no *o,o'*-isomer or *m,p'*-isomer (BRADLOW and VAN DER WERF 1947, RIEMSCHNEIDER 1950). This is due to the predominantly *p*-orienting effect of fluorobenzene, as technical DDT prepared by an analogous reaction contains up to 80% *p,p'*-isomer, 11 to 29% *o,p'*-isomer, and 0.1 to 1.0% *o,o'*-isomer (METCALF 1955). Pure *p,p'*-DFDT crystallizes from ethanol as white needles, m. 44—45°, with an odor of ripe apple. DFDT $b._9$ 177—178° has a vapor pressure about 15 times that of DDT (interpolated v.p. about 0.5 mm at 178°) (METCALF 1948). Therefore DFDT is much less residually persistent than DDT and SUMMERFORD (1950) states that a DFDT residue of 400 mg per sq. ft. on glass lost 95% of its weight in 9 weeks as compared to 15% for a similar deposit of DDT.

DFDT like DDT is unstable in the presence of alkali and dehydrochlorinates by an E_2 elimination reaction to form DFDE, 2,2-bis-(*p*-fluorophenyl)-1,1-dichloroethylene m. 45—46°. The velocity of the elimination reaction is dependent upon the relative availability of electrons at the C—H bond being ruptured and this is influenced by the substituents on the benzene rings of the DDT-type compound (CRISTOL 1945). Rate data for this reaction are given in Table 6 and dehydrochlorination takes place in the order of increasing electronegativity of the halogens I > Br > Cl > F > H.

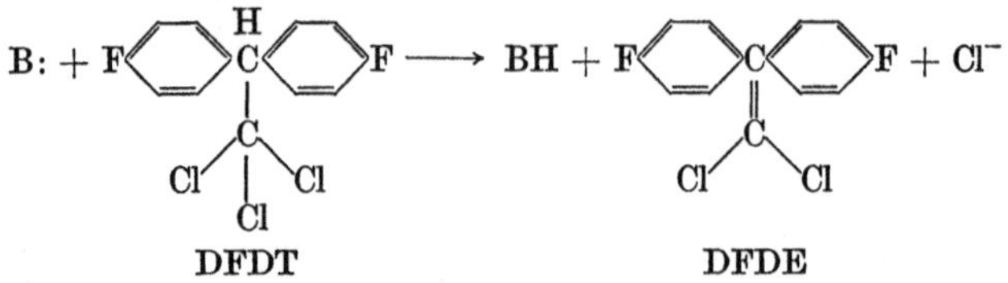

DFDT is much more soluble in common solvents than DDT as shown in Table 6.

Table 6. *Some properties of halogenated DDT derivatives*[1]

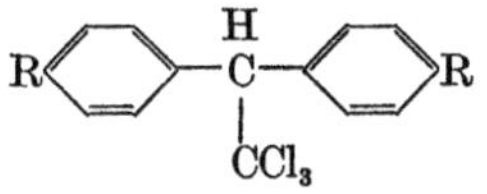

R	m.p. °C	Solubility g per 100 ml in					Hydrolysis rate constant 10^5 k liters/sec/mole at 37°
		Olive oil	Carbon tetrachloride	Xylene	Mineral oil	Dibutyl phthalate	
F	45	45	650	670	83	260	2,319
Cl	110	10.5	45	57	5	33	12,515
Br	141	2.0					18,760
I	179	0.5					19,800
H	65	33.7					272

[1] VON OETTINGEN and SHARPLESS (1946); METCALF (1948).

DFDT is about one-fifth as acutely toxic to the mouse and rat as DDT (VON OETTINGEN and SHARPLESS 1946, LEHMAN 1951) (Table 7) and is the least toxic of a number of DDT analogues to the fish *Gambusia* and *Carassius auratus*. However, like DDT it is stored in the perirenal fat of animals when fed in small amounts (NEGHERBON 1959).

a) Insecticidal action of DFDT

DFDT is considerably more rapid in its rate of action than DDT. HAMADA (1957) found the DFDT/DDT knockdown ratio for kerosene sprays to the house fly was 1.33. For residual applications where vapor pressure may be a factor the DFDT/DDT knockdown ratios for several insects were: *Drosophila melanogaster* 8, *Lucilia sericata* 9, *Cantharis consors* 16. In an extensive series of comparisons against 13 species of insects and one mite the two compounds were of roughly equal activity. DFDT was notably more toxic than DDT to the german cockroach *Blattella germanica* (METCALF 1948). The most careful comparisons available in the literature are presented in Table 7.

Table 7. *Comparative toxicity of halogenated DDT derivatives to several species of insects*[1]

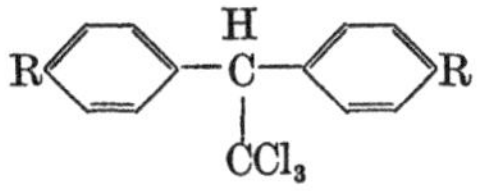

R	P. humanus LC_{50} %	C. lectularius LC_{50} %	M. sanborni relative LC_{50}	O. surinamensis relative LC_{50}	A. quadrimaculatus LC_{50}, ppm	H. haemorrhoidalis LC_{50} %	M. domestica LD_{50} γ/g	Rat oral LD_{50} mg/kg
F (DFDT)	1.4	5	1.01	4.4	0.007	0.006	5.0	1120
Cl (DDT)	0.3	0.53	1.0	1.0	0.002	0.001	1.65	200
Br (DBrDT)	0.6	1.4	1.6	1.1	0.0025	0.06	1.95	
H	7.5	12	16	—	1.0	1.0		

[1] METCALF (1955).

Little definitive information is available concerning the mode of action of DFDT. Like DDT, poisoned insects pass through a sequence of symptoms: (1) postural instability, (2) tremors, (3) hyperactivity, (4) convulsions, (5) paralysis, and (6) death, suggesting a direct effect on the neuromuscular system. Electrophysiological investigation demonstrated that in *Periplaneta americana* DFDT applied to the nerve axon produced a multiplication of the nerve impulse, each stimulus in the poisoned insect giving rise to a burst of impulses. Investigation in this field has been almost entirely carried out with DDT and is beyond the scope of this review. The physiological evidence (see METCALF 1955) seems to indicate that these compounds unstabilize the nervous system, possibly through adsorption on the axon and consequent depolarization. The typical locus of action is probably the sensory neurones such as the campaniform sensillae which become capable of repetitive discharges and thus bombard the neuromuscular system with a stream of afferent impulses. The violent disturbances which result may cause prostration and death by metabolic exhaustion, or through the accumulation of neurotoxic substances.

2. Analogues of DFDT

A number of these compounds have been evaluated as insecticides. The ratio of toxicity of the DFDT-isomers to the house fly was *p,p'*- 1.0, *m.p'*- ($b._{0.1}$ 113 to 116°) 0.7, and *o,p'*- ($b._4$ 125—127°) 0.02 (RIEMSCHNEIDER 1950). The DFDT-carbinol, *p*-fluorophenyl-trichloromethyl carbinol was 0.2 to 0.4 as active as DDT to *Drosophila* (BROWNING et al. 1948). The DFDT ethylene 2,2-bis-(*p*-fluorophenyl)-1,1-dichloroethylene, m. 45°, *p,p'*-difluorobenzophenone m. 106°, and *p,p'*-difluorobenzohydrol m. 47.3° were non-toxic to *Heliothrips haemorrhoidalis*. The 2,2-bis-(*p*-fluorophenyl)-1,1,1-trimethylethane m. 52° was non-toxic to *Oncopeltis fasciatus* and *Blattella germanica* (ROGERS et al. 1953) whereas 2,2-bis-(*p*-fluorophenyl)-1,1,1-tribromoethane m. 73.4° was about 0.25 as toxic as DFDT to *M. sanborni* but about 2 times as toxic to *O. surinamensis* (LORD 1948). The 3,3-bis-(*p*-fluorophenyl)-2,1,1-trichloropropene $b._{0.2}$ 149° was equally effective to *Calliphora vomitoria* and considerably more active than the corresponding *p,p'*-dichloro compound to *F. fusca*, *C. granaria*, *Drosophila*, and *Melophagus ovinus* (MÜLLER 1946, RIEMSCHNEIDER 1958).

The fluoro- analogue of DDD or TDE, 2,2-bis-(*p*-fluorophenyl)-1,1-dichloroethane m. 77°[1] was approximately 0.5 as toxic as DFDT to *H. haemorrhoidalis* (METCALF 1948) and about as toxic as DDT to *Drosophila*, *C. vomitoria*, *F. fusca*, and *Trogium pulsatorium* while 2-(2-fluorophenyl)-2-(4'-fluorophenyl)-1,1-dichloroethane was less toxic than DFDD (MÜLLER 1946). BLINN and GUNTHER (1950) have prepared DFDD ethylene or 2,2-bis-(*p*-fluorophenyl)-1-chloroethylene m. 33.5° and 2,2-bis-(*p*-fluorophenyl)-1,1,2-trichloroethane $b._4$ 142.5° but no toxicity data are given. COHEN et al. (1957) prepared 2,2-bis-(*p*-chlorophenyl)-2-fluoro-1,1-dichloroethane m. 103° and 2,2-bis-(*p*-chlorophenyl)-2-fluoro-1,1,1-trichloroethane m. 82°.

BERGMANN et al. (1957) prepared the following partially fluorinated DDT analogues which have been evaluated as insecticides by TAHORI et al. (1958), see Table 8: 2,2-bis-(*p*-chlorophenyl)-1,1-difluoro-1-chloroethane m. 54°[2] (treated with KOH this gave 1,1-bis-(*p*-chlorophenyl)-1,1-difluoroethylene $b._2$ 165°), 2,2-bis-(*p*-chlorophenyl)-1,1-dichloro-1-fluoroethane, m. 78° (treated with KOH this gave 2,2-bis-(*p*-chlorophenyl)-1-chloro-1-fluoroethylene, $b._3$ 165°), and 2,2-bis-(*p*-chlorophenyl)-1-fluoroethane, m. 54°.

Other analogues which have been investigated as insecticides to *Drosophila* are: 2,2-bis-(3-fluoro-4-methylphenyl)-1,1,1-trichloroethane (moderately active); 2,2-bis-(2-methyl-4-fluorophenyl)-1,1,1-trichloroethane (inactive); 2,2-bis-(2-methyl-5-fluorophenyl)-1,1,1-trichloroethane (inactive) (RIEMSCHNEIDER 1958).

KALUSZYNER (1960) has compared the cyclic DDT analogue 3-chloro-6-methoxy-9-trifluoromethyl fluorene (I) m. 95° (LD_{50} 75 γ per female fly) with

[1] This compound m. 43° stated by BRADLOW and VAN der WERF (1947) to have this identity was shown by BLINN and GUNTHER (1950) to be the DFDT ethylene.

[2] POUTERMAN and GIRARDET (1946) prepared a compound m. 90° by the antimony trifluoride fluorination of DDT, to which they assigned this structure.

Table 8. *Toxicity and synergistic activity of some fluorinated-DDT analogues to susceptible and DDT-resistant Musca vicina*[1]

	Topical LD_{50} γ per fly		Synergistic activity DDT to synergist, 10 : 1
	S-flies	R-flies	
$(p\text{-}ClC_6H_4)_2CHCCl_3$	0.7	140	1
$(p\text{-}ClC_6H_4)_2CHCF_3$	4	13	10.8
$(p\text{-}ClC_6H_4)_2CHCF_2Cl$	14	50	10
$(p\text{-}ClC_6H_4)_2CHCFCl_2$	5	115	4.7
$(p\text{-}ClC_6H_4)_2CHCHCl_2$	4	>140	1
$(p\text{-}ClC_6H_4)_2C(OH)CF_3$	5	6	15.6
$(p\text{-}ClC_6H_4)_2C(OH)CFCl_2$	6	5	10.7
$(p\text{-}ClC_6H_4)_2C(OH)CHCl_2$	1	4	9.3
$(p\text{-}ClC_6H_4)_2C(OH)CHFCl$	9	11	10.7
$(C_6H_5)_2C(OH)CHF_2$	52	70	2.1
$(p\text{-}ClC_6H_4)_2C(OH)CHF_2$	31	27	5.2
$(p\text{-}BrC_6H_4)_2C(OH)CHF_2$	27	31	4.5
$(p\text{-}ClC_6H_4)_2C(OOCCH_3)CF_3$	4	7	15.6
$(p\text{-}ClC_6H_4)_2C(OOCCH_3)CF_2Cl$	150	80	3.9
$(p\text{-}ClC_6H_4)_2C(OOCCH_3)CFCl_2$	>200	200	3.6

[1] TAHORI et al. (1958).

that of the free ring analogue 2-(*p*-chlorophenyl)-2-(*p*-methoxyphenyl)-1,1,1-trifluoroethane (II) m. 50° (LD_{50} 10–12 γ per female fly). The author suggests that the higher toxicity of the latter confirms the theory of RIEMSCHNEIDER (1958) that free rotation of the trihalomethylgroup is essential for high DDT-type toxicity to insects.

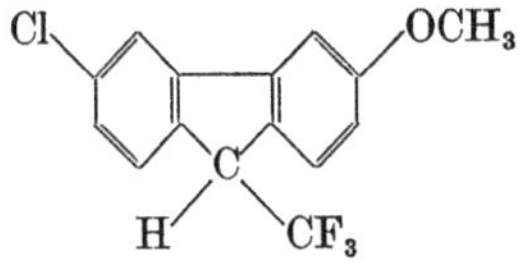

I

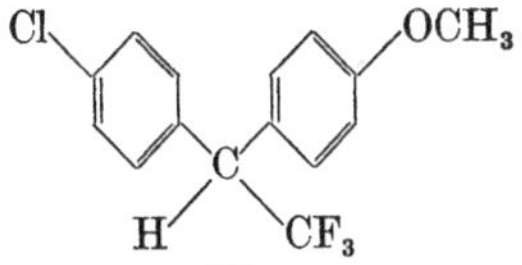

II

3. Diphenyl trifluoroethanes

KALUSZYNER et al. (1955) have synthesized a number of substituted phenyl trifluoroethanes and these have been evaluated as toxicants to the house fly and

Table 9. *Toxicity and synergistic activity of some fluorinated DDT analogues to DDT-resistant Musca vicina*[1]

Compound	Relative insecticidal activity	Synergistic activity, DDT to synergist 10 : 1
$(p\text{-}ClC_6H_4)_2CHCCl_3$	1	1
$(p\text{-}ClC_6H_4)_2CHCF_3$	0.33	0
$(p\text{-}BrC_6H_4)_2CHCF_3$	0.33	0
$(p\text{-}CH_3OC_6H_4)_2CHCF_3$	0	0
$(p\text{-}CH_3C_6H_4)_2CHCF_3$	0	0
$(p\text{-}ClC_6H_4)_2C(OH)CF_3$	0.33	15
$(p\text{-}FC_6H_4)_2C(OH)CF_3$	0.25	10
$(p\text{-}BrC_6H_4)_2C(OH)CF_3$	0.20	12
$(p\text{-}CH_3OC_6H_4)_2C(OH)CF_3$	0.16	5
$(p\text{-}CH_3C_6H_4)_2C(OH)CF_3$	0	0
$(p\text{-}ClC_6H_4)_2C(OH)CF_2CF_3$	0	0
$(p\text{-}ClC_6H_4)_2C(OH)CF_2CF_2CF_3$	0	0
$(p\text{-}ClC_6H_4)_2C(OOCCH_3)CF_3$	0.25	11

[1] TAHORI (1955).

as DDT-synergists by TAHORI (1955) as shown in Table 9. The compound 2,2-bis-(*p*-chlorophenyl)-1,1,1-trifluoroethane m. 64° synthesized by KIRKWOOD and DACY (1946) has been shown by KALUSZYNER et al. (1955) to be a rearranged compound 1,2-di-(*p*-chlorophenyl)-1,1,2-trifluoroethane. The authentic compound has a m. p. 44.5° and its insecticidal activity (Tables 8, 9) appears to invalidate some of the conclusions of KIRKWOOD and PHILLIPS (1946) regarding the inactivity of the trifluoromethyl group and its relation to fluoroform.

4. o-Fluoro-DDT and resistance to DDT and DFDT

Upon continuous selection with DDT, house flies and many other insects have appeared as resistant strains which may be virtually immune to the action of the insecticide. Two wild strains of house flies selected by the action of DDT and subsequently with lindane and dieldrin showed variable susceptibility to DFDT and other DDT analogues as shown in Table 10 (METCALF 1955). It is noteworthy that the DFDT was relatively much more active than DDT to the highly resistant $R_{Pollard}$ strain.

Table 10. *Cross tolerance of DDT-resistant house flies*

p,p'-disubstd. phenyl trichloro-ethanol	24 hr. topical LD_{50} γ per ♀[1]			Dehydrochlor-ination by DDT-ase[2]
	S_{Lab}	$R_{Bellflower}$	$R_{Pollard}$	
di-Cl	0.033	11	100	100
di-F	0.10	4.0	1.2	50
di-Br	0.039	40	—	100
di-CH_3	0.16	0.70	2.7	30
di-C_2H_5	0.11	1.2	2.7	—
di-CH_3O	0.068	0.96	1.4	20

[1] METCALF (1955).
[2] LIPKE and KEARNS (1960).

KEARNS and coworkers (LIPKE and KEARNS 1960) have isolated the enzyme "DDT-ase" which catalyzes the dehydrochlorination of DDT and its analogues in resistant house flies, forming

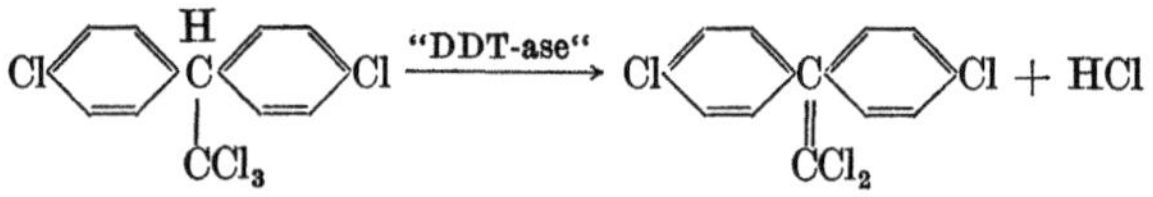

the inactive ethylene derivatives. *In vitro* studies with the purified enzyme showed that the initial rate of dehydrochlorination with DFDT was only one-half that of DDT.

o-Fluoro-DDT — HENNESSY et al. (1961) have investigated a particularly interesting fluoro analogue of DDT, 2-(4-chlorophenyl)-2-(2'-fluoro-4'-chloro-phenyl)-1,1,1-trichloroethane. MOOREFIELD et al. (1962) have also prepared the α-deutero analogue of this compound. Against DDT-resistant house flies, these compounds were surprisingly active as shown in Table 11 where they are compared with the corresponding *o*-chloro-DDT. The *o*-F-DDT was nearly as toxic to the susceptible flies as DDT,

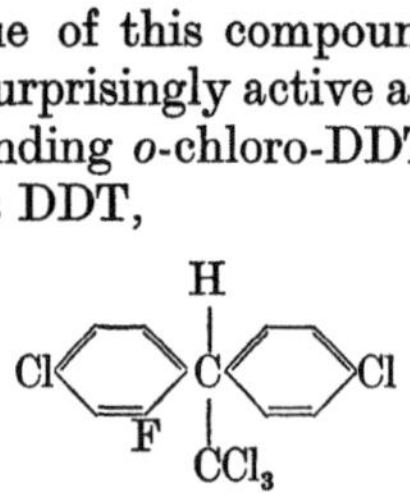

o-F-DDT

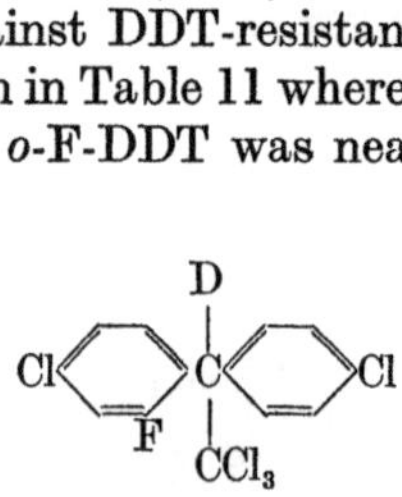

α-deutero-*o*-F-DDT

and was appreciably more toxic to the DDT-resistant flies than DDT and the α-deutero analogue was even more effective. The corresponding *o*-Cl-DDT although less toxic to the susceptible flies was equally toxic to the resistant strain. The presence of the *ortho*- substituent sharply decreased the rate of enzymatic dehydrochlorination of the DDT- analogue by DDT-dehydrochlorinase of resistant flies, and this resistance to dehydrochlorination increased with size of the *ortho*- substituent F < Cl < Br.

Table 11. *Activity of 2-fluoro-DDT and analogues against susceptible and resistant house flies*[1]

Compound	LD_{50} γ per ♀ fly	
	Susceptible	DDT-resistant
2,2-bis-(p-chlorophenyl)-1,1,1-trichloroethane *p,p'*-DDT . .	0.09	>20
α-deutero-DDT	0.06	>20
2-(4-chlorophenyl)-2-(2'-fluoro-4'-chlorophenyl)-1,1,1-trichloroethane *o*-F-DDT	0.1	14.0
α-deutero-*o*-F-DDT	0.1	1.5
2-(4-chlorophenyl)-2-(2',4'-dichlorophenyl)-1,1,1-trichloroethane *o*-Cl-DDT	0.6	0.8
α-deutero-*o*-Cl-DDT	0.6	0.7
2-(4-chlorophenyl)-2-(2'-chlorophenyl)-1,1,1-trichloroethane *o-p'*-DDT	6.2	30

[1] Hennessy et al. (1961), Moorefield et al. (1962).

5. Fluorocarbinols as DDT synergists

The dehydrochlorination of DDT both *in vivo* and *in vitro* can be competitively inhibited by a variety of structural analogues of DDT of which the carbinols such as 1,1-bis-(*p*-chlorophenyl)-ethanol (DMC) are among the most active. A number of substituted diphenyl trifluoroethanols of this type have been prepared by Kaluszyner et al. (1955) and evaluated as toxicants and as DDT synergists to DDT-resistant *Musca vicina* by Tahori (1955) as shown in Table 9. When comparisons were made against a considerably more resistant strain with several other well known DDT synergists, the following values were obtained for synergistic activity: 1,1-bis-(*p*-chlorophenyl)-2,2,2-trifluoroethanol 137; 1,1-bis-(*p*-chlorophenyl)-ethanol 46; 1,1-bis-(*p*-chlorophenyl)-ethane 79; and bis-(*p*-chlorophenyl)-chloromethane 93 (Tahori 1955).

Cohen and Tahori (1957) have studied the synergistic behavior of some of the substituted diphenyl-2,2,2-trifluoroethanols in the house fly. These carbinols penetrated into the insect more rapidly than DDT, perhaps because of their combination of hydrophilic and lipophilic groups. After 4 hours the following approximate per cent penetrations were recorded:

DDT 40,
1,1-bis-(*p*-chlorophenyl)-2,2,2-trifluoroethanol 80;
1,1-bis-(*p*-bromophenyl)-2,2,2-trifluoroethanol 82;
1,1-bis-(*p*-methoxyphenyl)-2,2,2-trifluoroethanol 57.

However, the synergists also decreased the rate of penetration of DDT so that a 10 to 1 ratio of DDT to synergist represented the best compromise between the synergistic effect and decreased penetration. The dramatic effects of the 1,1-bis-(*p*-chlorophenyl)-2,2,2-trifluoroethanol synergist in decreasing the *in vivo* dehydrochlorination of DDT in the house fly and in affecting mortality are shown in

Table 12. *In vitro* experiments performed with DDT-ase enzyme showed that the synergist used at 1 part to 100 parts of DDT produced 49% and at 1 part to 10 parts of DDT 87% inhibition of the detoxifying enzyme.

Table 12. *Inhibition of DDT-dehydrochlorination by 1,1-bis-(p-chlorophenyl)-2,2,2-trichloroethanol*[1]

γ per ♀ fly		Penetration DDT	Dehydro-chlorination DDT	Mortality
DDT	synergist	%	%	%
11	0	79	59	4
11	0.5	72	30	44
11	1.1	69	23	58
11	3.3	50	20	38
11	11	35	29	30
0	11	—	—	8

[1] Cohen and Tahori (1957).

A further exploration of the DDT-type fluorocarbinols as toxicants and DDT-synergists for house flies has been made centering about various 1,1-bis-(phenyl)-2,2-difluoroethanes and ethanols (Bornstein et al. 1957, Blum et al. 1959). The data which they obtained are given in Table 13 and indicates that the most active synergist found when used at a 1:5 ratio with DDT was 1,1-bis-(*p*-chlorophenyl)-2,2-difluoroethanol which was slightly more active than 1,1-bis-(*p*-chlorophenyl)-2,2-difluoroethane. The latter compound was about 0.125 as active as DDT to susceptible house flies.

Table 13. *Toxicity and synergistic action of diaryl difluoroethanes and difluoroethanols to Musca domestica*[1]

Compound	b.p. or m.p. °C	Topical LD_{50} γ per fly	
		compound alone	DDT (5) + Compound (1) (as DDT)
$(p\text{-}ClC_6H_4)_2CHCCl_3$ (DDT)		0.35	
$(p\text{-}ClC_6H_4)_2CHCHF_2$	m. 37.5—38.5	2.5	0.70
$(p\text{-}ClC_6H_4)_2CH(OH)CHF_2$	$b._{0.2}$ 130—136	3.7	0.62
$(p\text{-}ClC_6H_4)_2C(O_2CCH_3)CHF_2$	m. 86.0—86.8	9.2	1.62
$(p\text{-}ClC_6H_4)_2C{=}CHF$	m. 78.0—79.5	>10	11.90
$(p\text{-}BrC_6H_4)_2CHCHF_2$	m. 42.0—42.8	2.4	0.96
$(p\text{-}BrC_6H_4)_2CH(OH)CHF_2$	$b._{0.17}$ 153—164	4.8	0.71
$(p\text{-}BrC_6H_4)_2C(O_2CCH_3)CHF_2$	m. 80.0—80.5	9.3	1.70
$(p\text{-}BrC_6H_4)_2C{=}CHF$	m. 84.2—85.2	>10	7.20
$(p\text{-}FC_6H_4)_2CHCHF_2$	—	4.8	7.60
$(p\text{-}FC_6H_4)_2C(OH)CHF_2$	$b._{0.05}$ 99—100	8.7	3.48
$(p\text{-}FC_6H_4)_2C(O_2CCH_3)CHF_2$	$b._{0.1}$ 80° (mol. dist.)	>10	8.50
$(p\text{-}FC_6H_4)_2C{=}CHF$	m. 32—33	>10	>12
$(C_6H_4)_2CHCHF_2$	m. 38.5—39.5	>10	>12
$(C_6H_4)_2C(OH)CHF_2$	$b._{0.15}$ 110—111	>10	>12
$(C_6H_4)_2C(OOCCH_3)CHF_2$	m. 51.0—52.0	>10	>12
$(C_6H_4)_2C{=}CHF$	$b._{0.05}$ 77	>10	>12
$(p\text{-}ClC_6H_4)_2C(OH)CH_3$	—	—	3.70
$(p\text{-}ClC_6H_4)_2CHCH_3$	—	—	1.60
$(p\text{-}ClC_6H_4)_2C{=}CH_2$	—	—	4.4

[1] Bornstein et al. (1957), Blum et al. (1959).

6. Fluorocarbinols as oviposition inhibitors

Certain of the fluorocarbinol analogues of DDT have been shown to have the interesting property of inhibiting the oviposition of house flies when applied topically at 1 γ per female fly or by tarsal contact when the fly was exposed for 30 min to a residue of the compound at 1 g per M^2. The two most effective compounds investigated were 1,1-bis-(*p*-chlorophenyl)-2,2,2-trifluoroethanol and 1,1-bis-(*p*-chlorophenyl)-2,2,3,3,3-pentafluoropropanol. Neither compound was active when fed at 0.01 % in milk.

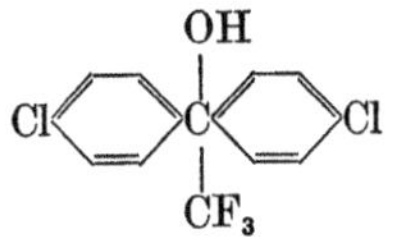

bis-(*p*-chlorophenyl)-trifluoroethanol

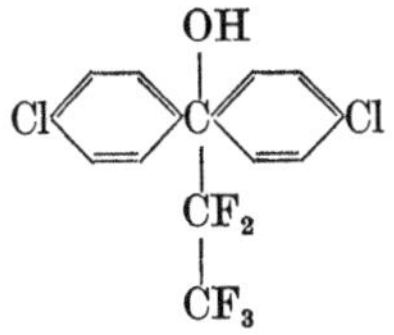

bis-(*p*-chlorophenyl)-pentafluoropropanol

1,1-bis-(*p*-chlorophenyl)-2,2,3,3,4,4,4-Heptafluorobutanol was much less active, as were

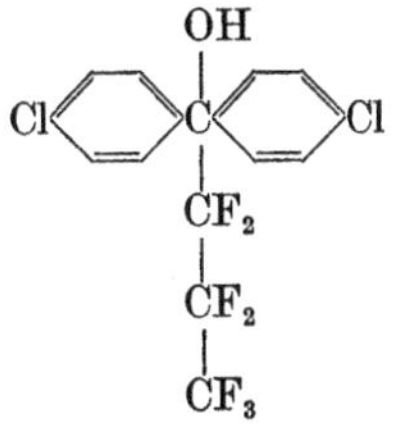

bis-(*p*-chlorophenyl)-heptafluorobutanol

the *p,p'*-dibromo analogue and 2,2,2-trichloro analogue of bis-(*p*-chlorophenyl)-trifluoroethanol. Replacement of the *p,p'*-chlorine atoms by methyl or methoxy yielded inactive compounds as did replacement of the 2,2,2-trifluoro group by hydrogen as in 1,1-bis-(*p*-chlorophenyl) ethanol.

Dissection of the ovaries of flies continuously exposed to the two active compounds mentioned above showed that motile spermatozoa were abundant in the spermathecae and the ovaries were of normal development and contained eggs. The action of the compounds described is therefore to produce "forced retention" (Ascher 1957). This author suggests that the activity of the fluorinated carbinols is due to their unusual stability. Thus 1,1-bis-(*p*-chlorophenyl)-2,2,2-trifluoroethanol remained unmetabolized in the house fly for six days while the inactive 1,1-bis-(*p*-chlorophenyl)-ethanol was metabolized very rapidly.

Ascher (1958b) found that 1,1-bis-(*p*-chlorophenyl)-2,2,2-trifluoroethanol reduced the mean number of eggs deposited by female *Aedes aegypti*, exposed for 40 min, from 61.0 to 27.2 per female.

7. Fluorinated acaricides

a) Fluorocarbinols

The acaricide 1,1-bis-(*p*-chlorophenyl)-2,2,2-trichloroethanol (Kelthane®) m. 77° is highly effective against all stages of most phytophagous mites. Its fluoro-analogue 1,1-bis-(*p*-fluorophenyl)-2,2,2-trichloroethanol m. 78.5° (its acetate melts at 135°) has been prepared by Bergmann and Kaluszyner (1958). This compound had a topical LD_{50} value to the house fly of 12 γ per fly as compared to 33 γ for Kelthane®. The compound 1,1-bis-(*p*-chlorophenyl)-2,2,2-trifluoroethanol, $b._{2.5}$ 150–160° (acetate m. 69.5°) which is the fluoro-analogue of both Kelthane® and 1,1-bis-(*p*-chlorophenyl) ethanol or DMC, was found to be effective against *Tetranychus telarius*, the two spotted spider mite, and had an LC_{50} of 250 p.p.m. as compared to 29 p.p.m. for Kelthane® and 450 p.p.m. for chlorobenzilate or ethyl *p,p'*-dichlorobenzilate.

BERGMANN et al. (1957) have prepared a number of related fluorocarbinols which were evaluated by TAHORI et al. (1958) as toxicants and DDT-synergists as shown in Table 8. We can find no published records of their evaluation as acaricides: 1,1-bis-(phenyl)-2,2-difluoroethanol, b.$_{0.16}$ 120°; 1,1-bis-(*p*-chlorophenyl)-2,2-difluoroethanol, b.$_{0.03}$ 140°; 1,1-bis-(*p*-bromophenyl)-2,2-difluoroethanol, b.$_{0.01}$ 150°; 1,1-bis-(*p*-chlorophenyl)-2,2-dichloro-2-fluoroethanol, m. 79°; 1,1-bis-(*p*-chlorophenyl)-2,2-difluoro-2-chloroethanol, b.$_{2}$ 175°; 1,1-bis-(*p*-chlorophenyl)-2-fluoro-2-chloroethanol, b.$_{0.15}$ 140°; and 1,1-bis-(*p*-chlorophenyl)-2-fluoroethanol, m. 75°.

b) Fluorobenside

The acaricide chlorobenside or *p*-chlorophenyl *p*-chlorobenzyl sulfide m. 72° v.p. 2.59×10^{-6} mm at 20° is used as a persisting acaricide for the control of orchard mites. Its fluoro analogue, fluorobenside or *p*-fluorophenyl *p*-chlorobenzyl sulfide m. 36°, v.p. 8.00×10^{-5} mm Hg at 20° is approximately 20 times as volatile. It is also more soluble in organic solvents (197 g in 100 g light petroleum oil at 20°, compared to 33 g per 100 g for chlorobenside) and has been favored for use in aerosol formulations applied in glasshouses where the greater volatility increases its effectiveness (CRANHAM and STEVENSON 1953). Rats tolerated an acute oral dosage of 3000 mg per kg for fluorobenside as compared to 10,000 mg per kg for chlorobenside. Chronically 100 p.p.m. of fluorobenside were tolerated in the diet of rats for two years without ill effects as compared to 1000 p.p.m. for chlorobenside. Both compounds are oxidized in air to the corresponding sulfoxides and sulfones which are also acaricidal and partially account for the residual activity of these materials (MARTIN 1961).

c) Fluorotedion

The acaricide Tedion® is 2,4,5,4′-tetrachlorodiphenyl sulfone m. 146°, a compound which is especially active as a persisting ovicide and larvicide for phytophagous mites. Its fluoro analogue 2,4,5-trichloro-4′-fluorodiphenyl sulfone was found to be of equivalent toxicity to the eggs and larvae of *Tetranychus urticae* (HUISMAN et al. 1958).

E. Fluorinated cyclohexanes

A number of fluorinated cyclohexanes have been investigated for insecticidal activity because of the structural relationship to lindane or γ-1,2,3,4,5,6-hexachlorocyclohexane which is a powerful insecticide.

RIEMSCHNEIDER (1950) evaluated fluorohexachlorocyclohexane b.$_{0.5}$ 116–125° and found it about 0.05 as active as lindane to *Drosophila melanogaster*. When correction is made for the percentage of active fluoro-isomer in the fluorinated mixture, it appears that the active component of the monofluoro analogue is about 0.5 as active as lindane. Fluoroheptachlorocyclohexane, m. 215° and fluoroheptabromocyclohexane, m. 256° were non-toxic.

The following fluoro-compounds were inactive when topically applied at 10 γ per female house fly (LD_{50} for lindane is 0.02 γ per female):

1,2,3,4,5,6-hexachloropentafluorocyclohexane, b.$_{0.5}$ 92°;
1,2,3,4,5,6-hexachlorohexafluorocyclohexane, m. 101°;
1 H,2 H,4 H-heptafluorocyclohex-1-ene, b. 106°;
1 Ha,2 Ha,4 He,5 He-octafluorocyclohexane, b. 118°;
1 H,4 H-octafluorocyclohex-1-ene, b. 84°;

1 Ha,2 Ha,4 Ha-nonofluorocyclohexane, m. 12°;
1 Ha,2 Ha,4 He-nonofluorocyclohexane, m. 44°; and
1 Ha,2 He,4 Ha-nonofluorocyclohexane, b. 107°.

The first two compounds were also inactive as synergists for lindane when evaluated at a 1:1 ratio with resistant flies (BLUM 1958).

F. Fluorinated cyclodienes

The cyclodiene insecticides, produced by the Diels-Alder reaction, include chlordane, heptachlor, aldrin, dieldrin and their analogues. Limited investigation described almost entirely in patent literature has been carried out on the introduction of fluorine atoms into various portions of these structures. RIEMSCHNEIDER (1956) described 4,5,6,7-tetrachloro-8,8-difluoro-3a,4,7,7a-tetrahydro-4,7-methanoindene m. 37°, a fluoro-analogue of chlordane. Heptachlor or 1,4,5,6,7,8,8-heptachloro-3a,4,7,7a-tetrahydro-4,7-methanoindene, m. 95°, is a well known insecticide which also occurs in technical chlordane. It readily oxidizes in insect, mammalian and plant tissues to heptachlor-2,3-epoxide of which two isomers m. 86° and 157° are known (METCALF 1955). *Fluoroheptachlor epoxide*, 1-fluoro-4,5,6,7,8,8a-hexachloro-2,3-epoxy-2,3,3a,4,7,7a-hexahydro-4,7-methanoindene, is also known as two isomers, m. 170.5°(α) and m. 220°(β). The comparative toxicity of these materials with heptachlor and heptachlor-epoxide is given in Table 14.

Table 14. *Comparative toxicity of heptachlor epoxide and fluoroheptachlor epoxide*[1]

	Topical LD_{50} Musca domestica	LC_{50} Culex pipiens quinquefasciatus		Oral LD_{50}
	γ per female	larva ppm	adult γ per cm^2	rat mg per kg
Heptachlor m. 95°	0.045	0.0056	0.065	90
Heptachlor epoxide m. 159°	0.02	0.0063	0.07	
Fluoroheptachlor epoxide m. 170.5°	0.29	0.14	0.74	465
Fluoroheptachlor epoxide m. 220°	0.017	0.0072	0.054	

[1] METCALF (1963).

G. Fluorinated carbamates

The carbamate insecticides are anticholinesterases like the organophosphorus insecticides discussed earlier in this chapter. Certain fluorinated carbamates have been evaluated for insecticidal action but none of these compounds has come into practical use.

Dimethylcarbamyl fluoride, $(CH_3)_2N\overset{O}{\overset{\|}{C}}F$, was evaluated as an insecticide by SCHRADER (1947a) and was found to be effective against aphids and house flies when sprayed at 0.2%. This compound was found by CASIDA et al. (1960) to have an intraperitoneal LD_{50} to the mouse of 0.17 mg per kg and a topical LD_{50} to the house fly of 45 mg per kg. Carbamylfluoride has been shown by WILSON et al. (1961) to be an irreversible inhibitor of cholinesterase, the fluorine atom serving as a displacable group and the dimethylcarbamoyl moiety "carbamylating" the active site on the enzyme surface as has been discussed for the analogous reaction of the phosphorofluoridates.

Other carbamyl fluorides which have been investigated as insecticides include: diethyl- $b._8$ 43°; di-2-chloroethyl, $b._3$ 103°; pyrrole *N*-carbonyl fluoride, $b._{12}$ 70°;

morpholine *N*-carbonyl fluoride, b.$_{12}$ 89°; and piperidine *N*-carbonyl fluoride, b.$_{12}$ 77°. The last three mentioned were of the same order of toxicity to aphids as dimethylcarbamyl fluoride (SCHRADER 1947a).

Other fluorinated phenyl *N*-methylcarbamates have been investigated for insecticidal activity by METCALF et al. (1962), as shown in Table 15. These compounds are much more stable than carbamyl fluoride and are competitive inhibitors of cholinesterase rather than irreversible inhibitors. The data shown in the table demonstrate the importance of the phenyl substituent in interacting with the anionic site of the cholinesterase molecule. Replacement of hydrogen by halogen has the greatest effect in the *ortho*-position, with less effect in the *meta*-position, and little or no effect in the *para*-position. The degree of interaction with the enzyme (inhibition) increases with the size of the substituent atom from F (VAN DER WAALS' radius 1.35 Å) to Cl (radius 1.80) to Br (radius 1.95) to I (radius 2.15).

Table 15. *Effects of fluorination on biological activity of phenyl N-methylcarbamates*[1]

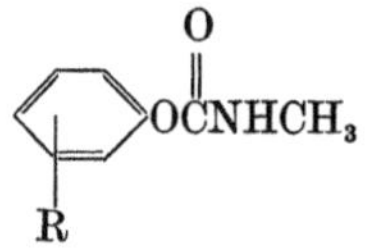

R	m.p. °C	I_{50} fly cholinesterase molar concn	Musca domestica ♀ topical LD_{50} γ per g — Alone	Musca domestica ♀ topical LD_{50} γ per g — 1:5 p.b.[2]	Estigmene acrea l. LC_{50} mg per leaf disc
H	85	2.0×10^{-4}	500	38	>10
o-F	75	1.6×10^{-5}	250	40	3—10
m-F	52	8.5×10^{-5}	390	60	1—3
p-F	101	2.3×10^{-4}	480	135	>10
o-Cl	90	5.0×10^{-6}	75	24	3—10
m-Cl	81	5.0×10^{-5}	>500	36	3—10
p-Cl	115	2.4×10^{-4}	>500	160	>10
o-Br	93	2.2×10^{-6}	60	19	3—10
m-Br	92	1.3×10^{-5}	170	28.5	3—10
p-Br	120	1.0×10^{-4}	>500	220	>10
o-I	105	8.0×10^{-7}	90	17.5	1—3
m-I	108	7.0×10^{-6}	260	29	1—3
p-I	130	8.8×10^{-5}	>500	500	>10
m-SF_5	86	1.4×10^{-5}	430	136	
m-CH_3	76	8.0×10^{-6}	50	27	0.1—0.3

[1] METCALF et al. (1962), METCALF and FUKUTO (1962).
[2] Piperonyl butoxide synergist.

H. Sulfonyl fluorides

Methyl sulfonyl fluoride (also called methanesulfonyl fluoride), CH_3SO_2F, has been used in Germany as a commercial fumigant (MARTIN and SHAW 1946). The compound is a clear liquid b. 122–124°, soluble in water to about 5% at 22° and stable in water solution. Methyl sulfonyl fluoride is used as a greenhouse fumigant and for the control of ectoparasites of animals by burning in pyrotechnic mixture. The vapor is non-inflammable and is stated to have produced no leaf injury to cineraria, fuchsia, geranium, tradescantia, and roses upon exposure for 15 hours at a dosage of 5 g per cubic meter.

As a fumigant methyl sulfonyl fluoride has been stated to be more toxic to insects than chloropicrin, five times as toxic to *Sitophilus granarius* and *Tribolium confusum* as ethylene oxide, and approximately as toxic to aphids as nicotine and hydrogen cyanide, a concentration of 100 to 200 mg per cubic meter producing 100% mortality in 15 hours exposure. However, methyl sulfonyl fluoride is readily absorbed by grain and produces hazardous residues. Such poisoned grain can in fact be used to kill field mice. The compound has a subcutaneous minimum lethal dosage of 3.5 mg per kg to mice, rats, dogs, 5.6 for guinea pigs, and 7.0 for apes. As a fumigant, a c.t. of 2800 mg per cubic meter per minute killed rats, but rabbits survived 3000 to 6000; and dogs 23,000.

MARTIN and SHAW (1946) quote SCHRADER as stating that other sulfonyl fluorides useful for fumigation include: ethyl- $b._{14}$ 38° which is less toxic to mammals with a subcutaneous minimum lethal dosage to mice of 10 mg per kg; propyl- $b._{26}$ 57°; butyl- $b._{14}$ 72°; chloromethyl- $b._{19}$ 42°; and chloroethyl- $b._{14}$ 65°. Others mentioned with weaker insecticidal action included iodomethyl-, fluoromethyl-, vinyl, dimethylaminoethyl-2-sulfonyl fluoride, and ethyl-1,2-bis-sulfonyl fluoride.

Aromatic sulfonyl fluorides such as phenyl-, *p*-chlorophenyl-, and *p*-nitrophenyl-, *o,m* and *p*-aminophenyl and 3,4-dichlorophenyl- were of very low insecticidal activity (SCHRADER 1947a).

I. Fluorosulfonates

Aromatic esters of fluorosulfonic acid have weak insecticidal properties. SCHRADER (1947a) investigated phenyl fluorosulfonate, *o*- and *p*-chlorophenyl fluorosulfonate, and 3,4-dichlorophenyl fluorosulfonate. These compounds had a strong inhibiting action on molds and were patented as wood preservatives. Phenyl fluorosulfonate was about 0.005 as toxic as methyl sulfonyl fluoride as a fumigant to *Sitophilus granarius* and about 0.06 as toxic to aphids (MARTIN and SHAW 1946).

J. Miscellaneous organofluorine compounds described as insecticides

A large number of fluorinated organic compounds have been patented as insecticides, largely for mothproofing, but little data are available for discussion. These include: fluorinated fatty acids, such as fluorosteric, fluoroleic and fluoroundecanoic acid and their esters and salts; fluorinated ethyl and phenyl silanes; sulfamyl fluorides, such as *N*-hexyl-*N*-methylsulfamyl fluoride, *N*-dodecyl-*N*-methylsulfamyl fluoride, *N,N*-bis-(2-cyanoethyl) sulfamyl fluoride; phenyltrifluoromethyl sulfone and its *p*-CH_3, *p*-Cl- and *p*-NO_2 derivatives (SUMMERFORD 1959).

MARTIN (1958) has reviewed in detail a large number of complex organic molecules which act as colorless direct dyes for wool and are fixed to the fiber by reactive sulfonic acid groups. Compounds containing fluorine and trifluoromethyl groups were very active against clothes moths, carpet beetles, and hide beetles. A large number of related molecules containing these groups has been evaluated and highest activity was found with acid amides containing halogenated or trifluoromethylated monosulfonic acids of the aromatic series (the Mitin FF®-type) as shown in Table 16 below.

V. Summary

Both inorganic and organic compounds of fluorine have been used for the control of insect pests. The inorganic fluorine compounds such as sodium fluoride and cryolite are effective principally as stomach poisons and very probably owe their activity to the inhibitory effects of fluoride ion on magnesium-containing enzymes.

Table 16. *Activity of fluorine-containing mothproofing agents*[1]

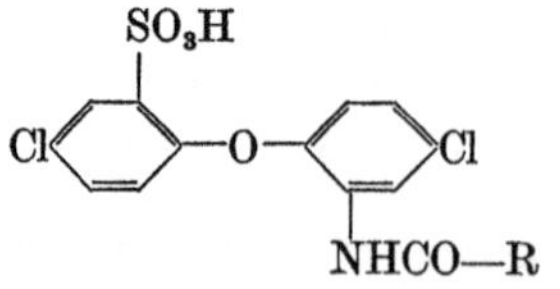

R	Toxicity to		
	Moth larva	Attagenus piceus	Anthrenus vorax
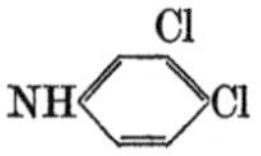	+++(+)	++++	+++
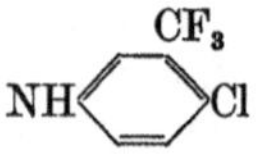	++++	++++	+++
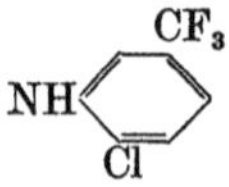	+++	++++	++++
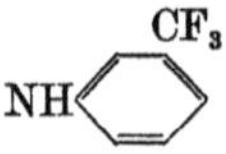	+++	++++	+++
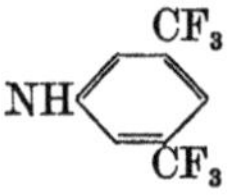	++++	++++	++++

[1] From MARTIN (1958).

A large variety of organofluorine compounds have insecticidal properties of all descriptions. In these materials fluorine is effective in one of three ways: (a) as a firmly fixed blocking atom which mimics hydrogen but does not participate in a vital enzymatic reaction, *e.g.* 2-fluoroethanols and α-fluoroacetic acid; (b) as a reactive or displaceable atom which permits the compound to undergo a chemical reaction with a vital enzyme, *e.g.* the phosphoro- and phosphono-fluoridates and phosphoramidofluoridates; and (c) as a typical halogen providing a stable lipophilic group with an aliphatic or aromatic nucleus, *e.g.* as fluoro-DDT or the trifluorocarbinols.

In addition to the utility of fluorocompounds as insecticides, the use of strategically fluorinated compounds has given valuable information in insect toxicology and biochemistry, particularly in regard to detoxication mechanisms involved in the mode of action of and resistance to insecticides.

References

ALDRIDGE, W. N.: Differentiation of true and pseudo cholinesterase by organophosphorus compounds. Biochem. J. **53**, 62—67 (1953).

ARTHUR, B. W., and J. E. CASIDA: Biological and chemical oxidation of tetramethyl phosphorodiamidic fluoride (Dimefox). J. Econ. Entomol. **51**, 49—56 (1958).

ASCHER, K. R. S.: Prevention of oviposition in the housefly through tarsal contact agents. Science **125**, 938 (1957).

— Insecticidal properties of N-substituted fluoracetamides. Riv. Parassitol. **19**, 229—231 (1958a).

ASCHER, K. R. S.: Reduced oviposition in *Aedes aegypti* following tarsal exposure to a fluorocarbon. Experienta (Basel) **14**, 8—9 (1958b).
— DDT-resistance-induced enhanced susceptibility towards cetyl fluoride and cetyl fluoracetate. XIII Intern. Congr. Entomol. Sec. 12, 557 (1960).
BARTLETT, G. R.: The mechanism of action of monofluoroethanol. J. Pharmacol. exp. Ther. **106**, 464—467 (1952).
BERGMANN, E. D., and A. KALUSZYNER: Bis (*p*-chlorophenyl) (trichloromethyl) carbinol and related compounds. J. Org. Chem. **23**, 1306—1308 (1958).
— P. MOSES, M. NEEMAN, A. KALUSZYNER, and S. REUTER: Methylfluorinated methyldiarylcarbinols and related compounds. J. Amer. chem. Soc. **79**, 4174—4178 (1957).
BIDSTRUP, P. L., J. A. BONNELL, and A. G. BECKETT: Paralysis following poisoning by a new organic phosphorus insecticide. Brit. med. J. **1953 I**, 1068—1072.
BLINN, R. C., and F. GUNTHER: Structure proof of 2,2-bis-(4-fluorophenyl)-1,1-dichloroethane. J. Amer. chem. Soc. **72**, 1399—1400 (1950).
BLUM, M. S.: The toxicities of fluorinated cyclohexanes to house flies. J. Econ. Entomol. **51**, 413—414 (1958).
— J. J. PRATT, and J. BORNSTEIN: Fluorinated analogues of DDT as toxicants and DDT synergists. J. Econ. Entomol. **52**, 626—628 (1959).
BORNSTEIN, J. ,M. S. BLUM, and J. J. PRATT: The synthesis and properties of some 2,2-difluoro-1,1-diarylethanols and 2-fluoro-1,1-diarylethanes. J. Org. Chem. **22**, 1210—1213 (1957).
BRADLOW, H. L., and C. VAN DER WERF: Preparation and chemical composition of difluorodiphenyltrichloroethane. J. Amer. chem. Soc. **69**, 662—664 (1947).
BROWNING, H. C., F. FRASER, S. SHAPIRO, I. GLICKMAN, and M. DUBRULE: Biological activity of DDT and related compounds. Canad. J. Res. **26** D, 282—300 (1948).
BUCKLE, F. S., R. HEAP, and B. C. SAUNDERS: Toxic fluorine compounds containing the C-F linkage. Pt. III. Fluoroacetamide and related compounds. J. chem. Soc. **1949**, 912 to 919.
CASIDA, J. E., K. B. AUGUSTINSSON, and G. JONSSON: Stability, toxicity, and reaction mechanism with esterases of certain carbamate insecticides. J. Econ. Entomol. **53**, 205 to 212 (1960).
CHADWICK, L. E., and D. L. HILL: Inhibition of cholinesterase by diisopropyl fluorophosphate, prostigmine, and hexaethyl tetraphosphate in the roach. J. Neurophysiol. **10**, 235—246 (1947).
CHEFURKA, W.: Oxidative metabolism of carbohydrate in insects. I. Glycolysis in the housefly *Musca domestica* L. Enzymologia **17**, 73—89 (1954).
COHEN, S., A. KALUSZYNER, and R. MECHOULAM: On the fluorination of DDT with hydrogen fluoride and mercuric oxide. J. Amer. chem. Soc. **79**, 5979—5981 (1957).
—, and S. TAHORI: Mode of action of di-(*p*-chlorophenyl)-(trifluoromethyl)-carbinol, as a synergist to DDT against DDT-resistant houseflies. J. Agr. Food Chem. **5**, 519—523 (1957).
CRANHAM, J. E., and B. A. STEVENSON: *p*-Chlorobenzyl *p*-chlorophenyl sulfide. Further aspects of field use. Chem. Ind. London **1953**, 1206.
CRISTOL, S. J.: A kinetic study of the dehydrochlorination of substituted 2,2-diphenylchloroethanes related to DDT. J. Amer. chem. **67**, 1494—1498 (1945).
DAVID, W. A. L., and B. O. C. GARDINER: Investigations on the systemic insecticidal action of sodium fluoroacetate and three phosphorus compounds on *Aphis fabae*. Ann. Appl. Biol. **38**, 91—110 (1951).
— — Fluoroacetamide as a systemic insecticide. Nature (Lond.) **181**, 1810 (1958).
— — The action of the systemic insecticide fluoroacetamide on certain aphids and on *Pieris brassicae*. Bull. Entomol. Res. **50**, 25—38 (1959).
DAVIES, D. R.: Cholinesterases and mode of action of some anticholinesterases. J. Pharm. Pharmacol. **6**, 1—26 (1954).
FAULKNER, P.: A hexose-1-phosphatase of silkworm blood. Biochem. J. **60**, 590—591 (1955).
FUKUTO, T. R.: The chemistry and action of organic phosphorus insecticides. *In:* R. L. METCALF, Ed., Adv. Pest Control Res. **1**, 147—218 (1957).
GILMOUR, D.: Biochemistry of Insects. New York: Academic Press 1961.
GRAHAM, K.: Respiratory enzyme mechanisms in an insect with reference to the qualitative and quantitative effects of inhibitors as an approach to insect toxicology. Trans. roy. Soc. Can. Sec. 5, **40**, 41—75 (1946).
GRIFFITHS, J. T., and O. E. TAUBER: Evaluation of sodium fluoride as a stomach poison and as a contact poison against the roach *Periplaneta americana*, L. J. Econ. Entomol. **36**, 536—540 (1943).
HAMADA, M.: Studies on the synthesis of DDT-type compounds and the relation of their chemical constitutions to insecticidal activities. 1—136 pp., privately printed (1957).

HANNA, A. D., E. JUDENKO, and W. HEATHERINGTON: Systemic insecticides for the control of insects transmitting swollen-shoot virus disease of cacao in the Gold Coast. Bull. Entomol. Res. **46**, 669—710 (1955).
HARRISON, I. R.: Control of bulb scale mite in narcissus. Plant Path. **5**, 127—129 (1956).
HEAL, R., and H. MENUSAN: A technique for the bloodstream injection of insects and its application in tests of certain insecticides. J. Econ. Entomol. **41**, 535—543 (1948).
HEAP, R., and B. C. SAUNDERS: Esters containing phosphorus. VII. Substituted diaminofluorophosphine oxides. J. chem. Soc. **1948**, 1313—1316.
HENNESSY, D. J., J. FRATANTONI, J. HARTIGAN, H. H. MOOREFIELD, and M. H. J. WEIDEN: Toxicity of 2-(2-halo-4-chlorophenyl)-2-(4-chlorophenyl)-1,1,1-trichloroethanes to resistant houseflies. Nature (Lond.) **190**, 341 (1961).
HOCKENYOS, G. L.: The mechanism of the absorption of sodium fluoride by roaches. J. Econ. Entomol. **26**, 1162—1169 (1933).
HOECHST Data sheet on fluoracetylphenyl urea. Farbwerke Hoechst (1963).
HOWARD, H.: Process for making artificial cryolite. U.S. Pat. 1,475,155 (1924).
HUISMAN, H. O., J. H. UHLENBROEK, and J. MELTZER: Preparation and acaricidal properties of diphenyl sulfones. Rec. Trav. Chim. T **77**, 103—122 (1958).
KALUSZYNER, A.: Cyclic analogues of DDT-like compounds. J. Org. Chem. **25**, 473 (1960).
— S. REUTER, and E. D. BERGMANN: Synthesis and biological properties of diaryl (trifluoromethyl)-carbinol. J. Amer. chem. Soc. **77**, 4164—4168 (1955).
KENAGA, E. E.: Some biological, chemical and physical properties of sulfuryl fluoride as an insecticidal fumigant. J. Econ. Entomol. **50**, 1—6 (1957).
KILGORE, L.: New German insecticides. Soap **21** (12), 138—139, 169—171 (1945).
KIRKWOOD, S., and J. DACEY: Synthesis of some analogues of 1,1-bis-(*p*-chlorophenyl)-2,2,2-trichloroethane (DDT). Canad. J. Res. **24** D, 69—72 (1946).
—, and P. H. PHILLIPS: The relationship between the lipoid affinity and the insecticidal action of 1,1-bis-(*p*-fluorophenyl)-2,2,2-trichloroethane and related substances. J. Pharmacol. expt. Ther. **87**, 375—381 (1946).
KÖRTING, A.: Untersuchungen über die insektizide Wirkung einiger Fluorverbindungen. Z. Pflanzenkrankh. Pflanzenschutz. **43**, (8/9), 502—516 (1933).
LANGE, W., u. G. VON KREUGER: Über Ester der Monofluorphosphorsäure. Ber. **65**, 1598 (1932).
LEHMAN, A. J.: The toxicology of the newer agricultural chemicals. Quart. Bull. Assoc. Food Drug Officials, U.S. **15**, 122 (1951).
LEWIS, S. F., and K. S. FOWLER: Effect of diisopropylphosphorofluoridate on the acetylcholine content of flies. Nature (Lond.) **178**, 919—920 (1956).
—, and B. N. SMALLMAN: The estimation of acetylcholine in insects. J. Physiol. **134**, 241—256 (1956).
LIPKE, H., and C. W. KEARNS: DDT-dehydrochlorinase. *In:* R. L. METCALF, Ed., Adv. Pest Control Res. **3**, 253—287 (1960).
LORD, K. A.: Toxicity of DDT analogues and BHC isomers to *M. sanborni* and *O. surinamensis*. Ann. Appl. Biol. **35**, 505—526 (1948).
— The effect of insecticides on respiration. II. The effects of a number of insecticides on the oxygen uptake of adult *Tribolium castaneum* Hbst. at 25° C. Ann. Appl. Biol. **37**, 105—122 (1950).
MARCOVITCH, S.: Studies on toxicity of fluorine compounds. Tenn. Agr. Exp. Sta. Bull. **139** (1928).
—, and W. W. STANLEY: Fluorine compounds useful in the control of insects. Tenn. Agr. Exp. Sta. Bull. **182** (1942).
MARTIN, H.: Chemische Konstitution und Wirkung sulfonsauregruppenhaltigen Mottenschutzmittel. Chimia **12**, 191—215 (1958).
— Guide to the chemicals used in crop protection. Research Branch, Canad., Dept. Agr., Publ. 1093, Ed. 4 (1961).
—, and H. SHAW: British Intelligence Objectives Rept. 1095. Item 22, 1946. H. M. Stationery Office, London.
MEIKLE, R. W., D. STEWART, and O. H. GLOBUS: Fumigant mode of action, drywood termite metabolism of Vikane fumigant shown by labelled pool technique. J. Agr. Food Chem. **11**, 226—230 (1963).
MENGLE, D. G., and J. E. CASIDA: Inhibition and recovery of brain cholinesterase activity in houseflies poisoned with organophosphate and carbamate compounds. J. Econ. Entomol. **51**, 750—757 (1958).
METCALF, C. L., W. P. FLINT, and R. L. METCALF: Destructive and Useful Insects, Ed. 4. New York: McGraw-Hill 1962.
METCALF, R. L.: Some insecticidal properties of fluorine analogues of DDT. J. Econ. Entomol. **41**, 416—421 (1948).
— Physiological basis for insect resistance to insecticides. Physiol. Revs. **35**, 197—232 (1955).

METCALF, R. L.: The role of systemic insecticides in world agriculture. Plant Protection Conference, 1956, p. 131—142. London: Butterworths Scientific Publications 1957.
— Unpublished data (1963).
—, and T. R. FUKUTO: Meta-sulfurpentafluorophenyl diethyl phosphate and meta-sulfurpentafluorophenyl N-methylcarbamate as insecticides and anticholinesterases. J. Econ. Entomol. **55**, 340—341 (1962).
— —, and M. Y. WINTON: Insecticidal carbamates: position isomerism in relation to activity of substituted phenyl N-methylcarbamates. J. Econ. Entomol. **55**, 889—894 (1962).
—, and D. L. LINDGREN: Insecticidal properties of elemental fluorine. J. Econ. Entomol. **41**, 522 (1948).
— R. B. MARCH, and M. MAXON: Substrate preferences of insect cholinesterase. Ann. Entomol. Soc. Amer. **48**, 222—228 (1955).
MOOREFIELD, H. H., M. H. J. WEIDEN, and D. J. HENNESSY: Relationship of the insecticidal and the free radical activities of DDT. Contrib. Boyce Thompson Inst. **21**, 481—486 (1962).
MORROW, J. E.: Insecticide and method of producing same. U.S. Patent 2,210,594 (1941).
MÜLLER, P.: Über Zusammenhänge zwischen Konstitution und insektizider Wirksamkeit. Helv. Chim. Acta **29**, 1560—1580 (1946).
NEGHERBON, W. O.: Handbook of Toxicology. Vol. III. Insecticides. Philadelphia, London: W. B. Saunders Co., 1959.
O'BRIEN, R. D.: Toxic Phosphorus Esters. New York, London: Academic Press 1960.
PERKOW, W.: Die Insektizide. Heidelberg: Alfred Huthy 1956.
PETERS, R. A., R. WAKELIN, P. BUFFA, and L. C. THOMAS: Biochemistry of fluoracetate poisoning. The isolation and some properties of the fluorotricarboxylic acid inhibitor of citrate metabolism. Proc. Roy. Soc. (B) **140**, 497—507 (1953).
PHILLIPS, M. A.: The fluoracetate series of pesticides. World Crops **7**, 480—482 (1955).
PILAT, M.: Histological researches into the action of insecticides on the intestinal tube of insects. Bull. Entomol. Res. **26**, 165—172 (1935).
POUTERMAN, E., and A. GIRARDET: Fluoration of DDT. Experientia (Basel) **2**, 459 (1946).
RIEMSCHNEIDER, R.: Zur Kenntnis der Kontakt-Insektizide. II. Pharmazie **9** (1), 651—800 (1950).
— Zur Chemie von Polyhalocyclopentadienen und verwandten Verbindungen. IV. Mitteilung: Thermische Spaltung und Oxydation des Adduktes $C_{10}H_6Cl_6$. Ber. **89**, 2697—2701 (1956).
— Chemical structure and activity of DDT analogues with special consideration of their spatial structures. *In:* R. L. METCALF, Ed., Adv. Pest Control Res. **2**, 307—350 (1958).
RIPPER, W.: Systemic insecticides. Paper read at 63rd International Congress of Crop Protection, Paris 1952.
— The status of systemic insecticides in pest control practices. *In:* R. L. METCALF, Ed., Adv. Pest Control Res. **1**, 305—352 (1957).
— R. M. GREENSLADE, and G. S. HARTLEY: Selective insecticides and biological control. J. Econ. Entomol. **44**, 448—459 (1951).
ROEDER, K., and N. K. KENNEDY: The effect of certain tri-substituted phosphine oxides on synaptic conduction in the roach. J. Pharmacol. exp. Ther. **114**, 211—220 (1955).
— —, and E. A. SAMSON: Synaptic conduction to giant fibers of the cockroach and the action of anticholinesterases. J. Neurophysiol. **10**, 1—10 (1947).
ROGERS, E., H. BROWN, I. RASMUSSEN, and R. HEAL: The structure and toxicity of DDT insecticides. J. Amer. chem. Soc. **75**, 2991—2999 (1953).
SACKTOR, B.: Investigations on the mitochondria of the housefly, *Musca domestica* L. I. Adenosinetriphosphatase. J. Gen. Physiol. **36**, 371—387 (1953).
SAUNDERS, B. C.: Some aspects of the chemistry and toxic action of organic compounds containing phosphorus and fluorine. Cambridge University Press, 1957.
SCHRADER, G.: The development of new insecticides. British Intelligence Objectives Subcommittee, Final Report 914. London, 1947 a.
— Synthetic insecticides. British Intelligence Objectives Sub-committee, Final Report 1808. London, 1947 b.
— Die Entwicklung neuer Insektizide auf Grundlage organischer Fluor- und Phosphor-Verbindungen. Angew. Chem., Monograph No. 62 (1952).
— Die Entwicklung neuer insektizider Phosphorsäure-Ester, Ed. 3. Weinheim: Verlag Chemie GmbH 1963.
SHAFER, G. D.: How contact insecticides kill. Mich. Tech. Bull. 15 (1915).
SHEPARD, H. H., and R. E. CARTER: The relative toxicity of some fluorine compounds as stomach insecticides. J. Econ. Entomol. **26**, 913 (1933).
SMALLMAN, B. N., and R. W. FISHER: Effect of anticholinesterases on acetylcholine levels in insects. Canad. J. Biochem. **36**, 575—586 (1958).
STEWART, D.: Sulfuryl fluoride — a new fumigant for control of the drywood termite *Kalotermes minor* Hagen. J. Econ. Entomol. **50**, 7—11 (1957).

SUMMERFORD, W. T.: Chemistry and toxicity of some organofluorine insecticides. Adv. Chem., Series 1, 160—174 (1950).

SWEETMAN, H. L.: Tests for toxicity of arsenicals and sodium fluoride to the American roach, *Periplaneta americana* L. Canad. Entomol. **73**, 31—34 (1941).

TAHORI, A.: Diaryl-trifluoromethylcarbinols as synergists for DDT against DDT-resistant houseflies. J. Econ. Entomol. **48**, 638—642 (1955).

— Selection for a fluoracetate resistant strain of houseflies and investigation of its resistance pattern. J. Econ. Entomol. **56**, 67—69 (1963).

— S. COHEN, and A. KALUSZYNER: DDT analogues as synergists for DDT. Experientia (Basel) **14**, 25—26 (1958).

VON OETTINGEN, W. F., and N. SHARPLESS: The toxicity and toxic-manifestations of DDT as influenced by chemical changes in the molecule. J. Pharmacol. exp. Ther. **88**, 400—413 (1946).

WARBURG, O., and W. CHRISTIAN: Isolation and crystallization of enolase. Biochem. Z. **310**, 384—421 (1942).

WILSON, I. B., M. A. HARRISON, and S. GINSBURG: Carbamyl derivatives of acetylcholine. J. biol. Chem. **236**, 1498—1450 (1961).

WINTERINGHAM, F. P. W., A. HARRISON, M. A. McKAY, and A. WEATHERLY: Biochemistry of diisopropylphosphorofluoridate poisoning in the adult housefly. Biochem. J. **65**, Proc. 49 (1957).

WOKE, P.: Effects of some ingested insecticides on the midgut wall of the southern armyworm larva. J. Agr. Res. **61**, 321—329 (1940).

Chapter 8

Monofluoro Aliphatic Compounds

By

F. L. M. PATTISON and R. A. PETERS

With 27 Figures

I. Introduction

In this chapter is given an account of the chemistry, biochemistry and pharmacology of monofluoro aliphatic organic compounds together with some account of their sources in Nature. Literature coverage extends to March, 1963[1]. For a review of the earlier work on the physiology and pharmacology, see CHENOWETH (1949). Other reviews have appeared (SAUNDERS 1957; PETERS 1957; and PATTISON 1959). The numbering of the enzymes is from a recent report[2].

These monofluoro compounds are of interest from more than one point of view; they are of especial pharmacological interest. Work started in the purely chemical field with SWARTS in 1896, who was the first to synthesize such substances. It was realized much later in Germany by commercial interests that the compounds might have value as insecticides; this work was not reported until after the second World War. During this latter period, some of these compounds, starting with fluoroacetate, were examined for their toxic effects[3]. Not long after, in South Africa, it was realized that a plant of the *Dichapetalum* genus made fluoroacetate, and that this was the source of its toxicity to animals; monofluorocarboxylic acids with a longer chain have also been found more recently in the seeds of *Dichapetalum toxicarium*. A third phase of interest started recently with the proof that the toxic principle of an Australian *Acacia* also contained fluoroacetate, important especially because it showed that the power of making the C–F bond was not confined to one genus. Fluoroacetate, as "Compound 1080," has been much used for the destruction of rodents and other pests, especially rabbits in Australia and New Zealand. There are indications that there might be plants in South America containing C–F compounds[4].

Hence in dealing with these compounds, we have to describe the pure chemistry, and then consider which compounds are present in Nature and why the compounds in question have biochemical and pharmacological effects. Finally we must give some account of those compounds which have been made synthetically, even though for the moment they have no place in Nature, as it may turn out that some of these may be pharmacologically important. It seems to be clear that any

---

[1] Manuscript submitted in final form, September 16, 1963.

[2] Report of the Enzyme Commission of the International Union of Biochemistry, pp. 1 to 159 (Pergamon Press).

[3] The terms "toxic" and "non-toxic" are arbitrarily assigned to LD_{50} values of < 25mg/kg and > 75 mg/kg respectively (intraperitoneal injection into mice). It follows of course that some "non-toxic" materials would be toxic when administered in large amounts.

[4] Added in proof: this has now been confirmed (OLIVEIRA 1963).

attempt to reverse toxicity with an antidote or otherwise must rest upon accurate knowledge of the whole biological action, from the biochemistry and physiology through the pharmacology and pathology to the living animal.

II. Occurrence in nature

Fluoroacetic acid (FCH_2COOH) occurs in Nature in various species of *Dichapetalum*, presumably as fluoroacetate at the pH of the cell sap. It is possible that it is sometimes present as a fluoroacetyl compound. The acid was first recognized as the toxic principle of Gifblaar *(Dichapetalum cymosum)* in brilliant work by MARAIS (1944) as a final result of earlier research by RIMINGTON (1935). Gifblaar had been long known to be very toxic to cattle in the Transvaal region of South Africa (THEILER 1902; STEYN 1928). The leaves are tempting to cattle when they come up in the Spring; they are more toxic when young. It is said (BADENHUIZEN, personal communication) that the leaves are actually the top shoots of the tree, the roots of which may penetrate into the soil for 15 metres, a fact which makes the poisonous plants difficult to eradicate.

A poisoning resembling that induced by fluoroacetate has been found with other species of *Dichapetalum* which grow in other parts of Africa (PETERS and HALL 1960a, b), though the specimens of leaves and roots examined were less toxic than those of *D. cymosum.*

More recently, fluoroacetate has been identified in an entirely different genus in Australia, in the Northern Territory and in Queensland, in the *Acacia georginae* (Gidyea), where it can be responsible for the loss of thousands of pounds worth of cattle in the large farms (MURRAY, MCCONNELL and WHITTEM 1961; OELRICHS and MCEWAN 1961). This discovery indicates that other plants can put together the C—F bond; a possibility reinforcing a view familiar to biochemists who often find that a biochemical reaction appearing in one part of Nature is also occurring in another.

Fluoro-oleic acid occurs in the seeds of *Dichapetalum toxicarium* (*Chailletia toxicaria*, Don) in the Sierra Leone district of Africa, the toxicity of which has been known for over 50 years. The ground seeds were used as a rodenticide, and extracts of the seeds were examined in England as long ago as 1906 by POWER and TUTIN[1]. The effect of the seeds as administered by the local doctors for various purposes is well described by RENNER (1904). He was summoned to a case, a native, who was suffering badly from pains in the legs and paralysis of the lower limbs. This condition, which was really a neuronitis, cleared off slowly. He recognized that he had seen the same signs before in young folk, and had not been able to diagnose them. Since this native had eaten some ground seeds of *D. toxicarium*, which had been prepared as a rat poison with fish, he was able to diagnose this case, and to draw the inference that the other cases which he had seen had been due to the administration by some "local" doctor of the ground seeds or their extract for various purposes. A full account of this is given by PATTISON (1959) in a quotation from the original paper of RENNER.

A reexamination of some of these seeds some 50 years later led to the discovery that, in addition to very small amounts of fluoroacetate, the main toxic principle was soluble in lipid solvents and consisted of fluorooleic acid (PETERS et al. 1960), together with traces of fluoropalmitic acid (HALL and WARD, unpublished results); this conclusion has been confirmed by synthesis (PATTISON and DEAR 1961; DEAR and PATTISON 1963), details of which are given on p. 397. Research has shown that the leaves of *D. toxicarium* contained no detectable C—F compounds, and that the

[1] Sir Henry Dale did the pharmacological work then.

seeds of *D. cymosum* had no fluoro-oleate (PETERS and HALL 1960a, b). From this it must be concluded that the long chain fluoro fatty acid is not an obligate component of seeds. The absence of fluoroacetate from the leaves of *D. toxicarium* may mean only that the specimen examined was free from toxicity. It is well known that the leaves of *D. cymosum* lose their toxicity and fluoroacetate as they get older (BADENHUIZEN and SLINGER 1954).

III. Chemistry

A. Introduction

The main purpose of this section is to present the chemistry of those monofluoro compounds, the biological effects of which are discussed later in the review; other compounds, of potential biological interest are also included. The section concludes with some chemical properties of the C—F bond. Much of the information provided has appeared fairly recently in a monograph dealing with toxic aliphatic fluorine compounds (PATTISON 1959). The world literature is now so extensive that in a review of this kind, devoted as it is to the more biological aspects of the subject, only representative references can be cited; in short, the treatment is not exhaustive.

B. Isolation of fluorine compounds from plants and animals

1. Fluoroacetic acid, FCH_2COOH

In 1943/44, MARAIS (1943, 1944) reported the isolation and characterization of the toxic principle of "gifblaar" [*Dichapetalum cymosum* (Hook) Engl.], one of the most poisonous plants of Southern Africa. This was proved to be fluoroacetic acid. Historical, ecological and toxicological aspects of the subject have been reviewed recently (PATTISON 1959). The following procedure was used in isolating the acid (MARAIS 1943). Ten kilograms of the dried and finely ground plant material were continuously extracted with 96% ethanol. The alcohol was removed by distillation under reduced pressure, and the syrupy residue was dissolved in dilute sulphuric acid. Filtration gave a clear, slightly brown solution. Ether extraction of this, followed by neutralization with aqueous potassium hydroxide gave an aqueous solution of crude potassium fluoroacetate. Concentration of the solution, acidification, and ether extraction gave an ethereal solution of fluoroacetic acid, which was decolorized (charcoal) and dried (sodium sulphate). The ether was removed and the residue distilled. The distillate was neutralized with potassium hydroxide and evaporated to dryness. The potassium salt was washed with acetone, dried at 100° and crystallized from 96% ethanol. It was named "potassium cymonate" pending identification.

In the subsequent report, MARAIS (1944) reported the unexpected discovery of fluorine in "potassium cymonate." Analysis of the potassium and calcium salts and of the *p*-nitrobenzyl and *p*-bromophenacyl esters gave the formula $C_2H_3FO_2$. Treatment of "potassium cymonate" with strong alkali gave glycollic acid, thus confirming the identity of the original material as the potassium salt of fluoroacetic acid. Synthesis of fluoroacetic acid from chloroacetic acid gave a material which was identical with the natural product.

Seventeen years later, in 1961, came announcements (OELRICHS and MCEWAN 1961, 1962; MURRAY et al. 1961) from Australia that the plant known as "gidyea" (*Acacia georginae* F. M. Bailey) also contained fluoroacetate. Similar in its action to gifblaar, gidyea causes heavy losses of cattle and sheep in Northern Territory and Queensland. The pods, seeds and leaves have all proved to be toxic.

To isolate the poison (OELRICHS and MCEWAN 1961), the seeds were extracted with ethanol and the extract was divided into acidic, neutral and basic fractions. The acid extract was purified by repetitive re-extraction from ether with sodium bicarbonate and finally by fractional distillation of the volatile acids so obtained. Silicic acid chromatography was used in later work (OELRICHS and MCEWAN 1962). The toxic factor was identified as the fluoroacetate ion by conversion to the butyl ester, and by gas chromatography and infrared spectroscopy. Toxicity tests with natural and synthetic samples gave identical results.

2. ω-Fluoro-oleic acid, $F(CH_2)_8CH{=}CH(CH_2)_7COOH$ (cis)

The isolation of ω-fluoro-oleic acid was made from the seeds of *Dichapetalum toxicarium* (West Africa). Seeds were received through the cooperation of the Tropical Products Association, London, (England) and of Sir JOHN SIMONSEN. The first thought that these seeds would contain fluoroacetate as the main toxic principle was not correct, though traces of fluoroacetate could be isolated from an aqueous extract of the seeds. The main toxic substance was found to be in the lipid fraction. After saponification and purification by precipitation of saturated long chain acids with cold acetone at −20° C, the fraction containing mainly unsaturated acids was studied by reversed phase chromatography. From preliminary studies, it was concluded that the main acid was a fluoro-octadecenoic acid (PETERS and HALL 1959). It was not found to be possible to separate larger amounts by increase of the scale of the cylindrical tubes (the oil did not run evenly); but by the use of a specially designed rectangular trough (HALL 1961) and of a marker (oil red 4 B), the acid was separated in large amounts from the main impurities which accompanied it; these were oleic acid and linoleic acid. After a further purification an oil was obtained; the purest specimen melted at 13.5° C.

Examination by infrared analysis showed that the spectrum resembled that of oleic acid, rather than elaidic acid. That the fluorine atom was in the ω-position was determined by nuclear magnetic resonance spectroscopy in comparison with synthetic 10-fluorodecanoic acid. Examination of the methyl ester by gas chromatography after ozonization gave two bands, which ran in the same region as the methyl esters of 9-fluorononanoic and azelaic acids (PETERS, HALL, WARD and SHEPPARD 1960). This identification was made possible by synthetic specimens of the ω-fluoro acids concerned, provided by one of us (F.L.M.P.).

It was found that for the rats in use in Cambridge, the lethal dose of ω-fluoro-oleic acid was 7—9 mg/kg; for mice, the LD_{50} by intraperitoneal injection was 2.4 mg/kg (DEAR and PATTISON 1963). The amounts of ω-fluoro-oleic acid producing citrate accumulation in preparations of kidney particles in the standard test were small; 1.25 μg of fluoro-oleic acid induced an accumulation of 2.6 μmoles of citrate; it was therefore much more powerfully activated in kidney than was fluoroacetate.

About the time that the unsaturated acid was isolated, it was noticed by R. J. HALL that a solid (m.p. 72°) separated out of the impure fractions. This compound had no double bond, a titration value for an equivalent weight of 286, and a higher content of fluorine (6.8%). It inhibited aconitase in kidney mitochondrial preparations and was toxic to animals. Further investigation has shown this to be ω-fluoropalmitic acid contaminated with traces of ω-fluoro-oleic acid (HALL and WARD 1962). At the same time the examination by gas chromatography of a cruder specimen of the oil has shown that there may be present in the seed in very small amounts most of the lower ω-fluorocarboxylic acids containing an even number of carbon atoms in their chain. This is interesting and suggests that the ω-fluoro-oleic acid is built up in steps of two carbon atoms from the lower fatty acids, the first acid to be added being fluoroacetate.

3. Fluorocitric acid, HOOCCHFC(OH) (COOH)CH_2COOH

This acid was first known from the chemical identification of the compound formed by enzymic action from fluoroacetate, which is inhibitory to citrate metabolism. The existence of a fluorotricarboxylic acid was surmised by LIÉBECQ and PETERS (1949) and by MARTIUS (1949) independently. The latter thought that the inhibitor might be fluorocitrate or fluoro*iso*citrate; though they considered a fluorotricarboxylic acid likely, LIÉBECQ and PETERS did not care to go beyond the fact that citrate metabolism was inhibited, because (a) the block might have been further on in the tricarboxylic acid cycle and (b) in 1948, citrate was thought to be out of the direct line of the reactions of the tricarboxylic acid cycle. Somewhat later BUFFA and PETERS (1950) found no accumulation of α-ketoglutarate, which suggested that the block causing accumulation was in one of the enzymes aconitase or isocitrate dehydrogenase. Direct investigation of this by LOTSPEICH et al. (1952) showed that "inhibitor fractions" from kidney (BUFFA, PETERS and WAKELIN 1951) had no effect upon isocitrate dehydrogenase from animal sources; but that these did inhibit aconitase.

The test used in the isolation of the inhibitor was essentially based on the effect upon the citrate metabolism of a homogenate prepared from guinea pig tissue. It was found that with about 150 mg of homogenized tissue and 10 μmoles of citrate, over 9 μmoles disappeared in thirty minutes at 38° in air. The concentration of inhibitor was judged by the amount of citrate left at the end of the test (PETERS 1952).

The enzymic synthesis of the inhibitor was made with homogenates of the kidneys of guinea pigs, rabbits, oxen and dogs in phosphate-potassium chloride solution, to which had been added fumarate, crude adenosine triphosphate and sodium fluoroacetate. The yields were low (PETERS, WAKELIN, BUFFA and THOMAS 1953). Figure 1 shows the scheme of isolation for the initial stages. It is to be noticed that it was found early in the work that the inhibitor was precipitated with the citrate fraction; but that it appeared to be more acidic than this. Advantage of this was taken at the lead stage; and later it was noticeable in a barium fractionation which was not used in the final isolation. This crude fraction was found to contain much less fluoride (analyzed by standard methods) than had been supposed, indicating that the citric inhibitor was much more active than seemed possible at first. It was still contaminated with citrate, and on paper chromatograms the inhibitor ran with the tricarboxylic fraction, being quite distinct from fluoroacetate. After removal of phosphate, treatment with ammonium hydroxide and propanol at pH 7.0, and a further treatment with lead, purification was accomplished by the use of Amberlite resin columns, IR 100 H to remove the last traces of metals, and then by adsorption on IRA 400. From this the citric acid was removed in fifteen, 5 ml samples with 0.02 N hydrochloric acid, after which the fluorocitric acid was removed with 0.1 N hydrochloric acid. The combined fluorocitric acid fractions were concentrated *in vacuo* below 43°, the procedure being stopped when the acid had been concentrated to 1—2 N hydrochloric acid. The whole was transferred to a vacuum desiccator at 0° containing phosphorus pentoxide and sodium hydroxide to remove volatile acid and water. The fluorocitric acid was then 25% pure. It was purified by adding 2 N hydrochloric acid (2.0 ml) and extracting with successive amounts of ether (10 ml) at

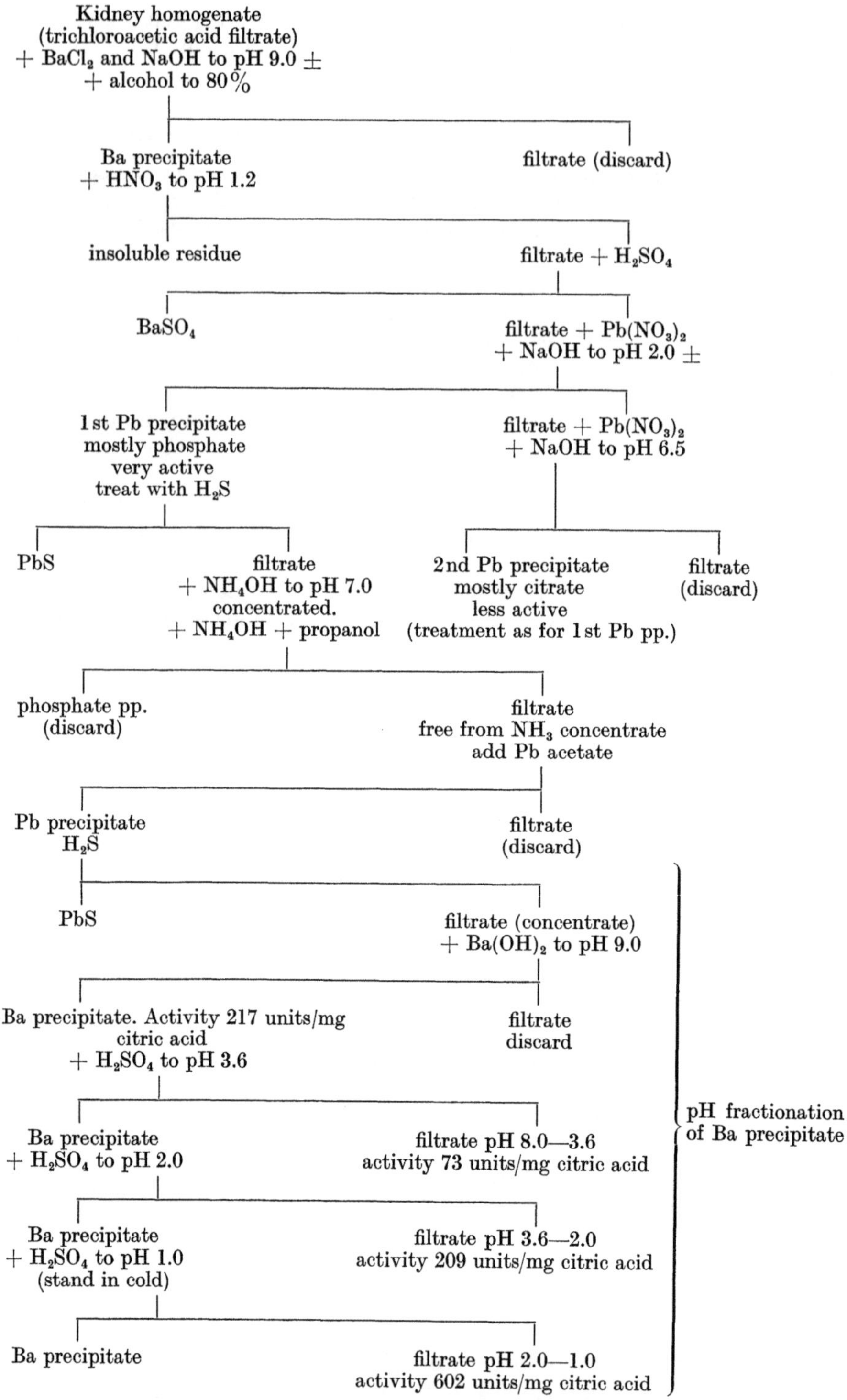

Fig. 1. Scheme of isolation of inhibitor (PETERS, 1952)

room temperature. The extracts were tested specifically for citrate inhibition in the standard test. The ether extracts 3 to 6 when evaporated *in vacuo* gave hydrated crystals and, when subsequently dried over phosphorus pentoxide, gave 7.1 mg of very hygroscopic crystals.

This method is given in detail because at the present time it is the only method of getting biologically synthesized fluorocitrate. The compound is very active; on average, 0.606 μg inhibited the metabolism of 1 μmole of citrate in the tests. The melting point was indeterminate between 90–120°. It did not give the reaction for citrate of PUCHER, SHERMAN and VICKERY (1936). If vanadium salts are used instead of permanganate as in TAYLOR's method (1953), care must be taken to cool, otherwise fluorocitrate is also estimated, presumably by removal of the fluorine atom (WARD and PETERS 1961). It titrated as for a tricarboxylic acid with one intensely acidic group. The fluorine content by an unequivocal spectrochemical method (GILLIESON and NEWCOMB 1951) gave F, 8.11%, theoretical F, 9.05%. On paper chromatograms, it travelled with the citric acid. Fluoro*cis*-aconitic acid was excluded by the chromatography and by the absence of unsaturation in the infrared spectrum (PETERS, WAKELIN, RIVETT and THOMAS 1953) and also by the absence of reaction with permanganate. The infrared spectrum excluded isocitric acid; but showed a band at 9.75 μ. The rotation $[(\alpha)_D]$ in presence of half the usual concentration of molybdate was −314°, L-malic acid being +725°. Owing to the length of this preparation, only some milligrams of the biosynthetic acid have been prepared; this has been carefully conserved for standard tests.

C. Preparative procedures

1. Methods for forming the C-F bond

The following procedures are particularly suitable for forming monofluoro aliphatic compounds. Examples of each are given, to show the scope of the reaction.

a) Halogen exchange

This, the most widely used procedure, involves the reaction of a chloro- or bromo-compound with a metal fluoride such as potassium fluoride:

$$ClCH_2COOCH_3 + KF \rightarrow FCH_2COOCH_3 + KCl$$

$$Cl(CH_2)_nCl + KF \rightarrow F(CH_2)_nCl + KCl$$

$$Br(CH_2)_nCN + KF \rightarrow F(CH_2)_nCN + KBr$$

$$Br(CH_2)_nCOOR + AgF \rightarrow F(CH_2)_nCOOR + AgBr$$

$$Br(CH_2)_nCOOR + KF \rightarrow F(CH_2)_nCOOR + KBr$$

$$Cl(CH_2)_nOH + KF \rightarrow F(CH_2)_nOH + KCl .$$

This general method as applied to monofluoro compounds has been described previously (PATTISON 1959). The choice of reaction conditions is dependent on the stability and reactivity of the reactant and product. It may be carried out under pressure in an autoclave (GRYSZKIEWICZ-TROCHIMOWSKI et al. 1947; JENKINS and KOEHLER 1948; SAUNDERS and STACEY 1948), or at normal pressure in a solvent such as diethylene glycol (HOFFMANN 1948, 1949, 1950; PATTISON, HOWELL, MCNAMARA, SCHNEIDER and WALKER 1956; PATTISON and HOWELL 1956a). Recently, sodium fluoride in solvents such as tetramethylene sulphone, acetonitrile or dimethyl-formamide has been found to be a satisfactory reagent (TULLOCK and COFFMAN 1960); other metallic fluorides have been used to a more limited extent. An excellent review covering all types of halogen exchange fluorinations has appeared very recently (BARBOUR et al. 1963).

b) From sulphonate esters

The conversion of sulphonates to fluorides, under conditions comparable to the halogen exchange reaction above, affords another convenient route to specific aliphatic fluorine compounds (EDGELL and PARTS 1955; PATTISON and MILLINGTON 1956; BERGMANN and SHAHAK 1958):

$$CH_3CH(OTs)COOR + KF \rightarrow CH_3CHFCOOR + TsOK \quad [Ts{=}CH_3C_6H_4SO_2^-]$$
$$CH_3(CH_2)_5OMs + KF \rightarrow CH_3(CH_2)_5F + MsOK \quad [Ms{=}CH_3SO_2^-]$$
$$MsOCH_2CH{=}CHCOOEt + KF \rightarrow FCH_2CH{=}CHCOOEt + MsOK$$
$$MsOCH_2COCH_3 + KF \rightarrow FCH_2COCH_3 + MsOK\,.$$

Sulphonates are usually prepared from alcohols; hence the preparation of fluorides by this procedure involves essentially the conversion of an alcohol to a fluoride; for certain types of alcohols, this can even be achieved in one reaction by a continuous process, and more generally by a semi-continuous process (PATTISON and MILLINGTON 1956).

c) Decomposition of α-fluorinated amines

An interesting procedure for converting alcohols to fluorides has been developed by YAROVENKO and RAKSHA (1959):

$$CF_2{=}CClF + R_2NH \rightarrow R_2NCF_2CHFCl$$

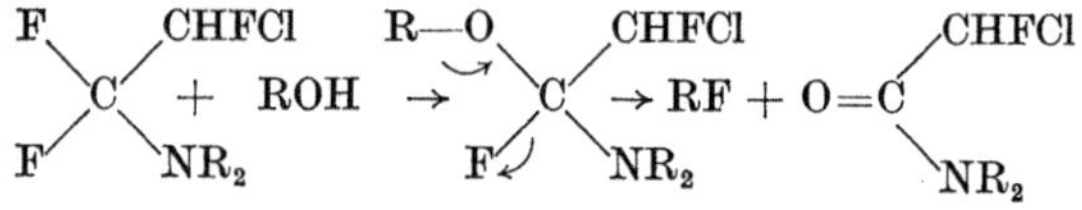

For example, n-butyl alcohol can be converted to n-butyl fluoride in 66.5% yield by this method.

d) Epoxides plus hydrogen fluoride

The opening of epoxides by hydrogen fluoride (KNUNYANTS et al. 1949a, b) is of less general scope, but is particularly convenient for forming 1,2-fluorohydrins:

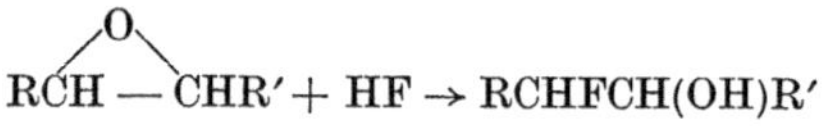

These in turn can be converted to α-fluoroketones by oxidation.

e) Diazoketones plus hydrogen fluoride

This procedure is restricted to the preparation of fluoromethyl ketones, FCH_2COR (OLAH and KUHN 1956; KNUNYANTS et al. 1956; FRASER et al. 1957; BERGMANN and IKAN 1957):

$$RCOCl + CH_2N_2 \rightarrow RCOCHN_2 + HF \rightarrow RCOCH_2F + N_2\,.$$

f) Reactions involving perchloryl fluoride

Monofluoro compounds can be prepared using perchloryl fluoride (INMAN et al. 1958) by a variety of methods (NEWTON and PATTISON 1961; DEAN and PATTISON 1963):

$$RCH(COOR)_2 \rightarrow RCF(COOR)_2$$

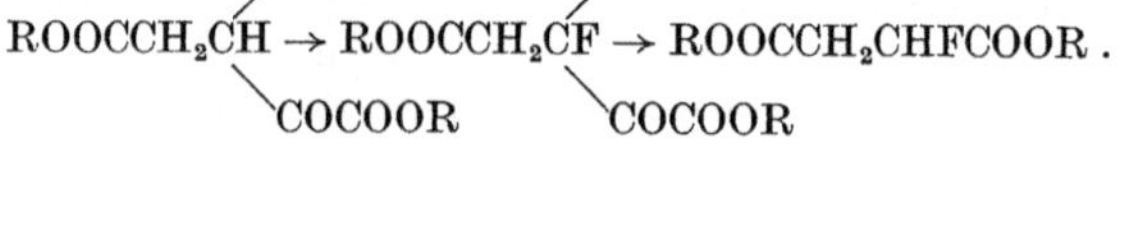

g) Addition of BrF

A useful procedure for adding the elements of BrF to unsaturated steroids has been described (Bowers 1959; Bowers et al. 1960); more recently it has been extended to the field of aliphatic compounds (Buchanan, Dean and Pattison 1962b). The method involves the treatment of an alkene with N-bromoacetamide and hydrogen fluoride.

$$RCH{=}CH_2 \xrightarrow[HF]{NBA} RCHFCH_2Br$$

The fluorobromides so formed are useful intermediates; for example, they can be converted to α-fluoroacids:

$$RCHFCH_2Br \rightarrow RCHFCH_2OAc \rightarrow RCHFCOOH$$

h) Miscellaneous procedures

Several procedures have been described recently which are more appropriate for forming polyfluoro aliphatic compounds. For example, lead tetrafluoride in effect adds fluorine to alkenes (Bowers et al. 1962), and sulphur tetrafluoride replaces oxygen by fluorine (Hasek et al. 1960):

$$RCH{=}CHR' \xrightarrow{PbF_4} RCHFCHFR'$$

$$RCOOH \xrightarrow{SF_4} RCF_3$$

$$RCOR' \xrightarrow{SF_4} RCF_2R'.$$

2. Fluoroacetates

Sodium fluoroacetate is readily available as a commercial chemical, because of its application in rodent control. Hence this material is an excellent starting point for preparing members of the fluoroacetate series. The commercial production has been described by Jenkins and Koehler (1948): essentially this involves the reaction of ethyl chloroacetate with potassium fluoride in an autoclave followed by hydrolysis of the resultant ethyl fluoroacetate.

$$ClCH_2COOC_2H_5 + KF \rightarrow FCH_2COOC_2H_5 + KCl$$

$$FCH_2COOC_2H_5 + NaOH \rightarrow FCH_2COONa + C_2H_5OH$$

Commercial sodium fluoroacetate ("Compound 1080") may be converted to fluoroacetic acid (Pattison, Stothers and Woolford 1956) or to fluoroacetyl chloride (Pattison, Fraser, Middleton, Schneider and Stothers 1956) easily and in high yield; these in turn are very useful in preparing other fluoroacetates.

Another important compound is 2-fluoroethanol. It may be prepared by halogen exchange methods (Hoffmann 1948; Saunders, Stacey and Wilding 1949), or by opening of ethylene oxide by hydrogen fluoride (Knunyants et al. 1949a, b).

Both fluoroacetic acid and 2-fluoroethanol undergo many of the reactions of their non-fluorinated analogues. Some of these procedures have been reviewed (Pattison 1959). For example, fluoroethanol and fluoroacetic acid under conditions of esterification form 2-fluoroethyl fluoroacetate (Saunders and Stacey 1949).

Of the biologically active compounds described later in this chapter, mention may be made of the following compounds.

a) Fluoroacetyl choline

Fluoroacetyl choline was prepared (BLOHM 1951; GRYSZKIEWICZ-TROCHIMOWSKI et al. 1953) from β-bromoethyl fluoroacetate and trimethylamine:

$$(CH_3)_3N + FCH_2COOCH_2CH_2Br \rightarrow (CH_3)_3\overset{+}{N}CH_2CH_2OCOCH_2F\ Br^-.$$

b) Fluoroacetyl coenzyme A

Fluoroacetyl coenzyme A has been reported by BRADY (1955). The mixed anhydride of ethyl formate and fluoroacetic acid ($FCH_2COOCOOEt$) was prepared from ethyl chloroformate and fluoroacetic acid in pyridine-ether. A slight excess of this was then added at 0° to an aqueous solution of reduced coenzyme A containing potassium bicarbonate (pH 7.5). The pH was adjusted to 6.1 with dilute hydrochloric acid, and the aqueous phase was extracted four times with ether saturated with water. Final traces of ether were removed by bubbling nitrogen through the aqueous solution at room temperature. Yield: 85–93%.

c) Fluoroacetyl phosphate

Fluoroacetyl phosphate was prepared (MARCUS and ELLIOTT 1958) from fluoroacetyl chloride and silver phosphate by the reaction:

$$FCH_2COCl + AgH_2PO_4 \rightarrow FCH_2CO{-}O{-}\underset{\displaystyle OH}{\overset{\displaystyle O}{\overset{\|}{\underset{|}{P}}}}{-}OH$$

d) 2-Fluoroacetohydroxamic acid

2-Fluoroacetohydroxamic acid has been prepared from fluoroacetate esters by reaction with hydroxylamine (GAL, PETERS and WAKELIN 1956; KNUNYANTS and SOKOL'SKII 1960):

$$FCH_2COOCH_3 + H_2NOH \rightarrow FCH_2CONHOH + CH_3OH$$

3. ω-Fluorocarboxylic acids

a) Saturated, unbranched acids, $F(CH_2)_nCOOH$

The available methods for forming ω-fluorocarboxylic acids or esters have been reviewed (PATTISON 1959). The following are representative and general:

(i) Alkyl esters.

α) $X(CH_2)_nCOOR + AgF \rightarrow F(CH_2)_nCOOR + AgX$
(BUCKLE, PATTISON and SAUNDERS 1949; PATTISON, HUNT and STOTHERS 1956)

β) $Br(CH_2)_nCOOR + KF \rightarrow F(CH_2)_nCOOR + KBr$
(PATTISON, HUNT and STOTHERS 1956; PATTISON, HOWELL, McNAMARA, SCHNEIDER and WALKER 1956)

γ) $F(CH_2)_nCN + H_2O + CH_3OH \rightarrow F(CH_2)_nCOOCH_3 + NH_3$
(PATTISON, HUNT and STOTHERS 1956; PATTISON, STOTHERS and WOOLFORD 1956)

δ) $F(CH_2)_nMgCl + ClCOOR \rightarrow F(CH_2)_nCOOR + MgCl_2$
(PATTISON, HUNT and STOTHERS 1956; HOWELL, COTT and PATTISON 1957)

ε) $F(CH_2)_nCOOH + HOOC(CH_2)_mCOOR \rightarrow F(CH_2)_{n+m}COOR + 2\,CO_2 + H_2$
(PATTISON, HUNT and STOTHERS 1956; PATTISON, STOTHERS and WOOLFORD 1956; PATTISON and WOOLFORD 1957b)

ζ) 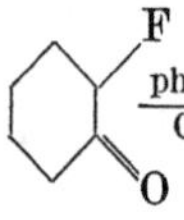 $\xrightarrow[CH_3OH]{\text{photolysis}} F(CH_2)_5COOCH_3$ (FERGUSON et al. 1963).

(ii) Free acids.

α) $\mathrm{F(CH_2)_nCH_2OH + 2\,O \rightarrow F(CH_2)_nCOOH + H_2O}$
(PATTISON, HUNT and STOTHERS 1956; PATTISON, STOTHERS and WOOLFORD 1956)

β) $\mathrm{F(CH_2)_nCN + 2\,H_2O \rightarrow F(CH_2)_nCOOH + NH_3}$
(PATTISON, HUNT and STOTHERS 1956; PATTISON, HOWELL, MCNAMARA, SCHNEIDER and WALKER 1956)

γ) $\mathrm{F(CH_2)_nCOOR + H_2O \rightarrow F(CH_2)_nCOOH + ROH}$
(PATTISON, HUNT and STOTHERS 1956; PATTISON, STOTHERS and WOOLFORD 1956)

δ) $\mathrm{F(CH_2)_nMgX + CO_2 + H_2O \rightarrow F(CH_2)_nCOOH + Mg(OH)X}$
(PATTISON, HUNT and STOTHERS 1956; PATTISON and HOWELL 1956b)

ε) $\mathrm{F(CH_2)_nCOOH \rightarrow F(CH_2)_nCH_2COOH}$ (Arndt-Eistert)
(BUCKLE, PATTISON and SAUNDERS 1949)

ζ) $\mathrm{F(CH_2)_nCH_2COOH \rightarrow F(CH_2)_nCOOH}$ (Barbier-Wieland)
(BUCHANAN and PATTISON 1962).

In addition to the above, special methods have been developed for certain individual members of the series; these have been reviewed (PATTISON 1959). Derivatives of these acids have been prepared (PATTISON, FRASER, O'NEILL and WILSHIRE 1956).

Because ω-fluoropalmitic acid has been shown to occur naturally (see p. 390), it is appropriate to mention the best method for its synthesis; this involves the total hydrogenation of 16-fluoro-9-octadecynoic acid, $\mathrm{F(CH_2)_6C{\equiv}C(CH_2)_7COOH}$, which in turn is prepared by a simple variation of the reaction scheme outlined for ω-fluoro-oleic acid (see below).

b) ω-Fluoro-oleic acid, $F(CH_2)_8CH{=}CH(CH_2)_7COOH$

ω-Fluoro-oleic acid has recently been synthesized (PATTISON and DEAR 1961; DEAR and PATTISON 1963) by the following series of reactions:

$$\begin{aligned}\mathrm{F(CH_2)_8Br + NaC{\equiv}CH} &\rightarrow \mathrm{F(CH_2)_8C{\equiv}CH + I(CH_2)_7Cl}\\ &\rightarrow \mathrm{F(CH_2)_8C{\equiv}C(CH_2)_7Cl + NaCN \rightarrow F(CH_2)_8C{\equiv}C(CH_2)_7CN}\\ &\rightarrow \mathrm{F(CH_2)_8C{\equiv}C(CH_2)_7COOH \rightarrow F(CH_2)_8CH{=}CH(CH_2)_7COOH}\ (\textit{cis}).\end{aligned}$$

The overall yield from 8-fluoro-octyl bromide was 36.5% of the theoretical. The synthetic product was shown to be identical with the naturally occurring material by physical and biological methods.

Other ω-fluoro unsaturated acids have also been synthesized (DEAR and PATTISON 1963), including ω-fluoroelaidic acid and ω-fluoropalmitoleic acid.

c) Branched ω-fluorocarboxylic acids

These have been obtained by various methods of which the following are typical:

(i) α-Methylcarboxylic acids.

α) $$\mathrm{F(CH_2)_nX + CH_3CH(COOEt)_2 \rightarrow F(CH_2)_n\underset{\displaystyle CH_3}{\underset{|}{C}}(COOEt)_2 \rightarrow F(CH_2)_n\underset{\displaystyle CH_3}{\underset{|}{C}}HCOOH}$$

(BUCHANAN and PATTISON 1962)

β) $$\mathrm{F(CH_2)_n\overset{\displaystyle CH_3}{\overset{|}{\underset{\displaystyle CH_3}{\underset{|}{C}}}}CH_2COOH \xrightarrow{\text{Barbier-Wieland}} F(CH_2)_n\overset{\displaystyle CH_3}{\overset{|}{\underset{\displaystyle CH_3}{\underset{|}{C}}}}COOH}$$

(BUCHANAN and PATTISON 1962).

(ii) β-Methylcarboxylic acids.

$$\alpha)\quad \mathrm{F(CH_2)_nCOOH + HOOCCH_2\underset{\displaystyle CH_3}{\underset{|}{C}}HCH_2COOEt \xrightarrow[\text{coupling}]{\text{anodic}} F(CH_2)_{n+1}\underset{\displaystyle CH_3}{\underset{|}{C}}HCH_2COOEt}$$

(Pattison and Woolford 1957a, b)

$$\beta)\quad \mathrm{F(CH_2)_nCOOH + HOOCCH_2\overset{\displaystyle CH_3}{\overset{|}{\underset{\displaystyle CH_3}{\underset{|}{C}}}}CH_2COOEt \rightarrow F(CH_2)_{n+1}\overset{\displaystyle CH_3}{\overset{|}{\underset{\displaystyle CH_3}{\underset{|}{C}}}}CH_2COOEt}$$

(Pattison and Woolford 1957b).

d) Other branched acids

Other branched acids were prepared by variations of the above. For example, ω-fluorotuberculostearic acid was prepared (Pattison and Woolford 1957a) as follows:

$$\mathrm{F(CH_2)_7COOH + HOOCCH_2\underset{\displaystyle CH_3}{\underset{|}{C}}HCH_2COOR \rightarrow F(CH_2)_8\underset{\displaystyle CH_3}{\underset{|}{C}}HCH_2COOR}$$

$$\rightarrow \mathrm{F(CH_2)_8\underset{\displaystyle CH_3}{\underset{|}{C}}HCH_2COOH + HOOC(CH_2)_7COOR}$$

$$\rightarrow \mathrm{F(CH_2)_8\underset{\displaystyle CH_3}{\underset{|}{C}}H(CH_2)_8COOR}\,.$$

4. Other fluoro acids and derivatives

a) Fluoropyruvic acid, $FCH_2COCOOH$

Fluoropyruvic acid may be obtained by two different methods:

(i) By hydrolytic decarboxylation of diethyl fluoro-oxalacetate (Blank, Mager and Bergmann 1955; Nair and Busch 1958):

$$\mathrm{EtOOCCH_2F + EtOOCCOOEt \rightarrow EtOOCCHFCOCOOEt \rightarrow FCH_2COCOOH}$$

(ii) By oxidation of ethyl fluorolactate using N-bromosuccinimide (Bergmann, Cohen and Shahak 1961):

$$\mathrm{FCH_2CH(OH)COOR \rightarrow FCH_2COCOOR}$$

b) Fluoromalonic acid and esters, $CHF(COOR)_2$

Several procedures are available for the preparation of fluoromalonic acid and its derivatives. Of these, the first is probably the most convenient.

(i) $\mathrm{EtOOC\bar{C}HF + ClCOOEt \rightarrow EtOOCCHFCOOEt + Cl^-}$
(Bergmann, Cohen and Shahak 1959; Buchanan, Dean and Pattison 1962a)

(ii) $\mathrm{EtOOCCOCHFCOOEt \xrightarrow[ROH]{K_2S_2O_8} ROOCCHFCOOEt}$
(Bergmann and Shahak 1961)

(iii) $\mathrm{CF_2{=}CFCN \xrightarrow{70\%\ H_2SO_4} CHF(COOH)_2}$
(La Zerte et al. 1956).

The ester is readily hydrolyzed to the free acid by treatment with potassium hydroxide in ethanol at room temperature, followed by acidification with concentrated hydrochloric acid (Buchanan and Pattison 1962).

c) *Fluoromalic acid, ROOCCHFCH(OH)COOR*

Dimethyl fluoromalate was prepared (TAYLOR and KENT 1954, 1956) by reduction of diethyl fluoro-oxalacetate with potassium borohydride:

$$\mathrm{EtOOCCHFCOCOOEt} \xrightarrow[\mathrm{CH_3OH}]{\mathrm{KBH_4}} \mathrm{CH_3OOCCHFCH(OH)COOCH_3}$$

This on treatment with ammonia in methanol formed fluoromalamide, $H_2NCOCHFCH(OH)CONH_2$, and on hydrolysis with aqueous sodium hydroxide at room temperature formed sodium fluoromalate, NaOOCCHFCH(OH)COONa.

In a more recent paper, KRASNA (1962) has proved the existence of two racemic mixtures of fluoromalic acid, identified with the threo- and erythro-configurations:

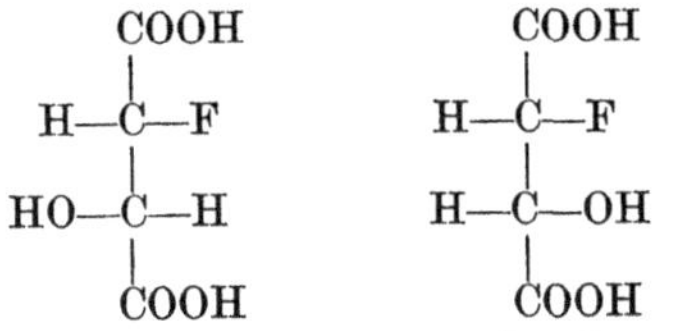

threo-form erythro-form

The enzymic synthesis of fluoromalic acid has been inferred (DIXON et al. 1960), from fluoroacetyl coenzyme A and glyoxalate.

Diethyl α,α-difluoromalic acid was obtained (RAASCH 1958a) from diethyl α,α-difluoro-oxalacetate (q.v.) by catalytic high-pressure hydrogenation, or by reduction with sodium borohydride. The ester was readily hydrolyzed to the free acid by dilute hydrochloric acid.

d) *Fluoroacetoacetates*

(i) Ethyl γ-fluoroacetoacetate, FCH_2COCH_2COOEt was prepared (FRASER and PATTISON 1955; FRASER, MILLINGTON and PATTISON 1957) from fluoroacetyl chloride by the following reactions:

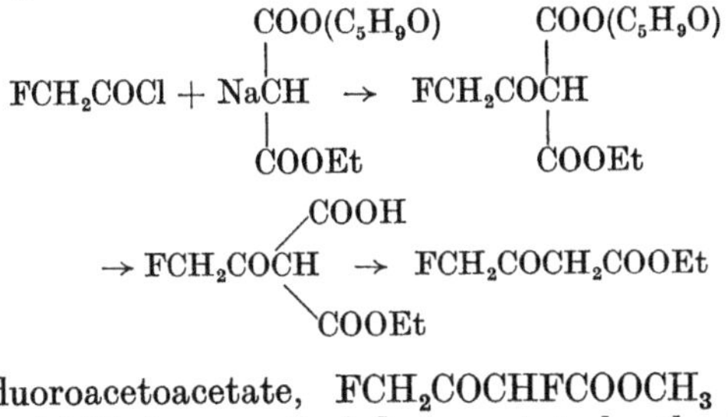

(ii) Methyl α,γ-difluoroacetoacetate, $FCH_2COCHFCOOCH_3$ was prepared (SAUNDERS and STACEY 1948) from methyl fluoroacetate by the Claisen condensation:

$$2\,\mathrm{FCH_2COOCH_3} \xrightarrow{\mathrm{Na}} \mathrm{FCH_2COCHFCOOCH_3} + \mathrm{CH_3OH}$$

The corresponding ethyl ester was prepared (McBEE et al. 1953) by essentially the same method, using sodium hydride as the condensing agent.

e) *Fluoro-oxalacetic acid and esters, ROOCCHFCOCOOR*

Diethyl fluoro-oxalacetate is readily prepared (RIVETT 1953; BLANK, MAGER and BERGMANN 1955) from ethyl fluoroacetate:

$$\mathrm{EtOOCCH_2F} + \mathrm{EtOOCCOOEt} \xrightarrow{\mathrm{KOEt}} \mathrm{EtOOCCHFCOCOOEt} + \mathrm{EtOH}$$

In an interesting study, KUMLER et al. (1962) showed by nuclear magnetic resonance analyses, that, whereas diethyl oxalacetate consists of 79% of the enol form, diethyl fluoro-oxalacetate exists only in the keto form (100%).

The free acid may be obtained from the ester under conditions favoring transesterification (KUN, GRASSETTI, FANSHIER and FEATHERSTONE 1959). The

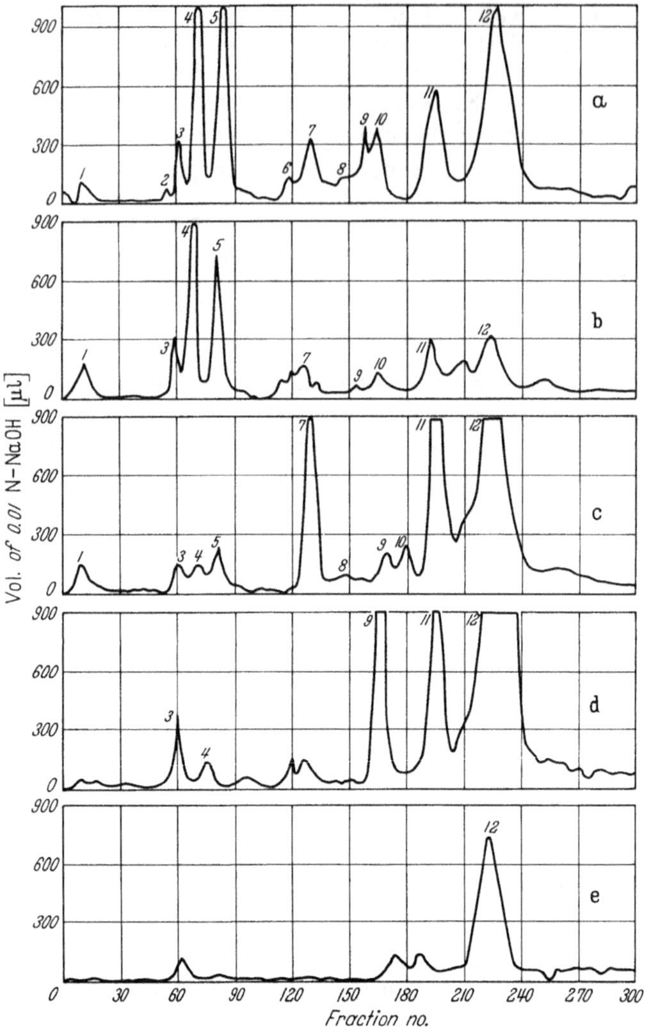

Fig. 2. Silicic acid-column chromatography of samples of fluorocitric acid. Sample (a): synthetic triethyl fluorocitrate hydrolyzed by 0.1 N NaOH at 20° for 24 hr. Sample (b): a second synthetic triethyl fluorocitrate hydrolyzed by 0.1 N NaOH at 20° for 48 hr. Sample (c): a third synthetic triethyl fluorocitrate hydrolyzed by N NaOH at 20° for 48 hr. Sample (d): a fourth synthetic triethyl fluorocitrate hydrolyzed by 3 N HCl at 100° for 6 hr. and precipitated as the barium salt. Sample (e): biosynthetic fluorocitric acid. Fraction volumes were 2.2 ml and eluting solvents were used as follows: fractions 1—48, butan-1-ol-chloroform (5:100, v/v); fractions 49—108, butan-1-ol-chloroform (15:100, v/v); fractions 109—157, butan-1-ol-chloroform (25:100, v/v); fractions 158—300, butan-1-ol-chloroform (35:100, v/v). From WARD and PETERS (1961)

ester is dissolved in glacial acetic acid, and concentrated hydrochloric acid is added. The mixture is kept at room temperature for three days, and then evaporated to dryness under reduced pressure at room temperature. Yield: 85%. The acid may be recrystallized from ether-petroleum ether.

In essentially the same way was prepared diethyl α,α-difluoro-oxalacetate (RAASCH 1958a), using sodium hydride as the condensing agent. The crystalline free acid was obtained by hydrolysis with 10% hydrochloric acid.

f) Fluorocitric acid and esters, HOOCCHFC(OH)(COOH)CH$_2$COOH

The first recorded synthesis of fluorocitric acid was that of RIVETT (1953), in which diethyl fluoro-oxalacetate was subjected to the Reformatski reaction:

$$\text{EtOOCCHFCOCOOEt} \xrightarrow[\text{BrCH}_2\text{COOEt}]{\text{Zn}} \text{EtOOCCHFC(OH)(COOEt)CH}_2\text{COOEt}$$

More recently, BROWN and SAUNDERS (1962) have obtained the di-ester as follows:

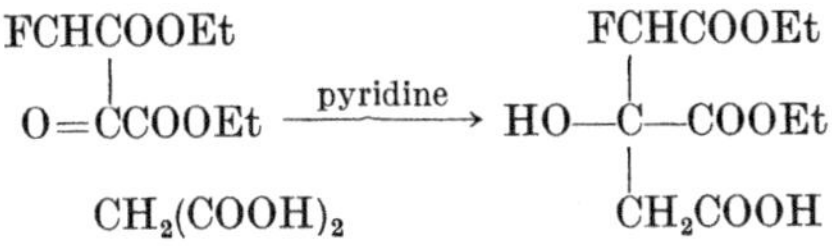

The triester of synthetic fluorocitrate has little toxicity, which is thought to be due to the fact that it does not come into contact with the esterases of the body. Hence for enzymic or animal experiments sodium fluorocitrate is required. Unfortunately simple hydrolysis gives a mixture of twelve or thirteen substances (WARD and PETERS 1961) as determined by the silicic column method of BULEN, VARNER and BURRELL (1952). Of these, peaks 11 and 12 (see Fig. 2) belong to the four isomers of the fluorocitric acids. Peak 12 contained the active inhibitor and this was approximately half as active as the biosynthetic sample. It is interesting that the two inactive components form a separate peak 11. Peaks 4 and 5 can be converted by treatment with alkali to peaks 11 and 12. Excess of alkali unfortunately breaks down even 11 and 12, converting these to peaks 10 and 7 respectively. It is believed that peaks 4 and 5 are partial esters. The best method found for ensuring full activity was to stand the sample of triethyl fluorocitrate at 20° for twenty-four hours in the presence of 6 g equiv. of sodium hydroxide (0.5 *N*), and then to neutralize with hydrochloric acid. RIVETT's use of acid hydrolysis followed by barium precipitation achieved some purification: but the alkaline treatment was better. At present the separation by the silicic acid column, though tedious, is the only known method of getting purified and active synthetic sodium fluorocitrate. The free acid is highly deliquescent; crystals have been observed in a desiccator, but outside the desiccator their life was but a few seconds.

The enzymic synthesis of fluorocitric acid from fluoro-oxalacetate and acetyl-coenzyme A has been reported by FANSHIER et al. (1962); the acid was isolated as the cyclohexylamine salt. Surprisingly, this material behaved differently with aconitase; this raises interesting stereochemical implications.

g) Triethyl α-fluoroaconitate, EtOOCCHFC(COOEt)=CHCOOEt

BERGMANN and SHAHAK (1960) have reported the synthesis of this ester as follows:

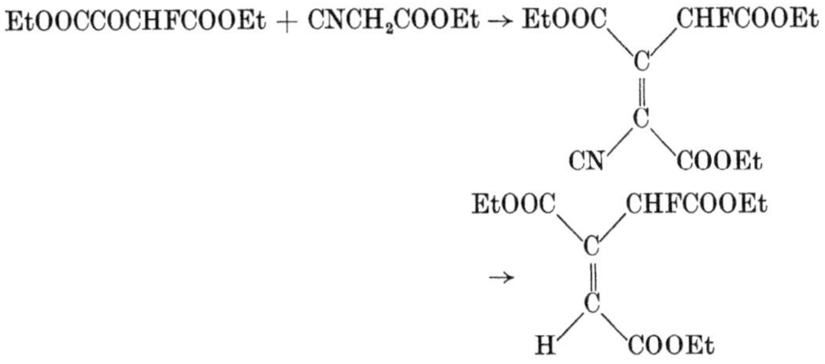

h) Fluoromevalonic acids

Three monofluoromevalonic acids have been described:

α-Fluoromevalonolactone

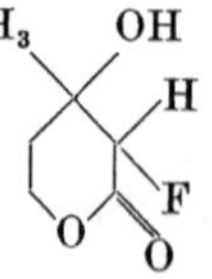

SCHMIDT and JAHN (1961)
BERGMANN and COHEN (1960)

γ-Fluoromevalonolactone

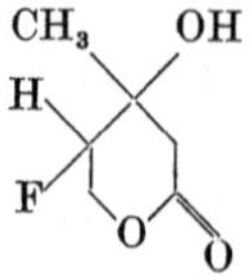

BERGMANN and COHEN (1960)
BERGMANN and COHEN (1961a)

Me-Fluoromevalonolactone

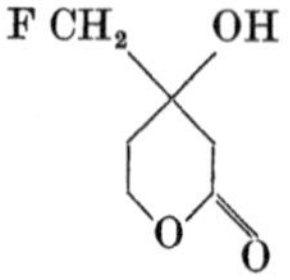

TSCHESCHE and MACHLEIDT (1960)
SINGER et al. (1959)

Much interesting chemistry is involved in these preparations; this can be seen from the following reaction schemes:

(i) α-Fluoromevalonolactone:

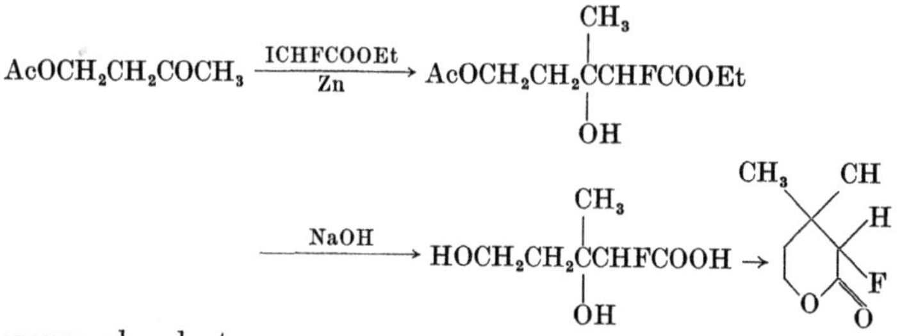

(ii) γ-Fluoromevalonolactone:

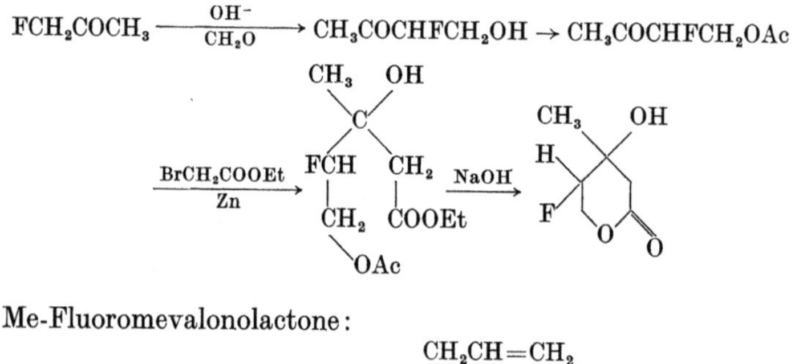

(iii) Me-Fluoromevalonolactone:

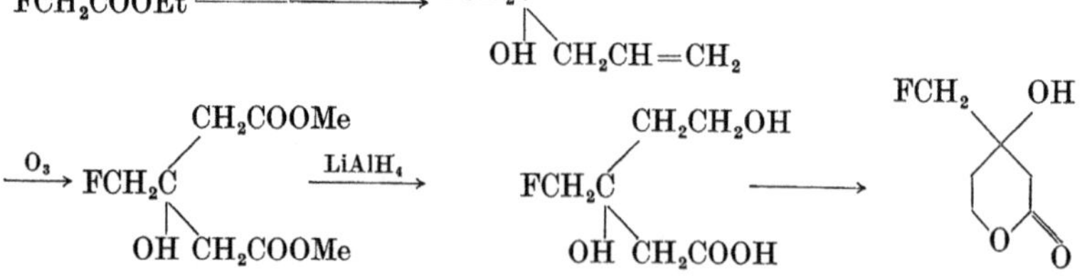

i) Fluorinated amino-acids

Several monofluorinated amino-acids have been prepared. The following will serve as representative examples:

(i) β-Fluoroalanine, $FCH_2CH(NH_2)COOH$ (Yüan et al. 1960):

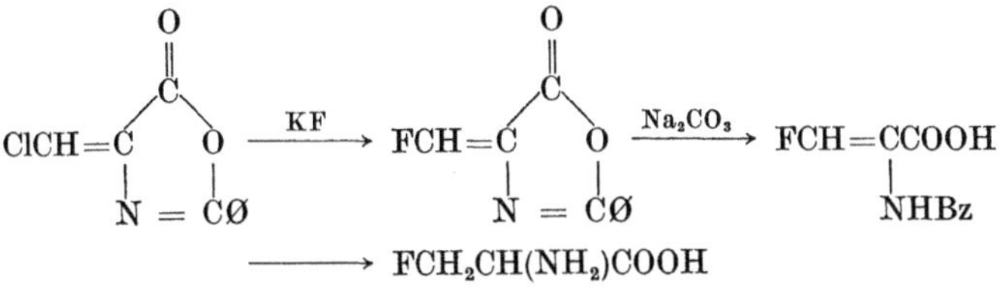

(ii) α-Fluoro-β-alanine, $H_2NCH_2CHFCOOH$ (Bergmann and Cohen 1961b):

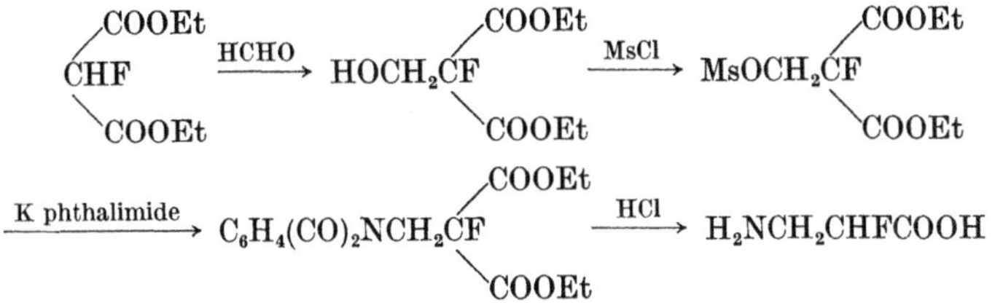

(iii) γ-Fluoroglutamic acid, $HOOCCH(NH_2)CH_2CHFCOOH$ (Hudlický 1961; Buchanan, Dean and Pattison 1962a):

$$(1)\ CH_2{=}CFCOOEt \xrightarrow{\text{Et acetamidomalonate}} (EtOOC)_2C(NHAc)CH_2CHFCOOEt$$

$$\xrightarrow{HCl} HOOCCH(NH_2)CH_2CHFCOOH$$

$$(2)\ CH_2{=}C(NHAc)COOEt \xrightarrow{CHF(COOEt)_2} EtOOCCH(NHAc)CH_2CF(COOEt)_2$$

$$\xrightarrow{HCl} HOOCCH(NH_2)CH_2CHFCOOH$$

(iv) 5-Fluoronorvaline and 6-fluoronorleucine (Raasch 1958b):

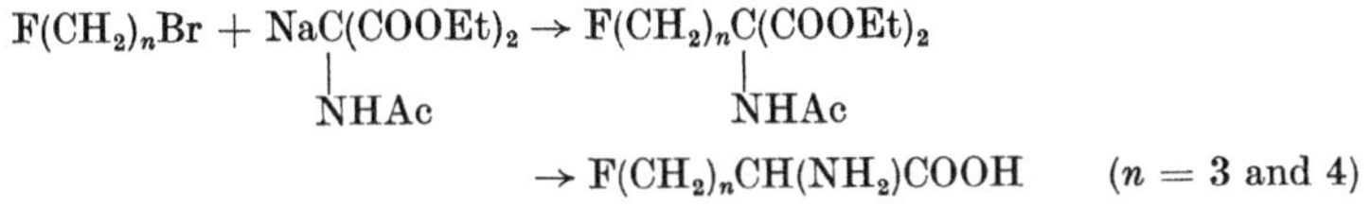

j) 2-Deoxy-2-fluoroglyceric acid, $HOCH_2CHFCOOH$

This acid was obtained (Kent et al. 1960) from 2-deoxy-2-fluoroglyceraldehyde (Taylor and Kent 1956) by oxidation with hypohalites:

$$HOCH_2CHFCHO \rightarrow HOCH_2CHFCOOH$$

5. Other ω-fluoro series

Many series of compounds containing an ω-fluorine atom have been prepared and reviewed (Pattison 1959). Their most interesting feature is that they give rise to an alternation of toxicity, depending on the number of carbon atoms in their chain; this is discussed in a later section (p. 440). The results provide a means of deducing the metabolic fate of the various functional groupings; that is, the fluorine atom is acting as a biochemical "tag." Among the series which give clearcut and explicable results are those listed below. The references cited are those which give both preparations and biological results; a more complete bibliography involving preparative details has been collected elsewhere (PATTISON 1959).

1-Fluoroalkanes, $CH_3(CH_2)_nF$ (PATTISON and NORMAN 1957)

ω,ω'-Difluoroalkanes, $F(CH_2)_nF$ (PATTISON and HOWELL 1956a)

ω-Fluoroalkynes, $F(CH_2)_nC{\equiv}CH$ (PATTISON and NORMAN 1957)

ω-Fluoroalkyl halides, $F(CH_2)_nX$ (PATTISON and HOWELL 1956a)

ω-Fluorocarboxylic acids (unbranched), $F(CH_2)_nCOOH$ (PATTISON, HUNT and STOTHERS 1956)

ω-Fluorocarboxylic acids (branched), $F(CH_2)_nCHMe(CH_2)_mCOOH$ (PATTISON and WOOLFORD 1957b)

ω-Fluoroalcohols, $F(CH_2)_nOH$ (PATTISON, HOWELL, MCNAMARA, SCHNEIDER and WALKER 1956), and derivatives (MILLINGTON and PATTISON 1956)

ω-Fluoroaldehydes, $F(CH_2)_nCHO$ (WILSHIRE and PATTISON 1956)

ω-Fluoroketones, $F(CH_2)_nCOR$ (FRASER, MILLINGTON and PATTISON 1957; PATTISON, COTT and HOWELL 1957)

ω-Fluoroalkyl ethers, $F(CH_2)_nOR$ (PATTISON, HOWELL and WOOLFORD 1957)

ω-Fluoronitriles, $F(CH_2)_nCN$ (PATTISON, COTT, HOWELL and WHITE 1956)

ω-Fluoro-ω'-nitroalkanes, $F(CH_2)_nNO_2$ (PATTISON, COTT, HOWELL and WHITE 1956)

ω-Fluoroalkylamines, $F(CH_2)_nNH_2$ (PATTISON, HOWELL and WHITE 1956)

ω-Fluoroalkyl thiocyanates, $F(CH_2)_nSCN$ (HOWELL, MILLINGTON and PATTISON 1956)

ω-Fluoroalkyl mercaptans, $F(CH_2)_nSH$ (HOWELL, MILLINGTON and PATTISON 1956)

ω-Fluoroalkanesulphonyl chlorides, $F(CH_2)_nSO_2Cl$ (MILLINGTON, BROWN and PATTISON 1956)

Miscellaneous nitrogen compounds (O'NEILL and PATTISON 1957).

The preparations of the above classes can be found in the cited references or in the review (PATTISON 1959). The fluorine was usually introduced by one of the methods listed in Section III C 1 (p. 393), and a variety of procedures was then adopted for the introduction of the other functional groups [Section III D 2 p. 408]. The following reactions are representative, and are taken from the literature sources quoted above.

$$2\,F(CH_2)_nCOOH \rightarrow F(CH_2)_{2n}F + 2\,CO_2 + H_2$$
$$F(CH_2)_nX + NaC{\equiv}CH \rightarrow F(CH_2)_nC{\equiv}CH + NaX$$
$$F(CH_2)_nOH + SOCl_2 \rightarrow F(CH_2)_nCl + SO_2 + HCl$$
$$F(CH_2)_{n-1}COOR \xrightarrow{LiAlH_4} F(CH_2)_nOH$$
$$F(CH_2)_{n-2}MgX \xrightarrow{(CH_2)_2O} F(CH_2)_nOH$$
$$F(CH_2)_nCH_2NO_2 \rightarrow F(CH_2)_nCH{=}N(\rightarrow O)ONa \rightarrow F(CH_2)_nCHO$$
$$F(CH_2)_nLi \xrightarrow{C_6H_5CN} F(CH_2)_nCOC_6H_5$$
$$F(CH_2)_nONa + IR \rightarrow F(CH_2)_nOR + NaI$$
$$F(CH_2)_nX + NaCN \rightarrow F(CH_2)_nCN + NaX$$
$$F(CH_2)_nCN \xrightarrow{LiAlH_4} F(CH_2)_nCH_2NH_2$$
$$F(CH_2)_nCOCl \rightarrow F(CH_2)_nCON_3 \rightarrow F(CH_2)_nNCO + N_2\,.$$

Monofluoroacetone, FCH_2COCH_3 has proved to be of biochemical interest. In addition to the earlier methods of preparation (PATTISON 1959), several new procedures have been described recently, of which the following two deserve special mention:

(1) $ClCH_2CH(OH)CH_3 \rightarrow FCH_2CH(OH)CH_3 \rightarrow FCH_2COCH_3$ (BERGMANN and COHEN 1958)

(2) $FCH_2COCl + (CH_3)_2Cd \rightarrow FCH_2COCH_3$ [84% yield] (VOONG et al. 1959)

Certain derivatives of glycerol have been found to have interesting biochemical properties; it is appropriate to mention their preparation at this point, although not all contain an ω-fluorine atom. TAYLOR and KENT (1956) have reported the preparation of 2-fluoro-1,3-propanediol (2-deoxy-2-fluoroglycerol) and 2-fluoro-3-hydroxypropanal (2-deoxy-2-fluoro-DL-glyceraldehyde) from diethyl fluoro-oxalacetate (q.v.) by the following reactions:

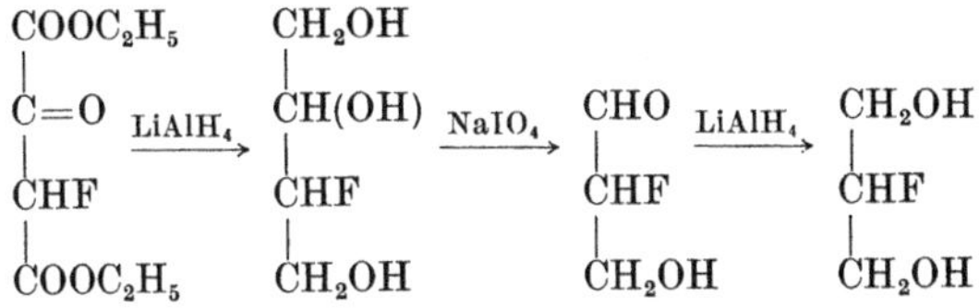

The isomeric compound, 3-fluoro-1,2-propanediol (DL-1-deoxy-1-fluoroglycerol) has been obtained (PATTISON and NORMAN 1957) from epifluorohydrin:

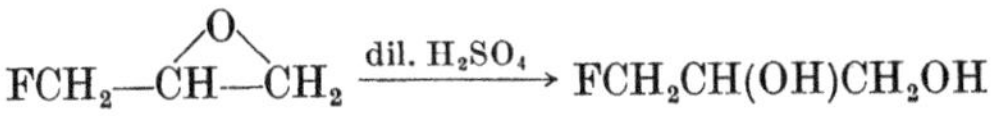

TAYLOR and KENT (1958) have prepared 6-deoxy-6-fluoro-α-D-galactose and 5-deoxy-5-fluoro-$\alpha\beta$-D-ribose by reaction of the appropriate methanesulphonate esters with potassium fluoride in hydroxylic solvents. The general procedure affords an elegant method for the introduction of fluorine into extracyclic positions of carbohydrate molecules.

D. Chemical properties

1. Stability of compounds containing the C-F bond

It has now been well established that, except in special cases involving the effect of neighbouring groups, the primary C—F bond is highly resistant to nucleophilic attack by such bases as hydroxide, alkoxide, malonate anion *etc.* Several fundamental studies attest to this assertion; a recent review (PARKER 1963) marshalls the evidence currently available. To compare the reactivity of the four halogen atoms, the relative rates of hydrolysis of the four methyl halides in water at 100° are significant (GLEW and MOELWYN-HUGHES 1952):

$$CH_3F : CH_3Cl : CH_3Br : CH_3I :: 1 : 25 : 300 : 100$$

HOFFMANN examined the action of sodium ethoxide and of potassium hydroxide on the following type pairs:

$Cl(CH_2)_nCl$ and $F(CH_2)_nF$ $[n = 2\text{—}6]$ (HOFFMANN 1949)

$Cl(CH_2)_nCl$ and $F(CH_2)_nCl$ $[n = 2\text{—}5]$ (HOFFMANN 1950)

$Br(CH_2)_nBr$ and $F(CH_2)_nBr$ $[n = 2\text{—}5]$ (HOFFMANN 1950)

The data obtained again proved that the primary fluorine is much more stable towards alkaline reagents than the corresponding chlorine and bromine atoms. CHAPMAN and LEVY (1952a) concluded, on the basis of a kinetic study, that, with ethanolic sodium ethoxide, primary alkyl fluorides undergo substitution at rates 10^3-10^4 times slower than those for the corresponding bromides. In short, there can be little doubt that the primary C—F bond is very much more stable than the C—Cl, C—Br and C—I bonds. The same conclusion can be extended to secondary and tertiary fluorides, which undergo elimination predominantly, at rates 10^5-10^6 times slower than those for the corresponding bromides (CHAPMAN and LEVY 1952a). In most instances, the greater stability of the C—F bond can be correlated with the considerable bond stretching necessary to attain the transition state.

The high solvation of the incipient fluoride ion in the transition state is undoubtedly a major factor in the breakage of the C–F bond, when it occurs; since this solvation is due to hydrogen bonding, it is reasonable to conclude that catalysis also by acids would be observed. This is indeed the case (PARKER 1963). The corresponding alkyl chlorides, on the other hand, do not show acid catalysis, because of the inability of chlorine to form strong hydrogen bonds. Several solvolytic reactions of alkyl halides which exhibit this acid catalysis have been shown to be autocatalytic, due to the influence of generated molecular hydrogen fluoride (CHAPMAN and LEVY 1952b).

The only well-established cases where alkyl fluorides appear to be more reactive than alkyl chlorides are in Friedel-Crafts alkylation and acylation reactions. This is well illustrated in the following reaction (OLAH 1963):

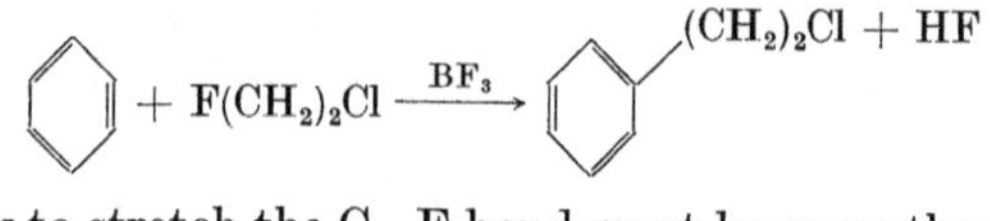

The extra energy necessary to stretch the C–F bond must be more than balanced by a greater gain of energy for the fluoride than the chloride; this probably arises from electrophilic catalysis by the Lewis acid. There is some evidence that fluorine is sometimes displaced in preference to other halogens in Grignard reactions of ω-fluoroalkyl halides; for example (PATTISON and HOWELL 1956b):

$$F(CH_2)_6Cl \xrightarrow[CO_2]{Mg} F(CH_2)_6COOH \quad \text{(predominant product); but}$$

$$F(CH_2)_6I \xrightarrow[CO_2]{Mg} I(CH_2)_6COOH \quad \text{(predominant product)}$$

The C–F bond is stable to catalytic hydrogenation at atmospheric pressure and low temperatures (HUDLICKÝ 1962); for example, 2-fluorohexyl nitrate is readily hydrogenolyzed (platinum) to 2-fluorohexanol in 67% yield (DEAN and PATTISON 1962). On the other hand, catalytic hydrogenation at high pressures and temperatures results in almost complete removal of the fluorine (PATTISON and SAUNDERS 1949; NEWMAN et al. 1948); for this reason, fluorinated alicyclic compounds are not available by catalytic hydrogenation of the corresponding fluorine-containing aromatic compounds. Nor is the reduction using active metals to be recommended: for example, Bouveault-Blanc reduction (NEWMAN et al. 1948) and lithium in liquid ammonia at room temperature (DEAR and PATTISON 1963) both result in considerable loss of fluorine. Zinc in propionic acid has been reported to convert 1,2-bromofluorocyclohexane to cyclohexene, a reaction analogous to that of other *vic*-dihalides (BOWERS et al. 1960). Of the metal hydrides, both sodium borohydride and lithium aluminum hydride have proved to be satisfactory (for example, see pp. 399, 409).

The structural environment of some covalently bonded fluorine atoms renders homolytic bond fission a relatively low energy process, in spite of the general stability of the C–F bond. For example, styrene fluorobromide, $C_6H_5CHFCH_2Br$ is readily hydrogenolyzed to ethylbenzene at room temperature and atmospheric pressure using platinum catalyst (DEAN and PATTISON 1962); the C–F bond scission is probably aided by the stability of the benzylic radical so formed. In contrast, 1,2-bromofluorocyclohexane under the same conditions is recovered unchanged. Again, α-fluoroesters lose fluorine under conditions of mild hydrogenation, aided by resonance stabilization of the intermediate $\left(-\dot{C}H-C{\overset{O}{\underset{OR}{\lessgtr}}} \leftrightarrow -C{=}C{\overset{O\cdot}{\underset{OR}{\lessgtr}}}\right)$;

however such stabilization is not possible with the α-fluorocarboxylate anion, and potassium 2-fluorohexanoate is unchanged under the same conditions.

The C—F bond is resistant to oxidative degradation under a wide variety of experimental conditions (see pp. 404, 408). Only in special cases has loss of fluorine been observed; for example, oxidation of styrene fluoronitrate, $C_6H_5CHFCH_2ONO_2$ gave benzoic acid. Such a transformation can again be correlated with resonance stabilization of the intermediate benzylic radical. This oxidative cleavage would be expected to be general for compounds possessing the C_6H_5CHF- grouping.

The presence and location of other groupings in the molecule can have a profound effect on the stability of the C—F bond. To take a simple example, the lower ω-fluorocarboxylic acids vary considerably in their behaviour to bases. Fluoroacetic acid, FCH_2COOH, being an α-fluoro acid, is susceptible to nucleophilic attack, and in fact loses its fluorine almost quantitatively on being heated with 30% aqueous sodium hydroxide for an hour (Mirosevic-Sorgo and Saunders 1959) or more (Peters and Shorthouse 1962). 3-Fluoropropionic acid, $F(CH_2)_2COOH$ readily undergoes β-elimination of hydrogen fluoride even with 10% sodium hydroxide. 4-Fluorobutyric acid, $F(CH_2)_3COOH$ and 5-fluorovaleric acid, $F(CH_2)_4COOH$ are unstable to alkali because of facile lactonization. But from this point on, 6-fluorohexanoic acid, $F(CH_2)_5COOH$ and higher ω-fluorocarboxylic acids are much more stable, approximating the behaviour of the alkyl fluorides discussed above.

Another example of the effect of an adjacent group centres around 2-fluoroethanol, $F(CH_2)_2OH$ (Bronnert and Saunders 1960). Because of the ready loss of hydrogen fluoride under nucleophilic conditions, ethylene oxide is transitorily formed, which in turn undergoes ring opening by the different reagents. For example, 2-fluoroethanol with phenylmagnesium bromide forms 2-phenylethanol, and with sodium phenate, 2-phenoxyethanol is formed.

The scission of the C—F bond by enzymes is being studied in different laboratories. There are two recorded instances of fluoride elimination from aromatic systems (Hughes and Saunders 1954; Ali et al. 1962), including such a simple molecule as *p*-fluorobenzoic acid. But of greater significance to the subject of this review is the report that the C—F bond in fluoroacetate is ruptured by soil microbes (Horiuchi 1962a) and by mammalian enzymes (Horiuchi 1962b). In the latter study, the excreta of the mouse dosed with sodium fluoroacetate (orally) contained four times the quantity of inorganic fluoride as those of the untreated mouse; in related work, the "rupture activity" of various mouse and rat organs was studied: the mouse had activity in the kidney, liver and intestine, whereas the rat had activity only in the intestine. These findings are not consistent with other work, and further study is required.

The instability of certain monofluoro compounds *per se* has recently been brought forcibly to the attention of one of us (Pattison 1962). It has been the practice to seal samples of all new, analytically pure, liquid fluorine compounds in glass ampoules and to store them in the dark; these were usually water-white. Now after some years, several of these have been exploding spontaneously, in some cases embedding glass in plaster walls twenty feet away. Clearly some kind of autocatalytic decomposition is occurring, in which hydrogen fluoride figures prominently. To show the diversity of compounds which have behaved in this way, the partial list below is given without further comment, other than the general warning that explosions of such highly toxic materials could be extremely dangerous.

1,2-Bromofluorocyclohexane, 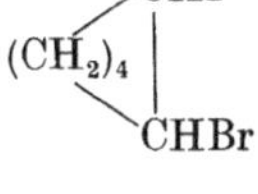

2-Fluoroethyl iodide, FCH_2CH_2I

2-Fluoroethyl oleate, $FCH_2CH_2OCOC_{17}H_{33}$

2-Fluoro-2-phenylethyl nitrate, $C_6H_5CHFCH_2ONO_2$ (very violent)

2-Fluoroethyl thiolacetate, $FCH_2CH_2SCOCH_3$

3-Fluoropropionyl chloride, FCH_2CH_2COCl (very violent)

1,4-Difluoro-2-butene, $FCH_2CH{=}CHCH_2F$

4-Fluorobutyl acetate, $F(CH_2)_4OCOCH_3$

4-Fluorobutanesulphonyl chloride, $F(CH_2)_4SO_2Cl$

4-Fluoro-4′-chlorodibutyl ether, $F(CH_2)_4O(CH_2)_4Cl$

5-Fluorovaleric acid, $F(CH_2)_4COOH$

2. Chemical reactions

In the above discussion, two points were stressed: (a) the C—F bond is much more stable than the C—Cl, C—Br and C—I bonds; and (b) neighbouring groups can have a considerable effect on the stability of the compound. Hence, it is relatively easy to predict the properties of most of the compounds described in this review.

In the fluoroacetate series, a wide variety of common organic reactions can be carried out without appreciable loss of fluorine. The α-fluorine atom of fluoroacetic acid is more prone to nucleophilic attack than the fluorine of the long-chain members, so some caution must be observed when employing strongly basic reaction conditions. Similarly, 2-fluoroethanol is less stable than the long-chain ω-fluoroalcohols, as mentioned above. Some of the many types of reactions which have been reported have been reviewed (Pattison 1959); these include oxidation, reduction, hydrolysis, substitution, dehydration, *etc.*

The C—F bond in the long-chain compounds can survive under a wide range of experimental conditions (Pattison 1959). The reactions below illustrate this point.

a) Halide substitution reactions

$$F(CH_2)_nX + KCN \rightarrow F(CH_2)_nCN + KX$$
$$F(CH_2)_nX + AgNO_2 \rightarrow F(CH_2)_nNO_2 + AgX$$
$$F(CH_2)_nX + AgNO_3 \rightarrow F(CH_2)_nONO_2 + AgX$$
$$F(CH_2)_nX + KSCN \rightarrow F(CH_2)_nSCN + KX$$
$$F(CH_2)_nX + MC{\equiv}CH \rightarrow F(CH_2)_nC{\equiv}HC + MX \quad (M{=}Na,\ Li\ etc.)$$
$$F(CH_2)_nX + AgOSO_2R \rightarrow F(CH_2)_nOSO_2R + AgX$$
$$F(CH_2)_nX + NaCH(COOEt)_2 \rightarrow F(CH_2)_nCH(COOEt)_2 + NaX\,.$$

b) Organometallic reactions

$$F(CH_2)_nX + Mg \rightarrow F(CH_2)_nMgX \rightarrow \text{acids, esters, ketones, alcohols, aldehydes } etc.$$
$$F(CH_2)_nX + \text{Li or } n\text{-BuLi} \rightarrow F(CH_2)_nLi \rightarrow \text{ketones, alcohols, } etc.$$

c) Anodic coupling reactions

$$2\ F(CH_2)_nCOOH \rightarrow F(CH_2)_{2n}F + 2\ CO_2 + H_2$$
$$F(CH_2)_nCOOH + HOOC(CH_2)_mX \rightarrow F(CH_2)_{n+m}X + 2\ CO_2 + H_2$$

d) Cyanoethylation

$$F(CH_2)_nOH + CH_2{=}CHCN \rightarrow F(CH_2)_nOCH_2CH_2CN\,.$$

e) Diels-Alder reactions

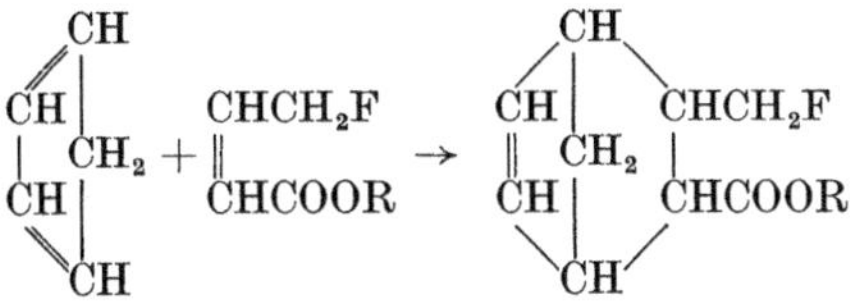

f) Lithium aluminium hydride reductions

$F(CH_2)_nCOOH \rightarrow F(CH_2)_nCH_2OH$

$F(CH_2)_nCOOR \rightarrow F(CH_2)_nCH_2OH$

$F(CH_2)_nCN \rightarrow F(CH_2)_nCH_2NH_2$

$F(CH_2)_nNO_2 \rightarrow F(CH_2)_nNH_2$

$F(CH_2)_nSCN \rightarrow F(CH_2)_nSH$

g) Barbier-Wieland degradation

$$F(CH_2)_nCH_2COOR \rightarrow F(CH_2)_nCH_2C(OH)(C_6H_5)_2 \rightarrow F(CH_2)_nCH{=}C(C_6H_5)_2 \rightarrow F(CH_2)_nCOOH$$

h) Arndt-Eistert synthesis

$$F(CH_2)_nCOOH \rightarrow F(CH_2)_nCOCHN_2 \rightarrow F(CH_2)_nCH{=}C{=}O \rightarrow F(CH_2)_nCH_2COOH$$

i) Acetylenic syntheses

$F(CH_2)_nC{\equiv}CH \rightarrow F(CH_2)_nCH{=}CH_2 \rightarrow F(CH_2)_nCH_2CH_3$

$F(CH_2)_nC{\equiv}CH \rightarrow F(CH_2)_nC{\equiv}CMgX \rightarrow F(CH_2)_nC{\equiv}CCOOH$, *etc.*

$F(CH_2)_nC{\equiv}CH \rightarrow F(CH_2)_nC{\equiv}CX$

$F(CH_2)_nC{\equiv}CH \rightarrow F(CH_2)_nC{\equiv}CR$

IV. Physiology and biochemistry

In the first sections we have described the major chemical compounds concerned in this field. We now take up the question how these compounds produce their effects *in vivo*.

A. The toxic signs

We may first ask the question what are the toxic effects of these compounds in the animal. The toxic signs, after a dose of fluoroacetate, are to be seen in the heart and in the central nervous system. The emphasis upon one or the other depends largely upon the animal. Table 1a gives an approximate idea of the doses which are toxic with different animals. Though there may be wide variation, such as for rats of different strains, there is seen to be a different order as between some of the animals. For instance the dog shows mainly an attack upon the central nervous system, whereas animals such as the sheep and the rabbit show cardiac effects. In the rat both are attacked. There is always a time interval before the signs appear. In the rat this is about 30 mins. One extraordinary feature is the variation in the level of dosage which induces toxic signs. In the dog, it is about 60 µg/kg, though there have been statements that some dogs are sensitive to 20 µg/kg (Miura et al. 1956). The sheep requires about 300 µg/kg, the rat about 5 mg/kg and the frog about 300 mg/kg. Even for one kind of animal there is

Table 1a. *Toxicity of methyl and sodium fluoroacetate (various estimates)*[1,2]

	Methyl fluoroacetate				Sodium fluoroacetate	
	LD_{50} mg/kg	Responses: cardiac	Responses: CNS	LD_{50} mg/kg	LD_{50} mg/kg	LD_{100} mg/kg
Group I						
rabbit	0.2—0.25 (iv)	ventricular fibrillation	none	0.5 (or), 0.5—1.0 (sc)	0.3	0.7—0.8
goat	0.6 (iv)	"	none	<1.0 (or, sc)	0.7	
horse	0.5—1.75 (im)	"	none		1.0	5.0
spider monkey	14.0 (iv)	"	none			
sheep						0.25—0.5
Group II						
cat	0.5 (iv)	slight	marked	<0.3 (or), 0.3 (sc)	0.3	
pig	0.4 (ip)	response heart	brain about equal		0.3	1.0
Rhesus monkey	4.0 (iv)	ventricular fibrillation	very slight	10—12 (or, sc)	5.0—7.5	
Group III						
dog	0.06 (iv)	none	marked	0.1—0.2 (or, sc)	0.1—0.2	
guinea pig	0.35 (ip)	none	marked	0.4 (or); 0.2 (sc)		
Group IV					5.0—7.0 albino rat	
rat	5.0 (im, sc), 4 (or)	atypical		3—4 (or), 2—3 (sc)	3.0—7.0 Norway rat 1.0—4.0 black rat	
hamster	2.5—5.0 (ip)	atypical				
Other species						
mouse				6—7 (or), 5 (sc)	8.0—10.0	
fowl					6.0—7.0	14.0
Source of data:	Chenoweth and Gilman (1946)			Foss (1948)	Meldrum et al. (1957)	

[1] See also Chenoweth (1949).
[2] iv, intravenous; or, oral; sc, subcutaneous; im, intramuscular; ip, intraperitoneal.

Table 1b. *Toxicity of methyl fluoroacetate, mortality of rabbits following intravenous injection*

Dose mg/kg	Total animals injected	Total animals dying	Per cent mortality
0.15	10	0	0
0.20	10	1	10
0.25	16	9	56
0.50	101	94	94

Data from Chenoweth and Gilman (1946), which show the steep rise in toxicity between 0.2 and 0.25 mg/kg.

variation (see Table 1b); and as in other animal tests, it is advisable to work out the lethal doses for the animals with which one is working, as they are likely to vary under different conditions. In the case of the rat, Fig. 3 shows the tetanic fit, which is induced by dosing with fluoroacetate, and the state upon coming from the fit. An animal may have several such fits before it succumbs. The object of biochemical research is to determine the nature of the biochemical lesion or lesions which give rise to these effects, and to explain the other peculiarities such as the variation in the response of the animals.

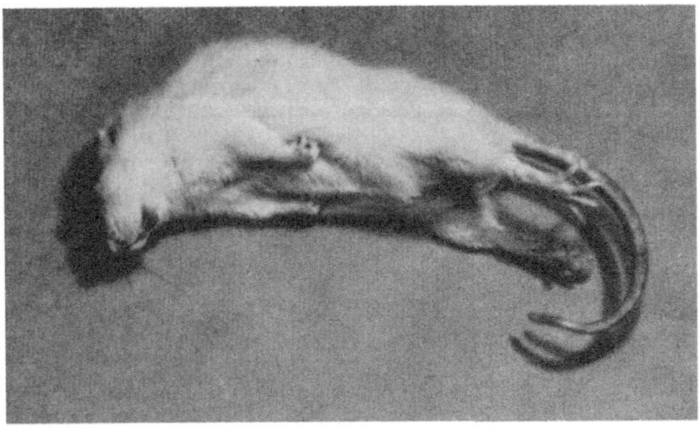

Fig. 3a

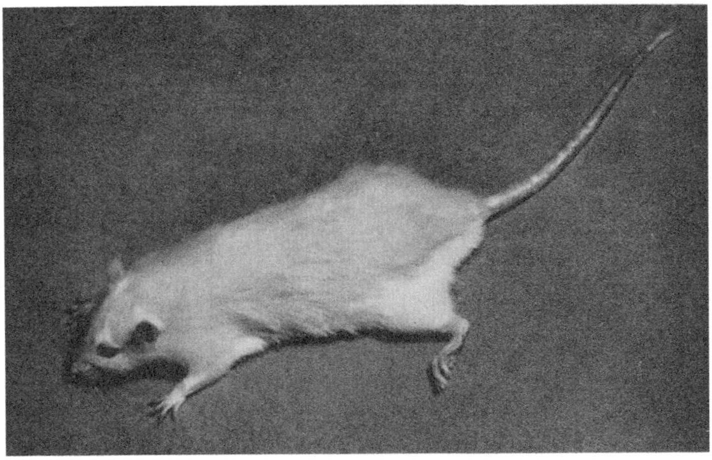

Fig. 3b

Fig. 3. Tetanic fit induced with fluoroacetate (PETERS, 1951). (a) fit: (b) recovering

B. The biochemistry

Early attempts were made in 1940–1941 (DIXON and NEEDHAM 1946) to find whether fluoroacetate had some effect upon enzymes in various preparations from tissues. These met with little success, and it became clear in 1947, that fluoroacetate as such had no effect at all upon isolated enzymes or those are organized in mitochondria (BARTLETT and BARRON 1947; KALNITSKY and BARRON 1947). The only exception known to this is that of the glyoxalate system, in a specialized bacterium (KORNBERG and ELSDEN 1961; GOTTO and KORNBERG 1961). At the same time it became evident that the effect of the compound is quite different from that of inorganic fluoride (LIÉBECQ and PETERS 1949). Table 2 gives a direct experiment upon this point. Rather earlier, the organic chemists as mentioned on p. 440 (BUCKLE, PATTISON and SAUNDERS 1949) had found the remarkable fact that in a series of ω-substituted fatty acids, there was alternation in toxicity, in the sense that even numbered carbon acids were toxic whereas acids of the odd numbered series, of which fluoropropionate is the lowest member, were either non-toxic or showed much less toxicity. This was exactly like the Knoop rule for the degradation of fatty acids, and suggested that it was the breakdown to the

Table 2. *Pigeon brain homogenate*

The effect of sodium fluoroacetate and sodium fluoride upon the oxygen uptake (in µl/bottle) of sodium pyruvate (9.1 mM) in the presence of sodium fumarate (3.3 mM).

Exp.		O_2 uptake (30 min)	
2631[1,2]	No inhibitor	426	
	NaF (24 mM)	262	38% inhibition
	NaFlAc (16.6 mM)	439	No inhibition
2643[3,4]	No inhibitor	99	
	NaFlAc (7.5 mM)	96.5	No inhibition

[1] Residual O_2 uptake not substracted.
[2] Dialysed preparation ($4^1/_2$ hr), completed with 0.19 mM adenylic acid and 1.33 mM Mg^{++}: 220 mg tissue.
[3] Residual O_2 uptake substracted.
[4] Undialysed preparation: 167 mg tissue.
Data of LIÉBECQ and PETERS (1949).

two-carbon product which was the toxic factor. In 1948, two sets of workers independently suggested that the toxic product was not fluoroacetate itself but a six-carbon acid derived from this. The experiments with thoroughly washed

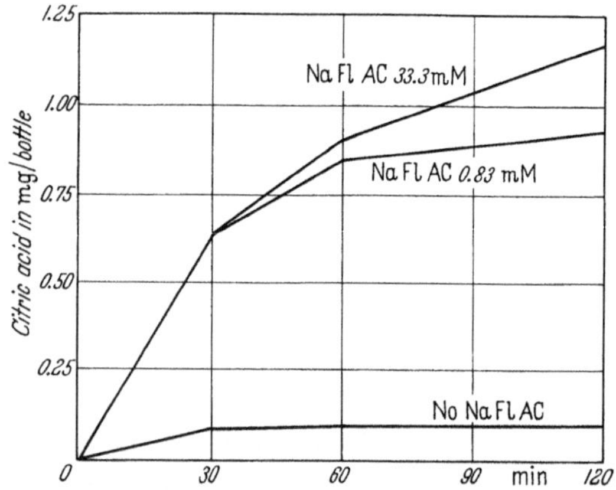

Fig. 4. Homogenate of cortex of guinea pig kidney, suitably reinforced with magnesium, phosphate and adenosine triphosphate. Kidney preparation thoroughly washed. Temp., 38° C. The curves show the accumulation of citrate in presence and absence of fluoroacetate. Data of LIEBECQ and PETERS (1949)

kidney particles (mitochondria) were especially convincing because other constituents of the cells had been eliminated (LIÉBECQ and PETERS 1949) (Fig. 4); but the other experiments were important in which it was shown that minced ox heart was blocked at the citric acid stage (MARTIUS 1949). This effect upon the metabolism of citrate was found to occur also *in vivo* (BUFFA and PETERS 1949) so that the biochemical lesion was evidently in the last stage of the metabolism concerned with citrate. A large rise in citrate concentration one to two hours after dosing was found in rats given a lethal dose of fluoroacetate, occurring in many organs of the body (Table 3.) These observations were confirmed and extended by POTTER and BUSCH (1950); the time course of citrate accumulation was also investigated by LINDENBAUM et al. (1951) in rats given sub-lethal doses of fluoroacetate. They found that a rapid increase in citrate occurred in the first hour after dosing followed by a slower rise to a maximum in 4 hours. After this the citrate levels subsided to the normal in approx. 24 hours.

Table 3. *Accumulation of citrate in the rat.* Data of BUFFA and PETERS (1949)

Tissue	Citric acid (µg/g wet tissue)					
	Controls			Poisoned		
	Animals tested	Average	Range	Animals tested	Average	Range
Blood	4	3	0—8	4	50	31—88
Brain	7	21	0—46	7	166	118—271
Heart	10	25	0—58	7	677	558—810
Kidney	8	14	0—48	8	1036	854—1220
Spleen	3	0	0	4	413	304—468
Liver	4	0.8	0—3	4	31	13—72
Lung	3	9	0—27	4	257	229—293
Stomach	3	37	19—53	4	386	297—457
Small intestine	3	36	25—53	4	368	157—535
Large intestine	3	21	10—38	4	248	193—338
Uterus[1]	3	217	179—276	4	207	158—300

[1] Virgin animals.

Dose NaFlAc, 5 mg/kg body weight, dissolved in 0.5 ml 0.9% NaCl; controls injected with 0.5 ml 0.9% NaCl. Animals killed 60 min after the injection.

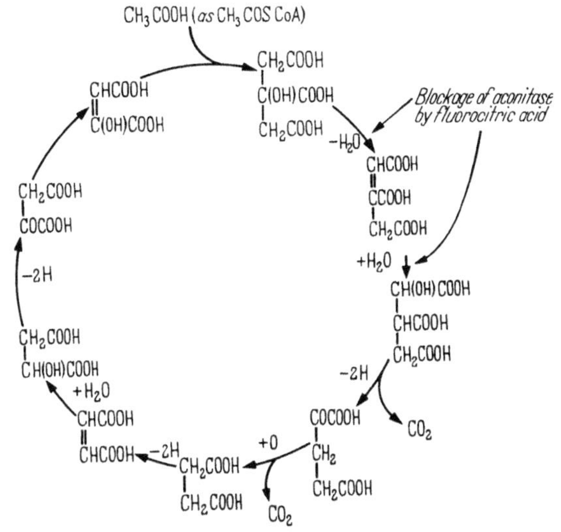

Fig. 5. The tricarboxylic acid cycle. Specific enzymes are not included. Although most of the reactions are reversible, the cycle is probably unidirectional in operation, and is shown as such in this simplified schematic representation. From PATTISON (1959)

The rise in citrate suggested to LIÉBECQ and PETERS and to MARTIUS independently that a synthesis had taken place to some fluoro compound from fluoroacetate via the citric acid cycle (Fig. 5). Proof of this idea of a synthesis required the isolation of the unknown fluoro-inhibitory substance formed from fluoroacetate.

The isolation of this factor took some time; but it was finally obtained from kidney particle preparations treated with fluoroacetate; it proved to be fluorocitrate (see p. 391). From this it became clear that the "condensing enzyme" which is responsible for combining acetyl CoA with oxaloacetate, was not distinguishing between acetate and fluoroacetate. The latter was being synthesized to fluorocitrate by combination with oxaloacetate in the tricarboxylic cycle of reactions. Once formed the fluorocitrate must be acting as a blocking agent. This process has been called "lethal synthesis" (PETERS 1952). It is illustrated in the diagram (Fig. 6). It is of course the opposite of the so-called protective synthesis, in which a synthesis in the body can induce detoxification of a foreign molecule. Fluorocitrate has now been synthesized (see page 401). As would be expected from its asymmetric centres, the synthetic fluorocitrate is not more than half as active as the biosynthetic product. Related work suggests that the stereochemistry may be even more complicated (KACSER 1955).

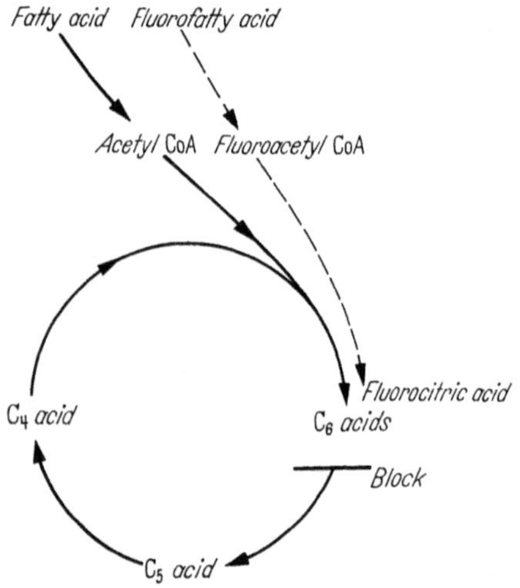

Fig. 6. Diagram illustrating the course of lethal synthesis of fluorocitrate via the citric acid cycle

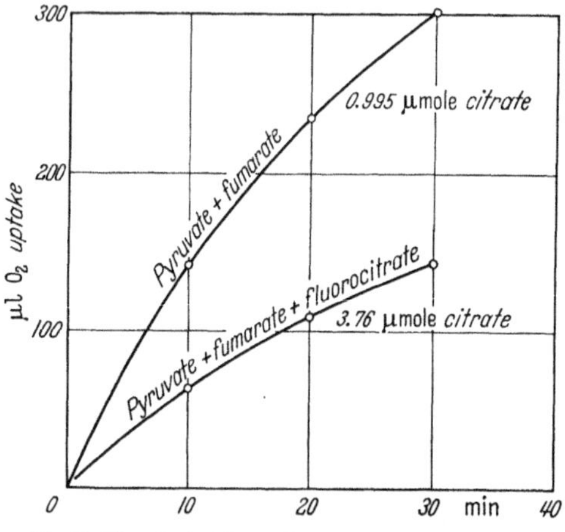

Fig. 7. The effect of fluorocitrate on the oxygen uptake and citrate accumulation in homogenates of pigeon brain. Tissue, approx. 200 mg/bottle. Temp. 38° C. Each bottle contained 27 µmole pyruvate, fumarate, ATP, magnesium chloride, phosphate buffer and potassium chloride with or without fluorocitrate. Data of PETERS and WAKELIN (1953)

One of the best proofs that fluorocitrate is the main active inhibitory substance comes from injection experiments into the brain. When introduced into the subarachnoid space of the pigeon's skull (under anaesthesia), fluorocitrate can produce convulsions and death in a few minutes, whereas much larger injections of fluoroacetate are without effect. Even as little as 11 µg of fluorocitrate has killed a pigeon. A similar state can be induced with fluorocitrate injections into the brains of young rats (DAWSON and PETERS 1955), or into the sub-arachnoid space in the rabbit (HASTINGS et al. 1953, 1955; PETERS, WAKELIN and HASTINGS 1953). At a more biochemical level, another experiment can be made which bears upon this proof of toxicity. With mitochondria prepared in potassium chloride solution from the brain of the pigeon, fluoroacetate has no effect upon the oxygen uptake in presence of pyruvate and fumarate, whereas fluorocitrate in small concentration causes a fall in oxygen uptake with an increased accumulation of citrate (Fig. 7) (PETERS and WAKELIN 1953).

Though fluorocitrate appears to be the main substance responsible for toxicity of fluoroacetate, there are probably small amounts of other substances made in the tissues. For example, PHILLIPS and LANGDON showed (1955) that some fluoride entered into the lipid substances in the liver after injections of fluoroacetate. The products have not been shown to be toxic.

In Table 4 a comparison is made between the effects of intraperitoneal injection of fluoroacetate and fluorocitrate, from which it is seen that fluorocitrate has a much larger effect on the citrate accumulation of liver tissue.

Table 4. *Effect of intraperitoneal injections of fluoroacetate and of fluorocitrate (synthetic) on the accumulation of citrate in male rats; animals sacrificed 2 hrs. after dosing.* Data of GAL, PETERS and WAKELIN (1956)

Tissue	Fluoroacetate dose 5 mg/kg	Fluorocitrate	
		dose 20 mg/kg	dose 80 mg/kg
Brain	178	151	364
Heart	798	108	365
Kidney	1020	1230	3060
Liver	33.5	812	1720
Spleen	596	510	635
No. of animals	(2)	(4)	(4)
Convulsions	+	None	+

Av. wt. of rats 50 ± 5 g. Results expressed as µg of citrate/g of wet tissue. Normal values are for brain 20 ± 6, kidney 29 ± 13 and liver 3.5 ± 0.4 mg/kg.

Note the difference between fluoroacetate and fluorocitrate.

C. Some practical applications

As mentioned, the rise in citrate concentration in the tissues takes place mainly in the first hour and is complete after 4 hours; after this time a gradual fall occurs, the return to the normal being practically complete in 24 hours (LINDENBAUM et al. 1951). This accumulation of citrate with sublethal doses has been found to protect against lead poisoning (FRIED et al. 1956) and more recently against the damage caused by radiation (BACQ et al. 1960; see also BACQ and ALEXANDER 1961). In the experiments of BACQ et al., if sodium fluoroacetate were injected into the peritoneum of mice in a dose of 4—5 mg/kg five hours before irradiation, the mortality produced by a dose of 650 to 675 r irradiating the whole body was reduced. At the same time the high levels of citrate in the poisoned animals returned to normal within 24 hours of this irradiation as compared with 48 hours required for non-irradiated control mice. Their interpretation of this was that the fluoroacetate induced accumulation of citrate in the mitochondria; this in turn protected the animals by complexing the magnesium ions required for the activity of deoxy ribonuclease (E.C. DNA-ase 3.1.4.5.), the activity of which they think is responsible for radiation damage (see also ORD and STOCKEN 1953).

D. Citrate accumulations in other animals

Though there has not been a complete investigation, where the effect of fluoroacetate has been tested, it has been found to induce citrate accumulations in other animals. The effect in frogs and toads is especially interesting, because these animals require enormous doses to cause death, of the order of 500 mg/kg. BUFFA and PETERS (1949) found that there was a slow rise in the citrate amounts in the central nervous system of the frog; the Japanese workers (MIURA et al. 1961), found a large increase in the liver, kidney and heart after oral doses of 500 mg/kg of fluoroacetate in the bull frog, *Rana catesbyana*. The rise occurred over a period of six hours. A similar rise occurred *in vitro* in liver enzyme preparations, though the amounts of fluoroacetate used *in vitro* were rather larger than the ones which were used with the kidneys of guinea pigs. They have established the essential similarity of the poisoning; but it still leaves the problem whether the effect is due to failure of lethal synthesis of fluorocitrate or to failure to synthesize enough fluorocitrate quickly. We have tested this (MURRAY and PETERS in unpublished experiments) by finding out the dose of fluorocitrate which will kill the animals. Using *Rana pipiens*, it was found in a few experiments that injections of fluoroacetate killed slowly; an injection of synthetic fluorocitrate (50 mg/kg) killed an animal within 24 hours. Such an amount of fluorocitrate is equivalent in terms of active fluorine to 4.5 mg/kg of fluoroacetate, so that it seems that the large doses required are due to failure of the frog to convert fluoroacetate sufficiently quickly to fluorocitrate. It was found in our experiments that fluoroacetate was not excreted. More work could be done on this problem with profit.

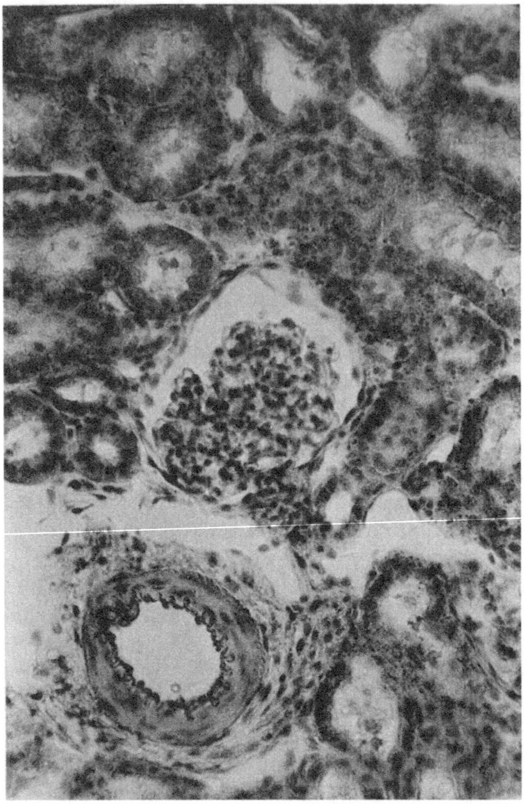

Fig. 8. Kidney of non-tumour bearing rat, acute death 2 hr after fluorocitrate 60 mg/kg, i.p., (containg 6.9 mg of active isomer). The tubule below the left glomerulus shows hyaline droplet. degeneration of the cells, with blockage of the lumen. There is exudate in the capsular spaces. Picro-Mallory. (Data of CATER and PETERS)

E. Effects on the kidney in vivo

All of these observations can be inferred to be due to the initial formation of fluorocitrate; and it is interesting to note that the direct injection of fluorocitrate in a lethal and impure dose (60 mg/kg of a synthetic specimen) is accompanied by profound changes in the kidney. This is equivalent to approximately 12 mg/kg of biosynthetic fluorocitrate. In animals dying in two hours the epithelium of the proximal convoluted tubules is stripped (CATER and PETERS 1961), and shed into the urine as casts. The condition resembles certain forms of poisoning by metals; Figs. 8, 9 show some of these changes and are to be compared with the normal kidney (Fig. 10). The condition will render the animals anuric, though the best information is that this would be unlikely in itself to cause the death of the animal, as uraemia kills slowly. Death is more likely to be due to the effect upon the heart.

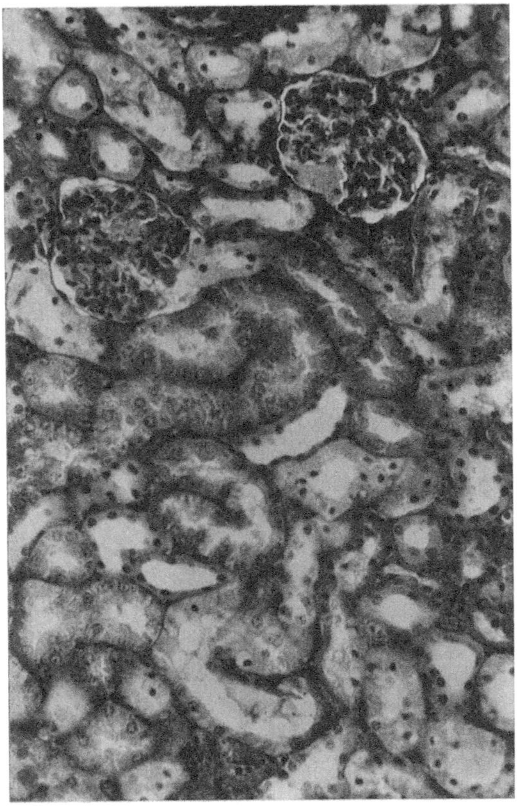

Fig. 9

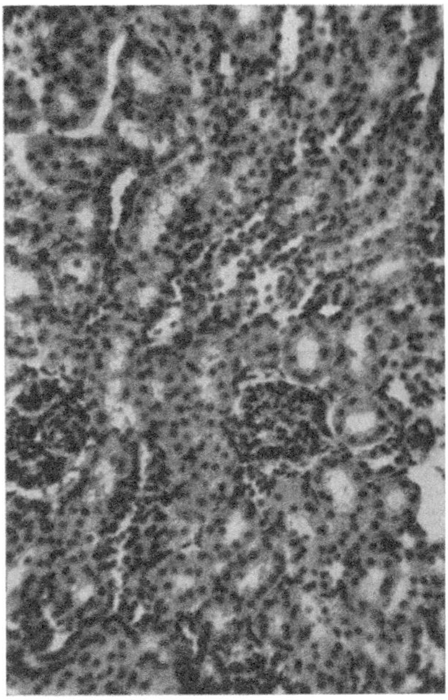

Fig. 10

Fig. 9. Kidney of hepatoma-bearing rat killed 24 hours after 4 doses of fluorocitrate, total 46 mg/kg (containing 5.3 mg/kg of active isomer). The small artery shows lipid in the muscular coat and all the tubular cells show numerous small lipid droplets. Frozen sections Scharlach R. (Data of CATER and PETERS)

Fig. 10. Normal kidney. Section frozen and stained with Scharlach R. Lower magnification than Figs. 8 and 9. From CATER and PETERS (1961)

F. The biochemical lesion

We come now to the question of the biochemical lesion induced by the lethal synthesis of fluorocitrate. Theoretically, there are several possibilities.

(1) Any interference along the enzymatic chains in the citric acid cycle might dam back the reactions at the aconitase stage. Alternatively,

(2) There might be a direct effect on the isocitrate dehydrogenase (L_s-isocitrate; NADP oxidoreductase, E.C. 1.1.1.42.). Finally,

(3) There might be a direct effect upon the enzyme aconitase (aconitate hydratase, E.C. 4.2.1.3.).

Though (1) cannot be excluded as a possibility, there are several arguments against it. For instance the poisoning of rat brain *in vivo* diminishes the amount of α-ketoglutarate present (DAWSON 1953). By direct tests, (2) has been excluded, and all the evidence now points to (3), that is, the direct inhibition of aconitase (Fig. 11).

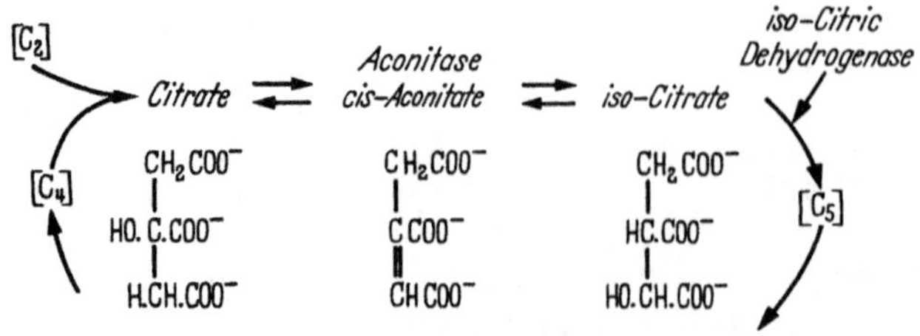

Fig. 11. The reactions of the tricarboxylic acid cycle effected by the enzymes aconitase and isocitric dehydrogenase. At equilibrium about 90 % is citrate. From PETERS (1963)

G. Reactions of aconitase

Early indications that all three stages of the reaction of aconitase were inhibited (LOTSPEICH et al. 1952) have been established thoroughly in later work (MORRISON 1954). Some remarks are required about aconitase, an enzyme characterized by MARTIUS (1938, 1937). This enzyme has a specific requirement for ferrous ion,

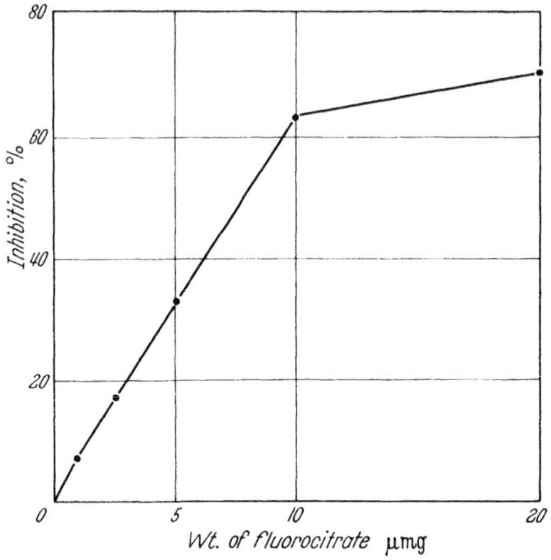

Fig. 12. Inhibition of aconitase by enzymic fluorocitric acid (activated). The enzyme was preincubated in the presence and absence of fluorocitrate for 10 min without isocitrate. The experiment was started by adding DL-isocitrate (2176 μmoles) and observing formation of *cis*-aconitate for 4 min. The ordinate scale represents the change in absorption at 240 mμ from 0.5—4.0 min, as percentage inhibition. From PETERS (1961)

(DICKMAN and CLOUTIER 1951). When purified it loses its Fe^{++} and can then be reactivated by treating with Fe^{++} and a reducing agent, preferably cysteine. MORRISON 1954 (following BUCHANAN and ANFINSEN 1949) succeeded in purifying it to a high activity. In this state the reactivated enzyme was inhibited by fluorocitrate so far as could be ascertained equally in all its reactions[1]. On the whole there was not the inhibition expected with enzymatic fluorocitrate, though there

[1] This has always been the experience of PETERS and colleagues with the soluble preparations of aconitase. From rats poisoned with fluoroacetate BUSCH and POTTER (1952) described an experiment in which there was a block in citrate metabolism in tissues separated from the animals, though not in *cis*-aconitate.

were results with synthetic fluorocitrate to be discussed below. In later work (PETERS 1961), it has been found that if the enzyme is used at a less highly purified stage it is much more sensitive to fluorocitrate; that is to say at a stage when about 50% is still in a state where it does not need reactivation with Fe^{2+} and cysteine. It will be seen from the results given in Fig. 12 that the enzyme is then nearly as sensitive as the cholinesterase to the phosphorus insecticide inhibitors. This means that there is a form of isolated and soluble aconitase which is at least as sensitive to fluorocitrate as is that of the aconitase in the kidney mitochondria. Again, using this preparation, the synthetic aconitase is about half as sensitive to the synthetic fluorocitrate as to the biosynthetic; it may be less.

At the same time there are still some experimental results which have not been explained. In their work with the purified enzyme requiring activation, MORRISON and PETERS (1954) got results in which synthetic fluorocitrate appeared to be more toxic than the biosynthetic. Even later than this when working with one synthetic preparation it was found that one peak from the silicic acid column (see page 400) was a very powerful inhibitor. This has not appeared again. It is possible that more recent work may ultimately explain the discrepancy. In an interesting paper, FANSHIER et al. (1962) have carried the information about the fluorocitrates further, though at the same time they introduced us to further complications. They have confirmed the fact that fluorocitrate is not estimated as citrate by the permanganate method of PUCHER et al. (1936), WARD and PETERS (1961) and also extended the finding of PETERS (1961) that a less pure preparation of the aconitase enzyme preparation is better inhibited by fluorocitrate than the more purified which requires activation by Fe^{++} and cysteine. They have studied the enzymatic synthesis of a fluorocitrate formed from β-fluorooxalacetate and acetyl-S-CoA. This enzymatic preparation is differently synthesized from that formed naturally upon exposure of fluoroacetate to kidney preparations, as in this latter case the fluorine atom is introduced to the condensing enzyme as fluoroacetyl CoA. Their enzymatic fluorocitrate, which we can designate as II, is only slightly inhibitory to the aconitase in their kidney mitochondrial preparation, made by freezing and extracting the mitochondria; but it is more inhibitory than their chemically synthesized fluorocitrate to the mixed enzymes in the preparation. It is to be noted that the inhibitions are induced by concentrations of 10^{-4} M fluorocitrate, whereas the soluble aconitase studied by PETERS (1961) was sensitive to inhibition down to 10^{-8} M. There is evidently much work to be done in this field; especially when the suggestion is considered that there will be more than 4 isomers, if it matters to the enzymatic chemistry whether the fluorine is introduced on the C_2 or C_4 fragment.

MORRISON and PETERS (1954) thought that the effect of fluorocitrate on aconitase was reversible when the amount of isocitrate was increased five times. This was illusory. Later work with the enzyme not requiring reactivation (PETERS 1961) showed that even a little *cis*aconitate formed from isocitrate (10 µg in the cuvettes, approx. 0.03 mM) was enough to inhibit the stage isocitrate-cisaconitate. When larger amounts of isocitrate were added *at the start* of the reaction, even a large excess of isocitrate did not reduce the inhibition to less than 8%. Hence it is not to be expected that it is easy to reverse a fluorocitrate inhibition *in vivo*.

H. Other reactions of fluoroacetate

As mentioned above, the lethal synthesis of fluorocitrate is not the only reaction of fluoroacetate in the animals *in vivo*. The observations of PHILLIPS and LANGDON (1955) on liver have been extended using radioactive fluoroacetate marked with

C^{14} in the FCH_2 group, and widened to include other organs (GAL et al. 1961). They found a small and variable amount of radioactive CO_2 excreted by the lungs in rats after injection of the labelled compound. This did not exceed 3%. The accompanying Table 5 shows the percentage recovery of the label from the various fractions of different tissues. It will be seen how the liver predominates, followed by the lungs which had about $^1/_3$ that of the liver. In the case of the liver, fractionation showed that the bulk of the label was in the steam volatile fraction; a small amount was recovered in the lipids and a trifling amount in the protein (0.1%). Much less fluorocitrate was recovered from the liver than from the kidney. It is to be noted that the amount of fluorocitrate excreted in the urine represented only 3% of the total radioactivity injected. One fact not known is the degree of incorporation into various glands other than the liver and thymus. This does not seem to have been studied in other organs except the thyroid, which is well known to have a high concentration of citrate. In some microorganisms (see page 434, 436), it is probable that fluoromalate can be made from fluoroacetate.

Table 5. *Distribution of radioactivity administered as fluoroacetate-2-C^{14} in organs at 4 hours.* Data of GAL, DREWES and TAYLOR (1961)

Tissue	Wet weight of tissue (g)	Radioactivity found (counts/min)	Percentage recovery	Concentration of label µg fluoroacetate per g wet weight
Brain	1.33	28,131	2.26	26.9
Heart	0.93	15,624	1.26	21.4
Kidneys	1.95	30,834	2.49	20.1
Liver	8.47	148,311	11.95	22.3
Lungs	3.82	50,306	4.05	16.8
Intestines and stomach	9.60	128,330	10.33	17.0
Carcass	115.00	740,523	59.70	8.2
Testes	2.50	28,325	2.28	14.4
Spleen	1.96	24,905	2.00	16.2
Urine		6,230	0.50	
Total			96.82	

Sodium fluoroacetate-2-C^{14} (1,241,300 counts/min or 10.53 mg/kg) was intraperitoneally given per animal. Results are averages of three animals.

I. Protection and antidotes

By "protection" is meant the injection of a substance before or at the same time as the administration of the poison; this would thus be before the formation of fluorocitrate, and therefore essentially would result in the prevention of the synthesis of fluorocitrate. Several attempts have been made in this direction over the years. In one series of experiments (TOURTELOTTE and COON 1949, 1951; HUTCHENS et al. 1949), it was claimed that alcohol was a good antidote, but this seems to be mainly confined to a few animals. More promising, is the effect of monoacetin, which was introduced by CHENOWETH and colleagues (CHENOWETH et al. 1951). This compound is stated to be effective as a protecting agent in the case of the rat, if given within 8 minutes after giving the poison.

It has been claimed by GITTER (1953, 1956) that acetamide in large doses has a similar protective effect, and GITTER has supported this opinion by the finding that it lowers the amount of citrate formed in rats and guinea pigs. However there seems to be some difficulty in the use of acetamide because L. R. Murray tells one of us that they have not been able (unpublished work) to repeat the cure of guinea pigs with acetamide in Alice Springs, Australia. The matter seems to merit further attention, because acetamide has been added to preparations of fluoroacetamide used for killing flies in the belief that the toxicity is so reduced.

Attempts to find a true antidote in the sense that it could reverse the effect of fluorocitrate once this has been formed have been tackled by one of us (R.A.P.) with colleagues over many years with tests at the level of the soluble aconitase

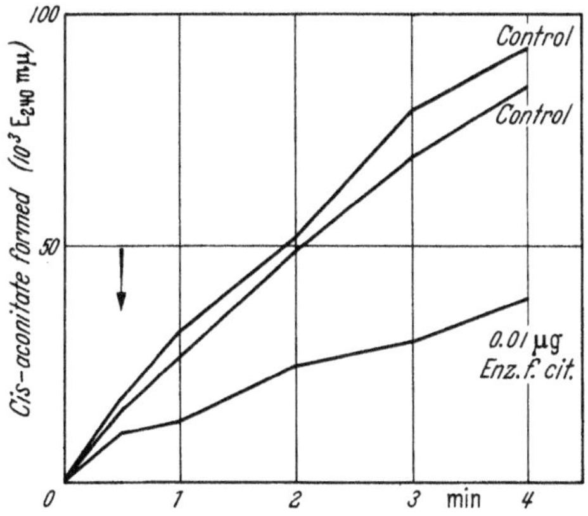

Fig. 13 a

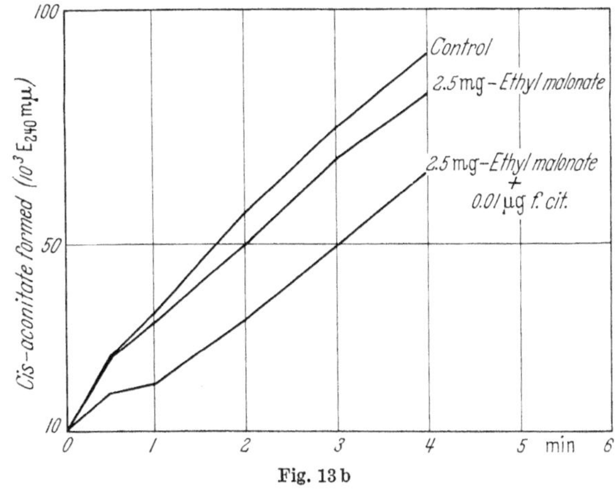

Fig. 13 b

Fig. 13. Aconitase. Reversal of the inhibitory effect of fluorocitrate by ethyl malonate. After previous preincubation with and without fluorocitrate, isocitrate was added and the reaction studied over 4 min, *iso*-citrate → *cis*-aconitate. Calculations were made over the period 0.5—4.0 min (PETERS and LEGGE, see PETERS, 1963). (a) shows the inhibition produced by 0.01 μg fluorocitrate; (b) shows the effect of addition of 2.5 mg ethyl malonate in reducing the inhibition of the fluorocitrate. Alone, ethyl malonate had little effect.

enzyme, the mitochondrial preparation and the whole animal. Most of this work has not been published; a very large number of substances, over 400, have been tried, and of these the most effective substances at the level of the soluble enzyme have been malonates. Fig. 13a, b gives such a result. When tried *in vivo* with some of these compounds we have succeeded in tiding the animal over the convulsive period. Eventually however the rats become quiescent as if they had been dosed with a barbiturate; they go steadily downhill, and die within 10 to 24 hours. The cause of this is not yet known.

J. The biochemical behaviour of fluoro-oleic and other long chain ω-fluoro fatty acids

Mention has been made already of the isolation of fluoro-oleic acid (page 390) and some other long chain fatty acids from natural sources, and of the synthesis and testing for toxicity of many fatty acids and allied compounds. In fact the capacity for inducing citrate accumulation is one method of exploring the pathway for the biochemical conversion of compounds like nitriles (see page 440).

1. Fluoro-oleic acid

This compound like other long-chain ω-fluoro fatty acids is more easily activated by mitochondrial preparations from the kidney of the guinea pig, than is fluoroacetate. Even a few micrograms in 3.0 ml *in vitro* are enough to produce a marked accumulation of citrate, from which a synthesis of fluorocitrate can be inferred (PETERS et al. 1959). In the testing of the long-chain fatty acids *in vitro*, one has to remember that fatty acids by themselves in sufficient concentration may be toxic, and therefore may interfere with the condensing enzyme necessary for the conversion of oxaloacetate and fluoroacetyl CoA (page 413) into fluorocitrate. For details of an experiment see Table 6. It is clear that the odd-even rule applies to the longer chain acids when acting *in vitro;* for instance the accompanying figure makes this clear (Fig. 14 for the C_{12} and C_{13} acids).

Table 6. *Non-specific effects of long chain fatty acids on the synthesis of citric acid from fumarate by mitochondria from guinea pig kidney.* Data of PETERS et al. (1959)

Mitochondria in 1.0% potassium chloride solution containing phosphate buffer were reinforced with magnesium chloride and adenosine triphosphate. Substrate sodium fumarate. Temp. 38° C. Time 40 min. Sodium fluorocitrate was added unless stated to block citrate metabolism.

Additions	Citrate synthesized (µmoles)
None	6.23
None (no fluorocitrate)	0.20[1]
Sodium palmitate (200 µg) . .	1.55
Sodium laurate (100 µg) . . .	0.28
Sodium oleate (50 µg)	0.56

[1] Citrate was metabolized further in absence of fluorocitrate.

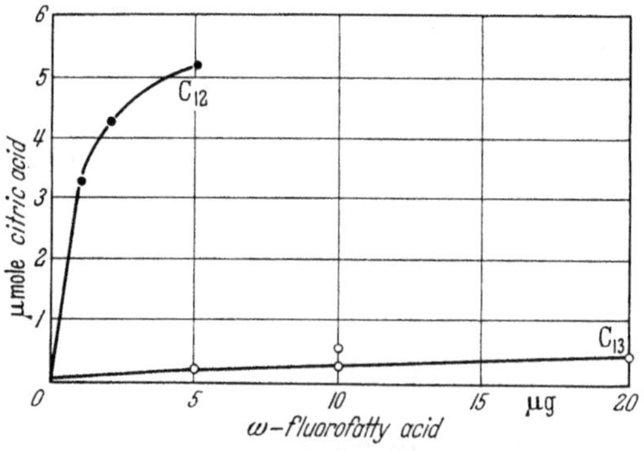

Fig. 14. Comparison of the inhibitory effect on citrate metabolism by kidney mitochondria of a C_{12} and C_{13} ω-fluorofatty acid. C_{12} blocked; C_{13} was without effect. The synthetic acids were supplied by one of us (FLMP). From PETERS (1958)

The clinical effects of the long-chain acids are different from those of fluoroacetate. Table 7 gives the citrate accumulations after dosing with ω-fluorodecanoic acid as compared with fluoroacetate, from which it will be seen that the amounts in heart and kidney are reversed. This indeed is in line with the effects

Table 7. *Comparative values for citrate accumulation in heart and kidney after dosing with fluoroacetate or fluorodecanoate, by intraperitoneal route.* Data of PETERS (1957)

	Citrate, μg/g tissue (wet)	
	Heart	Kidney
Fluoroacetate (5—10 mg/kg)	677	1000
Fluorodecanoate (10 mg/kg)	1070	240
Fluorodecanoate (5 mg/kg)	698	314

in vivo. With fluoro-oleic acid, the sheep/rabbit toxicity ratio is reversed as compared with fluoroacetate, and from observations the rabbit seems to die suddenly after dosing with the acid, with a typical heart attack. A similar sign can be observed in the sheep. For instance one animal in our experiments (PETERS and HALL 1960b) remained normal for 5 days and then suddenly died within three hours. The condition has been explained by J. H. WHITTEM (1963) who found evidence in the heart of the sheep of a cloudy swelling ranging to frank necrosis of the myocardial fibres. ANNISON et al. (1960) found that sheep given sublethal doses of fluoroacetate at intervals sometimes succumbed to a final small dose. In this case too, it may be due to a damage of the heart. One case of a rat poisoned by fluorodecanoate was studied by one of the authors (R.A.P.) with Sir Alan Drury. From the electrical responses of the heart it was found that the rate of the heart beat was more affected than the rhythm.

2. Other long-chain ω-fluoro fatty acids

$$F(CH_2)_nCOOH \quad (n \geqq 3)$$

Earlier in all this work CHENOWETH and colleagues (KANDEL and CHENOWETH 1952a, b; HENDERSHOT and CHENOWETH 1954, 1955), studied the behaviour of fluorobutyrate and of fluorohexanoate, finding that these were activated in a rather similar manner to fluoroacetate and that there might be an accumulation of citrate (see POTTER and BUSCH 1950). It was curious that monoacetin was not an effective antidote against fluorobutyrate, but that monobutyrin afforded protection. Presumably these deal with the appropriate stages in activation by the enzymes of the fatty acid cycle.

K. The actual activating substance

It would be expected that fluoroacetyl-CoA would be the actual substance which is condensed with oxaloacetate to form fluorocitrate; this has been proved by BRADY (1955) in a very clear piece of work. This being the case, it must be realized that it is not strictly accurate to speak of breakdown of the long-chain fatty acid to fluoroacetate; rather one should think in terms of formation of fluoroacetyl-CoA. When this is realized it becomes easier to understand the anomalous behaviour of a compound like fluoroacetyl fluoroacetate, where the preformed fluoroacetyl group may form fluoroacetyl-CoA more readily. BRADY found some interesting facts about the action of fluoroacetyl-S-CoA. With thiol transacetylase, fluoroacetylation of 2-mercaptoethanol by fluoroacetyl-S-CoA occurred. Using the condensing enzyme and oxaloacetate, the initial condensation to fluorocitrate was slower than that with acetyl-S-CoA (Fig. 15). But in a system arranged to synthesize acetoacetate, the reaction velocity again was more rapid with acetyl-S-CoA though the affinity for the condensing enzyme was greater.

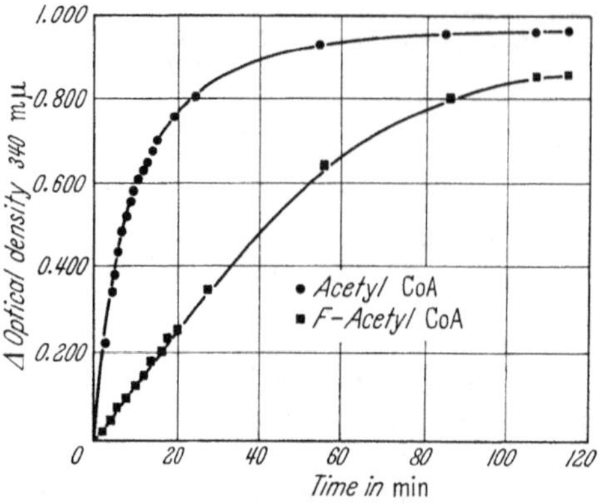

Fig. 15. The experiment shows the reaction of fluoro-acetyl-S-CoA with oxaloacetate in the presence of crystalline condensing enzyme. The oxaloacetate was supplied from L-malate and NAD (nicotinamide adenine dinucleotide) with malic dehydrogenase. The curves represent a spectrophotometric measurement of the reaction with acetyl CoA and fluoroacetyl CoA. Data of BRADY (1955)

L. Fluoroacetate activation

We can understand from the above facts how the reactions leading to fluorocitrate occur ultimately through fluoroacetyl-S-CoA, and that therefore the formation of fluorocitrate only shows that fluoroacetyl-S-CoA has been formed, whether this arises from a short chain fatty acid or by degradation of a long chain one. When we consider the conversion of fluoroacetate itself to fluoroacetyl-S-CoA we have to consider a special activation. It appears that the center which activates fluoroacetate is not the same as that which activates acetate, or rather the usual acetate activating center, because it has been shown by several workers (BRADY 1955, DOMINGUEZ et al. 1954, PETERS 1952, ROSE et al. 1954) that the usual acetate-activating system prepared from "acetoned" liver of a pigeon does not activate fluoroacetate. Yet there must be some connection with acetate activation because it has been established (PETERS 1955; PETERS and WAKELIN 1957) that in kidney homogenates acetate in $^1/_{20}$ molar concentration (Fig. 16) inhibits the synthesis of fluorocitrate *in vitro*. (The conditions for this proof were difficult to establish; they finally involved using pigeon brain homegenates to estimate the fluorocitrate formed from the kidney homogenates blocked with malonate.) Hence there must be some activating enzyme which can act both upon fluoroacetate and

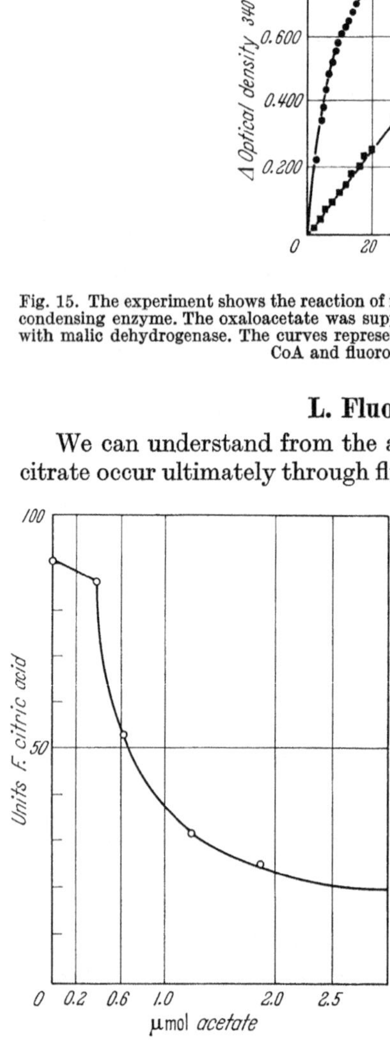

Fig. 16. Inhibitory effect of acetate upon the synthesis of fluorocitric acid by kidney particles as determined with kidney particles; substrate, malate and fluoroacetate 20 μmole/3 ml. From PETERS (1963)

acetate, which is different from the usual acetate-activating enzyme. Attempts by BRADY and by ourselves to isolate this enzyme have proved ineffective. We (TREBLE, SHAWDON and PETERS, unpublished work) have confirmed the observation of BRADY that cysteine must be present at the stage of dialysis to retain the activity of the enzyme, and we have also found activity in the sheep as well as in the rabbit kidney, but attempts to take the isolation further have not succeeded in our hands. The diagram (Fig. 17) represents the above facts. Whichever way we look at it, the main toxic reaction in the animal seems to be due to the conversion of the mono-fluoro compound to fluoroacetyl-S-CoA and the subsequent formation of fluorocitrate, via the condensing enzyme. This reaction can be used in two ways, both of them involving block of aconitase with the consequent accumulation of citrate. Either it can be used as mentioned to test whether a metabolite enters the citric acid cycle or whether in the course of its metabolism it passes through the stage of fluoroacetyl-S-CoA. From this angle one understands why there is no block in oxidative phosphorylation (JUDAH and REES 1953, 1954;

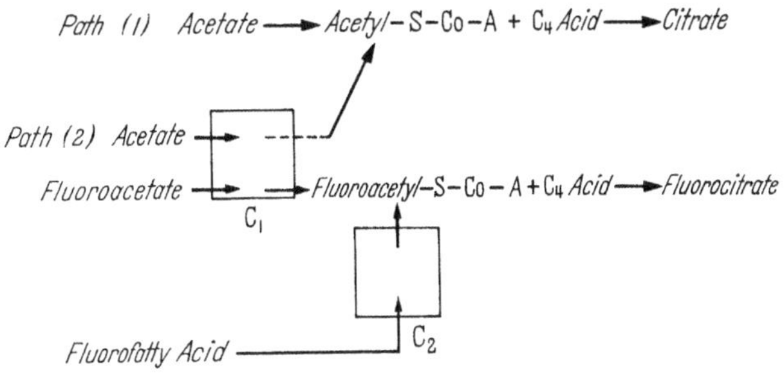

Fig. 17. Scheme suggested for the synthesis of fluorocitrate, showing the presence of one independent pathway (path 1) for acetate activation via the pigeon liver preparation. From PETERS (1963)

GAL 1960) unless this involves in some way the enzyme aconitase. It is a fact that *in vitro* in kidney homogenates, as the concentration of citrate is increased, there is increasing disappearance of citrate without an accompanying increase of uptake of O_2 (ELLIOTT and KALNITSKY, 1950). This fact may be explained by recent work on citrate cleavage (LOWENSTEIN 1963). With mammary gland, TERNER (1955) has extended to this the earlier results of LIÉBECQ and PETERS (1949), confirming for this tissue the main facts found for kidney, and at the same time adding new facts, among which was the interesting point that fluoroacetate had an inhibitory effect upon the metabolism of acetate. It appears that the situation with regard to acetate is analogous to the facts found by TREBLE (1962) for fluoroethanol (see page 438), where the identification of a second alcohol dehydrogenase in liver made clear that one enzyme was inhibited, and that the other oxidized fluoroethanol. In any case we have to explain why in some experiments acetate inhibits formation of fluorocitrate, and in others fluoroacetate inhibits acetate oxidation. In regard to intermediates in the formation of fluoroacetyl-S-CoA, MARCUS and ELLIOTT (1956) and ELLIOTT and MARCUS (1955, 1958, 1959) found that fluoroacetyl phosphate can react in the transacetylase and the acetokinase reactions.

M. Kidney and renal transport

Some of the above facts make it easier to interpret the excellent work by FARAH et al. (1953, 1955) on kidney *in vivo*. They found that in the anaesthetized dog sodium fluoroacetate reduced renal blood flow and the clearance of *p*-aminohippurate (PAH), creatinine and inulin, as well as reducing PAH and glucose transport maximum. If sodium acetate was infused, it protected against the effects of the fluorine compound on the PAH secretory mechanism. But once the fluoroacetate effects had occurred, acetate could not reverse them. The interpretation of this appears to be that acetate, as in the experiments of PETERS and WAKELIN (1957) *in vitro*, was preventing the synthesis of fluoroacetyl-S-CoA and so the formation of fluorocitrate which once formed was not then affected by acetate. In their experiments, protection was found with acetate, pyruvate, butyrate, valerate and monoacetin *in vitro*.

N. Effect on the whole animal

1. Effects upon ketone and glucose metabolism

When we come to the whole animal, the effect must be necessarily more complex. Not only have we to consider the accumulation of fluorocitrate in individual organs as revealed by the height of citrate accumulation, but also the more complex effects which depend upon changes in the circulation and upon blood vessels,

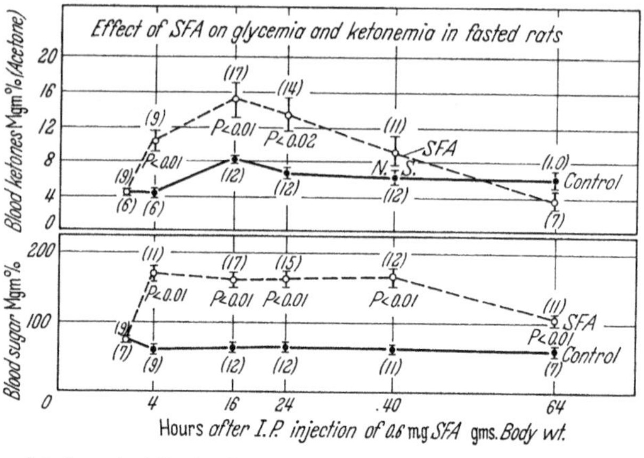

Fig. 18. Glycemia and ketonemia following intraperitoneal injection of 0.6 mg sodium fluoroacetate/100 g in fasted rats. From COLE et al. (1955)

and also the concomitant effects upon the endocrine glands. That there are these actions has been known for a long time. The ketonuria following the feeding of butyric acid was increased by fluoroacetate (BEATTY and WEST 1951), and in rats injections of fluorocitrate led to an appearance of ketone bodies in the urine (GAL et al. 1956). Also fluoroacetate increased the synthesis of acetoacetate *in vitro* in liver (BUSCH and POTTER 1952). On the side of glucose metabolism, fluoroacetate increased the level of the blood sugar *in vivo* (ELLIOTT and PHILLIPS 1954).

A more complete study of these interesting interrelationships has been made by ENGEL and colleagues (COLE et al. 1954, 1955; ENGEL et al. 1954). Their work showed how far-reaching may be the effects in the whole animal of a biochemical lesion in one enzyme, in this case "aconitase." Fig. 18 indicates the effects upon the blood levels of glucose and of blood acetone following the injection of 6 mg/kg of sodium fluoroacetate in fasted rats. They termed the glycaemia "SFA diabetes." The rise in ketone bodies (ketonaemia) took place rapidly, and the glycaemia appeared in 3 hours and lasted for 64 hours; there was also an increase in the lactate concentration in the blood. The administration of the fatty acid octanoate increased the ketonaemia, which was reduced by glycerol and monoacetin as also by a previous treatment with cortisone. They considered that the effects of the hyperglycaemia were "either secondary to the effects of sodium fluoroacetate on the tissues or to a more specific effect on insulin production by the beta cells of the pancreas," and that there might be a fall in the hexokinase activity with a

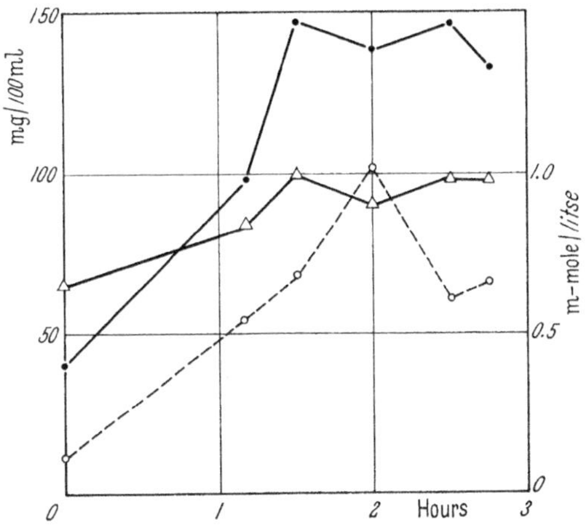

Fig. 19. Changes in some blood constituents in a sheep after giving a single lethal injection (intravenous, 0.4 mg/kg) of sodium fluoroacetate at time 0. Blood acetate (mM/l), △; blood glucose (mg/100 ml), ●; blood lactate (mg/100 ml), ○. Annison et al. (1960)

declining supply of high energy phosphate. Some other facts were obtained in sheep by Annison et al. (1960). Sublethal doses of fluoroacetate (0.1 mg/kg) were given to sheep at intervals of several days. After each of these there might occur

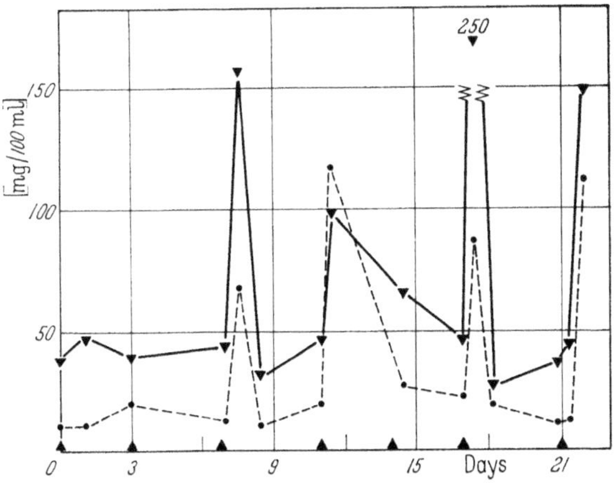

Fig. 20. Similar to Fig. 19 but showing changes following successive administration of a non-lethal dose of sodium fluoroacetate (0.1 mg/kg). Injection of sodium fluoroacetate, ▲; blood glucose, ▼; blood lactate, ●. From Annison et al. (1960)

(Fig. 19, 20) a sharp rise in the concentration of glucose and of lactate in the blood, these returning to normal within 12 hours. In the experiments in sheep quoted in this work there was not always a rise in concentration of ketone bodies in the blood, nor was there always a significant change in the blood in fatty acids and in non-esterified fatty acids. In other sheep subjected to a similar treatment, these striking rises in sugar and lactate did not occur. Hence it seems that the effects on the glycaemia and on the ketonaemia may vary with different animals. The ketonaemia in the sheep did not ever attain the high levels observed by COLE et al. (1955) in the rat. Since there was also a precipitous fall in the glycogen content of the liver and of the abdominal muscle, it is possible that the rapid mobilization of tissue glycogen could account for the glycaemia. D. B. LINDSAY (see ANNISON et al. 1960) has shown that in the sheep as in man (GORDON and CHERKES 1956), the injection of adrenalin may increase the amount of non-esterified fatty acids in the blood, and he has suggested that the glycaemia and lactic acidaemia may be due in fact in this animal to a release of adrenalin, perhaps owing to an intense sympathetic stimulation. From these interesting results we are forced to conclude that there is still more to learn about the effects of these compounds in the whole animal, effects which are very important, because it is well-known to workers in this field that the injection of fluoroacetate into rats is followed by profound shock-like effects in addition to the well known convulsive effects on the nervous system. Some of the shock may be possibly explained by the reduction of the rate of the heart beat and by the hypothermia (BUFFA et al. 1960a; STONER 1956; BACQ et al. 1960); but it seems that there may be effects upon the sympathetic system also, in view of the marked vasoconstriction usually seen in the ears of poisoned rats. In this same field there should be mentioned the isolation of mono-fluoroacetone from the livers of rats perfused with fluoroacetate (MIURA and HORI 1961).

In assessing the effects upon the formation of ketone bodies in the whole animal, one should not overlook the experiments of PEETERS et al. (1953, 1954) on the isolated and perfused udder of the cow. After poisoning with fluoroacetate, the perfusion of acetate with glucose led to an increase of 10 times in the amount of the acetoacetate formed, a fact consistent with the idea that a block in the citric acid cycle can lead to a diversion of acetyl-S-CoA into the metabolic pathway of the ketones.

O. Effects upon isolated muscle tissue

1. Smooth muscle from the rabbit intestine

Three groups of authors (FURCHGOTT and SCHORR 1946; FARAH et al. 1950; WEEKS and CHENOWETH 1949) agree that spontaneous contractions of the muscle strips are abolished by fluoroacetate in presence of acetate, pyruvate and oxalo-acetate. Spontaneous contractions may still occur in the presence of glucose. The observations other than on spontaneous contractions can be explained by the formation of fluorocitrate and its effect upon the energy supply. The spontaneous contractions in glucose solution may be due to reactions connected with the pentose-phosphate cycle.

An observation by CLARKE and RIKER (1950) has always been difficult to reconcile with the view that the main action of fluoroacetate was on "aconitase" after its conversion to fluorocitrate. They found (p. 126 of their paper) that caffeinated frog sartorius muscles, when stood for 2 hours in 0.001 M fluoro-acetate, formed much less lactate under aerobicc onditions than the controls, whereas a block in oxidation of pyruvate should have increased the lactate. This may be explained by some recent observations in Cambridge. GARLAND, NEW-SHOLME and RANDLE (personal communication to R.A.P.) have found that accumulations of citrate can block glycolysis by a feed-back mechanism at the phosphofructokinase stage. This would decrease the formation of pyruvate, and so of lactate.

2. Muscles poisoned in vivo

Comparison of respiration (in Krebs-pyruvate solution) of diaphragmatic muscles and dorsal muscles from the rat, together with citric formation with and without poisoning by fluoroacetate has been made by BUFFA et al. (1960b), with the results shown in Table 8. Though the citrate increased in both, only the dorsal muscle showed a diminution in Q_{O_2} with pyruvate. Oxidative phosphorylation was unaffected (see also FAIRHURST et al. *in vitro* 1958). In another study, it was

Table 8. *Respiration of rat muscles in Krebs-pyruvate solution with and without fluoroacetate.* Data of BUFFA et al. (1960b)

Wt., mg	Diaphragm			Dorsal		
	Control	FAc	Percentage decrease	Control	FAc	Percentage decrease
	Respiratory Quotient Q_{O_2}					
69	13.09	11.76	10	6.00	4.60	23
97	11.62	10.30	11.3	5.48	3.48	36.5
143	8.55	8.24	3.9	4.46	2.47	44.5
No change in P : O ratio, nor in oxidative phosphorylation						
	Citrate formation, μg/g tissue					
	30.5	574		16	253	

found that there was a gradual diminution in the amount of energy-rich phosphate compounds in muscle, though the phosphorylation capacity was not affected *in vivo*.

3. Cardiac muscle

Effects of fluoroacetate upon the heart-lung preparation of the dog have been studied by FAWAZ (1956); a cardiac insufficiency was induced, its severity depending upon the dose. While the citrate content of the muscle increased up to 20 times, no trace of this reached the blood. There was a lowering of the amount of creatine-phosphate, about 60%, but the change in the ATP was much less, under −10%. It is interesting that the heart can tolerate such large amounts of citrate, and suggests that it may be the slowed rate which causes death from heart failure. See also REILLY et al. (1953).

P. Studies on acids and other compounds related to the citric acid cycle

1. Fluoromalamide $H_2NCOCHFCH(OH)CONH_2$

It was found by GAL et al. (1956) (Table 9) that fluoromalamide (presumably converted to fluoromalate) at 300 mg/kg had little effect when it was injected into rats; diethyl fluorooxaloacetate at 150 mg/kg induced a slight rise in the citrate content of the kidney with no effect on the brain or the liver. Dimethyl fluoromalate had virtually no action at 150 mg/kg; but this experiment with esters needs repetition with Na salts, because it is now known that di- and tri-esters unlike monoesters are sometimes not converted to the corresponding acids in the body.

2. 2-Fluoroacetohydroxamic acid $FCH_2CONHOH$

2-Fluoroacetohydroxamic acid was interesting, because at 8.0 mg/kg a slight rise was found in the citrate content of the brain. There was no rise in the liver but a substantial increase in the kidney from 29 to 251 μg/g citrate in the tissues. Nevertheless this caused convulsions. The accumulation of citrate is consistent with the idea that the hydroxamate gives rise to fluoroacetate *in vivo*. The problem arises whether other monofluoro acids have any effects upon enzymes *in vitro*. Some of these compounds can be considered individually.

Table 9. *The effect of some fluorocompounds on citrate production in the rat*[1]

Formula	Compound	Dose mg/kg	Citric acid, μg/g		
			Brain	Kidney	Liver
$F\cdot CH_2\cdot COO^-$	Fluoroacetate[2,3]	5.0	180	1000	57
$F\cdot CH_2\cdot CO\cdot COO^-$	Fluoropyruvate[3]	80.0	36	42	23
$F\cdot CH\cdot COO^-$ | $CO\cdot COO^-$	Fluorooxaloacetate (as diester)	150.0	53	344	16
$F\cdot CH\cdot CONH_2$ | $HO\cdot CH\cdot CONH_2$	Fluoromalamide	300.0	46	125	62
$F\cdot CH\cdot COO^-$ | $HOC\cdot H\cdot COO^-$	Fluoromalate (as dimethyl ester)	150	43	48	16
$F\cdot CH_2\cdot CONH_2$	Fluoroacetamide[3]	10	120	247	20
$F\cdot CH\cdot COO^-$ | $HOC\cdot COO^-$ | $HCH\cdot COO^-$	Fluorocitrate[2,3] (synthetic)[4]	40	240	2500	1200
Control	None	—	39	45	52

[1] Data of GAL et al. (1956b).
[2] Inhibits citrate metabolism in rats.
[3] Causing convulsions.
[4] Fluorocitrate (synthetic), not purified. Rises of citrate seen in heart, which are usually greater than in the kidney.
Fluoroacetohydroxamic acid at 8.0 μg/kg, slight rise in kidney. Causes convulsions. Fluorolactate has been found non-toxic.

3. Fluoromalic acid HOOCCHFCH(OH)COOH

It was shown by GAL (1960) that fluoromalate inhibited the nicotinamide adenine dinucleotide phosphate (NADP) dependent malic dehydrogenase in liver from the pigeon and chicken; it required a thousand times higher concentration of fluorocitrate to do this (see also STICKLAND 1959)[1]. With liver preparations, the following results were obtained (Table 10):

Table 10. *Effects on the malic enzyme of purified particulate systems from liver. All flasks contained* 2.7×10^{-2} *M pyruvate and* 1.2×10^{-2} *M* $KHCO_3$. *Temperature, 37°.* Selected results from GAL (1960)

Inhibitor	Pigeon liver particles			Rat liver mitochondria		
	Q_{O_2} (N)	Ac Ac[1]	Citrate[1]	Q_{O_2} (N)	Ac Ac[1]	Citrate[1]
None	179	3.11	1.65	188	0.94	2.60
Fluorocitrate 3.3×10^{-5} M	110	3.91	3.26	125	2.94	1.64
Fluoromalate $6\cdot 6 \times 10^{-4}$ M	176	3.70	0.56	148	2.03	1.63

[1] Acetoacetate (AcAc) and citrate concentrations in μmoles/mg N. Flasks also contained O_2, 50 micromoles potassium phosphate buffer at pH 7.4, 4 micromoles magnesiun chloride, 230 micromoles potassium chloride, 4 micromoles ATP and 1 ml tissue suspension. At 6.6×10^{-3}, fluoromalate inhibits the respiration 50%.

[1] It is difficult to interpret this work, as there was no check upon the inhibitory power of the hydrolyzed triethylfluorocitrate upon aconitase (see page 432).

Fluorocitrate inhibited respiration, also citrate accumulation in the rat liver mitochondria under these conditions. Both fluorocitrate and fluoromalate increased formation of acetoacetate, over twice that with the rat tissue. The addition of fumarate increased the amount of citrate formed in the presence of fluorocitrate, and reversed the inhibitory effect of fluoromalate. The inhibition produced by fluorocitrate in the rat liver preparation could be overcome by adding glucose and hexokinase together with increased amounts of adenosine triphosphate (ATP) with some potassium fluoride.

The details given above show the difficulty of getting conditions in enzyme experiments to illustrate the effects and emphasizes the need for caution in applying results with enzymes to the whole animal.

Turning now to the *isolated enzymes*.

(a) With the NADP (nicotinamide-adenine dinucleotide phosphate) dependent malic dehydrogenase, the following results were obtained (Table 11):

Table 11. *Inhibition of malic dehydrogenase by fluoromalate and by fluorocitrate.* Data of GAL (1960)

Addition	Concn.	μmoles × 10 TPN reduced in 3 min	Per cent inhibition
Nil (control)	—	25.0	—
Fluoromalate	6.6×10^{-4}	10.0	60
Fluorocitrate	6.6×10^{-4}	19.5	22

The system contained tris buffer pH 7.4, 0.002 M; $MnCl_2$, 2.0×10^{-4} M; NADP, 1×10^{-4}M; malic enzyme (C, gel eluted), 0.1 ml (≡ 6.4 μg N by KJELDAHL); total vol., 3 ml; temp. 30° C. Malate, 5×10^{-5} M.

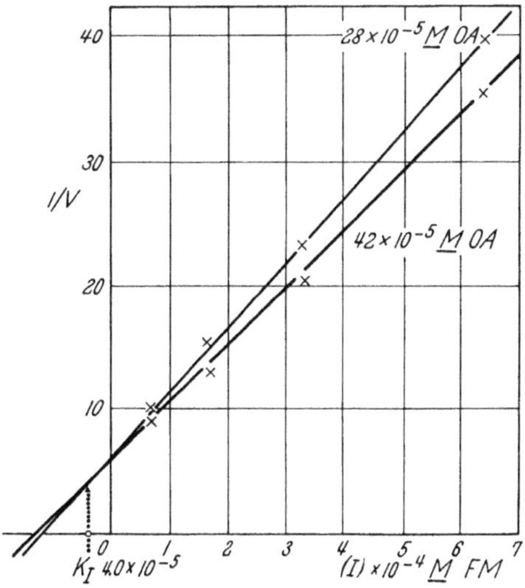

Fig. 21. Inhibition of NAD-dependent malic dehydrogenase. Graphical representation of the competition between oxaloacetate and fluoromalate; inhibition of oxaloacetate reduction by NADH. Enzyme, 4 μg protein; NADH, 0.3 μmole; Tris buffer, pH 7.4 (0.02 M); Temp. 27° C; volume, 3 ml. From GAL (1960)

From this it is evident that fluoromalate is a more powerful inhibitor of this enzyme than fluorocitrate. The inhibition by fluoromalate is competitive.

(b) Inhibition of NAD (nicotinamide-adenine dinucleotide) dependent malic dehydrogenase. A graphical plot of the competition between oxaloacetate and fluoromalate is given in Fig. 21. The reaction (from GAL 1960, p. 284) concerned is oxaloacetate + $NADH_2 \rightleftarrows$ malate + NAD.

At a concentration of 6.6×10^{-4} M, fluoromalate inhibited this to the extent of 80% (GAL 1960).

Fluoromalic acid can exist in several isomeric forms. Erythro and threo isomers have been separated after synthesis by KRASNA (1961, 1962). One isomer, obtained in sufficient yield, was found by him to be a competitive inhibitor of fumarate (approached from both ways) and of malic dehydrogenase.

From (a) and (b) we must conclude that the main inhibitory effect is on the malate systems. Not more than 20% inhibition was given by fluoromalate on the Mn^{++} activated oxaloacetate decarboxylation.

Note:

The large concentrations of fluorocitrate (1.0 mM) reported by STICKLAND (1959) to inhibit the malic enzyme seem to be outside the physiological range. In any case they are difficult to evaluate without information upon the effect of the hydrolyzed mixture which was used upon an isolated aconitase preparation or upon kidney mitochondria. The fluorocitrate used was obtained by heating the triester to 100° C for one hour in the presence of a theoretical amount of NaOH — a procedure which is likely to produce a mixture of substances (WARD and PETERS 1961).

4. β-Fluoro-oxaloacetic acid HOOCCHFCOCOOH

The free acid has been prepared from the diethyl ester by KUN et al. (1959) and its chemistry studied. With 20 μmoles/3 ml of oxaloacetate, 23.5 μmoles of fluorooxaloacetate caused a marked inhibition of the reduction to malate (in presence of reduced nicotinamide adenine dinucleotide ($NADH_2$), which was competitive. At the same time, the compound itself was found to be reduced slowly to fluoromalate. Subsequent work (KUN et al. 1960) showed that β-fluoro-oxaloacetic acid inhibited the glutamate-aspartate transaminase. A most interesting reaction took place on incubating aspartate and fluorooxaloacetate in presence of the enzyme, viz. a formation of oxaloacetate, ammonia and free fluoride. They believe the reaction is probably as follows:

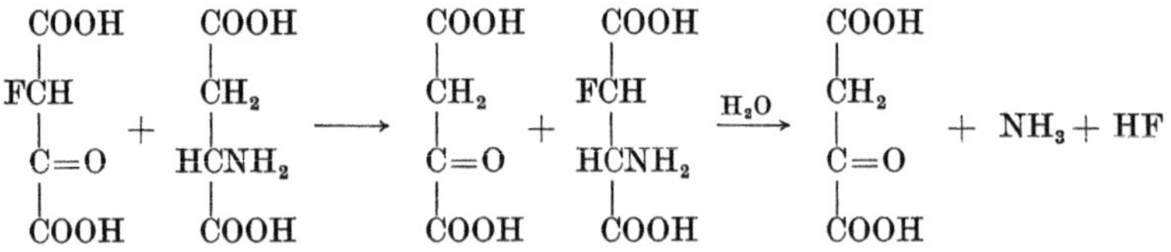

It would be most important if this reaction could occur *in vivo*. In further work β-fluoro-oxaloacetate in high concentrations was found to inhibit the malate dehydrogenase [(carboxylating) enzyme from chicken liver. (E.C.1.1.1.40. L-malate: NADP oxidoreductase)] (KUN and WILLIAMS-ASHMAN 1962).

5. Fluoroacetoacetates (2,4-difluoroacetoacetate $FCH_2COCHFCOOR$; 4-fluoroacetoacetate FCH_2COCH_2COOR)

Referring to the pigeon and rat liver systems used for fluoromalate (GAL 1960; see page 430), both these fluoro-compounds were markedly inhibitory of acetoacetate formation in rat liver mitochondria, the inhibition at a concentration of 3.3×10^{-3} M being complete. They had no influence on citrate formation or accumulation in the pigeon liver system, while they inhibited this in rat liver particles.

Using a pigeon liver system, the fluoroacetoacetates were markedly inhibitory to acetoacetate synthesis at a concentration of 1.3 mM, at which concentration fluoromalate had no effect (GAL 1960).

6. Fluoromalonate, HOOCCHFCOOH

This compound is clearly of interest in view of the behaviour of malonyl-CoA in fatty acid synthesis (BRADY 1958). It has been made in Palestine by CHARI-BITRON (1961), who recorded its toxicity as the potassium salt as LD_{50} 80 mg/kg for the mouse, against that of fluoroacetate as 15 mg/kg; that is to say about $^1/_5$th and for the guinea pig $^1/_8$th of the toxicity of fluoroacetate. This is in contrast to the findings of one of us (PATTISON, unpublished work) where the toxicities of the diethyl ester and the free acid were about the same as for fluoroacetate to mice. The effects observed were that the animal became lethargic in 15–20 mins. In 2 hours the rectal temperature decreased, and the animals were sprawled, showing periodic convulsions. The blood glucose concentration rose, but there were no ketone bodies excreted in the urine. At death there was a large increase of citrate in the kidney, and smaller accumulations in the heart, brain and diaphragm; none in liver. Like fluoroacetate there was no effect on particles from the pigeon brain, but a supernatant from kidney particles treated with fluoromalonate induced citrate increases in brain resembling those induced by fluorocitrate. Malonate reduced these effects. The compound therefore can be converted to fluoroacetyl-CoA somewhere in the body. When the diester was given, it had equally low toxicity to the rat, whereas to the mouse it was as toxic as fluoroacetate. In our experience, results with di- or tri-esters are apt to give variable results, which we attribute to variability in the way in which the animal happens to handle the esters. If converted slowly to the acids, they will give lower toxicity results. (In fact we have found that the triester of fluorocitrate may be relatively non-toxic upon injection.) The result with this diester of fluoromalonate may be interpreted to mean that the animal removes the ester group more quickly with a subcutaneous injection. On two occasions in the Cambridge author's laboratory, the diester of fluoromalonate, kindly given to us, was found to have little toxicity to a rat when given in alcohol intraperitoneally in a dose exceeding 150 mg/kg. More work with other routes of injection would be interesting. Toxicity in the mouse was associated with citrate accumulations in kidney, heart, brain and diaphragm, and liver. The administration of malonate immediately following the injection of fluoromalonate reduced the citrate accumulation in the heart and kidney.

7. Microorganisms

The reactions of C—F compounds are various and complicated in microorganisms, and are not yet understood completely (see PETERS 1957, p. 134). It has been reported recently by Japanese workers (HORIUCHI 1962a) that soil bacteria take fluoroacetate to pieces. This observation might help to answer the question of the fate of fluoroacetate synthesized in the leaves of the toxic plants.

Some points may be noted in regard to bacteria and yeast.

a) Bacteria

ELSDEN and ORMEROD (1956) have found that fluoroacetate at a concentration of 8×10^{-4} M strongly inhibited photometabolism by *Rhodospirillum rubrum* of the substrates acetate, pyruvate and oxaloacetate or H_2CO_3; with acetate, pyruvate and oxaloacetate citrate accumulated. In presence of propionate, DL-lactate, succinate, fumarate and DL-malate the effects were slight. In the dark, the oxygen uptake of all substrates, acetate, propionate, n-butyrate, succinate, fumarate and pyruvate was strongly inhibited, citrate arising from succinate, L-malate, fumarate or oxaloacetate. The fact that citrate sometimes accumulates with the poison suggests an action upon aconitase by fluorocitrate; but some of the other points are difficult to fit with this.

From the same laboratory, JAYASURIYA (1954, 1956) has investigated the effects of 0.001 M fluoroacetate upon cells of *Pseudomonas* OD_1 grown on lactate. With a preincubation the oxygen uptake was about 60% inhibited with glycine, glycollate and α-ketoglutarate, and 39% with oxalate; there was little effect when acetate or pyruvate were substrates.

Considering citrate accumulation, there was no extra citrate with acetate or oxalate; all the other substrates showed increased citrate, and also succinate, fumarate, malate and oxaloacetate, which had shown no appreciable decrease in oxygen uptake. The amounts of extra citrate were particularly marked with α-ketoglutarate and glycollate; in the latter case the extra citrate produced was directly proportional to the glycollate added. The author rightly points out that, though some of the facts are suggestive of a block in aconitase, there are others such as the inactivity with acetate which cannot be reconciled with this. Another instance of a discrepancy has been reported from Leeds (DAGLEY and WALKER 1956; CALLELY and DAGLEY 1959). Working with a vibrio grown on acetate, DAGLEY and his colleagues found that in the presence of fluoroacetate citrate accumulated when the medium contained acetate, octanoate, sebacate or benzoate. With malic, fumaric and succinic acid, pyruvate and not citrate accumulated. At first they suggested that there was a synthesis of fluoropyruvate in this latter case; they now think that it must be a lethal synthesis of monofluoromalate, because using an authentic sample of this compound at about 10^{-4} M, they can imitate the pyruvate accumulations observed with their vibrio. If the presence of monofluoromalate can be proved by isolation, it will raise the interesting point that in this organism two pathways may be blocked.

It can be inferred that fluoromalate can be synthesized as follows, from fluoroacetyl-S-CoA at 0.25 of the rate for acetyl-S-CoA by the malate synthetase (DIXON et al. 1960).

$$\text{Fluoroacetyl-S-CoA} + \text{glyoxalate} + H_2O \rightarrow \text{fluoromalate} + \text{CoA-SH}$$

Working with the same vibrio ALI et al. (1962) have shown that when grown on benzoic acid, the organism oxidizes *p*-fluorobenzoate with the elimination of F^- ions. The *m*-fluorobenzoate was attacked, but this stopped after the uptake of one O_2 per mole of benzoate (see also ICHAHARA et al. 1962).

b) Yeast

Matters become more complicated when we come to yeast. Using Fleishman's bakers yeast, BLACK and HUTCHENS (1948), following upon work by KALNITSKY and BARRON (1947), made their observations at pH 6.0 and 10^{-3} M fluoroacetate. If this was added 30 mins. before acetate, the usual oxygen uptake due to acetate was much delayed, perhaps 3 hours; but during this period an oxygen uptake was induced by adding ethanol, acetaldehyde, succinate and succinic semialdehyde. With a smaller concentration of fluoroacetate, 2.0×10^{-6} M (2 μM) in experiments lasting 1 hour, the O_2 uptake in acetate was much reduced as the acidity of the medium was increased from pH 6.24 to 3.80 (97 to 16% of the control value).

Challenging problems are raised by these observations, which have been much extended and studied by ALDOUS and colleagues (ALDOUS and ROZEE 1956, 1958) using the same yeast. They pointed out that even at pH 4.0, only 5% of fluoroacetic acid would be in the undissociated state, calculating this from the pK of

2.66. Hence the results of BLACK and HUTCHENS could not be due to the decreased dissociation of the fluoroacid. Nevertheless ALDOUS and ROZEE found that the reduction in O_2 uptake followed the concentration of undissociated fluoroacetic acid, there being a 90% inhibition when the concentration of the undissociated

Table 12. *Reversal of the fluoroacetic acid-induced inhibition of oxygen consumption by pH in yeast cells.* Data of ALDOUS and ROZER (1956)

Treatment after poisoning by fluoroacetic acid	0 Consumption, µl/15 min		Percentage inhibition
	Control	Fluoroacetic acid	
Unwashed pH (2.1)	55.1	1.5	97.3
Washed at pH 2.1	53.5	14.2	73.5
Washed at pH 2.8	53.0	24.4	54.0
Washed at pH 5.0	58.9	56.3	4.4

Yeast cells were originally exposed to 5×10^{-3} M fluoroacetic acid at pH 2.1 for 30 min; they were then washed and resuspended at the same or more alkaline pH values.

fluoroacetic acid was 4.0×10^{-3} M. The behaviour of yeast cells exposed to 5 mM fluoroacetic acid at pH 2.1 was studied by washing in buffer-glucose at different pH with the results given in Table 12. The surprising fact appears that the inhibition is lifted at pH 5.0; and it was even more surprising to find that the cells now

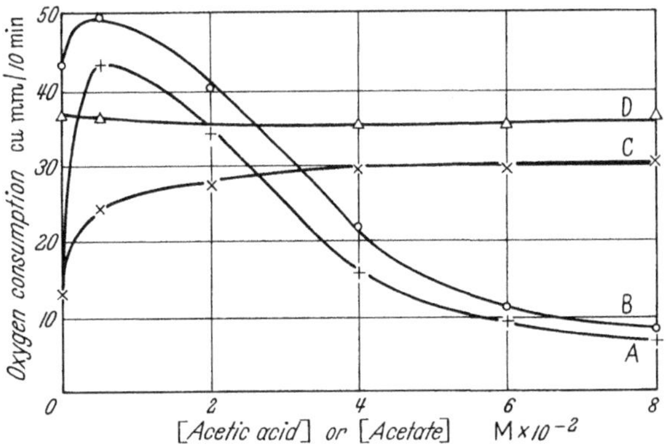

Fig. 22. Oxygen consumption of fed yeast cells as a function of the concentration of undissociated acetic acid or ionized acetate in the environment and the effect of these concentrations upon the subsequent utilization of glucose. Curve A, buffer pH 2.7 containing acetic acid in concentrations indicated on abscissa. Curve B, the same, one hour later, after the addition of glucose to give a final concentration of 1%. Curve C, same as A, but at pH 6.7 (ionized acetate). Curve D, same as B, but at pH 6.7. From ALDOUS and ROZEE (1958)

relieved from their inhibition showed the inhibition when replaced in the medium at pH 2.2. As pointed out, the results show that the fluorinated acid remains inside the cell in a form resistant to washing, though in view of the buffered internal pH at 6.3 (CONWAY and O'MALLEY 1946) it seems that any effects of pH will be effects upon the surface of the cells. It was thought that the metabolic reactions might be changing with changes of pH to which the cells were exposed.

Following up these results, the authors have shown (Fig. 22) that the oxygen uptake of yeast cells in acetate medium plus glucose depends upon the state of the acetic acid; at pH 2.7 increasing amounts of undissociated acetic acid decrease the O_2 uptake, whereas at pH 6.7 the rate is independent of ionized acetate concentration until concentrations of 20 mM are reached. Additions of glucose increase the respiration, and at pH 6.7 the O_2 uptake is the same as without acetate.

The effect of fluorocitric acid poisoning was studied in yeast cells treated in glucose at pH 2.2, subsequently washed and then placed in acetate buffer pH 2.2 and 6.7. The behavior in the rate of acetate oxidation was approximately the same at the two hydrogen ion concentrations, showing that the block in acetate oxidation was not lifted at the more alkaline pH. When exposure to the poison was done in glucose at pH 6.7, there was virtually no poisoning either of glucose or acetate oxidation when exposed to pH 2.2 and 6.7.

The authors were led to the view that the living yeast cell had two routes for oxidizing glucose, one at a pH more acid than pH 4.5 involving the citric acid cycle.

In unpublished work by ALDOUS, an attempt was made to isolate fluorocitrate from yeast cells exposed to fluoroacetate; no fluorocitrate was found, and this turned attention to other possibilities.

Since the effects of pH appear to be exerted on the surface of the cell and since ROTHSTEIN (1954) showed that the inhibitory action of H^+ ion on glucose fermentation could be antagonized by the K^+ ion, the effect of addition of K^+ ion was tried, and was found to increase the amount of citrate formed from glucose at pH 2.2 (about 40%) (ALDOUS personal communication).

A further detailed study made in Halifax[1] of the respiratory characteristics and changes in intracellular citrate of viable but non-dividing yeast cells suggests that fluoroacetic acid does not produce its toxic effect in the classical manner, *i.e.* by being converted to fluorocitrate and thereby blocking the citric acid cycle. The evidence which supports this conclusion is as follows: yeast cells may be irreversibly poisoned with fluoroacetic acid at any pH between 2 and 6, when the external substrate is acetate. These particular environmental conditions should induce operation of the glyoxalate cycle (KORNBERG and ELSDEN 1961). The cells may also be poisoned by fluoroacetic acid in 5% glucose provided the pH is maintained between 2 and 3 — conditions which in normal cells result in virtually no poisoning; and these particular environmental conditions result in a low intracellular citrate. Above pH 3.5 however, exposure to fluoroacetic acid in 5% glucose results in virtually no poisoning; and these particular environmental conditions result in a high concentration of intracellular citrate in normal cells. This increase in intracellular citrate in normal cells is due to an effect of pH on glucose metabolism; but it is not, in itself, a factor responsible for the failure to poison cells with fluoroacetic acid, *i.e.* there is no evidence for competition between this and citrate.

The authors suggest that exogenous acetate may condense with glyoxalate giving rise to malate, and in the case of exposure to fluoroacetic acid to fluoromalate where further reactions of the cycle are inhibited. When environmental conditions favour the operation of the glyoxalate cycle, *i.e.* when acetate is the exogenous substrate or when glucose is oxidized at pH 2 to 3, then an inhibition of oxidative activity appears. If the cells metabolize glucose at a pH greater than 3.5, the oxidative reactions no longer involve this cycle but proceed probably via the citric acid cycle where there is no metabolic block. The apparent "recovery" of the oxygen consumption of fluoroacetic acid treated cells respiring in a glucose medium at pH 5.5, and the failure to find fluorocitrate in such cells are consistent with the above explanation.

Q. Other compounds of interest

1. Deoxyfluoroglycerols

The 1- and 2-deoxyfluoroglycerols behave differently. They both cause death with the accumulation of citrate, but they do this in different ways and must be considered separately (O'BRIEN and PETERS 1958a, b).

[1] We are indebted to Prof. J. G. ALDOUS for this personal communication of work not yet published.

a) 1-Deoxy-1-fluoroglycerol, $FCH_2CH(OH)CH_2OH$

When this compound is given intraperitoneally, rats become immobile and catatonic, and die with accumulation of citrate, but without convulsions. The path by which the fluoroacetyl fragment is formed is still incertain. It can be proved *in vivo* by suitable ligatures that the compound giving rise to accumulation is formed in the liver; this was confirmed by perfusion experiments in which the heart and liver were perfused in circuit. When the fluoroglycerol was perfused through the liver, there was poisoning of the heart with an accumulation of citrate; but when the liver was out of circulation, then there was no accumulation of citrate in the heart, or poisoning of this. Hence the heart does not contain the necessary enzymes to perform the initial metabolic step. This suggests that it should be possible to make the fluoroacetyl fragment with liver homogenates or at any rate with slices. So far however it has not been possible to do this, even with considerable variation of the medium in which the slices are suspended. The situation seems much like that with fluoroethanol (see below). After perfusion of the liver it was possible to demonstrate the presence of some compound which behaved like fluoroacetate on a silicic acid column (Bulen, Varner and Burrell 1952).

b) 2-Deoxy-2-fluoroglycerol, $HOCH_2CHFCH_2OH$ and 2-Deoxy-2-fluoroglyceraldehyde, $HOCH_2CHFCHO$

Experiments with the aldehyde showed that there was a liberation of acid from respiring kidney particle preparations treated with this. At first this was thought to be due to the formation of a phosphoester. Further work however showed that this was due to a combination of the aldehyde with an –SH group

2-deoxy-2-fluoroglycerol → 2-deoxy-2-fluoroglyceraldehyde
→ 2-deoxy-2-fluoroglycerate → fluoroacetyl → tricarboxylic acid cycle
[serine hydroxymethylase]

Fig. 23. Scheme suggested for the conversion of 2-deoxy-2-fluoroglycerol to fluorocitrate

in cysteine. The aldehyde was nevertheless converted in the kidney to something which caused a citrate accumulation. The following steps have been suggested by Treble and Peters (1961, 1962) for the metabolism of 2-deoxy-2-fluoroglycerol (Fig. 23). In explanation of this, it may be said that there are three possibilities for the conversion of the fluoroglyceric acid to fluoroacetate.

(1) Decarboxylation to fluoroethanol. This step is ruled out because fluoroethanol is not toxic to kidney particles (p. 438).

(2) Oxidation to fluoromalonate. This was suggested by Pattison (1959) on chemical grounds as a direct step from the glycerol. However, the fluoroethanol is not oxidized to fluoroacetate, which appears to be against the oxidation of the $-CH_2OH$ in the glycerol.

(3) Direct conversion of fluoroglycerate to fluoroacetate by the serine hydroxymethylase. Evidence was obtained for this reaction, and it was supported by the fact that the L-fluoroglycerate was more toxic than the D-isomer. These latter compounds were kindly sent by Dr. P. W. Kent, as were also the two fluorocarbohydrates described below.

2. Fluorocarbohydrates

Treble investigated (in unpublished work) 5-deoxy-5-fluororibose. This proved quite non-toxic to rats at a dose level of 170 mg/kg.

6-Deoxy-6-fluorogalactose was also investigated. It had no toxicity when injected at a level of 147 mg/kg in rats. No rise in citrate levels was found in heart, kidney or liver. The fluorogalactose had no effect on *Saccharomyces fragilis*, which readily metabolizes galactose via glucose. Similarly the ability of *Pseudomonas saccharophylla* to oxidize galactose was not significantly affected by the presence of 0.02 M of the fluorogalactose.

3. Fluoroethanol, FCH_2CH_2OH

This is an interesting compound; it has the same order of toxicity for the rat as fluoroacetate, but in general it acts more slowly. Out of 9 rats studied by TREBLE (1962) with an intraperitoneal dose of 10 mg/kg fluoroethanol, only one died in 2 hours; 5 died in $5^1/_2$ to $8^1/_2$ hours, and 3 were killed at 8 hours in moribund condition. The rats showed lassitude and coma, but not convulsions; and there was a lowered heart rate. The average citrate accumulations at death are given in Table 13. The citrate accumulations and altered heart rate indicated that fluoroethanol is synthesized to fluorocitrate in the heart; yet earlier reports (KILBY and CARPENTER 1944), made it clear that fluoroethanol had no effect on the perfused heart of the rabbit. Hence, this appeared to be acting similarly to 1-deoxy-1-fluoroglycerol. If the liver is converting the fluoroethanol to a FC_2 fragment, it should be possible to show the effect on liver enzymes. Indeed TREBLE (1962) found that liver slices from the rat oxidized 2-fluoroethanol to a

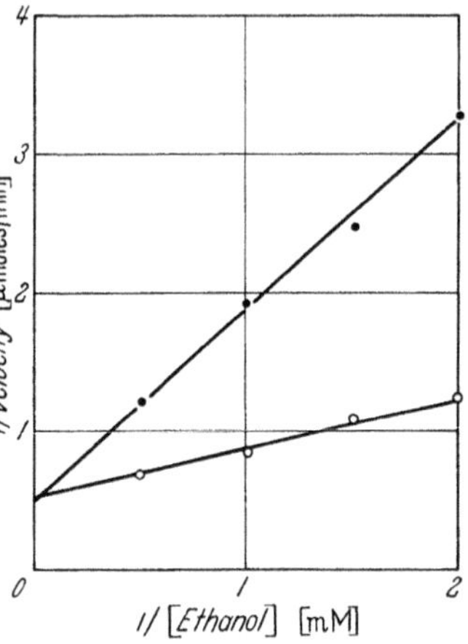

Table 13. *Effect of fluoroethanol on rats receiving 10 mg/kg of compound intraperitoneally.* Data of TREBLE (1962)

Time to death, hrs.	No. of rats	Citrate content, mg/kg wet wt.		
		Heart	Liver	Kidney
2	1	688	33	154
$5^1/_2$—$8^1/_2$	5	1079	359	969
Over 8	3	2542	1401	3220
Normal	4	95	27	38

Fig. 24. Inhibition of liver alcohol dehydrogenase by 2-fluoroethanol. Complete system: NAD, 1 mg; DL-cysteine, 0.5 mg; semicarbazide. HCl, 2 mg; sodium pyrophosphate, 0.1 M adjusted to pH 9 with HCl; total volume, 3.3 ml ○, Ethanol; ●, ethanol plus 5 mM 2-fluoro-ethanol. Dialyzed liver alcohol dehydrogenase (0.01 ml) was added with stirring to start the reaction. Each point is the average of three determinations. The reaction velocity was measured by determining the rate of increase of extinction at 328 mμ. From TREBLE (1962)

compound which then induced accumulation of citrate in the presence of kidney mitochondria, whereas fluoroethanol itself did not have this effect. Fluoroethanol was found by TREBLE to be a competitive inhibitor of crystalline liver alcohol dehydrogenase Fig. 24; but BARTLETT (1952) had reported that crude liver dehydrogenase could oxidize fluoroethanol. Further work showed that there was a second alcohol dehydrogenase precipitated at a lower concentration of ammonium sulphate, and this would oxidize fluoroethanol.

4. Fluoropyruvate, FCH_2COCOO^-

This compound was long wanted by workers in the fluoroacetate field, because it was thought that it would readily form the FC_2 fragment for condensation to citrate, as happens with pyruvate. MAGER and BLANK (1954) first succeeded in obtaining fluoropyruvic acid; they stated that it inhibited the growth of *E. coli* and *A. aerogenes*, and that it killed rats without convulsions when given in large doses, and with little change in citrate in the tissues. These latter facts were confirmed in Oxford (GAL et al. 1956); a dose of 80 mg/kg killed rats with no accumulation of citrate, and with occasional convulsions after 4 hours. This dose reduced the amount of expiratory CO_2 formed from C_2-C^{14} acetate *in vivo*. The level of pyruvic acid in the blood was lowered from 1.32 mg/100 ml to 0.88 mg showing that the fluoro-compound did not block pyruvate oxidation *in vivo*. Injections of glucose, thiamine-HCl and pyruvate did not reverse the poisoning. Experiments *in vitro* (GAL et al. 1956) with kidney particle preparations showed that fluoropyruvate blocked the formation of citrate from fumarate, but did not inhibit the disappearance of citrate, that is to say that the enzyme aconitase was not attacked (Table 14).

Table 14. *The effect of fluoropyruvate upon (a) the synthesis of citrate from fumarate, and (b) the metabolism of citrate by kidney mitochondria.* Data of GAL et al. (1956)

Kidney mitochondria (guinea pig) were suspended in KCl-buffer solution and reinforced with MgCl and ATP. Fumarate was added to (a) and Na citrate to (b). (a) also contained fluorocitrate to block the further metabolism of citrate synthesized, and (b) contained malonate to block the metabolism of citrate at the succinate stage. 30 min, temp. 38° C.

Blocking agent	Addition	μmoles citric acid	
		Accumulated	Disappearing
(a) Fluorocitrate	Fumarate alone	7.52	—
	Fumarate fluoropyruvate (3.14 mM)	0.76	—
	Fumarate fluoropyruvate (6.29 mM)	0.58	—
(b) Malonate (no fluorocitrate)	Citrate (10 μmoles)	—	9.83
	Citrate fluoropyruvate (3.14 mM)	—	9.92
	Citrate fluoropyruvate (6.29 mM)	—	9.93

The accompanying curve (Fig. 25) shows the inhibition of pyruvate oxidation by fluoropyruvate at varying concentrations (mitochondria from pigeon brain). This compound at 16.3 mM also inhibited by 63% the carboxylase of yeast. Hence it has a powerful effect on enzymes concerned with pyruvate metabolism. These facts point to quite a different action, as compared with fluoroacetate, and it was found by AVI-DOR and MAGER (1956a) that the compound reacted somewhat like iodoacetate, with —SH groups in compounds like cysteine (DIXON 1948). This was accompanied by a rapid splitting off of fluoride, a fact confirmed by PETERS and HALL (1957) using the method of HALL (1960) for measurement of the fluoride removed.

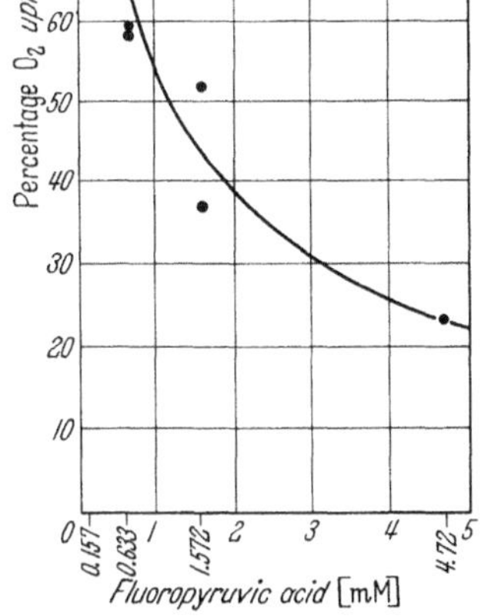

Fig. 25. Inhibition of pyruvate oxidation by fluoropyruvate in pigeon brain particles; points at 0.633 mM with centrifuged particles, the rest with uncentrifuged particles. The total volume of 3.0 ml contained in 1.0 ml of fumarate (10 μmoles), pyruvate (27 μmoles), Mg^{2+} (4.0 μmoles $MgCl_2$), ATP (1.2 μmoles), KCl (0.134 M); and in the remaining 2.0 ml of brain particles in KCl (0.134 M) and 0.1 M phosphate buffer (pH 7.2). Citric acid accumulations were also determined, and gave, as compared with the control (100%): at 0.157 mM 87%; 0.633 mM 31, 50, 53, 68, 79%; at 1.572 mM 29, 34%; at 4.72 mM 29%. From GAL et al. (1956)

Though the compound is rapidly reduced by the lactate dehydrogenase, it causes a number of rather unspecific effects, which can mostly be attributed to the action on $-SH$ groups, such as the inhibition of the NADH oxidase activation of heart muscle. Further investigation (CHARI-BITRON and AVI-DOR 1959), showed that fluoropyruvate imitated the action of iodoacetate on the swelling, phosphorylating activity and respiration of guinea-pig mitochondria. The rate of swelling was accelerated, the latent adenosine triphosphatase was activated, and the oxidation of the nicotinamide adenine nucleotide linked substrates of the citric acid cycle was inhibited.

An interesting reaction has been investigated by AVI-DOR (1960), which he believes to be brought about by the γ-glutamyl transpeptidase in microsomes from rat kidney. The compound formed from the reaction of glutathione and fluoropyruvate which contains no fluoride, upon reaction with microsomes gives a compound behaving like cysteinyl-glycine pyruvate with a concomitant transfer of a glutamyl moiety. This work underlines the complications set up with $-SH$ substances when they combine with fluoropyruvate (see also MAGER et al. 1955, GAL et al. 1956). As a final point it should be mentioned that the compound can be used to estimate $-SH$ groups, according to the following equation (AVI-DOR and MAGER 1956b):

$$RSH + FCH_2COCOOH \rightarrow RSCH_2COCOOH + HF$$

5. Synthetic ω-fluoro compounds

The development of other series of toxic ω-fluoro compounds followed quickly from the discovery of the unique biological activity of the fluoroacetates. Thus, the *ω-fluorocarboxylic esters*, $F(CH_2)_nCOOR$ were shown by 1945 to give rise to a remarkable alternation in toxicity on ascent of the series (SAUNDERS 1947; BUCKLE, PATTISON and SAUNDERS 1949); if the total number of carbon atoms in the acid moiety is even, the compound is toxic and produces symptoms in animals similar to those produced by fluoroacetate, whereas if the total number is odd, the compound is non-toxic. The free acids follow the same pattern (PATTISON, HUNT and STOTHERS 1956). This pronounced alternation in toxicity has been correlated with the β-oxidation of fatty acids (PATTISON and SAUNDERS 1949); thus only the even members can give rise to fluoroacetyl coenzyme A, which in turn forms fluorocitrate, the actual enzyme poison.

The homologous series of *ω-fluoroalcohols*, $F(CH_2)_nOH$ was next examined (PATTISON, HOWELL, MCNAMARA, SCHNEIDER and WALKER 1956). The same type of alternation in toxicity soon became apparent, with the same generalizations regarding the odd and even members; this fact confirms, in a novel way, the biological oxidation of alcohols to acids. Not surprisingly, the *ω-fluoroaldehydes*, $F(CH_2)_nCHO$ gave rise to a similar effect (WILSHIRE and PATTISON 1956).

The consistency of these results led us to examine other series of compounds containing an ω-fluorine atom (PATTISON 1953, 1954, 1957). Thus, aliphatic amines are known to be converted *in vivo* to the corresponding aldehydes and then to acids, as follows:

$$RCH_2NH_2 + O_2 \xrightarrow{\text{amine oxidase}} RCH{=}NH + H_2O_2$$
$$RCH{=}NH + H_2O \rightarrow RCHO + NH_3$$
$$RCHO + O \rightarrow RCOOH$$

Since there is no loss of carbon in this process, it would be expected that the *ω-fluoroalkylamines*, $F(CH_2)_nNH_2$, if catabolized by the same process, would form the corresponding acids, and again give rise to an alternation of toxicity. Such was indeed the case (PATTISON, HOWELL and WHITE 1956), as can be seen from the results below (Table 15):

Table 15. *Toxicity of ω-fluoroalkylamines*

Compound	Formula	LD_{50} (mice, I.P.) mg/kg
5-Fluoroamylamine	$F(CH_2)_5NH_2$	50
6-Fluorohexylamine	$F(CH_2)_6NH_2$	0.9
7-Fluoroheptylamine	$F(CH_2)_7NH_2$	50
8-Fluoro-octylamine	$F(CH_2)_8NH_2$	0.76

In a more recent study, RAASCH (1958b) has described two adjacent members of the *ω-fluoro-α-aminoacid* series, $F(CH_2)_nCH(NH_2)COOH$ (see p. 403). 5-Fluoronorvaline ($n = 3$) and 6-fluoronorleucine ($n = 4$) had LD_{50} values (intraperitoneal injection in mice) of 1.08 mg/kg and >215 mg/kg respectively. These clear-cut results may be explained by a degradative mechanism akin to that of the amines described above, involving first oxidative deamination and then oxidative decarboxylation; for example:

$$\underset{\text{toxic}}{F(CH_2)_3CH(NH_2)COOH} \rightarrow F(CH_2)_3COCOOH \rightarrow \underset{\text{toxic}}{F(CH_2)_3COOH}$$

Verification of such a mechanism, which postulates the intermediate formation of an α-ketoacid, could readily be accomplished by preparing and examining the two corresponding ω-fluoro-α-ketoacids, $F(CH_2)_nCOCOOH$ ($n = 3$ and 4).

It thus soon became apparent that the ω-fluorinated "tail" acts as a "tag" for deducing or confirming the metabolism of the functional "head". In short, the ω-fluorine atom, with its characteristic toxicological properties, may be considered as a new tool for the elucidation of biochemical processes. The type of reasoning used may be illustrated by a consideration of the nitrile grouping (—CN). It has been shown (PATTISON, COTT, HOWELL and WHITE 1956) that ω-fluoronitriles containing an *odd* number of carbon atoms (that is, including the carbon of the —CN) are toxic, and those containing an even number are non-toxic. The figures below (Table 16) illustrate this statement:

Table 16. *Toxicity of ω-fluoronitriles*

Compound	Formula	LD_{50} (mice, I.P.) mg/kg
5-Fluorovaleronitrile	$F(CH_2)_4CN$	1.0
6-Fluorohexanonitrile	$F(CH_2)_5CN$	50
7-Fluoroheptanonitrile	$F(CH_2)_6CN$	2.7
8-Fluoro-octanonitrile	$F(CH_2)_7CN$	>100

Listed below are three possible modes of degradation which might occur to an organic chemist:

(a) *Hydrolysis:* $RCN \rightarrow RCOOH$

e.g. $$\underset{\text{toxic}}{F(CH_2)_4CN} \rightarrow \underset{\text{non-toxic}}{F(CH_2)_4COOH}$$

(b) *Reduction:* $RCN \rightarrow RCH_2NH_2$

e.g. $$\underset{\text{toxic}}{F(CH_2)_4CN} \rightarrow \underset{\text{non-toxic}}{F(CH_2)_4CH_2NH_2}$$

(c) *C—CN cleavage:*

$$RCH_2CN \rightarrow RCOOH + HCN$$

$$\underset{\text{toxic}}{F(CH_2)_4CN} \rightarrow \underset{\text{toxic}}{F(CH_2)_3COOH} + HCN$$

It can be seen that neither hydrolysis nor reduction is consistent with the facts, whereas the C—CN cleavage provides a satisfactory explanation of the observed toxicity data. Such a conclusion is in conformity with earlier work on nitriles (LANG 1894). *ω-Fluoroalkyl mercaptans*, $F(CH_2)_nSH$ provide another example of a simple series in which the ω-fluorine atom confers profound changes in properties (HOWELL, MILLINGTON and PATTISON 1956). By reference to the well-known transthiolation reaction (RSH → ROH), it was considered likely that these compounds would exhibit the same alternation in toxicity as that of the ω-fluoroalcohols. That the two- and four-carbon members were acetylated was probably unimportant because of the widespread occurrence of deacetylating enzymes. The toxicity results shown below (Table 17) conform to the expected pattern and thus provide *a priori* evidence for the transthiolation *in vivo* of simple aliphatic mercaptans.

Table 17. *Toxicity of ω-fluoroalkyl mercaptans*

Compound	Formula	LD_{50} (mice, I.P.) mg/kg
2-Fluoroethyl thiolacetate	$F(CH_2)_2SAc$	56
3-Fluoropropyl mercaptan	$F(CH_2)_3SH$	>100
4-Fluorobutyl thiolacetate	$F(CH_2)_4SAc$	1.8
5-Fluoropentyl mercaptan	$F(CH_2)_5SH$	>100
6-Fluorohexyl mercaptan	$F(CH_2)_6SH$	1.25

The method can equally well be used for *predicting* the metabolism of compounds of which the mode of breakdown is not known. The rationale, based merely on crude toxicity figures, resides in the characteristic toxicological behaviour of the ω-fluorocarboxylic acids. In the study of the metabolic fate of any grouping Z in an aliphatic compound, the first task is the preparation of a few adjacent members of the series $F(CH_2)_nZ$; thereafter, the examination of the toxicity pattern allows of the interpretation of the results.

To illustrate the value of the ω-fluorine atom in the elucidation of the intermediary metabolism of unknown or little known processes, mention may be made of alkyl halides. Little is known regarding the metabolism of members containing more than two carbons; even the two carbon members (ethyl chloride, bromide and iodide) vary markedly in their behaviour *in vivo* (KOCHMANN 1923; BLUMGART et al. 1931; MILLER and HAGGARD 1943). To deduce the action of the higher members, the series $F(CH_2)_nX$ (X=Cl, Br or I) were examined (PATTISON and HOWELL 1956a). It was argued that, if there were an alternation in toxicity, this would imply hydrolytic scission of the C—X bond, with resultant formation of the corresponding ω-fluoroalcohols; on the other hand, lack of toxicity in adjacent members would suggest that the C—X bond was stable *in vivo*. The figures shown in Table 18 do indeed show a pronounced alternation, indicating the formation of the fluoroalcohols, which in turn may be oxidized to the corresponding ω-fluorocarboxylic acids; bromides result in a similar alternation. It is not unreasonable to extend these results to non-fluorinated halides, and hence to arrive at the conclusion that alkyl halides are likely to be metabolized by the biochemical hydrolysis of the C—X bond.

Table 18. *Toxicity of ω-fluoroalkyl chlorides*

Compound	Formula	LD_{50} (mice, I.P.) mg/kg
2-Fluoroethyl chloride	$F(CH_2)_2Cl$	>100
4-Fluorobutyl chloride	$F(CH_2)_4Cl$	1.2
5-Fluoropentyl chloride	$F(CH_2)_5Cl$	32
6-Fluorohexyl chloride	$F(CH_2)_6Cl$	5.8
7-Fluoroheptyl chloride	$F(CH_2)_7Cl$	>100
8-Fluoro-octyl chloride	$F(CH_2)_8Cl$	2.3
9-Fluorononyl chloride	$F(CH_2)_9Cl$	>100
10-Fluorodecyl chloride	$F(CH_2)_{10}Cl$	5.0

This method and reasoning has been applied to many other series, such as those listed on p. 404. These series, with one exception, are unbranched compounds. The exception concerns branched ω-fluorocarboxylic acids, $F(CH_2)_nCHMe(CH_2)_mCOOH$, the results of which are perhaps worth describing. Branched-chain fatty acids occur in synthetic fats, and consequently their metabolism is of some medical importance. What would be the effect of a branch methyl group on the breakdown of a fatty acid? An answer has been obtained from an examination of the corresponding ω-fluoro compounds.

Considering the general formula $CH_3(CH_2)_nCHMe(CH_2)_mCOOH$, the following initial degradation seems very probable:

(a) *m* odd:

$$\xrightarrow{\beta\text{-oxn.}} CH_3(CH_2)_nCHMeCH_2COOH$$

(b) *m* even:

$$\xrightarrow{\beta\text{-oxn.}} CH_3(CH_2)_nCHMeCOOH$$

Thus the problem appeared to be reduced to the metabolism of the α- and β-methyl derivatives.

Several ω-fluorocarboxylic acids containing a branch methyl group were prepared (Pattison and Woolford 1957b), the toxicity results of which clearly indicated the following answer to the problem:

(a) α-methyl acid:

$$RCH_2CHMeCOOH \rightarrow RCOOH \quad \text{(loss of 3 C fragment)}$$

(b) β-methyl acid:

$$RCH_2CHMeCH_2COOH \rightarrow RCOOH \quad \text{(loss of 4 C fragment).}$$

To confirm this answer, and to determine the effect of *gem*-dimethyl groups at the α- and β-positions, all possible variations of methyl branching were examined in the adjacent C_8 and C_9 ω-fluoro acids (Pattison and Woolford 1957b; Buchanan and Pattison 1963). The various *gem*-dimethyl derivatives were expected to be non-toxic because of inhibition of β-oxidation. The results are shown below (Table 19).

The success in predicting the effects of the various branches provides confirmation of the earlier work, and in turn answers the problem of the catabolism of branched methyl carboxylic acids in general.

It should be mentioned that all the toxic members of the different ω-fluoro series examined gave rise to typical fluoroacetate symptoms *in vivo*. Moreover, in the limited number of compounds examined, it was observed (Parker and Walker 1957; Walker and Parker 1958) that the toxic members resulted in a pronounced accumulation of citric acid in the body, whereas the non-toxic members caused none. This therefore provides indirect evidence of the ultimate formation of fluoroacetate, as explained elsewhere in this review; the fluoroacetate

Table 19. *Toxicity of ω-fluorocarboxylic acids containing a branch methyl group*

Compound	Prediction	Found: LD_{50} (mice, I.P.) mg/kg
8-Fluoro-octanoic acids		
$F(CH_2)_7COOH$	toxic	0.64
$F(CH_2)_6CHMeCOOH$ (α-Me)	toxic	1.1
$F(CH_2)_6CMe_2COOH$ (α-Me_2)	non-toxic	>100
$F(CH_2)_5CHMeCH_2COOH$ (β-Me)	non-toxic	118
$F(CH_2)_5CMe_2CH_2COOH$ (β-Me_2)	non-toxic	121
9-Fluorononanoic acids		
$F(CH_2)_8COOH$	non-toxic	>100
$F(CH_2)_7CHMeCOOH$ (α-Me)	non-toxic	>100
$F(CH_2)_7CMe_2COOH$ (α-Me_2)	non-toxic	>100
$F(CH_2)_6CHMeCH_2COOH$ (β-Me)	toxic	4.5
$F(CH_2)_6CMe_2CH_2COOH$ (β-Me_2)	non-toxic	185

must have been formed from the original ω-fluoro compounds by one of the natural detoxication processes, followed by β-oxidation. Throughout these biological transformations, the fluorine apparently remains intact. No toxicity results with humans have been recorded for any of the compounds discussed in this section.

In conclusion, mention may be made of a rule which has been formulated for predicting the toxicity of new or unknown long-chain ω-fluoro compounds (PATTISON 1959). Considering the general formula $F(CH_2)_nCH_2CH_2Z$ (where Z is any grouping), the toxicity is largely dependent on the fate of the $-CH_2CH_2Z$ grouping in the body. It is convenient to consider this under two classes:

(1) Z is removed ($-CH_2CH_2Z \rightarrow -CH_2COOH$).

(2) Z promotes removal of the adjacent methylene group ($-CH_2CH_2Z \rightarrow \rightarrow -COOH$).

If the fate of Z can be equated with one of these classes, the following simple rule emerges for any compound $F(CH_2)_nZ$:

Class of Z	n in $F(CH_2)_nZ$	Predicted effect
1	odd	non-toxic
1	even	toxic
2	odd	toxic
2	even	non-toxic

R. Fluoroacetate and convulsions

The toxic convulsions induced by fluoroacetate in the rat have been mentioned already. That these are not due to fluoroacetate itself can be shown in the rat, the pigeon and the rabbit, by introducing this compound into the subarachnoid space, under ether anaesthesia. Relatively large doses, so injected, have no effect, though some convulsions are asphyxial in origin due to heart failure (CHENOWETH and GILMAN 1946). Fluorocitrate itself is very toxic. As little as 11 μg of the "enzymically" synthesized fluorocitrate is enough to start a convulsion in a pigeon, when injected into the subarachnoid space, and 1.5 μg in a rat of approximately 50 g. It is fairly certain that much of this does not reach the active centres so that the amount of fluorocitrate, which is causing convulsions probably does not exceed 1 μg/g tissue (wet) and may well be less. In rat experiments, it was found in Oxford (Dawson and Peters 1955; Gal et al. 1956) that there was a rise in citrate content of the brain tissue (up to 170 mg/g of rat tissue); generally speaking the only other organ to show any rise in citrate after brain injections was the kidney; this was variable and can be explained as a leakage from the skull. These negative effects with fluoroacetate and positive ones with fluorocitrate are in agreement with the fact that pigeon brain tissue *in vitro* does not convert fluoroacetate to fluorocitrate (see p. 414). It might be thought that the immediate stimulus for the convulsions was the accumulation of citrate, which could well immobilize Ca^{++} ions. It is well-known that citrate injected into the skull through the foramen magnum can induce convulsions in dogs which are relieved by restoring the Ca^{++} (Mullin et al. 1938).

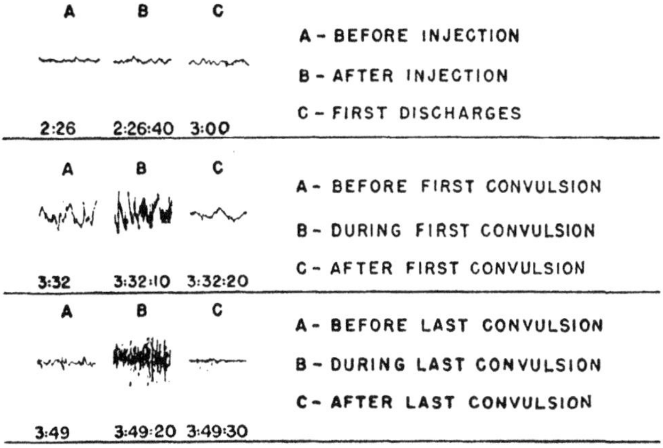

Fig. 26. Electric discharges following intracranial injection of fluorocitrate into a rabbit under nembutal anesthesia. Time below waves. Data of Hastings and Peters in Peters (1963)

One cannot be certain that the accumulation of citrate in tissues does not immobilize divalent ions; at the same time any effects due to this seem to be secondary. In the rabbit indeed, it was found (Hastings et al. 1953, 1955) after an injection of 2 μmoles of an impure, synthetic fluorocitrate preparation, that in 10 minutes there were mild signs of excitation which were reduced quickly by an injection of Ca^{++} (Fig. 26). However when the severe convulsions appeared there was no effect of a further injection of Ca^{++}. Chenoweth (1949) has always stated that there is no relation between citrate accumulation and excitation and it was found by Bannister and Foulkes (see Peters 1952) that the heart beat of *Xenopus* was not affected by the presence of increased citrate in the tissue. The situation seems to be analogous to that of thiamine deficiency, where there is no evidence that the accumulating pyruvate is itself toxic.

Accepting the view that citrate is not the initiator of the electrical disturbance, we have to face the question what is the biochemical lesion and how does this lower the potential of the membrane concerned, so as to produce an excitation. That this excitation can spread from one brain centre has been proved by Hendershot and Chenoweth (1955) in a crucial experiment. They used cerebral cortex of the dog, isolated *in vivo*, but arranged so that the circulation was intact. Simultaneous recordings could be taken for periods up to 3 hours from the isolated piece of tissue and 3 control areas. The injection of 8.6 to 20.0 μg/g tissue of either fluoroacetate or fluorobutyrate into the isolated area gave after 31 to 217 minutes convulsive electroencephalic patterns and increased citrate levels, varying from 3 to 6 times control pieces (Fig. 27).

The seizures spread to adjacent cortical areas without an increase of citrate in these areas; but the citrate picture was complicated by the fact that brains protected from fluorobutyrate by a previous injection of monobutyrin had an accumulation of citrate. Since the convulsions are presumably induced by fluorocitrate synthesis, it would appear that the brain of the dog (unlike the other brains) must be capable of synthesizing fluorocitrate. Alternatively the local blood vessels may do this. The matter needs clarifying by experiment. The synthesis if it occurs is evidently a slow one.

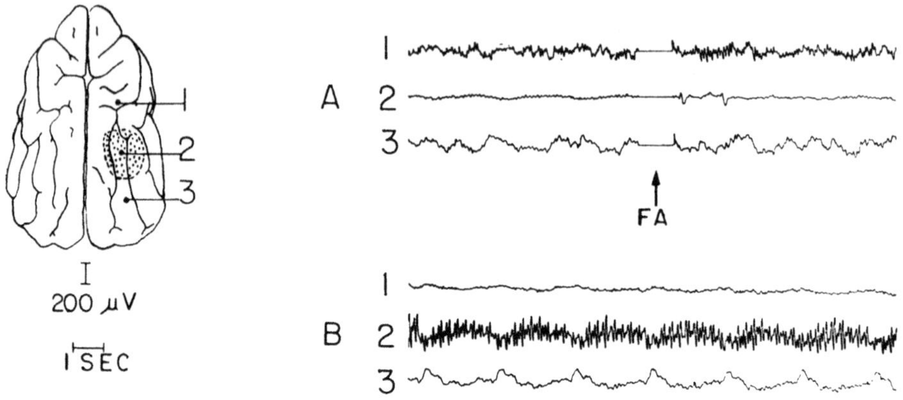

Fig. 27. Spiking type of electroencephalographic convulsive activity in isolated cerebral cortex of the dog. A. State of activity immediately before and immediately after the injection of 15 μg of sodium fluoroacetate into isolated piece (stippled). B. Appearance of spiking activity (10 per second) in isolated section (lead 2) but not in control areas (leads 1 and 3) 217 min after fluoroacetate injection. From HENDERSHOT and CHENOWETH (1955)

The initial changes in phosphoesters appear to be slight (DAWSON and PETERS 1955), though a continuation of convulsions leads to increased changes (PSCHEIDT et al. 1954). It has often been suggested that convulsions are due to the ammonium ion; but the large increase here seems to occur after the start of the convulsions (BENITEZ et al. 1954).

If we accept the working hypothesis that the biochemical lesion is due to an action of fluorocitrate upon aconitase, we are still faced with the question how a failure in aconitase is translated into a lowering of membrane potential (? failure of sodium pump). This leads first to the question of where the aconitase is in the mitochondria; from which it follows that there will be mitochondria in close association with the membrane concerned. There is no information on this known to the authors. Yet, it can well be imagined that blocking the citric acid cycle would cause a profound upset in the supply of the energy needed (? ATP) to maintain the integrity of the cell reactions. Again more work is needed. It is not due to change in CO_2 concentration because BULLWINKLE et al. (1955) found no change in p CO_2 concentration.

1. Fluoroacetylcholine, $Me_3\overset{+}{N}CH_2CH_2OCOCH_2F$

It has been repeatedly (and naturally) thought that the convulsions arise through a block in the acetylcholine system. Indeed the synthesis of fluoroacetylcholine has been proved to occur in brain tissue from the ox, from fluoroacetate and fluorocitrate (WOLLEMAN and FEUER 1957). However even if formed *in vivo* there is no evidence that there is any significant effect of fluoroacetylcholine as such. It has been proved to be degraded by cholinesterase (MEHLER and CHANG 1956), and to have essentially no more toxicity than an equal amount of fluoroacetate and acetylcholine, as SALLE (1952) showed in the earliest research on this question. One of us with colleagues (BUFFA and PETERS 1949) has tried to find changes in acetylcholine after dosing with fluoroacetate; however no change has been found.

V. Concluding remarks

So far as the biochemical pharmacology of these carbon-fluorine compounds is concerned, there seems little doubt that the main toxicity is due to the biochemical lesion in aconitase produced by the lethal synthesis of fluorocitrate from fluoroacetyl-CoA and oxaloacetate. Fluoropyruvate is an exception to this. Other reactions can take place in the liver to form fluoro-lipid substances, but this does not appear to be the main route of toxicity. It also appears that in yeast especially and perhaps other microorganisms, there may be a conversion to fluoromalate.

Why some animals receive their main attack on the nervous system and others in the heart is still a matter of speculation, as also is the great difference between doses needed to kill animals of different species. Based upon known facts, a hypothesis can be enunciated (a) that animals vary in their capacity for converting the carbon-fluorine compounds to fluoroacetyl-CoA, and (b) that the differently sited tissue reaction is due to a more ready penetration to heart or elsewhere, as the case may be.

There are still one or two unexplained facts, as mentioned. It is not clear yet where the fluoroacetyl-CoA is synthesized to make the fluorocitrate which causes excitation in the brain. In the sheep, JARRETT and PACKHAM (1956) found that animals which were dosed with 0.2 mg fluoroacetate daily behaved differently upon different diets. In particular a diet of lucerne or wheat chaff plus gluten protected them from fluoroacetate. The experiment was interesting, and the different effects on different diets may possibly be connected with a change in microorganisms in the rumen.

Though CATER and PETERS (1961) had no success in the treatment of hepatomas in rats with 1-deoxy-1-fluoroglycerol, it would appear that there is a field worth further exploration in the effects of these carbon-fluorine compounds. α-Fluoromevalonate for instance has been found to be a powerful inhibitor for the conversion of acetate to cholesterol (SINGER et al. 1959). This effect has been explored in its complicated stereochemical aspects in a most interesting paper by KIRSCHNER et al. (1961) using radioactive labels. One form of the fluoromevalonic acid stops the synthesis of squalene from mevaldinic acid. Their analysis showed that α-fluoromevalonic acid (Form B) inhibited the phosphorylation of mevalonic acid. With ATP, this form was phosphorylated to the 5-phospho- and to the 5-pyrophospho-2-fluoromevalonic acid. The fluoro-substituted compound then forbids the conversion to the intermediary product Δ^3-isopentenyl pyrophosphate, a reaction catalyzed by the enzyme pyrophosphomevalonate-decarboxylase. Hence the fluoro-compound interferes in more than one stage in a most interesting manner, inducing a final biochemical lesion in a specific enzyme.

Though not in the monofluoro aliphatic field, attention should be drawn to the exciting possibilities opened up by the use of 5-fluorouracil and similar fluorinated compounds by HEIDELBERGER and his colleagues. This work is summarized in a report in which it is shown that the main ultimate attack is upon the thymidylate synthesis (HARTMANN and HEIDELBERGER 1961). The possible applications to malignant disease are being pursued with vigour.

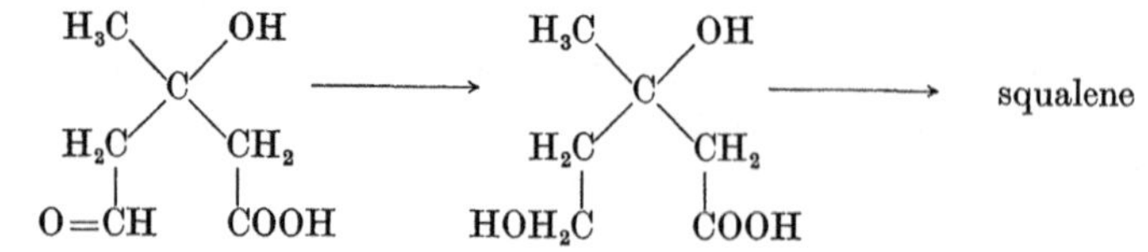

mevaldinic acid mevalonic acid

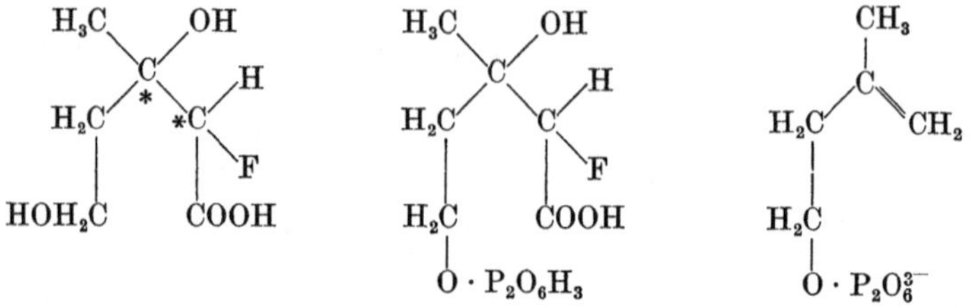

α-fluoromevalonic acid 5-pyrophospho-2-fluoromevalonic acid Δ^3-isopentenyl pyrophosphate

Nothing has been said in this review about the toxicity of these fluorine compounds to man. The information is scanty, as it must be based necessarily on unfortunate cases of accidental human poisoning. The toxic dose probably lies between 5 and 20 mg/kg for fluoroacetate; nothing is known about the other fluorocompounds. Detailed notes of the behaviour and the treatment of some of these human cases is to be found in the book by one of us (PATTISON 1959). Similarly only passing reference has been made to the uses of fluoro aliphatic compounds; these include pest control agents, insecticides, anaesthetics and convulsants. An account of these and other uses has been given in the aforementioned book and in other parts of this present volume.

References[1]

ALDOUS, J. G., and K. R. ROZEE: The effect of pH on the toxicity of fluoroacetic acid. Biochem. J. **62**, 605—610 (1956).
— — The metabolic characteristics of yeast cells treated with fluoroacetic acid; evidence of the regulation of glucose oxidation by pH. J. cell. comp. Physiol. **52**, 43—58 (1958).
ALI, D. A., A. G. CALLELY, and M. HAYES: Ability of a vibrio grown on a benzoate to oxidize *p*-fluorobenzoate. Nature (Lond.) **196**, 194—195 (1962).
ANNISON, E. F., K. J. HILL, D. B. LINDSAY, and R. A. PETERS: Fluoroacetate poisoning in sheep. J. comp. Path. **70**, 145—155 (1960).
AVI-DOR, Y.: A study of the effect of particle-bound γ-glutamyl transpeptidase on the product of interaction of fluoropyruvate with glutathione. Biochem. J. **76**, 370—374 (1960).
—, and J. MAGER: The effect of fluoropyruvate on the respiration of animal-tissue preparations. Biochem J. **63**, 613—618 (1956a).
— — A spectrophotometric method for determination of cysteine and related compounds. J. biol. Chem. **222**, 249—258 (1956b).
BACQ, Z. M., and P. A. ALEXANDER: Fundamentals of radiobiology, 555 pp., 2nd Ed. Oxford: Pergamon Press 1961.
— S. LIÉBECQ-HUTTER, and C. LIÉBECQ: Protection against irradiation afforded by sodium fluoroacetate. Radiat. Res. **13**, 286—297 (1960).
BADENHUIZEN, N. P., and J. SLINGER: Detection of monofluoroacetic acid in Gifblaar. (*Dichapetalum cymosum* (Hook) Engl.). S. Afr. J. Sci. **50**, 269—270 (1954).

[1] Addendum see p. 458.

BARBOUR, A. K., L. J. BELF, and M. W. BUXTON: The preparation of organic fluorine compounds by halogen exchange. *In:* M. STACEY, J. C. TATLOW and A. G. SHARPE, Eds. Advances in Fluorine Chemistry, Vol. 3, 181—270. London: Butterworths 1963.

BARTLETT, G. R.: Mechanism of action of 2-fluoroethanol. J. Pharmacol. exp. Ther. **106**, 464—467 (1952).

—, and E. S. G. BARRON: The effect of fluoroacetate on enzymes and on tissue metabolism. Its use for the study of the oxidative pathway of pyruvate metabolism. J. biol. Chem. **170**, 67—82 (1947).

BEATTY, C. H., and E. S. WEST: The effect of substances related to the tricarboxylic acid cycle upon ketosis. J. biol. Chem. **190**, 603—610 (1951).

BENITEZ, O., G. R. PSCHEIDT, and W. E. STONE: Formation of ammonium ion in the cerebrum in fluoroacetate poisoning. Amer. J. Physiol. **176**, 488—492 (1954).

BERGMANN, E. D., and S. COHEN: Organic fluorine compounds. Part IX. The preparation of fluoroacetone and 1:3-difluoroacetone. J. chem. Soc. **1958**, 2259—2262.

— — Organic fluorine compounds. Fluorine derivatives of mevalolactone. Tetrahedron Letters, No. 8, 20—22 (1960).

— — Organic fluorine compounds. Part XXII. Fluorine analogues of mevalonic acid. J. chem. Soc. **1961a**, 3457—3460.

— — Organic fluorine compounds. Part XXVI. Synthesis of α-fluoro-β-alanine. J. chem. Soc. **1961b**, 4669—4671.

— —, and I. SHAHAK: Organic fluorine compounds. Part XII. Preparation and reactions of diethyl fluoromalonate. J. chem. Soc. **1959**, 3286—3289.

— — — Organic fluorine compounds. Part XX. Some reactions of 1-chloro-3-fluoropropan-2-ol and epifluorohydrin. J. chem. Soc. **1961**, 3448—3452.

—, and R. IKAN: The reaction of diazoketones with anhydrous hydrofluoric acid. Chem. and Ind. (London) **1957**, 394.

—, and I. SHAHAK: Transformation of toluene-*p*-sulphonates into fluorides. Chem. and Ind. (London) **1958**, 157.

— — Triethyl α-fluoroaconitate. Nature (Lond.) **185**, 529—530 (1960).

— — A simple preparation of fluoromalonic acid esters. Chem. and Ind. (London) **1961**, 591.

BLACK, S., and J. O. HUTCHENS: The oxidation of acetate by yeast in the presence of fluoroacetate. Arch. Biochem. **17**, 211—223 (1948).

BLANK, I., J. MAGER, and E. D. BERGMANN: Studies of organic fluorine compounds. Part IV. Synthesis of esters of fluoro-oxaloacetic and of fluoropyruvic acid. J. chem. Soc. **1955**, 2190—2193.

BLOHM, T. R.: Fluoroacetylcholine bromide and some other choline ester salts. J. Amer. chem. Soc. **73**, 5445—5446 (1951).

BLUMGART, H. L., D. R. GILLIGAN, and J. H. SCHWARTZ: The elimination of ethyl iodide after inhalation and its relation to therapeutic administration. J. clin. Invest. **9**, 635—650 (1931).

BOWERS, A.: Steroids. CXXIX. A new general route to fluorinated steroids. J. Amer. chem. Soc. **81**, 4107—4108 (1959).

— P. G. HOLTON, E. DENOT, M. C. LOZA, and R. URQUIZA: Steroids. CLXXXVIII. New fluorination procedures. Part 3. cis-Addition of fluorine to a steroid olefin. A new route to 6 α-fluoro-Δ^4-3-ketones. J. Amer. chem. Soc. **84**, 1050—1053 (1962).

— L. C. IBÁÑEZ, E. DENOT, and R. BECERRA: Steroids. CXXXIX. New fluorination procedures. Part I. The addition of Br—F and I—F to cyclohexene and a variety of unsaturated steroids. J. Amer. chem. Soc. **82**, 4001—4007 (1960).

BRADY, R. O.: Fluoroacetyl coenzyme A. J. biol. Chem. **217**, 213—224 (1955).

— Enzymic synthesis of fatty acids by aldol condensation. Proc. Nat. Acad. Sci. (Wash.) **44**, 993—998 (1958).

BRONNERT, D. L. E., and B. C. SAUNDERS: Toxic fluorine compounds containing the C—F link. XI. Lability of the fluorine atom in 2-fluoroethanol. Tetrahedron **10**, 160—163 (1960).

BROWN, P. J., and B. C. SAUNDERS: A new synthesis of monofluorocitric acid. Chem. and Ind. (London) **1962**, 307—308.

BUCHANAN, J. M., and C. B. ANFINSEN: Partial purification of aconitase. J. biol. Chem. **180**, 47—54 (1949).

BUCHANAN, R. L., F. H. DEAN, and F. L. M. PATTISON: γ-Fluoroglutamic acid. Canad. J. Chem. **40**, 1571—1575 (1962a).

— — — The synthesis of α-monofluorocarboxylic acids. Preprints of the Second International Symposium on Fluorine Chemistry, Estes Park, Colorado, July, pp. 385—390 (1962b).

—, and F. L. M. PATTISON: Unpublished results (1962).

— — Unpublished results (1963).

BUCKLE, F. J., F. L. M. PATTISON, and B. C. SAUNDERS: Toxic fluorine compounds containing the C—F link. Part VI. ω-Fluorocarboxylic acids and derivatives. J. chem. Soc. **1949**, 1471—1479.

BUFFA, P., G. F. AZZONE, E. CARAFOLI e U. MUSCATELLO: Modificazione biochimiche mitocondriali e tessutali in relazione ad alcune ipo-ed i perterermie sperimentali del ratto. Sperimentale **110**, 79—107 (1960a).

— E. CARAFOLI e U. MUSCATELLO: Differenze metaboliche tre diaframma e muscolo grande dorsale del ratto rivelate dall intossicazione da fluoroacetato. Accad. Naz. dei Lincei. XXVIII Fase 6. Serie (iii) pp. 929—936 (1960b).

—, and R. A. PETERS: The *in vivo* formation of citrate induced by fluoroacetate and its significance. J. Physiol. (Lond.) **110**, 488—500 (1949).

— —, and R. W. WAKELIN: Biochemistry of fluoroacetate poisoning. Isolation of an active tricarboxylic acid fraction from poisoned kidney homogenates. Biochem. J. **48**, 467—477 (1951).

BULEN, W. A., J. E. VARNER, and R. C. BURRELL: Separation of organic acids from plant tissues. Anal. Chem. **24**, 187—190 (1952).

BULLWINKLE, R., R. H. FALLON, T. C. FLEMING, and A. B. HASTINGS: Note on the acid-base balance of the blood of rabbits following the intracerebral injection of fluorocitrate. Quart. J. exp. Physiol. **40**, 269—271 (1955).

BUSCH, H., and V. R. POTTER: Localisation of the enzymatic block in kidneys of rats treated with fluoroacetate. Proc. Soc. exp. Biol. (N. Y.) **81**, 172—175 (1952).

CALLELY, A. G., and S. DAGLEY: A possible lethal synthesis of monofluoromalonate. Biochem. biophys. Acta (Amst.) **35**, 256—257 (1959).

CATER, D. B., and R. A. PETERS: The occurrence of renal changes resembling nephrosis, in rats poisoned with fluorocitrate. Brit. J. exp. Path. **42**, 278—289 (1961).

CHAPMAN, N. B., and J. L. LEVY: Nucleophilic displacement of fluorine from organic compounds. Part II. Kinetics of the reactions of alkyl fluorides with ethanolic sodium ethoxide. J. chem. Soc. **1952a**, 1673—1677.

— — Nucleophilic displacement of fluorine from organic compounds. Part III. Acid-catalysed solvolysis of alkyl fluorides in aqueous ethanol. J. chem. Soc. **1952b**, 1677—1682.

CHARI-BITRON, A.: A study on the toxicity and the biochemical effects of monofluoromalonate. Biochem. Pharmacol. **6**, 169—176 (1961).

— and Y. AVI-DOR: Effect of fluoropyruvate on the swelling, phosphorylation and respiration of guinea pig liver mitochondria. Biochem. J. **71**, 572—578 (1959).

CHENOWETH, M. B.: Monofluoroacetic acid and related compounds. Pharmacol. Rev. **1**, 383—424 (1949).

—, and A. GILMAN: Studies on the pharmacology of fluoroacetate. 1. Species response to fluoroacetate. J. Pharmacol. exp. Ther. **87**, 90—103 (1946).

— A. KANDEL, L. B. JOHNSON, and D. R. BENNETT: Factors influencing fluoroacetate poisoning. Practical treatment with glycerol monoacetate. J. Pharmacol. exp. Ther. **102**, 31—54 (1951).

CLARKE, D. A., and W. F. RIKER: The effect of fluoroacetate on the sartorius muscle of the frog. J. Pharmacol. exp. Ther. **99**, 118—131 (1950).

COLE, B. T., F. L. ENGEL, and J. FREDERICKS: Sodium fluoroacetate diabetes: Correlations between glycemia, ketonemia and tissue citrate levels. Endocrinology **56**, 675—683 (1955).

— —, and K. HEWSON: Some metabolic effects of sodium fluoracetate poisoning in the rat. Fed. Proc. **13**, 28 (1954).

CONWAY, E. J., and E. O'MALLEY: The nature of the cation exchanges during yeast fermentation with formation of 0.02 N H ion. Biochem. J. **40**, 59—67 (1946).

DAGLEY, S., and J. R. L. WALKER: Accumulation of citrate and pyruvate during growth of a vibrio in the presence of fluoroacetate. Biochem. biophys. Acta (Amst.) **21**, 441—447 (1956).

DAWSON, R. M. C.: Cerebral amino acids in fluoroacetate poisoned, anaesthetised and hypoglycaemic rats. Biochim. biophys. Acta (Amst.) **11**, 548—552 (1953).

—, and R. A. PETERS: Observations upon the behaviour of some phosphate esters in brain at the start of convulsions induced by fluorocitrate and fluoroacetate. Biochim. biophys. Acta (Amst.) **16**, 254—257 (1955).

—, and D. RICHTER: Effects of stimulation on the phosphate esters of the brain. Amer. J. Physiol. **160**, 203—211 (1949).

DEAN, F. H., and F. L. M. PATTISON: Unpublished results (1962).

— — Monofluorosuccinic acid. Canad. J. Chem. **41**, 1833—1836 (1963).

DEAR, R. E. A., and F. L. M. PATTISON: Toxic fluorine compounds. XVIII. The synthesis of the toxic principle of *Dichapetalum toxicarium* (18-fluoro-*cis*-9-octadecenoic acid) and related ω-fluoro unsaturated acids. J. Amer. chem. Soc. **85**, 622—626 (1963).

DICKMAN, S. R., and A. A. CLOUTIER: Factors affecting the activity of aconitase. J. biol. Chem. **188**, 379—388 (1951).
DIXON, G. H., H. L. KORNBERG, and P. LUND: Purification and properties of malate synthetase. Biochim. biophys. Acta (Amst.) **41**, 217—233 (1960).
DIXON, M.: Biochem. Soc. Symposia. No. 2. p. 42. On the Biochemical Reactions of Chemical Warfare Agents. Cambridge Univ. Press (1948).
—, and D. M. NEEDHAM: Biochemical research on chemical warfare agents. Nature (Lond.) **158**, 432—438 (1946).
DOMINGUEZ, A. M., F. E. SHIDEMAN, H. R. MAHLER, and H. HIFT: Effects of monofluoroacetic, 4-fluorobutanoic and 6-fluorohexanoic acids on fatty acid and Krebs cycle oxidations. Fed. Proc. **13**, 1149 (1954).
EDGELL, W. F., and L. PARTS: Synthesis of alkyl and substituted alkyl fluorides from *p*-toluenesulfonic acid esters. The preparation of *p*-toluenesulfonic acid esters of lower alcohols. J. Amer. chem. Soc. **77**, 4899—4902 (1955).
ELLIOTT, W. B., and G. KALNITSKY: A mechanism for fluoroacetate inhibition. J. biol. Chem. **186**, 487—493 (1950).
—, and A. MARCUS: Enzymatic reactions of fluoroacetyl phosphate. J. biol. Chem. **234**, 1011—1014 (1959); also Fed. Proc. **14**, 201 (1955).
— — Fluoroacetyl phosphate, preparation and properties. J. Amer. chem. Soc. **80**, 4287 (1958).
—, and A. H. PHILLIPS: Effect of fluoroacetate on glucose metabolism *in vivo*. Archiv. Biochem. **49**, 389—395 (1954).
ELSDEN, S. R., and J. G. ORMEROD: The effect of monofluoroacetate on the metabolism of *Rhodospirillum rubrum*. Biochem. J. **63**, 691—701 (1956).
ENGEL, F. L., K. HEWSON, and F. T. COLE: Carbohydrate and ketone metabolism in the sodium fluoroacetate-poisoned rat. S.F.A. Diabetes. Amer. J. Physiol. **179**, 325—332 (1954).
FAIRHURST, A. S., R. E. SMITH, and E. M. GAL: The effects of fluoro-compounds on oxidative phosphorylation. Biochem. Pharmacol. **1**, 273—279, 280—287 (1958).
FANSHIER, D. W., L. K. GOTTWALD, and E. KUN: Enzymic synthesis of monofluorocitrate from β-fluoro-oxaloacetate. J. biol. Chem. **237**, 3588—3596 (1962).
FARAH, A., G. GRAHAM, and F. KODA: The action of sodium fluoroacetate on the renal tubular transport of para-aminohippurate and glucose in the dog. J. Pharmacol. exp. Ther. **108**, 410—423 (1953).
— F. KODA, and M. FRAZER: The action of fluoroacetate on the *p*-aminohippurate uptake by the renal slices of the dog. J. Pharmacol. exp. Ther. **113**, 169—177 (1955).
— T. C. WEST, and R. ANGEL: The action of sodium fluoroacetate on intestinal smooth muscle. J. Pharmacol. exp. Ther. **98**, 234—244 (1950).
FAWAZ, G.: Die Wirkung von Fluoressigsäure auf Leistung und Stoffwechsel des Herzlungenpräparates des Hundes. Naunyn-Schmiedebergs Arch. exp. Path. u. Pharmak. **228**, 377—386 (1956).
FERGUSON, H. G., P. DE MAYO, F. L. M. PATTISON, and T. TABATA: The photolysis of some α-substituted cyclohexanones. Canad. J. Chem. **41**, 2099—2100 (1963).
FOSS, G. L.: The toxicology and pharmacology of methyl fluoroacetate (MFA) in animals, with some notes on experimental therapy. Brit. J. Pharmacol. **3**, 118—127 (1948).
FRASER, R. R., J. E. MILLINGTON, and F. L. M. PATTISON: Toxic fluorine compounds. XV. Some ω-fluoro-β-ketoesters and ω-fluoroketones. J. Amer. chem. Soc. **79**, 1959—1961 (1957).
—, and F. L. M. PATTISON: Ethyl ω-fluoroacetoacetate. Nature (Lond.) **176**, 696 (1955).
FRIED, J. F., M. W. ROSENTHAL, and J. SCHUBERT: Induced accumulation of citrate in therapy of experimental lead poisoning. Proc. Soc. exp. Biol. (N. Y.) **92**, 331—333 (1956).
FURCHGOTT, R. F., and E. SCHORR: Sources of energy for intestinal and smooth muscle contractions. Proc. Soc. exp. Biol. (N. Y.) **61**, 280—286 (1946).
GAL, E. M.: Studies of enzyme inhibition by fluoromalate and fluoroacetoacetates. Arch. Biochem. **90**, 278—287 (1960).
— P. A. DREWES, and N. F. TAYLOR: The metabolism of fluoroacetic acid 2-C^{14}, in the intact rat. Arch. Biochem. **93**, 1—14 (1961).
— A. S. FAIRHURST, R. E. SMITH, and R. A. PETERS: Inhibition of oxidative mechanism by 3-fluoropyruvate. Biochem. biophys. Acta (Amst.) **20**, 583—584 (1956a).
— R. A. PETERS, and R. W. WAKELIN: Some effects of synthetic fluoro compounds on the metabolism of acetate and citrate. Biochem. J. **64**, 161—168 (1956b).
GILLIESON, A. H. C. P., and R. A. NEWCOMB: The application of the hollow cathode source to spectrochemical analysis. Part II. The micro-determination of organically bound fluorine. A.E.R.E. (Harwell) Report C/R 764, Ministry of Supply, Great Britain, 1951.
GITTER, S.: The influence of acetamide on citrate accumulation after fluoroacetate poisoning. Biochem. J. **63**, 182—187 (1956).

GITTER, S., I. BLANK, and E. D. BERGMANN: Organic fluorine compounds. I. Influence of acetamide on fluoroacetate poisoning. Koninkl. Ned. Acad. Wetenschap. Proc. Ser. C. **56**, 423—426 (1953).

GLEW, D. N., and E. A. MOELWYN-HUGHES: The kinetics of the acid and alkaline hydrolysis of methyl fluoride in water. Proc. Roy. Soc., A, **211**, 254—265 (1952).

GORDON, R. S., and A. CHERKES: Unesterified fatty acid in human blood plasma. J. clin. Invest. **35**, 206—212 (1956).

GOTTO, A. M., and H. L. KORNBERG: Properties of a glycerate-forming enzyme from *Pesudomonas ovalis* (Chester). Biochem. J. **79**, 9 P (1961).

GRYSZKIEWICZ-TROCHIMOWSKI, E., O. GRYSZKIEWICZ-TROCHIMOWSKI et R. LÉVY: Recherches sur les composés organiques fluorés dans la série aliphatique. VII. Note sur la préparation de l'acide monofluoroacétique et sur plusieurs de ses dérivés. Bull. Soc. chim. Fr. **1953**, 462—465.

— A. SPORZYNSKI et J. WNUK: Recherches sur les composés organiques fluorés dans la série aliphatique. I. Méthode genérale de préparation des composés organiques fluorés. Rec. Trav. chim. Pays-Bas **66**, 413—418 (1947).

HALL, R. J.: The determination of microgram amounts of fluorine by diffusion. Analyst. **85**, 560—563 (1960).

— An apparatus for large scale preparative chromatography with especial application to the separation of a long chain fluoro-fatty acid. J. Chromatogr. **5**, 93—97 (1961).

—, and P. F. V. WARD: Unpublished results (1962).

HARTMAN, K.-U., and C. HEIDELBERGER: Studies on fluorinated pyrimidines. XIII. Inhibition of thymidylate synthetase. J. biol. Chem. **236**, 3006—3013 (1961).

HASEK, W. R., W. C. SMITH, and V. A. ENGELHARDT: The chemistry of sulfur tetrafluoride. II. The fluorination of organic carbonyl compounds. J. Amer. chem. Soc. **82**, 543—551 (1960).

HASTINGS, A. B., R. A. PETERS, and R. W. WAKELIN: A study of the influence of the inorganic ion environment on the convulsions induced in pigeons by fluorocitrate. J. Physiol. (Lond.) **120**, 50 P (1953).

— — — The effect of subarachnoid injection of fluorocitrate into cerebrospinal fluid of rabbits. Quart. J. exp. Physiol. **40**, 258—268 (1955).

HENDERSHOT, L. C., and M. B. CHENOWETH: Antagonism of three homologous monofluorinated fatty acids by several fatty acids. J. Pharmacol. exp. Ther. **110**, 344—351 (1954).

— — Fluoroacetate and fluorobutyrate convulsions in the isolated cerebral cortex of the dog. J. Pharmacol. exp. Ther. **113**, 160—168 (1955).

HOFFMANN, F. W.: Preparation of aliphatic fluorides. J. Amer. chem. Soc. **70**, 2596—2597 (1948).

— Aliphatic fluorides. I. ω,ω'-Difluoroalkanes. J. Org. Chem. **14**, 105—110 (1949).

— Aliphatic fluorides. II. 1-Halogeno-ω-fluoroalkanes. J. Org. Chem. **15**, 425—434 (1950).

HORIUCHI, N.: C—F bond rupture in monofluoroacetate. Seikagaku **34**, 92—98 (1962a). [J. Jap. Biochem. Soc., in Japanese.]

— Studies on the rupture activity in the animal body to the C—F bond of FCH_2COONa. Kogyo Kagaku Zasshi **65**, 1177—1179 (1962b). [J. Chem. Soc. Japan, Ind. Chem. Section, in Japanese.]

HOWELL, W. C., W. J. COTT, and F. L. M. PATTISON: Organometallic reactions of ω-fluoroalkylmagnesium chlorides. II. Reactions of ω-fluoroalkylmagnesium chlorides. J. Org. Chem. **22**, 255—259 (1957).

— J. E. MILLINGTON, and F. L. M. PATTISON: Toxic fluorine compounds. VII. ω-Fluoroalkyl thiocyanates and ω-fluoroalkyl mercaptans. J. Amer. chem. Soc. **78**, 3843—3846 (1956).

HUDLICKÝ, M.: Organic compounds of fluorine. II. Fluorinated amino acids. Coll. Czech. Chem. Comm. **26**, 1414—1421 (1961).

— Chemistry of Organic Fluorine Compounds. New York: MacMillan 1962.

HUGHES, G. M. K., and B. C. SAUNDERS: Studies in peroxidase action. Part IX. Reactions involving the rupture of the C—F, C—Br and C—I links in aromatic amines. J. chem. Soc. **1954**, 4630—4634.

HUTCHENS, J. O., H. WAGNER, B. PODOLSKY, and T. M. MCMAHON: The effect of ethanol and various metabolites on fluoroacetate poisoning. J. Pharmacol. exp. Ther. **95**, 62—70 (1949).

ICHIHARA, A., K. ADACHI, K. HOSOKAWA, and Y. TAKEDA: The enzymatic hydroxylation of aromatic carboxylic acids; substrate specificities of anthranilate and benzoate oxidases. J. biol. Chem. **237**, 2296—3202 (1962).

INMAN, C. E., R. E. OESTERLING, and E. A. TYCZKOWSKI: Reactions of perchloryl fluoride with organic compounds. II. Fluorination of certain active methylene compounds. J. Amer. chem. Soc. **80**, 6533—6535 (1958).

JARRETT, J. G., and A. PACKHAM: Response of the sheep to sublethal doses of fluoroacetate. Nature (Lond.) **177**, 580—581 (1956).

JAYASURIYA, G. C. N.: Citrate accumulation from glycollate by an oxalate-decomposing organism. Biochem. J. **56**, xli (1954); **58**, xxxi (1954).
— The oxidative properties of an oxalate-decomposing organism, *Pseudomonas* ODI with particular reference to the synthesis of citrate from glycollate. Biochem. J. **64**, 469—477 (1956).
JENKINS, R. L., and H. C. KOEHLER: Making 1080 safe. A case study in the safe manufacture and distribution of a hazardous chemical. Chem. Ind. **62**, 232—235 (1948).
JUDAH, J. D., and K. R. REES: Activation of fatty acid oxidation by kidney and liver mitochondria. Biochem. J. **55**, 664—668 (1953).
— — A note on the action of fluoroacetate. Biochem. J. **57**, 374—376 (1954).
KACSER, H.: The stereochemical relations of the four fluorocitrate isomers. Disc. Faraday Soc. **20**, 283—286 (1955).
KALNITSKY, G., and E. S. G. BARRON: The effect of fluoroacetate on the metabolism of yeast and bacteria. J. biol. Chem. **170**, 83—95 (1947).
KANDEL, A., and M. B. CHENOWETH: Metabolic disturbances produced by some fluoro fatty acids: relation to the pharmacologic activity of these compounds. J. Pharmacol. exp. Ther. **104**, 234—247 (1952a).
— — Tolerance to fluoroacetate and fluorobutyrate in rats. J. Pharmacol. exp. Ther. **104**, 248—252 (1952b).
KENT, P. W., G. HEBBLETHWAITE, and N. F. TAYLOR: Fluorocarbohydrates. Part II. Characterization of (±)-2-deoxy-2-fluoroglyceric acid and its quinine salts. J. chem. Soc. **1960**, 106—108.
KILBY, B. A., and K. J. CARPENTER: Unpublished report (1944).
KIRSCHNER, K., V. HENNING, and F. LYNEN: Zur Biosynthese der Terpene. XIII. Die Hemmung der biologischen Squalensynthese durch 2-Fluormevalonsäure. Ann. **644**, 48—64 (1961).
KNUNYANTS, I. L., O. V. KIL'DISHEVA, and E. BYKHOVSKAYA: The reaction of aliphatic oxides with hydrogen fluoride. II. J. Gen. Chem. U.S.S.R. **19**, 93—103 (1949a) [Engl. translation].
— —, and I. P. PETROV: The reaction of aliphatic oxides with hydrogen fluoride. I. J. Gen. Chem. U.S.S.R. **19**, 87—91 (1949b) [Engl. translation].
— Ya. M. KISEL', and E. G. BYKHOVSKAYA: Reaction of hydrogen fluoride with diazo ketones. Izvest. Akad. nauk. S.S.S.R., Otdel. Khim. nauk, 377—378 (1956) [Russ.].
—, and G. A. SOKOL'SKII: A new rearrangement of trihaloacetohydroxamic acids. Doklady Akad. Nauk S.S.S.R. **132**, 602—605 (1960) [Russ.]. Chem. Abstracts **54**, 24366 g (1960).
KOCHMANN, M.: Inhalation anesthesia. *In* HEFFTER's Handbuch der exp. Pharm. **1**, 133—261 (1923).
KORNBERG, H. L., and S. R. ELSDEN: The metabolism of 2-carbon compounds by microorganisms. Advanc. Enzymol. **23**, 401—470 (1961).
KRASNA, A. I.: The inhibition of fumarase and malic dehydrogenase by DL-β-fluoromalic acid. J. biol. Chem. **236**, 749—753 (1961).
— The stereochemical configuration of DL-β-fluoromalic acid. J. biol. Chem. **237**, 1418—1420 (1962).
KUMLER, W. D., E. KUN, and J. N. SHOOLERY: The enolization of oxaloacetic acid, diethyl oxaloacetate and diethyl fluorooxaloacetate as determined by NMR analyses. J. Org. Chem. **27**, 1165—1167 (1962).
KUN, E., D. W. FANSHIER, and D. R. GRASSETTI: Interaction between β-fluorooxaloacetate and glutamate-aspartate transaminase of heart mitochondria. J. biol. Chem. **235**,416—419 (1960).
— D. R. GRASSETTI, D. W. FANSHIER, and R. M. FEATHERSTONE: The reaction of malic dehydrogenase with α-keto-β-fluorosuccinic (β-fluoro-oxaloacetic) acid. Biochem. Pharmacol. **1**, 207—212 (1959).
—, and H. G. WILLIAMS-ASHMAN: The influence of β-fluoro-oxaloacetate on the malate dehydrogenase (decarboxylating). Biochem. biophys. Acta (Amst.) **59**, 719—722 (1962).
LANG, S.: Über die Umwandlung des Acetonitrils und seiner Homologen im Thierkörper. Naunyn-Schmiedebergs Arch. exp. Path. Pharmak. **34**, 247—258 (1894).
LA ZERTE, J. D., D. A. RAUSCH, R. J. KOSHAR, J. D. PARK, W. H. PEARLSON, and J. R. LACHER: Perfluoroacrylonitrile and its derivatives. J. Amer. chem. Soc. **78**, 5639—5641 (1956).
LIEBÉCQ, C., and R. A. PETERS: The toxicity of fluoroacetate and the tricarboxylic acid cycle. Biochim. biophys. Acta (Amst.) **3**, 215—230 (1949).
LINDENBAUM, W., M. R. WHITE, and J. SCHUBERT: Citrate formation *in vivo* induced by non-lethal doses of fluoroacetate. J. biol. Chem. **190**, 585—593 (1951).
LOTSPEICH, W. D., R. A. PETERS, and T. H. WILSON: The inhibition of aconitase by "inhibitor fractions" isolated from tissues poisoned with fluoroacetate. Biochem. J. **51**, 20—25 (1952).

LOWENSTEIN, J. M.: See KORNACKER, M., and J. M. LOWENSTEIN: The relation between the rates of citrate cleavage and fatty acid synthesis in rat liver preparations. Biochem. J. **89**, 27 P (1963).
MAGER, J., and I. BLANK: Synthesis of fluoropyruvic acid and some of its biological properties. Nature (Lond.) **173**, 126 (1954).
— J. GOLDBLUM-SINAI, and I. BLANK: Effect of fluorocitric acid and allied fluoroanalogues on the growth of *Escher. coli*. J. Bact. **70**, 320—325 (1955).
MARAIS, J. S. C.: The isolation of the toxic principle "potassium cymonate" from "Gifblaar," *Dichapetalum cymosum* (Hook) Engl. Onderstepoort J. Vet. Sci. Animal Ind. **18**, 203—206 (1943).
— Monofluoroacetic acid, the toxic principle of "Gifblaar," *Dichapetalum cymosum* (Hook) Engl. Onderstepoort J. Vet. Sci. Animal Ind. **20**, 67—73 (1944).
MARCUS, A., and W. B. ELLIOTT: Enzymatic reactions of fluoroacetate and fluoroacetyl coenzyme A. J. biol. Chem. **218**, 823—830 (1956).
— — Fluoroacetyl phosphate; preparation and properties. J. Amer. chem. Soc. **80**, 4287 to 4291 (1958).
MARTIUS, C.: Über den Abbau der Citronensäure. Z. physiol. Chem. **247**, 104—110 (1937).
— Der intermediare Stoffwechsel der Citronensäure. Z. physiol. Chem. **257**, 29—42 (1938).
— Über die Unterbrechung des Citronensäure-Cyklus durch Fluoressigsäure. Ann. **561**, 227—232 (1949).
MCBEE, E. T., O. R. PIERCE, H. W. KILBOURNE, and E. R. WILSON: The preparation and reactions of fluorine-containing acetoacetic esters. J. Amer. chem. Soc. **75**, 3152—3153 (1953).
MEHLER, A. H., and Y. T. CHANG: Biological reactions of fluoroacetyl choline. Arch. Biochem. **62**, 293—298 (1956).
MELDRUM, G. K., J. T. BIGNELL, and I. ROWLEY: The use of fluoroacetate (compound 1080) for the control of the rabbit in Tasmania. Austral. Vet. J. **33**, 186—196 (1957).
MILLER, D. P., and H. W HAGGARD: Intracellular penetration of bromide as a feature in the toxicity of alkyl bromides. J. industr. Hyg. **25**, 423—433 (1943).
MILLINGTON, J. E., G. M. BROWN, and F. L. M. PATTISON: Toxic fluorine compounds. VIII. ω-Fluoroalkanesulfonyl chlorides and fluorides. J. Amer. chem. Soc. **78**, 3846—3847 (1956).
—, and F. L. M. PATTISON: Toxic fluorine compounds. XII. Esters of ω-fluoroalcohols. Canad. J. Chem. **34**, 1532—1541 (1956).
MIROSEVIC-SORGO, P., and B. C. SAUNDERS: Toxic fluorine compounds containing the C—F link. X. Rupture of the C—F link by alkali and other reagents. Tetrahedron **5**, 38—43 (1959).
MIURA, K., and T. HORI: Studies on the metabolism of fluoroacetate in the liver of a rat. Part II. Isolation and identification of monofluoroacetone bodies. Agr. biol. Chem. (Tokyo) **25**, 94—99 (1961).
— S. OTSUKA, and K. HONDA: Studies on the abnormal metabolism in animals poisoned with sodium fluoroacetate. Bull. Agric. Chem. Soc. (Japan) **20**, 219—222 (1956).
— T. UCHIYAMA, and K. HONDA: Studies on the metabolism of monofluoroacetate in the liver of a frog. Agr. biol. Chem. (Tokyo) **25**, 83—87 (1961).
MORRISON, J. F.: The purification of aconitase. Biochem. J. **56**, 99—105 (1954).
—, and R. A. PETERS: Biochemistry of fluoroacetate poisoning: the effect of fluorocitrate on purified aconitase. Biochem. J. **58**, 473—479 (1954).
MULLIN, F. J., A. B. HASTINGS, and W. M. LEES: Neuromuscular responses to variations in calcium and potassium concentrations in the cerebrospinal fluid. Amer. J. Physiol. **121**, 719—727 (1938).
MURRAY, L. R., J. D. MCCONNELL, and J. H. WHITTEM: Suspected presence of fluoroacetate in *Acacia georginae*, F. M. Bailey. Aust. J. Sci. **24**, 41—42 (1961).
NAIR, P. V., and H. BUSCH: Improved synthesis of monofluoro- and monochloropyruvic acids. J. org. Chem. **23**, 137—139 (1958).
NEWMAN, M. S., M. W. RENOLL, and I. AUERBACH: Synthesis and reduction of difluorodecanoic acid derivatives. J. Amer. chem. Soc. **70**, 1023—1024 (1948).
NEWTON, J., and F. L. M. PATTISON: Unpublished results, 1961.
O'BRIEN, R. D., and R. A. PETERS: The biochemistry of 2-deoxy-2-fluoro-DL-glyceraldehyde with a note on the toxicity of 2-deoxy-2-fluoroglycerol. Biochem. Pharmacol. **1**, 1—18 (1958a).
— — The metabolism of DL-1-deoxy-1-fluoroglycerol. Biochem. J. **79**, 188—195 (1958b).
OELRICHS, P. B., and T. MCEWAN: Isolation of the toxic principle in *Acacia georginae*. Nature (Lond.) **190**, 808—809 (1961).
— — The toxic principle of *Acacia georginae*. Queensland J. Agric. Sci. **19**, 1—16 (1962).
OLAH, G. A.: Unpublished results, cited in: G. A. OLAH, Ed. Friedel-Crafts and related reactions, Vol. I, 40. New York: Interscience Publishers 1963.

OLAH, G., u. S. KUHN: Darstellung und Untersuchung organischer Fluorverbindungen. XXI. Darstellung von Fluoracetaldehyd und aliphatischen Fluormethylketonen. Chem. Ber. **89**, 864—865 (1956).
OLIVEIRA, M. M.: Chromatographic isolation of monofluoroacetic acid from *Palicourea marcgravii* St. Hil. Experientia **19**, 586—587 (1963).
O'NEILL, G. J., and F. L. M. PATTISON: Toxic fluorine compounds. XIV. Some ω-fluoroalkyl nitrogen compounds. J. Amer. chem. Soc. **79**, 1956—1958 (1957).
ORD, M. C., and L. A. STOCKEN: Sex differences in effect of radiation and fluoroacetate poisoning on liver metabolism. Proc. Soc. exp. Biol. (N. Y.) **83**, 695—697 (1953).
PARKER, J. M., and I. G. WALKER: A toxicological and biochemical study of ω-fluoro compounds. Canad. J. Biochem. **35**, 407—417 (1957).
PARKER, R. E.: Mechanisms of fluorine displacement. *In:* M. STACEY, J. C. TATLOW and A. G. SHARPE, Eds. Advances in Fluorine Chemistry, Vol. 3, 63—91. London: Butterworths 1963.
PATTISON, F. L. M.: Toxic fluorine compounds. I. Nature (Lond.) **172**, 1139—1141 (1953).
— Toxic fluorine compounds. II. Nature (Lond.) **174**, 737—741 (1954).
— From war to peace: toxic aliphatic fluorine compounds. Chem. Canada **9**, 27—33 (1957).
— Toxic Aliphatic Fluorine Compounds. Amsterdam: Elsevier 1959.
— Unpublished results, 1962.
— W. J. COTT, and W. C. HOWELL: Organometallic reactions of ω-fluoroalkyl halides. III. ω-Fluoroalkyllithium compounds. J. org. Chem. **22**, 464—465 (1957).
— — —, and R. W. WHITE: Toxic fluorine compounds. V. ω-Fluoronitriles and ω-fluoro-ω'-nitroalkanes. J. Amer. chem. Soc. **78**, 3484—3487 (1956).
—, and R. E. A. DEAR: Synthesis of the toxic principle of *Dichapetalum toxicarium* (18-fluoro-*cis*-9-octadecenoic acid). Nature (Lond.) **192**, 1284—1285 (1961).
— R. R. FRASER, E. J. MIDDLETON, J. C. SCHNEIDER, and J. B. STOTHERS: Esters of fluoroacetic acid and of 2-fluoroethanol. Canad. J. Technol. **34**, 21—28 (1956).
— — G. J. O'NEILL, and J. F. K. WILSHIRE: Toxic fluorine compounds. X. ω-Fluorocarboxylic acid chlorides, anhydrides, amides and anilides. J. org. Chem. **21**, 887—889 (1956).
—, and W. C. HOWELL: Toxic fluorine compounds. IV. ω-Fluoroalkyl halides. J. org. Chem. **21**, 748—753 (1956a).
— — Organometallic reactions of ω-fluoroalkyl halides. I. Preparation of ω-fluoroalkylmagnesium halides. J. org. Chem. **21**, 879—882 (1956b).
— — A. J. MCNAMARA, J. C. SCHNEIDER, and J. F. WALKER: Toxic fluorine compounds. III. ω-Fluoroalcohols. J. org. Chem. **21**, 739—747 (1956).
— —, and R. W. WHITE: Toxic fluorine compounds. VI. ω-Fluoroalkylamines. J. Amer. chem. Soc. **78**, 3487—3489 (1956).
— —, and R. G. WOOLFORD: Toxic fluorine compounds. XIII. ω-Fluoroalkyl ethers. Canad. J. Chem. **35**, 141—148 (1957).
— S. B. D. HUNT, and J. B. STOTHERS: Toxic fluorine compounds. IX. ω-Fluorocarboxylic esters and acids. J. org. Chem. **21**, 883—886 (1956).
—, and J. E. MILLINGTON: The preparation and some cleavage reactions of alkyl and substituted alkyl methanesulphonates. Canad. J. Chem. **34**, 757—768 (1956).
—, and J. J. NORMAN: Toxic fluorine compounds. XVII. Some 1-fluoroalkanes, ω-fluoroalkenes and ω-fluoroalkynes. J. Amer. chem. Soc. **79**, 2311—2316 (1957).
—, and B. C. SAUNDERS: Toxic fluorine compounds containing the C—F link. Part VII. Evidence for the β-oxidation of ω-fluoro-carboxylic acids *in vivo*. J. chem. Soc. **1949**, 2745—2749.
— J. B. STOTHERS, and R. G. WOOLFORD: Anodic syntheses involving ω-monohalocarboxylic acids. J. Amer. chem. Soc. **78**, 2255—2259 (1956).
—, and R. G. WOOLFORD: (±)-18-Fluoro-10-methyloctadecanoic acid (Fluorotuberculostearic acid). J. Amer. chem. Soc. **79**, 2306—2308 (1957a).
— — Toxic fluorine compounds. XVI. Branched ω-fluorocarboxylic acids. J. Amer. chem. Soc. **79**, 2308—2311 (1957b).
PEETERS, G., R. COUSSENS, and G. SIERINS: Metabolism of fatty acids in the isolated and perfused bovine mammary gland. Intern. Colloquium Bioch. Problems Lipiden. 293—298 (1953).
— — — Sodium monofluoroacetate and the isolated lactating cow udder. Arch. int. Pharmacodyn. **98**, 288—301 (1954).
PETERS, R. A.: Lethal synthesis. [Croonian lecture.] Proc. roy. Soc. B, **139**, 143—170 (1952).
— Dohme Lectures. Biochemistry of some toxic agents. Bull. Johns Hop. Hosp. **97**, 1—42 (1955).
— Mechanism of the toxicity of the active constituent of *Dichapetalum cymosum* and related compounds. Advanc. Enzymol. **18**, 113—159 (1957).

PETERS, R. A.: The comparison of the effect of an odd and even unsaturated fluorofatty acid on kidney particles. Biochem. Pharmacol. **1**, 354—355 (1958).
— Further experiments on the inhibition of aconitase by enzymically prepared fluorocitric acid. Biochem. J. **79**, 261—268 (1961).
— Biochemical lesions and lethal synthesis, pp. 1—132 (p. 113). Oxford: Pergamon Press 1963.
— Applications of chemical defence research in medicine. Edinb. med. J. **48**, 197—213 (1951).
—, and R. J. HALL: Note upon the reaction of fluoropyruvate with some —SH substances. Biochim. biophys. Acta (Amst.) **26**, 433—439 (1957).
— — Further observations upon the toxic principle of *Dichapetalum toxicarium*. Biochem. Pharmacol. **2**, 25—36 (1959).
— — Fluorine compounds in Nature; the distribution of carbon — fluorine compounds in some species of *Dichapetalum*. Nature (Lond.) **187**, 573—575 (1960a).
— — The toxicity to rabbits and some other animals of the fluorofatty acid present in the seeds of *Dichapetalum toxicarium*. J. Sci. Food Agr. **1960b**, 608—612.
— — P. F. V. WARD, and N. SHEPPARD: The chemical nature of the toxic compounds containing fluorine in the seeds of *Dichapetalum toxicarium*. Biochem. J. **77**, 17—23 (1960).
—, and M. SHORTHOUSE: Unpublished results, 1962.
—, and R. W. WAKELIN: Pyruvate oxidate system in brain tissue. J. Physiol. (Lond.) **119**, 421—427 (1953).
— — Synthesis of fluorocitric acid and its inhibition in acetate. Biochem. J. **67**, 280—286 (1957).
— — A. J. P. MARTIN, J. WEBB, and F. T. BIRKS: Observations upon the toxic principle in the seeds of *Dichapetalum toxicarium*. Separation of a long chain fatty acid containing fluorine. Biochem. J. **71**, 245—248 (1959); also Biochem. J. **58**, xl (1954).
— — P. BUFFA, and L. C. THOMAS: Biochemistry of fluoroacetate poisoning. The isolation and some properties of the fluorotricarboxylic acid inhibitor of citrate metabolism. Proc. roy. Soc. (Lond.) B, **140**, 497—507 (1953).
— —, and A. B. HASTINGS: Proc. xix. Inter. Congress of Physiology. p. 674 (1953).
— — D. E. A. RIVETT, and L. C. THOMAS: Fluoroacetate poisoning: comparison of synthetic fluorocitric acid with the enzymically synthesized fluorotricarboxylic acid. Nature (Lond.) **171**, 1111—1112 (1953).
PHILLIPS, A. H., and R. G. LANGDON: Incorporation of monofluoroacetic acid into the non-saponifiable lipids of the rat liver. Arch. Biochem. Biophys. (Amst.) **58**, 247—249 (1955).
POTTER, V. R., and H. BUSCH: Citric acid content of normal and tumor tissues *in vivo* following injection of fluoroacetate. Cancer Res. **10**, 353—356 (1950).
POWER, F. B., and F. TUTIN: Chemical and physiological examination of the fruit of *Chailletia toxicaria* (A West African poison). J. Amer. chem. Soc. **28**, 1170—1183 (1906).
PSCHEIDT, G. R., D. BENITEZ, L. B. KIRSCHNER, and W. E. STONE: Effects of fluoroacetate poisoning on citrate, lactate and energy-rich phosphates in the cerebrum. Amer. J. Physiol. **176**, 483—487 (1954).
PUCHER, G. W., C. C. SHERMAN, and H. B. VICKERY: A method to determine small amounts of citric acid in biological material. J. biol. Chem. **113**, 235—245 (1936).
RAASCH, M. S.: α,α-Difluoro-substituted acids of the tricarboxylic acid cycle, their salts, amides and esters. U.S. Patent 2,824,888 February 25 (1958a).
— 5-Fluoronorvaline and 6-fluoronorleucine. J. org. Chem. **23**, 1567—1568 (1958b).
REILLY, J., W. F. RIKER, W. C. WHITEHOUSE, and K. KURIAKI: The action of methyl fluoroacetate on the papillary muscle of the cat with comparative experiments on the action of methyl chloroacetate. J. Pharmacol. exp. Ther. **108**, 393—409 (1953).
RENNER, W.: A case of poisoning by the fruit of *Chailletia toxicaria* (ratsbane). Brit. med. J. **1904 I**, 1314.
RIMINGTON, C.: Chemical investigation of the Gifblaar, *Dichapetalum cymosum* (Hook) Engl. 1. Onderstepoort J. Vet. Sci. Animal Indust. **5**, 81 (1935).
RIVETT, D. E. A.: The synthesis of monofluorocitric acid. J. chem. Soc. **1953**, 3710—3711.
ROSE, I. A., M. GREENBERG-MANAGO, S. R. KOREY, and S. OCHOA: Enzymatic phosphorylation of acetate. J. biol. Chem. **211**, 737—756 (1954).
ROTHSTEIN, A.: Symposia Soc. Exp. Biol. No. viii, pp. 165—201. Cambridge: Univ. Press 1954.
SAUNDERS, B. C.: Toxic properties of ω-fluoro-carboxylic acids and derivatives. Nature (Lond.) **160**, 179—181 (1947).
— Phosphorus and fluorine, p. 212. Cambridge: Univ. Press 1957.
—, and G. J. STACEY: Toxic fluorine compounds containing the C—F link. Part I. Methyl fluoroacetate and related compounds. J. chem. Soc. **1948**, 1773—1779.

— — Toxic fluorine compounds containing the C—F link. Part IV. (a) 2-Fluoroethyl fluoroacetate and allied compounds. (b) 2:2′-Difluorodiethyl ethylene dithioglycol ether. J. chem. Soc. **1949**, 916—919.

— —, and I. G. E. Wilding: Toxic fluorine compounds containing the C—F link. Part II. 2-Fluoroethanol and its derivatives. J. chem. Soc. **1949**, 773—777.

Salle, J.: Sur les propriétés du bromure de fluoroacétylcholine (F.ACH). Arch. int. Pharmacodyn. **91**, 339—349 (1952).

Schmidt, G., u. H. Jahn: Synthese der α-Fluor-mevalonsäure. Ann. **644**, 43—47 (1961).

Singer, F. M., J. P. Januszka, and A. Borman: New inhibitors of *in vitro* conversion of acetate and mevalonate to cholesterol. Proc. Soc. exp. Biol. (N. Y.) **102**, 370—373 (1959).

Steyn, D. G.: Gifblaar poisoning. A summary of our present knowledge in respect of poisoning by *Dichapetalum cymosum*. 13th and 14th Reports of the Director of Veterinary Education and Research (Onderstepoort Laboratories), Part I, 187—194 (1928).

Stickland, R. G.: Some properties of the malic enzyme of pigeon liver. (1) Conversion of malate into pyruvate. (2) Synthesis of malate from pyruvate. Biochem. J. **73**, 646—659 (1959).

Stoner, H. B.: The mechanism of toxic hepatic necrosis. Brit. J. exp. Path. **37**, 176—198 (1956).

Swarts, F.: Sur l'acide fluoroacétique. Bull. Acad. roy. Belg. [3] **31**, 675—688 (1896).

Taylor, N. F., and P. W. Kent: Synthesis of (±) methyl fluoromalate. Nature (Lond.) **174**, 401 (1954).

— — The synthesis of 2-deoxy-2-fluorotetritols and 2-deoxy-2-fluoro-(±)-glyceraldehyde. J. chem. Soc. **1956**, 2150—2154.

— — Fluorocarbohydrates. I. The synthesis of 6-deoxy-6-fluoro-α-D-galactose and 5-deoxy-5-fluoro-αβ-D-ribose. J. chem. Soc. **1958**, 872—875.

Taylor, T. G.: A modified procedure for the microdetermination of citric acid. Biochem. J. **54**, 48—49 (1953).

Terner, C.: The metabolism of citric acid in the mammary gland. The effect on the synthesis of citric acid in fluoroacetate-blocked homogenates. Biochem. J. **60**, 95—101 (1955).

Theiler, A.: Quoted by Steyn, D. G. 1928 (q.v.) (1902).

Tourtellotte, W. W., and J. M. Coon: Treatment of fluoroacetate poisoning in mice and dogs. J. Pharmacol. exp. Ther. **101**, 82—91 (1951).

— — Synergistic effect of sodium acetate and ethanol in antagonizing sodium fluoroacetate (1080) poisoning in mice. Fed. Proc. **8**, 339 (1949).

Treble, D. H.: The metabolism of 2-fluoroethanol. Biochem. J. **82**, 129—134 (1962).

—, and R. A. Peters: The metabolism of 2-deoxy-2-fluoroglyceraldehyde. Biochem. J. **80**, 15—16 P (1961).

— — Metabolism of 2-deoxy-2-fluoroglyceraldehyde. Biochem. Pharmacol. **11**, 891—899 (1962).

Tschesche, R., u. H. Machleidt: Synthesen von substituierten β-Hydroxy-β-methyl-glutarsäuren und Mevalonsäuren. Ann. **631**, 61—76 (1960).

Tullock, C. W., and D. D. Coffman: Synthesis of fluorides by metathesis with sodium fluoride. J. org. Chem. **25**, 2016—2019 (1960).

Voong, Sing-Tuh, and Teh-Chang Chiang: Syntheses and polymerization of several α-fluoromethylvinyl monomers. Hua Hsüeh Hsüeh Pao **24**, 155—161 (1958) [Chinese]. Chem. Abstracts **53**, 6064 (1959).

Walker, I. G., and J. M. Parker: Further toxicological and biochemical studies on ω-fluoro compounds. Canad. J. Biochem. **36**, 339—345 (1958).

Ward, P. F. V., and R. A. Peters: The chemical and biochemical properties of fluorocitric acid. Biochem. J. **78**, 661—668 (1961).

Weeks, J. R., and M. B. Chenoweth: Separation by fluoroacetate of energy sources for smooth muscle contraction. Fed. Proc. **8**, 345 (1949).

Whittem, J. H.: Communication with L. R. Murray to Austral. Vet. Assoc. Annual Conf., May 1963.

Wilshire, J. F. K., and F. L. M. Pattison: Toxic fluorine compounds. XI. ω-Fluoroaldehydes. J. Amer. chem. Soc. **78**, 4996—4998 (1956).

Wolleman, W., and G. Feuer: Die Entstehung von Fluorazetyl-Coenzyme A und Fluorazetylcholin aus Fluoressigsäure und Fluorozitronensäure in Gehirnextracten. Acta physiol. Hung. Acad. Sci. **11**, 165—171 (1957).

Yarovenko, N. N., and M. A. Raksha: Fluorination by means of α-fluorinated amines. J. Gen. Chem. U.S.S.R. **29**, 2125—2128 (1959) [Engl. translation].

Yüan, Ch'êng-Yeh, Ch'un-Nien Chang, and I-Fang Yeh: Chemotherapy of cancer. III. Synthesis of fluorine-containing amino acids. Yao Hsüeh Hsüeh Pao **7**, 237—244 (1959) [Chinese]. Chem. Abstracts **54**, 12096 (1960).

Addendum

Since the completion of the literature search for this review, some interesting further work has appeared. The reader is referred to the following papers:

AMIN, J. H., J. NEWTON, and F. L. M. PATTISON: A new synthesis of alkyl fluorides. The pyrolysis of 2-alkylpseudouronium fluorides and fluoroborates. Canad. J. Chem. **43**, 3173—3177 (1965).

BUCHANAN, R. L., and F. L. M. PATTISON: Preparation of α-fluoro-γ-aminoacids. Canad. J. Chem. **43**, 3466—3468 (1965).

FANSHIER, D. W., L. K. GOTTWALD, and E. KUN: Studies on specific enzyme inhibitors. VI. Characterization and mechanism of action of the enzyme-inhibiting isomer of monofluorocitrate. J. biol. Chem. **239**, 425—435 (1964).

LAHIRI, S., and J. H. QUASTEL: Fluoroacetate and the metabolism of ammonia in the brain. Biochem. J. **89**, 157—163 (1963).

McEWAN, T.: Isolation and identification of the toxic principle of *Gastrolobium grandiflorum*. Nature (Lond.) **201**, 827 (1964).

PATTISON, F. L. M., and R. L. BUCHANAN: Toxic fluorine compounds. 20. The use of the ω-fluorine atom in the study of the metabolism of branched-chain fatty acids. Biochem. J. **92**, 100—105 (1964).

PETERS, R. A., and M. SHORTHOUSE: Fluoride metabolism in plants. Nature (Lond.) **202**, 21—22 (1964).

PETERS, R. A., M. SHORTHOUSE, and L. R. MURRAY: Enolase and fluorophosphate. Nature (Lond.) **202**, 1331—1332 (1964).

WARD, P. F. V., R. J. HALL, and R. A. PETERS: Fluoro-fatty acids in the seeds of *Dichapetalum toxicarium*. Nature (Lond.) **201**, 611—612 (1964).

WILLIAMSON, J. R., E. A. JONES, and G. F. AZZONE: Metabolic control in perfused rat heart during fluoroacetate poisoning. Biochem. Biophys. Research Comm. **17**, 696—702 (1964).

Chapter 9

The Mammalian Toxicology of Organic Compounds Containing Fluorine

By

J. Wesley Clayton jr.

With 1 Figure

I. Introduction

A. Definitions and objectives

The objective of this chapter is to present the toxicology for mammals of certain organic compounds which contain fluorine in the molecule. The class of organic compounds under consideration is commonly known as the "fluorocarbons," although elements other than carbon and fluorine are often part of the molecule. They may also be referred to as poly- or multi-fluorinated organic compounds, since the majority of them contain more than one fluorine atom. However, even if other elements are present, the properties of the compound are largely governed by the fluorine moiety, and therefore the term "fluorocarbon" would apply.

Fluoroplastics, *i.e.*, plastics based on resins made by the polymerization or copolymerization of monomers containing on the average one or more atoms of fluorine per monomer unit, are not included in this review. The polymeric forms will be covered in Volume II of this series.

The toxicology of the fluoroester analogues of fluoroacetate and other monofluorinated compounds which are metabolized in the mammal to monofluoroacetate, is treated in chapter 8. Reference to these materials, acting by the now classic "Lethal Synthesis" described by R. A. Peters (1952), is made in the present chapter when it bears on the mechanism of action of the fluorocarbons.

It should also be noted that there are functional classifications of the fluorocarbon compounds which are based on chemical or biological properties. Examples are the fluoro-solvents, pesticides, fumigants, anesthetics, sterols, certain polycyclic aromatic hydrocarbons which are carcinogenic for animals, diuretics, antiemetics, ataractics, and a variety of others. In these schemes the compounds may contain one, two, or more fluorine atoms, and the fluoro-grouping may or may not influence the activity, depending upon the position of substitution or the inherent activity of the site in the molecule.

B. Historical aspects

The establishment of fluorocarbon chemistry and applications has been relatively recent when it is realized that metallic fluorides were recognized and used in the Sixteenth Century, and hydrogen fluoride was made and studied by Scheele in 1771. It was not until 1886 that Moissan separated elemental fluorine from ore, and forty years later tetrafluoromethane (CF_4), the simplest perfluorocarbon was prepared (Le Beau and Damiens, 1926). The properties of CF_4 were published by Ruff and Keim (1930). Following this unpretentious beginning, three main developments stimulated the technology of fluorochemistry and the consequent appearance of numerous fluorocarbons. The first of these was the advent of mechanical refrigeration in the 1920's with the requirement for compounds that not only provided the proper pressure-temperature behavior but also the requisite low inhalation toxicity in order to permit safe refrigeration units in the household[1]. The second trend followed in the late 1920's and is marked by the preliminary pharmacological evaluation by Lehmann (1928) of compounds containing the trifluoromethyl group $-CF_3$. This was followed in subsequent years by the investigation of a number of fluorinated compounds possessing pharmacological activity. Finally, there was the development, initiated during World War II, of ω-fluoroacetate derivatives as chemical warfare agents and pesticides. (Saunders, 1957; Pattison, 1959). In the last two decades, as an extension of these early efforts, a plethora of fluorocarbon compounds have been synthesized. These have diverse physiological properties and the toxicities run the gamut between the highly toxic fluoroacetate and the relatively inert perfluoroalkanes such as CF_4, CF_3-CF_3, and $\underline{CF_2CF_2CF_2CF_2}$.

Toxicological data, of course, accumulated concurrently with the three major developments, but the demonstration of the low order of toxicity of one of the early refrigerant compounds, dichlorodifluoromethane, CCl_2F_2, is dramatic and persuasive enough to deserve separate comment. The compound was introduced at the 1930 meeting of the American Chemical Society by Thomas Midgley who inhaled CCl_2F_2 into his lungs and upon exhalation extinguished a burning candle (Midgley and Henne, 1930). This striking performance fortunately did not establish a precedent, and subsequently animal exposures were employed to evaluate the biological effects of this class of fluorocarbons (Nuckolls et al., 1933).

C. Uses of fluorocarbons

Within the chemical industry, a variety of fluorocarbons serve as fluorinating compounds, oxidizing agents and intermediates (Hamilton, 1963), although most applications of polyfluoro-carbons exploit the stability conferred upon the molecule by the carbon to fluorine bond. Thus, enhanced thermal stability, nonflammability, and low chemical reactivity have supported a number of uses and stimulated a significant penetration into the market place. In addition, the temperature-pressure characteristics which prompted the use of various fluorocarbons as refrigerants was followed by their use as aerosol propellents, based on harnessing the high vapor pressure in a closed container. Fluorocarbons also serve as dielectric materials, high temperature lubricants, fire extinguishing agents, selective solvents, surface-active agents, and a number of thermally stable polymers with a wide range of utilization. The use of these compounds as anesthetic agents is reflected by Krantz and Rudo in Chapter 10. The pharmacological usefulness of various trifluoromethyl-containing compounds has been reviewed by Yale (1959) and Buu-Hoi (1961); and while a number of compounds have been obtained which show promise as inhalation anesthetics, ataractics, antiemetic agents,

[1] Fluorinated refrigerant compounds as well as the fluorinated propellants which came into vogue during World War II with the "bug bomb" are methanes and ethanes. These are known by several common trademarks and the chemical formulae have been reduced to a numerical expression following the trademark in order to simplify the cumbersome chemical names. The system of nomenclature is detailed by Hamilton (1963).

convulsants, diuretics, and anthelmintics (CLAYTON et al. 1964), there are others which possess no useful pharmacologic activities or are toxic to various degrees.

In addition to their major uses as summarized above, a number of minor uses are worthy of citation. For example, 1,1,2-trichloro-1,2,2-trifluoroethane forms an azeotrope with 2,2,2-trifluoroethyl vinyl ether; and although it does not impair the anesthetic activities of the ether, it does reduce its flammability, SARANGI et al. (1962). Trichlorotrifluoroethane (CCl_2FCClF_2) has been employed to extract nucleic acids from animal tissues, STANSLY and RAMSEY (1960). The lamprecidal activity of 3-trifluoromethyl-4-nitrophenol is a recent example of the development of a selective toxin containing a fluoro-grouping, APPLEGATE et al. (1958). As agricultural control agents, fluorocarbons have enjoyed only limited exploration. One example is the control of fruit and petiole abscission in apples by 2-chloro-4-fluorophenoxyacetic acid, EDGERTON and HOFFMAN (1961). The original dichloro analogue, 2,4-D, was effective in some varieties of apples but, because of a rapid decarboxylation, not in others. Evidently the substitution of a fluorine for a chlorine in the 4 position impedes the rate of decarboxylation so that the compound can exert its anti-abscissive action over a longer period. Another biomedical application is the use of CF_3I^{131} to measure regional blood flow in the brain (SOKOLOFF, 1957). Although the compound may be considered "inert" toxicologically, its distribution in the brain, perhaps due to its fat solubility, demonstrates that CF_3I^{131} is not wholly biologically inactive.

II. Toxicology

A. Fluoroalkanes — acute inhalation toxicity

A summary of the acute inhalation toxicity of several members of this group is presented in Table 1. Much of this work was carried out in the 1930's. The test design featured exposures of short duration, up to two hours, because the compounds were being developed as fire extinguishing agents or refrigerants. The

Table 1. *Inhalation toxicity of fluoromethanes*

Group	Structure	Exposure Concn. %	Exposure Hours	Fatal + or —	U.L.[1] class	TLV[2]
A	$CHCl_3$	2.0	2	+	3	50
	$CHCl_2F$	10.0	1	+	4—5	1000
	$CHClF_2$	20.0	2	—	5a	(1000)
	CHF_3	20.0	2	—	6[3]	(1000)
B	CCl_4	2.0	1	+	3	10
	CCl_3F	10.0	2	—	5a	1000
	CCl_2F_2	20.0	2	—	6	1000
	$CClF_3$	20.0	2	—	6[3]	(1000)
	CF_4	20.0	2	—	6[3]	(1000)
C	CH_3Cl	2.0	2	+	4	100
	CH_2Cl_2	5.0	2	+	4—5	500
	$CHCl_2F$	10	1	+	4—5	1000
	CCl_2F_2	20	2	—	6	1000

[1] U.L. signifies Underwriters' classification. The higher the value the lower the toxicity.
[2] TLV = Threshold Limit Value assigned by the American Conference of Governmental Industrial Hygienists, 1964 Values. Figures in parentheses indicate provisional values.
[3] Based on data from Haskell Laboratory.
From: Underwriters' Laboratories Reports MH Nos. 2360, 2375, and 3134, and from Haskell Laboratory's unpublished reports.

principal hazard to the public was a short exposure, because the total charge in a refrigeration unit or fire extinguisher would not be large, relative to the enclosure; and the duration of exposure would not ordinarily be prolonged. Emerging from this work was a classification which was developed by the Underwriters' Laboratories based upon the results of inhalation studies with guinea pigs. In Table 1, the column headed "U. L. Class" shows the relative standing of the fluoromethanes subjected to this kind of test. Some of the assignments to a class are based on work from the Haskell Laboratory. The higher the class number, the lower is the acute inhalation toxicity of the compound. It should be noted that not all of the experiments included in Table 1 employed the guinea pig as the test species. In the studies at Haskell Laboratory, rats were used; and in yet others, both rats and guinea pigs were exposed, *e.g.*, with CF_4, $CClF_3$. There were no major differences in the results where both species were exposed, and thus it is concluded that the classification may be based on data from either rat or guinea pig.

Summarizing the classification in order to highlight the differences among the various compounds illustrated: Class 3 includes compounds which are lethal or produce serious injury in animals freely inhaling the vapors for one hour at a concentration of 2 to 2.5% by volume, *e.g.*, CCl_4 and $CHCl_3$. Class 6, the least toxic category established is defined by compounds which do not produce injury in two hours' exposure to 20% by volume, *e.g.*, CCl_2F_2 and $CClF_2{-}CClF_2$. It is noteworthy that the fluoromethanes included in Table 1 are in the class range 4—5 to 6, denoting low toxicity. The extreme righthand column headed TLV in Table 1 also calls attention to the low order of toxicity of the compounds. The TLV or Threshold Limit Value is a hygienic guide to be applied to industrial exposures to the compounds. While all of the standards which are current do not have the same basis, the figure of 1000 ppm which is acceptable by the American Conference of Governmental Industrial Hygienists (ACGIH) for the fluoromethanes listed in Table 1 is commensurate with the low order of toxicity for this group. Only one chemical on the ACGIH list has a higher standard, viz., CO_2 at 5000 ppm; and it is a matter of history in the first list (Cook, 1945) proposing acceptable atmospheric levels for the industrial environment, that the fluoromethanes and fluoroethanes were assigned values from 5000 ppm ($CHCl_2F$) up to 100,000 ppm (CCl_2F_2). The present upper limit of 1000 ppm is in accord with good engineering practice, and the lowering to this current value was not dictated by toxicity data which have contradicted the first work conducted on these materials. On the contrary, further experimental results as well as a long history of safe use have confirmed the conclusions of low toxicity first reported (Nuckolls et al., 1933, 1940, 1941).

Table 1 discloses a general principle relating the chemical constitution with the toxicity of many of the fluoroalkanes, namely, a lower toxicity is associated with an increasing number of fluorine atoms in the molecule. Even where only one fluorine replaces a chlorine atom (compare $CHCl_3$ with $CHCl_2F$), there is a vast difference in toxicity as shown by the exposures listed. It is notable thereafter that subsequent replacement of the remaining chlorine by fluorine continues to show that toxicity is further decreased as indicated by the ability of animals to survive two-hour exposures to high concentrations of $CHClF_2$ and CHF_3. The same trend is evident in the series (B) in which hydrogen is absent from the molecule. The last group (C) indicates a reduction in toxicity when hydrogen is replaced either by chlorine or fluorine. Again, the effective reduction is greater when fluorine is one of the replacement atoms. For example, in comparison with dichloromethane, CH_2Cl_2, cited in Table 1, difluoromethane, CH_2F_2, according to Henne

(1937), is not toxic for guinea pigs inhaling 20% by volume for hours. Similarly, fluorochloromethane, CH_2ClF, is tolerated by guinea pigs at a lower concentration, *i.e.*, a few per cent in air. Thus, the order of toxicity would be:

$$CH_2Cl_2 > CH_2ClF > CH_2F_2$$

When the other halogens bromine and iodine are considered in relation to fluoro-substituted methanes, the same general principle emerges, namely, that replacement of the bromine with fluorine results in a decrease in toxicity and an increase in chemical stability. For example, studies summarized by VON OETTINGEN (1955), conducted on three bromo compounds, which included fluorine or chlorine revealed the following order of toxicity: $CBr_2F_2 > CBrClF_2 > CBrF_3$, Table 2.

Table 2. *Lethal concentrations of several fire extinguishing agents*

Compound	Species	Time of exposure, min	Lethal concn., %[1]
CCl_4	Rat	10	2.8
	Guinea pig	10	2.0
CH_2BrCl	Rat	15	2.9—3.2
	Mouse	15	2.7—2.9
CBr_2F_2	Rat	15	5.5
$CBrClF_2$	Rat	15	32
$CBrF_3$	Rat	15	83

[1] Vapor mixed with air in all exposures.

From: COMSTOCK and OBERST (1952, 1953). COMSTOCK et al. (1950).

Among the various chemical fire extinguishing agents are several fluoromethanes. In considering the safety of a fire extinguishing agent, it is important to consider the toxicity of the undecomposed agent and its decomposition products generated during use in extinguishing a fire. As indicated earlier in this chapter, toxicological investigations of fire extinguishing compounds feature primarily single exposures for short periods of time in view of the usual application of these compounds to fires which required quick extinguishment, such as in aircraft or various wartime situations. Studies of biological effects resulting from repeated exposures are also important but for a different reason, namely, the protection of personnel who may be subjected to repeated exposures which could be encountered in the manufacture and handling of the compound.

To highlight the effect of fluorine in the molecule of several fire extinguishing compounds, a summary of the acute inhalation toxicity evaluated by short exposure periods not exceeding 15 minutes, is given in Table 2. The association of low acute toxicity with a high degree of fluorination of the molecule is apparent as with the alkanes already cited. It is particularly notable in the last three compounds, viz., CBr_2F_2, $CBrClF_2$, and $CBrF_3$, where the total halogenation is the same. The comparison between CBr_2F_2 and $CBrClF_2$ would seem to indicate a significant reduction of toxicity when chlorine replaces bromine.

Tables 3 through 11 present in some detail the toxicity studies conducted on various fire extinguishing agents (NUCKOLLS, 1933; MATSON and DUFOUR, 1945, 1948; COMSTOCK and OBERST, 1953; GAGE, 1954; COMSTOCK and OBERST, 1952; COMSTOCK et al., 1950; TREON et al., 1957). In the studies reported by COMSTOCK et al. (1950), the vapor of the test compound was mixed with air, therefore anoxic effects at high concentrations cannot be excluded. Since anoxia can be experienced in fire fighting, the experimental exposure conditions employed by these authors simulated the actual human hazard.

Emerging from this work is the fact that among the several compounds examined, bromotrifluoromethane, $CBrF_3$, presents the least hazard in use. Table 3 presents a favorable toxicity picture for $CBrF_3$ when guinea pigs inhaled thermal decomposition products from different kinds of fire extinguishing agents

Table 3. *Mortality of guinea pigs exposed for thirty minutes to the thermal decomposition products of several halogenated fire extinguishing agents*

Compound	Type of fire			
	Gas flame	Gasoline	Ethanol	Wood
CCl_4	2/2	—	—	—
CH_2BrCl	3/3 3/3	3/3 0/3[1]	2/3 0/3	3/3
CBr_2F_2	0/3	0/3 0/3	0/3 0/3	0/3
$CBrClF_2$	1/3	0/3 0/3	0/3 0/3	0/3
$CBrF_3$	1/3	0/3 0/3[1]	0/3 0/3	0/3

[1] 0.4 lbs agent applied.
Ratios: no. of animals dying/no. of animals exposed. Each ratio signifies an exposure.
From: Nuckolls (1933), Matson and Dufour (1945, 1948).

employed. This is again shown by the toxicities arrayed in Table 4 for the undecomposed agent. Paulet (1962) in inhalation studies on several mammalian species has shown that $CBrF_3$ has a low degree of biologic activity. The acute and chronic toxicities are both of a very low order, Tables 5 and 6. Reaction of the

Table 4. *Toxicities of various gases encountered in fire fighting*

Compound	Formula	U.L. class	ALC[1] % Vol.	ALC decompn. prod. % Vol.
Bromotrifluoromethane	$CBrF_3$	6	83.2	1.4 2.0
Carbon dioxide	CO_2	5a	65.7	—
Difluorodibromomethane	CBr_2F_2	4	5.5	0.2
Bromochloromethane	CH_2BrCl	3	6.52	0.4
Carbon tetrachloride	CCl_4	3	2.86	.032
Carbon monoxide	CO	2	1.5	—
Methyl bromide	CH_3Br	2	0.59	1.6

[1] ALC = Approximate Lethal Concentration in 15-minute rat exposure; vapors mixed with air in all exposures.
From: Comstock and Oberst (1953).

nervous system was dominant. Histology was not reported by this author. When he heated $CBrF_3$ to 1000° C and exposed rats, mice, and guinea pigs for 30 minutes to the pyrolyzed gas, the animals succumbed to a concentration of 10,000 ppm of total gas (decomposed and undecomposed). The response of animals under these conditions of exposure was consistent with irritation of the respiratory tract, Table 7. Histology disclosed pulomonary edema. Scholz and Weigand (1964) have demonstrated the low order of inhalation toxicity of $CBrF_3$. In animal experiments, concentrations as high as 60% vol. produced no behavioral changes, and medical examination of 30 workers engaged in the manufacture of $CBrF_3$ revealed no damage to health. The concentrations of carbon monoxide and

Table 5. *Mortality and clinical response of animals exposed for two hours to bromotrifluoromethane*

Concentration	Rabbit		Mice		Guinea pig		Rat	
% Vol.	Mortality	Response	Mortality	Response	Mortality	Response	Mortality	Response
30	N.C.	—	0/10	None	0/10	None	0/10	None
40	N.C.	—	0/10	None	N.C.	—	N.C.	—
50	0/2	None	0/10	Hypoactivity. Slight change in behavior. Respiration slow and deep	0/10	Only slight initial reaction, then normal	0/10	Only a slight initial reaction, then normal
60	N.C.	—	0/10	Hypoactivity. Slight change in behavior. Respiration slow and deep	N.C.	—	N.C.	—
80 (20% O_2)	0/2 0/2	Exophthalmos, mydriasis, tremors, brief convulsions, ataxia	0/10	Hypoactivity. Dyspnea, fine tremors. Effect on equilibrium and gait. Awkwardness	0/10	Somnolence, fine tremors, hind leg weakness	0/10 0/10	Somnolence, gait difficulty
85 (15% O_2)	N.C.	—	6/10 8/10	Oppression. Prostration, tremors	1/10 2/10	Nervousness. Fine tremors. Effect on equilibrium. Somnolence	N.C.	—

Paulet, G.: Arch. Mal. Prof., t. 23, (6), pp. 341—347 (June 1962).
N.C. = Not conducted.

Table 6. *Response of mice, rats, and guinea pigs repeatedly exposed to bromotrifluoromethane*
Exposure: 50% vol., 2 hrs/day, 15 days.

Species	Mortality No. dying/No. exposed	Response
Mice	1/20[1]	No signs of toxicity Body weight constant
Rats	0/10	No signs of toxicity. Body weight gain
Guinea pigs	1/10[1]	No signs of toxicity. Body weight constant

[1] Mortality not attributable to exposure.
Paulet, G.: Arch. Mal. Prof., t. **23**, (6), pp. 341 to 347 (June 1962).

carbonyl halides (COX_2) from various fire fighting candidates as shown by Table 8, place $CBrF_3$ in a preferred position. The biological responses denoted in Table 9 suggest that $CBrF_3$ would produce no serious systemic injury. Table 10 indicates the high degree of safety of bromotrifluoromethane in rapid and slow fire extinguishing procedures and the low evolution of carbonyl halides which Comstock and Oberst (1953), state to be a trace, viz., <1 ppm, *cf*. Table 8. Table 11 summarizes a number of exposures employing several species of animals inhaling $CBrF_3$ at room temperature, 2000° F, and 1300° F. Only at 2000° F did the decomposition products produce significant fatalities. Data in Table 12 constitute a general summary of the status of various halogenated alkanes considered for

Table 7. *Mortality and response of several mammalian species to pyrolyzed bromotrifluoromethane*
Exposure: Pyrolysis temperature 1000° C, 30 minutes.

Species	No. animals	Concentration[1] % Vol.	Mortality %	Animal response	Pathology
Mice Rats Guinea pigs	10 10 5	50	100	Initial agitation, somnolence, effect on equilibrium, dyspnea, prostration	Pulmonary edema
Mice Rats Guinea pigs	10 10 5	2.5	100	Slight agitation, dyspnea	Pulmonary edema
Mice Rats Guinea pigs	10 10 5	1.0	100	Few reactions, slight dyspnea. Death in 48 hours	Pulmonary edema
Mice Rats	10 10	0.75	90 20	No reactions	Pulmonary edema in animals succumbing
Mice Rats	10 10	0.50	50 0	Death occurred in mice within 3 days after exposure	Pulmonary edema in mice succumbing

[1] Based on air mixed with decomposed and undecomposed $CBrF_3$.
Paulet, G.: Arch. Mal. Prof., t. **23**, (6), pp. 341—347 (June 1962).

Table 8. *Comparison of the toxicities of halogenated fire extinguishing agents*

Agent	Concn., Mg/M³	Concn. of compds. after discharge of 3 lbs. of extinguishing agent			
		CO Mg/M³	COX_2 Mg/M³	% Mortality, 14 days	
				Mice	Rats
CCl_4	18	1.1	.04	10	33
	30	1.1	.05	10	33
CH_2BrCl	82	1.1	.02	20	8
	47	1.1	.03	32	29
CBr_2F_2.	43	1.1	.02	37	0
	20	1.6	.06	100	9
$CBrF_3$	11	1.1	< 1 ppm	0	0
	14	1.1	< 1 ppm	5	3

$X_2 = Br_2$, Cl_2, or F_2.
From: Comstock and Oberst (1952).

fire extingushing agents. Here it is observed as noted above that the order of toxicity is related to the halogen components of the molecule, being low on the toxicity scale with an increase in number of fluorine atoms and higher on the scale with increase in the number of chlorine and/or bromine atoms. The total number of halogens would seem to have little influence on toxicity of these compounds.

Low toxicity and a high degree of fluorination is also evident in the alkanes of longer chain length. The acute inhalation toxicity of various polyfluoroethanes is summarized in Table 13. The inclusion of $CClF_2{-}CHF_2$ (Nuckolls et al., 1940) illustrates that hydrogen appeared to have little or no effect on toxicity when there are four fluorine atoms. An interesting point with regard to isomers is evident from work reported recently by Clayton et al. (1964), who compared the asym-

Table 9. *Halogenated fire extinguishing agents*
Minimal concentrations (ppm) required to produce characteristic reactions in rats.

Reactions	Chlorobromo-methane CH_2BrCl	Trifluorobromo-methane $CBrF_3$	Difluorodi-bromomethane CBr_2F_2	Tetrafluorodi-bromoethane $CBrF_2 \cdot CBrF_2$	Carbon tetrachloride CCl_4
Incoordination	4,750 (26 min)[1]			3,400	9,000 (14 min)
Drowsiness	4,750 (26 min)	500,000 (26 min)	10,000 (14 min)		9,000 (20 min)
Limb twitching and slight body tremors			15,000 (10 min)	13,500 (14 min)	15,500 (12 min)
Convulsions and acute body tremors			30,000 (11—13 min)	27,000 (9 min)	
Deep narcosis	19,000 (17 min)				18,000 (9—11 min)
Delayed death (about 36 hours)					18,000
Liver damage					18,000
Death during exposure	39,000 (30 min)				27,000

[1] Times of onset of reactions in parentheses.
From: GAGE (1954).

Table 10. *Toxicities of fire extinguishing agents*

1. Rapid fire extinguishing[1]

$$CBr_2F_2 > CH_2BrCl > CBrF_3$$

2. Slow fire extinguishing[1]

$$CBr_2F_2 > CH_2BrCl > CBrF_3$$
$$CCl_4$$

3. Evolution of carbonyl halides (slow extinguishment)

$$CCl_4 > CH_2BrCl > CBrF_3$$

[1] Gasoline fire.
From: COMSTOCK and OBERST (1953).

Table 11. *Inhalation toxicity of bromotrifluoromethane*

Thermal state of compound	Concn., % Vol.	Duration, No. × Hrs.	Mortality ratio: Cat	Guinea Pig	Mice	Rabbit	Rat	Total
Room temp.	32.7	1 × 7	0/1	0/6	0/10	1/4	0/10	1/31
Room temp.	17.6	2 × 7	0/1	0/5	0/10	0/4	0/10	0/30
1300° F	2.0	1 × .3	0/1	0/5	0/10	0/3	0/10	0/29
1300° F	0.75	1 × .3	0/1	0/6	0/10	0/4	0/10	0/31
2000° F	2.0	1 × .3	1/1	6/6	10/10	4/4	10/10	31/31
2000° F	0.75	1 × .3	1/1	6/6	10/10	2/4	8/10	27/31

From: TREON et al. (1957).

Table 12. *Summary of acute inhalation toxicity of various halogenated alkanes with reference to chemical constitution*

Order of toxicity → Decreasing								
ALC[1], % Vol.	CCl_4	CH_2BrCl	$CBrClF-CBrF_2$	CBr_2F_2	$CBrF_2-CBrF_2$	$CBrClF_2$	$CBrF_3$	CF_4
	2.8	2.9—3.2	2.5	5.5	13	33	83	90
Halogenation	Number of halogen atoms							
Cl	4	1	1	0	0	1	0	0
Br	0	1	1	2	2	1	1	0
F	0	0	3	2	4	2	3	4

[1] ALC = Approximate Lethal Concentration in 15-minute rat exposure, vapors mixed with air in all exposures.

From: COMSTOCK and OBERST (1953).

Table 13. *Acute inhalation toxicity of several fluoroethanes*

Structure	Approximate lethal concentration			Source
	% Vol.	Hrs exp.	Species	
CCl_2F-CCl_2F	1.5	4	Rat	CLAYTON et al. (1964)
$CClF_2-CCl_3$	1.5	4	Rat	CLAYTON et al. (1964)
$CCl_2F-CClF_2$	10	6	Rat	Haskell Laboratory, unpublished
$CClF_2-CClF_2$	>20	8	Guinea pig	YANT et al. (1932)
$CClF_2-CHF_2$	>20	2	Guinea pig	NUCKOLLS et al. (1940)
$CClF_2-CF_3$	>80[1]	4	Rat	CLAYTON et al. (1965)
CHF_2-CF_3	>10	4	Rat	Haskell Laboratory, unpublished
CF_3-CF_3	>80[1]	4	Rat	Haskell Laboratory, unpublished

[1] 80% fluorocarbon and 20% O_2.

metric and symmetric isomers of tetrachlorodifluoroethane, viz., $CClF_2-CCl_3$ and CCl_2F-CCl_2F respectively. Clinical and histologic responses of rats to single inhalation exposures to these two isomers were similar. The similarity is further evidenced by the first two ALC values listed in Table 13. Table 17 gives a more complete comparison of the toxicity of the two isomers.

When bromine is added to the ethane structure replacing chlorine, the resultant toxicity is greater although still of a low order. ROBBINS (1946), for example, lists the following lethal concentrations for four partially halogenated ethanes. His paper should be consulted for data on a large number of other fluorinated compounds.

Structure	Mouse ALC/10 min exposure
1. CH_2Cl-CF_3	25.0% by volume
2. $CH_2Cl-CHF_2$	7.5% by volume
3. CH_2Br-CF_3	11.7% by volume
4. $CH_2Br-CHF_2$	4.6% by volume

Comparison of compound 1 with compound 2 and compound 3 with compound 4 illustrates the apparent contribution of hydrogen to the toxicity when hydrogen replaces fluorine in a molecule in which degree of fluorination is relatively low. Comparison of 1 with 3 and 2 with 4 shows a relative increase in toxicity when bromine replaces chlorine.

The acute inhalation toxicity of various fluorinated propanes as determined by 10-minute mouse exposures is illustrated in Table 14. It is concluded that these have a low order of inhalation toxicity, and that again the number of fluorine atoms in the molecule is related inversely to this property. As with the methane and ethane compounds cited, an increase in toxicity is related to replacement of chlorine with bromine. Investigation of the acute inhalation toxicity of 2-chloroheptafluoropropane, which contains no hydrogen, disclosed an order of toxicity lower than that of the hydrogen-containing fluoropropanes of Table 14, indicating

Table 14. *Toxicity of several fluoropropanes for mice exposed for 10 min*

Structure	Anesthetic concn., %	Approx. lethal concn., %
$HCF_2—CF_2—CClF_2$	10	20
$HCF_2—CF_2—CBrF_2$	4	10
$HCF_2—CF_2—CHClF$	2.5	3
$HCF_2—CF_2—CHCl_2$	0.5	2
$CClF_2—CF_2—CH_2F$	10	15
$CClF_2—CF_2—CHF_2$	10	20

From: Unpublished data of Haskell Laboratory.

a role of hydrogen in the biologic activity of this group. Rats survived a four-hour exposure to 20% by volume of 2-chloroheptafluoropropane without clinical evidence of anesthesia, toxic effects, or pathologic change. Addition of chlorine increases the toxicity of the perhalogenated propanes as illustrated by 1,1,1-trichloropentafluoropropane which is lethal to rats exposed four hours to 3.0% by volume in contrast to the foregoing mono-chloro analogue which is not lethal at 20% by volume.

The toxicology of the polyfluorobutanes follows in sequence in a similar way as noted for the lower members of the series, with increasing fluorination of the chain resulting in a reduction in toxicity. The series of butanes culminates in decafluorobutane.

Rats exposed to 80% C_4F_{10} and 20% oxygen for four hours showed only slight effects on respiration, but no pathological changes when sacrificed (Clayton 1958). In a study conducted by Allied Chemical Corporation, two mice were exposed in a 22-liter exposure system to a mixture of approximately 76% (vol) C_4F_{10} and 20% (vol) oxygen, the remainder nitrogen. Two exposures were made (separate animals), one of 16 hours and the other of $14^1/_2$ hours. No sign of anesthetic or other toxic effect were noted during or following the exposure. Pathology was not carried out. The early toxicity study on C_4F_{10} reported by Struck and Plattner (1940), is complicated because only one mouse was used and the purity of the sample may be questioned in light of the subsequent studies of Banks et al. (1954).

The perfluorinated member of the cyclic butanes, octafluorocyclobutane (OFCB), has been subjected to intensive animal tests because of its proposed use as a food propellent (Clayton et al., 1960). A summary of inhalation studies is presented in Table 15. Acute exposures with mice and rats show OFCB to have an extremely low order, if not complete lack of toxicity. Four-hour exposures of rats, and fifteen-minute exposures of mice to 80% OFCB and 20% oxygen in a rotating exposure chamber designed to determine the point of anesthesia disclosed no signs of toxicity or anesthesia. As discussed below under chronic toxicity, repeated exposures of a variety of species to concentrations of 1.0% to 10% OFCB did not result in toxic effects.

Table 15. *Toxicity studies on octafluorocyclobutane (OFCB)*

Exposures		No. of exposures	Species	Toxic effects
OFCB concn. % Vol.	Duration hrs.			
80[1]	0.25	1	Mice	None
80[1]	4	1	Rats	None
1.0	6	19	Rats	None
10	6	4	Rat, mice, guinea pig, dog	None
10	6	90	Rats, mice, rabbit, dog	None

[1] 80% OFCB + 20% oxygen.
From: CLAYTON et al. (1960).

B. Fluoroalkanes — acute toxicity: oral, skin and eye

The preceding account has dealt exclusively with the acute inhalation toxicity of the fluoroalkanes. Its importance is to be expected since the first developed compounds were gases at room temperature when used as refrigerant or fire extinguishing compounds and the hazard was from inhalation. However, with the expanding uses for fluoroalkanes, it is apropos to consider the toxicity by other routes of administration. As shown in Table 16, the several fluoroalkanes illustrated show a low order of acute oral toxicity for the rat. Rats have been repeatedly dosed by gastric intubation with dichlorodifluoromethane (CCl_2F_2) dissolved in peanut oil. The average daily dose during ten daily treatments was 430 mg/kg. The six rats survived and showed no clinical signs of toxicity. A similar experiment with the symmetrical dichlorotetrafluoroethane ($CClF_2$—$CClF_2$) was carried out at a daily dosage of 1300 mg/kg and there were no deaths or clinical signs of toxicity. QUEVAUVILLER (1965) reported that a daily oral dose of 2000 mg/kg of dichlorotetrafluoroethane was tolerated by rats for a period of 23 to 33 days.

Table 16. *Acute oral toxicity of various fluoroalkanes*

Compound	ALD, mg/kg[1]	Source
CCl_2F_2	> 1,000[2]	Haskell Laboratory, unpublished
$CHCl_2CClF_2$	7,500	Haskell Laboratory, unpublished
CCl_2FCCl_2F	> 25,000	CLAYTON et al. (1964)
$CClF_2CCl_3$	> 25,000	CLAYTON et al. (1964)
$CClF_2CCl_2F$	45,000 (LD_{50} = 43,000)	ODOU (1963)
$CClF_2CClF_2$	> 2,250[2]	Haskell Laboratory, unpublished

[1] Rats, 10—14 day survival period.
[2] Maximum feasible dose of fluorocarbon dissolved in peanut oil.

The symmetric and asymmetric isomers of tetrachlorodifluoroethane have been compared for toxicity (CLAYTON et al., 1964). Several routes of administration were included in this study; the results are summarized in Table 17. The two isomers were shown by this work to have a low order of acute oral, dermal, and inhalation toxicity (*cf.* preceding section). The Approximate Lethal Dose for rats by the oral route was >25,000 for both isomers. On skin application, rabbits exhibited local irritation, but did not succumb nor exhibit a systemic response to either isomer, although a maximum feasible dose was applied (>7500 mg/kg of CCl_2F-CCl_2F; >11,000 mg/kg of $CClF_2-CCl_3$). Application of the symmetric isomer, CCl_2F-CCl_2F, to the skin of guinea pigs produced mild irritation but no skin sensitization. It was mildly irritating to the rabbit eye without damaging the cornea or iris. Washing the eye with water reduced the duration of irritation.

Table 17. *Comparison of the toxicity of the symmetric and asymmetric isomers of tetrachlorodifluoroethane*

Symmetric isomer CCl_2F—CCl_2F "Freon-112"	Asymmetric isomer $CClF_2$—CCl_3 "Freon-112a"
Oral toxicity	
Approximate lethal dose (rat)	
> 25,000 mg/kg	> 25,000 mg/kg
Diarrhea, weight loss at 11,000 mg/kg and above. Liver and major organs normal histologically.	Diarrhea, weight loss at 11,000 mg/kg and above. Slight increase in liver weight at 25,000 mg/kg. Liver and kidney normal histologically.
Ten-day repeated (rat)	
5,000 mg/kg daily	5,000 mg/kg daily
Mortality: 1/5; diarrhea; initial body weight loss; tremor inactivity; slight increase in liver weight; slight reversible histological change in liver.	Mortality: 0/6; diarrhea; initial body weight loss; tremor inactivity; slight increase in liver weight; liver normal histologically.
Dermal toxicity	
Approximate lethal dose (rabbit)	
> 7500 mg/kg	> 11,000 mg/kg
Skin erythema; no signs of systemic toxicity; no histological changes in major organs.	Severe skin irritation in ethanol; weight loss; histological change in skin musculature, none in major organs.
Inhalation toxicity	
Approximate lethal concentration (rat)	
15,000 ppm (vol.)	15,000 ppm (vol.)
Respiratory and CNS effects; slight liver change histologically.	Respiratory and CNS effects; slight to moderate liver changes histologically.

From: Clayton et al. (1964).

These experiments demonstrated that the biological action of the two isomers was similar at the same dose levels. Orally, the two compounds acted on the gastrointestinal tract and produced a mild liver reaction at high doses without causing histological injury. Repeated oral doses of both isomers, 5000 mg/kg daily, for 10 days, also act similarly. These resulted in a slight, reversible liver response, as judged histologically.

Trichlorotrifluoroethane, $CCl_2F-CClF_2$, as indicated by rat studies in Table 16 has a low order of oral toxicity with an LD_{50} of 43,000 mg/kg. Odou (1963) has administered a massive oral dose to a female dog lightly anesthetized with sodium pentobarbital. The total dose given was 92,000 mg/kg; death occurred in 1.5 hours. Some dogs have survived oral doses of this magnitude, and recently Odou (1963) reported that a human under anesthesia accidently received about one liter of cold $CCl_2F-CClF_2$ in the stomach. This produced immediate but transient cyanosis. The individual survived and reported only severe rectal irritation and diarrhea for 3 days thereafter.

Trichlorotrifluoroethane, $CCl_2F-CClF_2$, is also low in toxicity as judged by skin contact studies with rabbits. Application of $CCl_2F-CClF_2$ to the skin of rabbits gave an ALD of $>11{,}000$ mg/kg. The only effect was a local irritation of the skin at the site of application, and histology disclosed alterations in the dermis and adjacent connective tissues. There were no systemic changes attributable to treatment. Applications of $CCl_2F-CClF_2$ at a very high dose of 5000 mg/kg each day for 5 days resulted in fluctuations in weight and damage to the skin evident grossly and histologically. Slight liver changes were observed microscopically but no other systemic changes were disclosed. When instilled undiluted into the eyes of 3 rabbits and washed out with water 20 seconds later, $CCl_2F-CClF_2$ produced mild, transient conjunctivitis in one rabbit only; the others showed no reaction. Instillation into rabbit eyes without water washing produced minimal corneal dullness only in one rabbit and this subsided in 48 hours.

Similar results from eye studies on dichlorodifluoromethane were reported by Downing and Madinabeitia (1960), citing work conducted at Haskell Laboratory. In this work a 50% solution of CCl_2F_2 in refined mineral oil was sprayed into rabbits' eyes from a distance of about six inches. Controls consisted of rabbits receiving mineral oil alone. The animals receiving the fluorocarbon with mineral oil in the eye showed the same eye reaction as the controls did. In both groups, slight conjunctival irritation developed, but this had disappeared in 24 hours.

Chloropentafluoroethane, $CClF_2-CF_3$, dissolved in cottonseed oil, was administered orally to rats five times a week for two weeks. Five ml of test solution was given at each treatment, and the individual daily doses were in the range of 140–172 mg/kg. A group of control rats received the oil alone. During the treatment period, there were no differences between the test and control rats with respect to appearance and rate of weight gain. This was also true of a recovery period of two weeks. Test and control rats were killed four hours and fourteen days after the tenth dose. Gross and microscopic examination of major tissues revealed no change attributable to $CClF_2-CF_3$. Therefore under the conditions of this experiment there was no evidence of cumulative toxic effects exerted by $CClF_2-CF_3$, an observation supported by repeated inhalation studies reported in the next section.

Quevauviller et al. (1964) and Quevauviller (1965) have investigated the effects of various fluoroalkanes on the skin, tongue, soft palate, and auditory canal of rats; the eye of the rabbit; and the speed of healing of wounds and burns in the rat. Five materials were evaluated by these tests, namely, CCl_3F, CCl_2F_2, CCl_3F, and CCl_2F_2 mixed; CCl_3F and $CHClF_2$ mixed; and $CClF_2-CClF_2$. The animals were treated one or two times a day, five days a week for 5 or 6 weeks. In the case of wounds and burns, the treatment was continued until healing was complete. The compounds or mixtures were released from pressurized containers for 5 or 10 seconds from a distance of 10 cm to 20 cm onto the experimental site.

The skin of the rats became irritated evincing an edema and a slight inflammatory reaction. The reactions were most marked with the $CCl_3F/CHClF_2$ mixture and $CClF_2-CClF_2$. Older rats were more severely affected than younger rats.

The application of the five test substances to the tongue, soft palate, and auditory canal of rats produced no significant abnormalities. In one rat treated with $CClF_2-CClF_2$ the auditory canal showed desquamation of the epithelium and inflammation.

The rabbit eye responded to the five materials by a hyperemia and lacrimation. There was an inflammatory reaction of the eyelid noted in rabbits exposed to CCl_3F and $CClF_2-CClF_2$. There were no other histologic alterations.

The healing of wounds and burns experimentally made on the skin of rats was retarded compared to controls. There appeared to be little if any differences in this retardation among these five compounds or mixtures evaluated.

C. Fluoroalkanes — chronic inhalation toxicity

Summaries of studies in which animals were exposed repeatedly to several of the fluoroalkanes are given in Tables 18, 19 and 20. It is notable that comparatively few such experiments have been conducted and those that are cited here have shown an evolution of increasing complexity. This reflects the expanding use and the changing hazards associated with these compounds. In the 1930's single exposures usually yielded sufficient information upon which to gauge toxicity, and in fact hygienic standards such as the Threshold Limit Values of the American Conference of Governmental Industrial Hygienists were initially based on these single exposures (Cook, 1945). Lately, however, because of new uses such as food propellents or novel conditions of exposure such as in nuclear-powered submarines or space vehicles, toxicity investigations have become extended in scope.

Illustrative of the enlarged experimental design among the fluorinated methanes is the recent work on dichlorodifluoromethane (Siegel, 1964). This work is in agreement with that reported by Yant et al. (1932) on this material in disclosing a low order of toxicity. Neither work necessitates a change in the Threshold Limit Value of 1000 ppm (8-hour, time-weighted concentration) established by the ACGIH and based on single exposures of animals.

The potential use of octafluorocyclobutane (Clayton et al., 1960) and chloropentafluoroethane (Clayton et al., 1965) as food propellents when enclosed in pressurized containers required a demonstration that the compounds would be safe for humans ingesting them in foods. In view of the obvious inadequacy of feeding these two compounds which are gases at room temperature, it was decided to conduct repeated inhalation exposures at 100,000 ppm. The results showed a low order of toxicity under conditions which in all probability would not obtain even under conditions of abuse of the food articles as finally packaged.

There has been some criticism that the repeated studies on the fluoroalkanes do not provide comprehensive enough data upon which a safe working concentration can be based. For example, Caujolle (1963), states that a vast field of investigations is open before *absolute harmlessness* can be claimed. This is no doubt true, but recent studies have abvanced a considerable distance over earlier work. Lifetime studies on at least two species are eminently desirable to approach the evanescent goal of harmlessness; however, the studies summarized, together with long experience in handling would not seem to jeopardize the current hygienic standards. On the other hand as new uses are developed for this class of compounds, toxicity studies commensurate with the hazard should be carried out.

D. Fluoroalkanes — cyclic compounds

Toxicity experiments have been conducted on various fractions of fluorocyclohexanes and fluorocyclohexadienes resulting from fluorination of benzene, a process which was associated with minor toxic symptoms, headache and diarrhea in workers. In an acute exposure to a high concentration there was unconsciousness in an individual engaged in research on these materials (Ensor, 1960). The

Table 18. *Summary of repeated inhalation*

ALC % Vol. Species, time	Exposure			Animals				Observations
	Conc. ppm	Hrs/day	Days	Kind	Sex	No.	Mortality ratio	
								Trichlorofluoro-
6.6 Rats 4-hr.	12,000	4	10 +11 Recovery	Rats	M	4	0/4	Resp. slight increase in depth and rate; chewing motions, slight twitching; quick recovery after exposure
	4,000	6	28 +15 Recovery	Rats	M	6	0/6	No significant clinical signs of toxicity in any species
				Rats	F	6	0/6	
				Mice	M	4	0/4	
				Mice	F	4	0/4	
				GPigs	M	2	0/2	
				Rabbit	M	1	0/1	
	25,000	3.5	20	Cats	?	2	0/2	No signs of toxicity
				GPigs	?	3	0/3	
				Rats	M	5	0/5	
	12,500	3.5	20	Dogs	?	2	0/2	No signs of toxicity
								Dichlorodifluoro-
≧ 20 GPig 8-hr; ≧ 80 4—6 hr. Rats	200,000	7—8	52	Dog		2	0/2	*Dogs and monkeys:* Tremors, staggering gait. Decrease in severity with time. *GPigs:* No toxic signs. No abnormal foetuses
			35—52	Monkeys		2	0/2	
			3.5—56	GPigs		26	10/26	
	100,000	3.5	20	Cats	?	2	0/2	No signs of toxicity
				GPigs	?	3	0/3	
				Rats	M	5	0/5	
				Dogs	?	2	0/2	
	810	24 (cont. expos. except for 51 hours)	92	Rats		15	2/15	No signs of toxicity related to CCl_2F_2
				GPigs		15	1/15	
				Rabbits		3	0/3	
				Monkeys		3	0/3	
				Dogs		2	0/2	
	840	8	30	Rats		15	1/15	No signs of toxicity related to CCl_2F_2
				GPigs		15	0/15	
				Rabbits		3	0/3	
				Monkeys		3	0/3	
				Dogs		2	0/2	
								CCl_3F/CCl_2F_2 (50:50)
	5,000	2	100	Mice	M	5	0/5	No toxic signs or narcosis
				Mice	F	5	0/5	
	15,000	2	100	Rats	M	5	0/5	
				Rats	F	5	0/5	
	50,000	2	100	GPigs	M	5	0/5	
				GPigs	F	5	0/5	
								Chlorotrifluoro-
> 20 GPig 2-hr	10,000	6	20	Rats	M	6	0/6	No clinical signs of toxicity

exposures of several fluoromethanes

Body weight change	Hematology	Clinical chemistry; urinalysis	Pathology	Ref.
methane CCl_3F				
Normal	ND[1]	ND[1]	Brain: Neuronal edema, neuroglial vacuol.; Lungs: Emphysema, edema. Liver: Vacuolation of cells; Spleen: Increased hematopoiesis	1
Normal for all species	*Rats:* No significant change at the end of the exposure or 15 days later in rbc, wbc, hemoglobin or hematocrit	ND	No histological changes attributable to CCl_3F in any species sacrificed after 28th exposure or 15 days later	2
Normal all species	Normal rbc, wbc, differential white count, hemoglobin	Normal urinary protein and sediment	No changes in heart, lungs, liver, kidney, and spleen	3
Normal	Same as above	Same as above	Same as above	
methane CCl_2F_2				
Initial slight weight depression	Initial slight increase rbc and Hb; slight increase in polymorphs; lymphocytes decreased	ND	No gross changes attributable to CCl_2F_2	4, 4a
Normal all species	Normal rbc, wbc, differential white count, hemoglobin	Normal urinary protein and sediment	No changes in heart, lungs, liver, kidney, and spleen	3
Normal	Normal limits for: hematocrit, hemoglobin, WBC, and differential white counts. Bone marrow counts normal in rats	ND	*GPigs:* Liver cell vacuolation (15/15), focal necrosis (4/15). Monkeys: Liver cell vacuolation (2/3)	5
Normal	Normal limits for: hematocrit, hemoglobin, WBC, and differential white counts. Bone marrow counts normal in rats	ND	*GPigs:* Focal liver necrosis (2/8). Monkeys: Pigment deposit in liver, spleen and kidney	
and (10:90)				
Normal all species	Normal all species	ND	No effects attributable to exposure on liver or other organs	6
methane $CClF_3$				
Normal	No significant changes in red and white cell counts, hemoglobin, hematocrit and differential white cell count	ND	No gross or micropathological changes. Organ weights within normal range	7

Table 18

ALC % Vol. Species, time	Exposure: Conc. ppm	Hrs/day	Days	Animals: Kind	Sex	No.	Mortality ratio	Observations
								Chlorodifluoro-
40% Vol. Mice 2-hr	14,200	6	10 mos.	Rabbits Rats Mice	? ? ?	7 36 30	No record of any deaths	*Mice:* Lowered endurance in swimming test. *Rats:* Decrease in O_2 consumption, increase in the number of subthreshold impulses to produce reflex. *Mice:* Increase in the number of trials needed to establish conditioned reflex
	1,980	6	10 mos.	Rats Mice	?	30 30	No deaths recorded	Observation on O_2 consumption, swimming, endurance, formation of conditioned reflexes and number of subthreshold impulses needed to evoke a reflex were all similar to the controls
								Bromotrifluoro-
> 80 2-hr Mice Rats GPigs Rabbits	500,000	2	15	Mice Rats GPigs	M M M	20 10 10	1/20 0/10 1/10	No signs of toxicity in any species
	23,000	6	90	Rats Dogs	? ?	30 3	No deaths	No signs of toxicity

[1] Not done.

References:

1. Unpublished Haskell Laboratory report.
2. Haskell Laboratory report.
3. Scholz, J.: Fortschr. d. Biol. Aerosol-Forsch. **4**, 420—429 (1957—1961).
4. Sayers, R. R., W. P. Yant, J. Chornyak, and H. W. Shoaf: U. S. Bureau of Mines report No. 3013, May, 1930.

toxicity studies on various fractions implicated $C_6H_4F_8$ as the most toxic. A summary of the acute toxicity tests is given in Table 21. The author concludes that the toxicity of the fluorinated cyclohexanes tends to vary inversely with the fluorine content. The least toxic was $C_6H_2F_{10}$ which produced no toxic effects in the maximum doses employed in the intraperitoneal, subcutaneous, and oral tests. However, the results also show that the three isomers of $C_6H_4F_8$ differ measurably in toxicity, thus suggesting that the biological activity is related to properties of the molecule other than the degree of fluorination, which seemingly influence toxicity. It is postulated that compounds having less than 8 fluorine atoms would be even more toxic than $C_6H_4F_8$, b.p. 133° C.

(continued)

Body weight change	Hematology	Clinical chemistry; urinalysis	Pathology	Ref.
methane $CHClF_2$				
Mice decrease	*Rabbits:* Decrease in red count, hemoglobin, lymphocytes, reticulocytes. Increase in neutrophiles and eosinophiles	*Rabbits:* Decrease in blood cholinesterase; serum albumin decreased; globulin increased	Changes in lungs leading to emphysema, exudate alveolar septal thickening. Degenerative changes in heart, liver, kidney and nervous system	
Normal	No changes	No changes	No effects attributable to exposure	8
methane $CBrF_3$				
Constant Gain Constant	ND	ND	ND	9
Normal	No changes	No changes	No effects attributable to exposure	10

4a. LESTER, D., and L. A. GREENBERG: A.M.A. Arch. Ind. Hyg. and Occup. Med. **2**, 335—344 (1950).
5. SIEGEL, J.: Personal communication from U.S. Navy Toxicology Unit.
6. KÜBLER, H.: J. Soc. Cosmetic Chemists **14**, 341—351 (1963).
7. Unpublished Haskell Laboratory report.
8. KARPOV, B. C.: Tr. Leningr. Sanit.-Gigien. Med. Inst. **75**, 231—240 (1963).
9. PAULET, G.: Arch. Mal. Prof., t. **23**, 341—347 (1962).
10. COMSTOCK, C. C., J. KERSCHNER, and F. W. OBERST: Chemical Corps Medical Labs. Research Report No. 180, AD-11, 563 (1953).

E. Fluoroalkanes — biological action

Generally speaking, the low chemical reactivity of the fluoroalkanes is matched by their biological inertness. This feature is clear from the foregoing account where it has been repeatedly demonstrated that toxicity is inversely related to the number of fluorine atoms contained in the molecule. In this section, the action of the fluoroalkanes on the central nervous system and on the liver will be examined, and a similar association between the degree of fluorination and biologic activity will be shown.

The notable chemical stability in this group of materials is related to the CF_3- or $-CF_2$-groups which are not only stable themselves but also confer stability

Table 19. *Summary of repeated inhalation exposures of*

ALC % Vol. Species, time	Exposure			Animals				Observations
	Conc. ppm	Hrs/day	Days	Kind	Sex	No.	Mortality ratio	
1,1,2,2-Tetrachloro-1,2-di-								
~ 1.5 (Rats) 4-hr	3,000	4	10 +10 Recovery	Rats	M	4	0/4	Prostrate and incoordinate during 1st exposure. Rapid and shallow resp. Hyperresponsive during each expos. Immediate recovery after expos.
	1,000	6	31	Rats Rats Mice GPigs Rabbit	M F F M M	8 8 10 2 1	0/8 0/8 0/10 0/2 0/1	No clinical signs of toxicity
	1,000	18	16	Rats		6	0/6	No clinical signs of toxicity
1,1,2-Trichlorotrifluoro-								
8.69 Rats 4-hr	2,520 (2,075 to 2,885)	7	30	Rats Rats	M F	10 11	0/10 0/11	No clinical signs of toxicity
	5,000	7	30	Rats		12	0/12	Not given
	12,500	3.5	20	Cats Dogs	? ?	2 2	0/2 0/2	No signs of toxicity
	25,000	3.5	20	GPigs Rats	? M	3 5	0/3 0/5	No signs of toxicity
Dichlorotetrafluoro-								
> 20 GPigs 24-hr	200,000	8 8	4 2	GPigs GPigs		6 10	0/6 0/10	Slight tremors and convulsive jerks of the body
	141,600	8	21	GPigs		6	1/6	Died 3 days after termination of exposure from generalized infection. No abnormal symptoms observed
< 14.2 > 20 Dogs 8-hr	200,000	8 8	3—4 4	Dogs Dog		2 1	2/2 1/1	Marked generalized tremors and convulsions in dogs and death after 3 to 4 daily periods
< 20 Dogs 16-hr		8	4.03	Dog		1	1/1	
	141,600 141,600	8 8	3 21	Dog Dogs		1 2	0/1 0/2	Marked incoordination with generalized tremors and occasional convulsions. Tolerance developed after 3 to 5 days of exposure

several fluoroethanes and octafluorocyclobutane

Body weight change	Hematology	Clinical chemistry; urinalysis	Pathology	Ref.
fluoroethane CCl_2F—CCl_2F				
Slight wt. loss 1st day normal thereafter	ND[1]	ND[1]	No change after 10th expos.; tracheitis in 1 rat 10 days after last exposure	1
Normal for all species	Female rats: significant decrease in leucocyte count. Male rats: suggestive decrease in leucocyte count. Not statistically significant, however	ND	Male rats: liver and kidney wts. greater than controls. No gross or micropathological changes for other species. Micro.: transient liver reactions in rats	
Normal	ND	ND	None reported	2
ethane CCl_2F—$CClF_2$				
Normal	ND	ND	No gross or microscopic pathology	3
Did not gain normally	ND	ND	Three rats showed slightly pale livers; others normal. Kidneys normal	4
Normal all species	Normal, rbc, wbc, differential white count, hemoglobin	Normal urinary protein and sediment	No changes in heart, lungs, liver, kidney, spleen	5
ethane $CClF_2$—$CClF_2$				
Normal	ND	ND	Occasional slight fatty degeneration of the liver. No gross changes otherwise	6
Not given	ND	ND	Same as above	
Weight loss	Increased hemoglobin RBC's and younger forms of polymorphonuclear leucocytes. Platelets decreased	ND	Congestion throughout all the organs	6
Decrease first 5 days, increase thereafter	Same as above. All counts were normal 15—17 days after exposure	ND	No gross pathology noted	

Table 19

ALC % Vol. Species, time	Exposure Conc. ppm	Hrs/day	Days	Animals Kind	Sex	No.	Mortality ratio	Observations
								Dichlorotetrafluoro-
> 20 GPig 24-hr	100,000	3.5	20	Cats	?	2	0/2	No signs of toxicity
				GPigs	?	3	0/3	
				Rats	M	5	0/5	
				Dogs	?	2	0/2	
								Chloropentafluoro-
> 80 Rats 4-hr	100,000	6	90	Rats	M	10	0/10	No clinical signs of toxicity in any species related to $CClF_2—CF_3$
				Rats	F	10	0/10	
				Mice	F	10	0/10	
				Rabbits	M	2	0/2	
				Rabbits	F	2	0 2	
				Dogs	M	4	0/4	
								Octafluorocyclo-
> 80 Rats 4-hr	100,000	6	90	Rats	M	10	0/10	No clinical signs of toxicity. Behavior, blood pressure, heart rate and rectal temperature of dogs were normal
				Rats	F	10	0/10	
				Mice	F	10	0/10	
				Rabbits	M	2	0/2	
				Rabbits	F	2	0/2	
				Dogs	M	4	0/4	
	10,000	6	19	Rats	M	6	0/6	No clinical signs of toxicity

[1] Not done.

References:

1. Clayton et al. (1964).
2. Greenberg, L. A., and D. Lester: A.M.A. Arch. Ind. Hyg. and Occup. Med. **2**, 345—347 (1950).
3. Unpublished Haskell Laboratory Report.
4. U.S.N. Report NS-041-001.

on adjacent carbon atoms and attendant halogens. It was natural, therefore, that the chemical stability along with the volatility and nonflammability of many of the fluoroalkanes of short chain length, prompted investigations of these materials as anesthetics. While the property of anesthesia *per se* is discussed by Krantz and Rudo in Chapter 10 of this monograph, it is necessary to intersperse the ensuing chronological discussion here with several of the studies on fluorinated anesthetics in order to document the central nervous reaction to the fluoroalkanes.

(continued)

Body weight change	Hematology	Clinical chemistry; urinalysis	Pathology	Ref.
ethane $CClF_2$—$CClF_2$ (continued)				
Normal all species	Normal rbc, wbc, differential white count, hemoglobin	Normal urinary protein and sediment	No changes in heart, lungs, liver, kidney, spleen	7
ethane $CClF_2$—CF_3				
Normal for all species	*Rats and Dogs:* Normal rbc, wbc, differential white cell count, hemoglobin, hematocrit, and cell size	*Rats and Dogs:* Normal urine, normal ranges in dog bloods for: sugar, urea nitrogen, cholesterol, cholinesterase BSP retention. Slight increase in alkaline phosphatase in 3/4 dogs	Organ weights normal; no histopathologic change attributable to exposure in any species	8
butane CF_2—CF_2—CF_2—CF_2 (cyclic)				
Normal	No significant changes in red and white cell counts, hemoglobin, hematocrit, or differential white cell counts in rats and dogs	In dogs, normal ranges for blood sugar, BUN, cholesterol, cholinesterase, BSP, alkaline phosphatase. Normal urine analysis in rats and dogs	No gross or microscopic pathology noted. Organ weights within normal range	9
Normal	No significant changes in red and white cell counts, hemoglobin, hematocrit, or differential white cell counts	ND	Same as above	10

5. Scholz, J.: Fortschr. d. Biol. Aerosol-Forsch. **4**, 420—429 (1957—1961).
6. Yant, W. P., H. H. Schrenk, and F. A. Patty: U.S. Bureau of Mines Report No. 3185, Oct. 1932.
7. Scholz, J.: Fortschr. d. Biol. Aerosol-Forsch. **4**, 420—429 (1957—1961).
8. Clayton, J. W., D. B. Hood, M. S. Nick, and R. S. Waritz: "Inhalation Studies on Chloropentafluoroethane ('Freon-115')." In press (1965).
9. Clayton, J. W., M. A. Delaplane, and D. B. Hood: Amer. Indust. Hyg. Assoc. J. **21**, 382—388 (1960).
10. Unpublished Haskell Laboratory Report.

Sayers et al. (1930), in repeated exposures of dogs, monkeys and guinea pigs to CCl_2F_2, observed tremors and staggering gait in dogs and monkeys at 20% (Table 18), but no signs of toxicity in guinea pigs. Booth and Bixby (1932) exposed mice to $CHCl_2F$ and $CHClF_2$, and reported that concentrations of 4% and 16% caused convulsions and that 20% and 49% were lethal. Yant et al. (1932) reported incoordination and tremors in dogs but not in guinea pigs exposed 8, 16, and 24 hours at 15% $CClF_2$–$CClF_2$. In a series of repeated exposures to 14.2%

Table 20. *Effects of repeated exposures to fluorinated ethanes on rats*

Compound	% Vol.	Hrs/day	Days	Observations	Liver histology	Reference
CHF_2—CH_3	10	16	60	No toxic signs; no gross pathological change; mild round cell infiltration in lung	Normal	LESTER and GREENBERG (1950)
$CClF_2$—CH_3	10	16	9	Lethal; lung edema and hemorrhage; other organs normal	Normal	LESTER and GREENBERG (1950)
$CClF_2$—CH_3	1	16	60	No toxic signs; no gross pathological change; mild round cell infiltration in lung	Normal	LESTER and GREENBERG (1950)
$CClF_2$—$CHClF$	6	1	5	Anesthesia; no toxic signs reported; kidney histology normal	Normal	BURN et al. (1959)
$CClF_2$—$CHClF$	4	1	5	Anesthesia; no toxic signs reported; growth normal; kidney histology normal	Normal[1]	BURN et al. (1959)
CCl_2F—CCl_2F	0.1	18	16	No deaths; no toxic signs	Normal	GREENBERG and LESTER (1950)
$CClF_2$—CCl_3	0.1	18	17	No deaths; no toxic signs; no lung irritation	Normal	GREENBERG and LESTER (1950)
CCl_2F—CCl_2F	0.2	ca. 1	7	No deaths; no toxic signs	Normal	Haskell Laboratory, unpublished
$CClF_2$—CCl_3	0.2	ca. 1	5	No deaths; no toxic signs	Normal	Haskell Laboratory, unpublished
CCl_2F—CCl_2F	0.24 to 0.34	6	43	No deaths; no toxic signs	Normal	Haskell Laboratory, unpublished
CCl_2F—CCl_2F	0.5	4	6	Discomfort; muscular incoordination; slight narcosis	Not conducted	GAGE (1957)
	0.25	5.5	14	Same as above but milder; some weight loss; normal histologic picture in lungs, kidney and spleen	Normal	
CCl_2F—$CClF_2$	0.25	7	30	No clinical signs of toxicity; normal histology	Normal	Haskell Laboratory, unpublished
CCl_2F—$CClF_2$	0.50	7	30	Slight depression in growth; kidney grossly normal	Slightly pale grossly	USN Report NS-041-001 (1952)

[1] A moderate amount of mitotic activity observed in 1/4 rats, slight in 3/4.

$CClF_2$–$CClF_2$, 8 hours daily, these authors observed no signs in guinea pigs exposed for 21 days, but dogs displayed tremors, incoordination, and some convulsions for 3–5 days and thereafter appeared to have developed a tolerance which continued for the 21-day period. At 20% $CClF_2$–$CClF_2$, 8 hours daily, 2–4 days, guinea pigs showed tremors and convulsions; dogs exhibited marked convulsions, and all died within 4 days (Table 19). NUCKOLLS (1933), studying

Table 21. *Acute toxicity of several fluorinated cyclohexanes*

Compound	$C_6H_2F_{10}$	$C_6H_3F_9$	$C_6H_4F_8$	$C_6H_4F_8$	$C_6H_4F_8$
Boiling pt.		124° C	125° C	133° C	136° C
		LD_{50} in mg/kg			
Route					
Subcutaneous	> 2820[1]	24.03	24.05	15.37	32.40
Intraperitoneal	> 1410[1]	—	—	3.4	—
Oral	> 2820[1]	25.0	30.7	6.3	33.3

[1] All animals survived at the indicated dosages.
Animals used: Subcutaneous and oral tests, rats; intraperitoneal tests, rabbits.
From: Ensor (1960).

several fluorinated alkanes, noted loss of coordination in guinea pigs in 2-hour exposures to CCl_3F at a level of about 5%. A concentration of 10% caused severe tremors, loss of coordination, narcosis, and convulsions. Similar, but less marked, signs of nervous system reaction were encountered in 2-hour exposures with CCl_2F_2 up to 30%, and none with $CClF_2{-}CClF_2$ up to about 5%.

Robbins (1946) investigated anesthetic response by mouse exposures of twelve fluorinated derivatives of methane and ethane. He found anesthetic activity in nearly all of these and recommended clinical testing on four. The others were unsatisfactory because of undesirable nervous reactivity. Following Robbins work, a highly successful fluorinated anesthetic, halothane ($CHClBr{-}CF_3$) was developed. The account of its discovery is given by Suckling (1957) and Ferguson (1964).

Lester and Greenberg (1950) have studied five fluorinated alkanes, CCl_2F_2, $CH_3{-}CHF_2$, $CH_3{-}CClF_2$, CCl_3F, and $CH_2Br{-}CBrF_2$, and have shown that the dominant clinical response in rats exposed for 30 minutes was narcosis as evidenced by a disappearance of various reflexes with increasing concentrations. Death appeared to be a result of respiratory failure. None of these fluoroalkanes were satisfactory anesthetics as tested, because tremors and pulmonary irritation were encountered.

Burn (1959) and Burn et al. (1959) have studied the anesthetic properties of three fluoroethanes: $CCl_2F{-}CCl_2F$, $CClF_2{-}CCl_2F$ and $CClF_2{-}CHClF$. The first two produced initial excitement and convulsions in mice during anesthesia. Exposures were for fifteen minutes' duration, and the concentrations employed were 1.0 to 2.0% for $CCl_2F{-}CCl_2F$ and 5.0–12.0% for $CClF_2{-}CCl_2F$. The third compound, $CClF_2{-}CHClF$ (note the presence of a single hydrogen), did not produce untoward nervous activity in mice exposed to concentrations up to 7% for one hour.

Dishart (1961) reporting on several fluorinated propanes, has shown a lowered anesthetic potency in mice for derivatives which have more than four fluorine atoms. With these compounds, high concentrations were required to produce anesthesia, but it was accompanied by convulsions. In fluoropropanes which produced satisfactory anesthesia, two of the four fluorine atoms had to be situated centrally in the molecule, a position which conferred stability toward alkali and lack of toxic effects on the central nervous system of mice, for example, $HCF_2CF_2CH_2Cl$ and $HCF_2CF_2CH_2Br$. A higher degree of fluorination as in $HCF_2CF_2CH_2F$, $HCF_2CF_2CF_2Cl$, and $HCF_2CF_2CF_2Br$ or a lower chemical stability as in $CF_3CHBrCF_3$ provoked convulsant activity in mice in 10-minute exposures or toxic effects possibly related to the instability of the compound in the body. Karpov (1963) studied effects on the status of central nervous system function by chronic exposures of rabbits, rats, and mice, 6 hours a day for 10 months to

$CHClF_2$ at 14,200 ppm or 1980 ppm. Effects on the reactivity of the nervous system were evident at the higher concentration only — Table 18.

At Haskell Laboratory, exposures of rats to dichlorofluoromethane, $CHCl_2F$, yielded an LC_{50} of 5.0% (3.9–6.3%) by volume for 4-hour exposures. Rats showed evidence of central nervous system response and respiratory changes. The reactions were proportionate to exposure concentration with recovery shortly after exposure.

Other examples of the kind of response to various fluoroalkanes may be noted in Tables 9, 18, and 19. When death has occurred, the principal anatomic finding has been pulmonary injury. In order to study pulmonary effects, Quevauviller et al. (1953), exposed mice for 24 hours to 10,000 ppm of the following fluoroalkanes, CCl_3F, CCl_2F_2, $CClF_2{-}CClF_2$, plus a mixture of CCl_3F/CCl_2F_2 (50 : 50) and $CCl_3F/CHClF_2$ (37.5 : 62.5). All mice survived exposure showing no behavioral changes. On histological examination of the lungs, a similar development of localized congestion of the alveolar walls with leucocytic infiltration was found in controls and mice exposed to the $CCl_3F/CHClF_2$ mixture, but exposure to CCl_3F alone caused interalveolar thickening and a lymphocytic infiltration. Mice exposed to CCl_2F_2 showed a degree of congestion and leucocytic invasion greater than controls and a serous exudate into the bronchioles. The CCl_3F/CCl_2F_2 mixture was associated with extravasation, sometimes with complete alveolar obstruction by the red blood cells. The most severe effect of all was found in mice exposed to $CClF_2{-}CClF_2$ which apparently produced alveolar hemorrhage with emphysema and desquamation of the alveolar epithelium.

These results are in marked contrast to experience at Haskell Laboratory. They appear to conflict with Kubler's (1963) assessment of $CClF_2{-}CClF_2$ as one of the least toxic of the fluoroalkanes and to differ from the early work on these fluoroalkanes by various authors as summarized in Tables 18 and 19. Any strict comparison, however, would depend on a knowledge of the sample purity and identification of contaminants thereof. Overall, the evidence from animal experiments and human experience indicates that the fluoroalkanes do not present a major hazard under conditions of normal use. In summary, pulmonary effects have been observed, usually at high concentration, and the reactions in the central nervous system which the clinical signs indicated appear to be related inversely to the degree of fluorination of the alkane molecule. For example, it is possible from the data in Table 19 to follow the trend of a decline in nervous system reactivity as the number of fluorine atoms in the molecule increases from two in $CCl_2F{-}CCl_2F$ to eight in $\underline{CF_2{-}CF_2{-}CF_2{-}CF_2}$.

A number of halogenated alkanes are noted for their hepatotoxicity. Outstanding for this activity are the chlorinated alkanes, carbon tetrachloride (Adams et al., 1952), chloroform (Kylin et al., 1963), 1,2-dichloroethane (Spencer et al., 1951) and symmetrical tetrachloroethane (see von Oettingen, 1955 for references). On the other hand fluorinated alkanes would not be considered significant hepatotoxins. For example, the fluorinated methanes, namely, CCl_3F, CCl_2F_2, $CClF_3$, and CF_4 which have exhibited a low order of acute inhalation toxicity (Table 1) may be cited.

Lester and Greenberg (1950) exposed rats to varying concentrations (5–80%) of CCl_3F and CCl_2F_2 for 30 minutes and, in addition, to the latter for four and six hours. Liver injury was not observed in rats exposed to either compound, even when CCl_2F_2 was inhaled at 80% for four and six hours. Other fluoroalkanes were considered by these authors, namely, $CH_3{-}CHF_2$ and $CH_3{-}CClF_2$ (both lethal at 50%, 30-minute exposures), and $CH_2Br{-}CBrF_2$ (lethal at 0.5% in 18-hours exposure); in no case was the liver of exposed rats damaged. The primary site of injury was the lung.

The compounds CCl_3F, $CClF_3$ and CF_4 have been studied at Haskell Laboratory by way of single four-hour rat or guinea pig exposures, and repeated exposures. Rats exposed to vapors of CCl_3F in the range 3.6% to 11.8% (ALC = 6.6%) exhibited a non-injurious vacuolation of the liver cells, a change which has been observed in stock rats. Repeated exposures with CCl_3F, as outlined in Table 18, disclosed no significant liver change in several species. With $CClF_3$, twelve guinea pigs were exposed to 20% for two hours with no effects on the hepatocytes. Repeated exposures of rats as summarized in Table 18 for $CClF_3$ did not provoke a liver reaction. A single, 2-hour exposure of twelve guinea pigs to a concentration of 20% CF_4 produced no signs of toxicity or liver change.

Probably the fluoromethane which has received the most attention is CCl_2F_2. Lester and Greenberg's (1950) work has already been summarized. Preceding this was the work of Nuckolls (1933) on guinea pigs. These workers discovered no liver injury in guinea pigs in 2-hour exposures in concentrations up to 30%. Repeated exposures are summarized in Table 18. Sayers et al. (1930) found no gross liver alterations in dogs, monkeys, or guinea pigs; however, histology was not reported. Siegel (1964) in his work did observe hepatocyte vacuolation and focal necrosis, but not in all species or all animals exposed.

Emerging from these data is a picture of low biological activity for the fluoromethanes as far as the liver is concerned. The same inference may be drawn from the work done on the fluoroethanes as summarized in Table 19 and in Table 20. In the latter, special attention is given to the histology of the liver of exposed rats. One experiment which is of interest because it compares two fluorinated ethanes with chloroform, a well-known liver toxin, is that of Burn et al. (1959). These authors have compared $CClF_2{-}CHClF$ and $CF_3{-}CHBrCl$ (halothane) with chloroform for histological reactions in view of the potential use of the first compound as an anesthetic. Four groups of four rats each were exposed one hour per day for five successive days. The concentrations were: 4% $CClF_2{-}CHClF$ (Table 20), 1.25% $CF_3{-}CHBrCl$ and 1.0% $CHCl_3$. One group was exposed to air alone. At the end of the exposure period histology of rats exposed to $CClF_2{-}CHClF$ disclosed a moderate degree of mitotic activity in the liver but no fatty change. The rats exposed to $CF_3{-}CHBrCl$ showed similar changes with one area of focal necrosis observed in addition. Rats exposed to $CHCl_3$ showed marked fatty change. The slight effect in the liver exerted by $CClF_2{-}CHClF$ is highlighted by the exposure of rats one hour a day, for five days, to 6%. In this work the histology of the liver revealed no alteration attributable to the exposure.

Stephen and Little (1961) have reviewed the studies on the hepatotoxic potential of halothane anesthetic citing the work of Raventos (1956), Virtue et al. (1958), Gibson (1959), Jones et al. (1958), Stephen et al. (1958) and Haley and Wyant (1959). It was concluded that prolonged inhalation exposure (employing several mammalian species) to anesthetic concentrations of halothane is capable of inducing transitory histologc changes in the liver but that these are short of the frank necrosis produced by chloroform. Gastric intubation of halothane also produces these changes. Reports of liver injury in several humans anesthetized with halothane, Bunker and Blumenfeld (1963), out of several million patients anesthetized with this drug emphasizes its low hepatotoxicity. The possible influence of a fluoroalkene contaminant in halothane is discussed in the next section of this chapter.

The effects of the longer chain fluoroalkanes may be illustrated by decafluorobutane C_4F_{10}, and octafluorocyclobutane $\underbrace{CF_2CF_2CF_2CF_2}$. In single four-hour exposures of rats to 80% of each of these compounds there was no histologic change in the liver. Repeated exposures to octafluorocyclobutane of several species of animals (Table 19) disclosed no morphologic alteration of the liver resulting from exposure.

The reasons at the cellular level for the low activity of the fluoroalkanes on the liver, especially in compounds where there is a high degree of fluorination, is not apparent from the investigations cited. This remains as an important area for further studies in this group.

F. Fluoroalkenes

With the introduction of a double bond into the fluorocarbon structure there is an increase in the chemical reactivity, and the toxicity is generally greater than for the comparable saturated compound. However, there are notable exceptions to this generality, and there is a wide range of biological activity among the fluoroalkenes which have been studied. Reports on the toxicity of some fluoroalkenes have been made by ZAPP et al. (1955) and by HOOD et al. (1956). A summary of these results and those from more recent studies is given in Table 22 along with

Table 22. *Acute toxicity of several halogenated alkenes*

Structure	No. of F atoms	No. of Cl atoms	Acute inhalation ALC, ppm	Toxicity for rats[1] LC_{50}, ppm
$CH_2=CHF$	1	0	> 800,000[2]	—
$CF_2=CH_2$	2	0	128,000	—
			> 800,000[3]	—
$CF_2=CF_2$	4	0	—	40,000
$CF_3—CF=CF_2$	6	0	—	3,000
$(CF_3)_2—C=CF_2$	8	0	—	0.5, 0.76[4]
$CCl_2=CH_2$	0	2	32,000	—
$CHCl=CCl_2$	0	3	8,000	—
$CCl_2=CCl_2$	0	4	4,000	—
$CCl_2=CF_2$	2	2	1,000	—
$CClF=CF_2$	3	1	—	1,000

[1] Exposures are 4 hours' duration except where noted.
[2] 80% $CH_2=CHF$, 20% O_2; 12.5 hours' exposure.
[3] 80% $CH_2=CF_2$, 20% O_2; 19 hours' exposure.
[4] 0.5 ppm exposure was for 6 hours, the 0.76 ppm exposure was for 4 hours.
From: CARPENTER et al. (1949), LESTER and GREENBERG (1950), Haskell Laboratory, unpublished.

the data from CARPENTER et al. (1949) and LESTER and GREENBERG (1950). From these observations, any relationship between toxicity and the fluorine complement of the molecule must be conjectural. It seems unlikely, for example, that the high toxicity of perfluoroisobutylene (PFIB) is due entirely to the 8 fluorine atoms, and that the alkenes with fewer than 8 fluorines are thereby less toxic. The relationship to toxicity is probably dependent on molecular reactivity conferred by the double bond, and independent of the degree of fluorination *per se*.

One conclusion, recalling similar observations made on the fluoroalkanes, is that the chloro analogues are more toxic than the fluorine-containing alkenes. Compare in this regard $CF_2=CF_2$ (LC_{50}, 40,000 ppm) with $CCl_2=CCl_2$ (ALC, 4,000 ppm) and $CF_2=CH_2$ (ALC, 128,000 ppm) with $CCl_2=CH_2$ (ALC, 32,000 ppm). In addition, it would appear that there is an increase of toxicity with an increasing number of chlorine atoms. The order of toxicity for the three chlorine-containing compounds noted in Table 22 is:

$$CCl_2{=}CCl_2 > CHCl{=}CCl_2 > CCl_2{=}CH_2$$

All of the fluoroalkenes presented here act as pulmonary irritants at concentrations in the lethal range. Perfluoroisobutylene (PFIB) is many times more active in this property, as shown in Table 23. Rats succumbing to PFIB exposures died as a result of progressing pulmonary edema, and without evidencing an

Table 23. *Summary of single exposures of rats to perfluoroisobutylene*

Nominal concn., ppm by vol.	Time of exposure, hours : min	Mortality ratio, No. dead/No. exposed	Clinical signs	Pathological changes
1.0	4:15 5:20	2/2	Dyspnea, cyanosis, gasping convulsions	Acute pulmonary edema
0.5	6:00	2/2	Slight dyspnea after exposure. Both died overnight	Acute pulmonary edema
0.3	6:00	0/2	None during exposure. Slight increase in respiration rate and weight loss next day. Recovered thereafter	None observed. 9 days after exposure

From: Haskell Laboratory, unpublished.

effect on other organ systems. What mechanism is involved in this action of PFIB remains to be elucidated. It has been compared to phosgene on the basis of its primary effect on the lung.

Repeated exposures of four male rats to 0.1 ppm PFIB were not lethal. During the exposures, the rats were occasionally restless and had respiratory impairment. The latter was not severe, although it sometimes proceeded to cyanosis; and two rats developed moist rales. There were occasional losses of body weight by two rats during the first week of exposure only, but these were not marked; and the curve of body weights was close to normal. Pathology disclosed no tissue change assignable to PFIB, and the weights of the major organs were not altered by the exposure.

The action of PFIB in rats is similar to that of phosgene, and the data suggest that, for rats, PFIB is about ten times as toxic as phosgene (LCT_{50} = 25—40 ppm-hours for phosgene as 3 ppm-hours for PFIB).

Exposures of rats and mice to PFIB are reported by Danishevskii and Kochanov (1961). In two-hour exposures all rats succumbed to a concentration of 1.8 ppm (vol) (3.7 ppm-hours) and the maximum tolerated concentration was 1.6 ppm. Mice tolerated a concentration of 0.6 ppm while 1.2 ppm (2.4 ppm-hours) and 1.8 ppm (3.7 ppm-hours) were the minimum lethal and absolute lethal concentrations, respectively. Histology disclosed pulmonary hemorrhages and edema and degenerative changes in the kidney, viz., albuminous, granular dystrophy and plasmolysis of the cells of tubules. Degenerative changes, sometimes fatty, in the liver were also reported. A relationship between the degree of the histologic reaction and the level of exposure is not delineated by these authors.

The less toxic alkenes, tetrafluoroethylene, hexafluoropropylene, and chlorotrifluoroethylene are pulmonary irritants, but in addition, can cause renal injury in rats (Zapp et al., 1955 and Hood et al., 1956). Single exposures of rats to varying concentrations of chlorotrifluoroethylene (CTFE) have produced physiological evidence of kidney dysfunction. This is illustrated by experiments conducted by E. P. RADFORD and reported by ZAPP (1959). Figure 1 compares the effect of CTFE with mercuric chloride, a well-known nephrotoxin. The urine solute concentration of the rat exposed to various levels of CTFE and mercuric chloride is plotted against the exposure concentration or dose administered. It is observed that functional impairment of the kidney is evident as a lowering of the urine osmolality following a four-hour exposure to CTFE, at approximately one-tenth the LC_{50} value, viz., 100 ppm. The complexity of the biologic action of CTFE was revealed by long-term exposures of several mammalian species, HOOD et al. (1956). In this work, dogs inhaling from 15–150 ppm experienced changes in the central nervous system, blood pressure effects, leucopenia, erythrocytosis and increased plasma cholesterol. Rats in the same exposure series showed no clinical signs of toxicity, but kidney damage was observed microscopically.

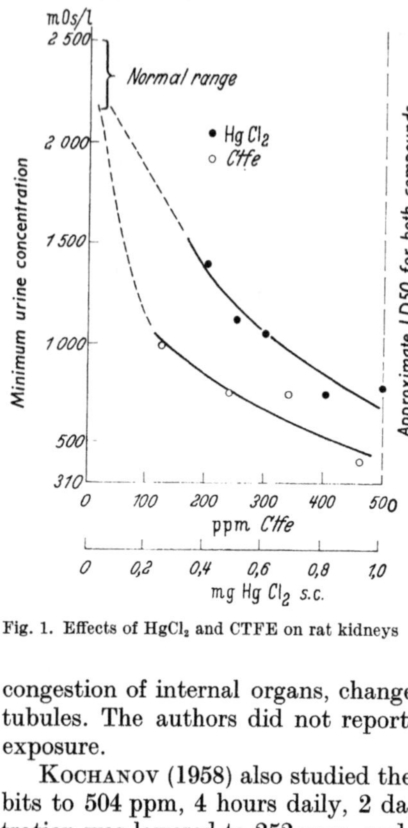

Fig. 1. Effects of $HgCl_2$ and CTFE on rat kidneys

KOCHANOV (1958) exposed groups of rats and rabbits for 2 hours each to various concentrations of CTFE. The LC_{50} for both rats and rabbits was determined as 5040 ppm. The concentrations resulting in death of all animals from the 2-hour exposure were 5544 ppm and 7560 ppm for rabbits and rats respectively. The animals became apathetic and inactive during exposure. There was also impairment of coordination at the highest concentration of approximately 10,000 ppm. Deaths occurred during the first few days after exposure. The rabbits appeared more sensitive to CTFE than the rats. Histology of animals that died disclosed congestion of internal organs, changes in the brain, and necrosis of the kidney tubules. The authors did not report on the histology of animals that survived exposure.

KOCHANOV (1958) also studied the chronic effects of CTFE by exposing 7 rabbits to 504 ppm, 4 hours daily, 2 days a week. After 58 exposures, the concentration was lowered to 252 ppm, and the exposure time was increased to 6 hours a day. Three rabbits died in 16, 29, and 30 days, and the remaining four completed 81, 99, 130 (2) days of exposure. Slight effects were noted in surviving rabbits, namely, a depression in the body weight curve, lowered respiration rate, a decrease in phosphatase and cholinesterase activity, and congestion of liver, spleen, and kidneys. Necrosis of kidney tubules apparently was not observed. A second experiment was conducted on five rabbits and ten rats exposed 6 hours a day, 6 days a week for 110 days (rabbits) and 70 days (rats). The concentration of CTFE was 252 ppm. There was a depression in the rate of weight gain; a decline in the ability to integrate subliminal impulses; an increase in the heart rate in the upright position; an increase in oxygen consumption; hypochromic anemia and leucopenia. Histology of the animals of the second series was not reported.

Danishevskii and Kochanov (1961) report studies on rats exposed to hexafluoropropylene, tetrafluoroethylene and chlorotrifluoroethylene. The following lethal levels were reported for two-hour exposures: hexafluoropropylene 3,240 to 13,365 ppm, tetrafluoroethylene 25,000 ppm, and chlorotrifluoroethylene 7,560 ppm. Histology of rats which died after exposure to these three fluoroalkenes showed pulmonary congestion and edema with degenerative changes in liver and kidney.

Investigating the toxicity of tetrafluoroethylene, Zhemerdei (1958) exposed rats and rabbits for two hours each to concentrations in the range of 0.5% to 10% by volume. The lowest lethal concentration for the rats exposed was 2.5%. The time of death of the rats was in direct proportion to the concentration and varied from 3 hours after exposure to 16 days and more. Rats exposed to 0.5% showed no signs of toxicity. At higher concentrations, there was inactivity, rapid respiration and somnolence. After exposure ended, there was depression, slow respiration, inactivity, and occasional tetanic convulsions elicited by external stimuli. For rabbits, the lowest lethal concentration was 4.0%. At 1.0%, there were no signs of toxicity; above 1.0%, there was inactivity and a decrease in respiration rate. After exposure, the rabbits appeared apathetic, lost appetite, and the rate of respiration increased. Rabbits which succumbed experienced a convulsion before death. Pathology of rats and rabbits disclosed congestion of organs, especially the brain, hemorrhage of the lungs and spleen, and degenerative changes in the kidneys. Considering probable differences in the kind and quantity of contaminants in the various samples, the work reported by Danishevskii and Kochanov (1961) and Zhemerdei (1958) reveals the same order of toxicity for the several fluoroalkenes as observed in the studies conducted at Haskell Laboratory.

An example of a fluoroalkene of low toxicity is vinyl fluoride, $CH_2{=}CHF$. Lester and Greenberg (1950) reported that a mixture of 80% by volume of $CH_2{=}CHF$ and 20% oxygen was not lethal to rats exposed for twelve and one-half hours. Repeated exposures of male and female rats were carried out at Haskell Laboratory (Limperos, 1956). The animals were exposed to a nominal concentration of 10% by volume, seven hours a day, five days a week, for a total of thirty exposures. None of the rats died, and there were no signs of toxic effect as determined by behavior, weight gain, and pathology. Vinylidene fluoride, $CH_2{=}CF_2$, would seem to be in the same class; Lester and Greenberg (1950) found that a concentration of 80% by vol. with 20% oxygen was not lethal for rats exposed for 19 hours.

Bunker and Blumenfeld (1963) have reported cases of human hepatic necrosis following administration of the anesthetic halothane, $CF_3CHBrCl$. Investigating the role of possible contaminants, Cohen et al. (1963) observed that the alkene, 2,3-dichloro 1,1,1,4,4,4-hexafluorobutene-2, (DCHFB) increased severalfold in concentration upon storage in a "copper kettle" vaporizer. The compound is one of several minor contaminants in commercial samples of halothane anesthetic, usually present in undiluted halothane at a level of 100 ppm by volume or at a concentration of 2 ppm by volume in gaseous anesthetic mixtures employing halothane. The reported concentration increase of tenfold prompted an inquiry into the toxicity of this alkene impurity. Cohen et al. (1963) reviewed the known toxicity of the butene showing that it was acutely toxic for a dog in anesthetic concentrations. Delayed onset of anesthesia was observed and this was followed by convulsions and death in one hour. The authors do not state what the concentration was. Another study reported by Chenoweth (1963) showed that

$CF_3-CCl=CCl-CF_3$ was lethal for rats in a four-hour exposure at 100 ppm, but that some rats survived 100 ppm exposure of 1 or 2 hours' duration. Response of the rats in the lethal exposures was consistent with pulmonary irritation. Pulmonary congestion and edema were observed post-mortem. Gross changes in the kidney and liver were also observed. In another study, this author also observed fatalities in rats from severe injury to lungs, liver, and kidney on inhaling this fluoroalkene for four hours at 50 ppm. In experiments conducted by COHEN et al. (1964), 85 male rats were exposed to $CF_3-CCl=CCl-CF_3$ in a dynamic system for 3-hour periods. Results indicated an LD_{50} for this exposure of approximately 50 ppm, with 100% fatalities at 105 ppm. The respiratory deaths occurring in 6 to 24 hours at 840 ppm, and the delayed deaths in 4 to 14 days resulting from exposures as low as 52 ppm were of interest. The latter group lost weight, slowly becoming lethargic, and expired. The rats exposed to the higher concentrations of $CF_3-CCl=CCl-CF_3$ showed acute hemorrhagic changes in the lungs, while the groups exposed to 105–210 ppm showed a healing interstitial pneumonitis and central lobular necrosis of the liver.

Studies of the effects of $CF_3-CCl=CCl-CF_3$ on dogs included induction of anesthesia with thiopental (150–200 mg) followed by a 3-hour inhalation of 1% halothane with added increments of the butene. Vaporization of the anesthetic was with 100% oxygen. Following insertion of the endotracheal tube, ventilation was supported with a Harvard respirator. Electrocardiogram, arterial blood pressure, and the electroencephalogram were monitored and intermittent determinations of pH, P_{O_2} and P_{CO_2} were made. Initially, control animals were paired with the experimental group, and the former maintained on 1% halothane without added DCHFB. The LD_{50} determined in the dog was 200 ppm for a three-hour exposure, decreasing to 150 ppm for a similar anesthesia repeated on four consecutive days. Post-mortem examinations showed only occasional renal tubular damage. The LD_{50} for the rhesus monkey was calculated by the method of maximum likelihood to be 54 ppm for a three-hour exposure. Death occurred within four to nine days. Convulsive disorders appeared in the two animals exposed to 350 and 400 ppm. Pathology revealed severe pulmonary changes in all animals. Grossly, areas of pneumonic consolidation were present, and microscopically the alveolar walls were edematous with occasional areas of necrosis and covered with a thick exudative layer. Animals living past the fifth day evidenced liver damage, the extent of which appeared related to the concentration of $CF_3-CCl=CCl-CF_3$. At the lowest fatal concentration the liver showed atrophic changes and an increase in lipid content, while at the highest concentration the animal showed central lobular necrosis of the liver.

A study at Haskell Laboratory of the acute inhalation toxicity of a related butene, $CF_3-CF=CH-CF_3$, showed that 200 ppm was the Approximate Lethal Concentration for a four-hour exposure of rats. Observations indicated that the compound acts predominantly on the central nervous or respiratory systems. Rats became sedated during exposure; after exposure, there were weight losses, polypnea, and quivering. Death occurred in 2–3 days. Necropsy was not conducted.

Comparing the two butenes cited above, it is noted that the chlorinated compound apparently is the more toxic of the two. Effects on the liver were reported in rats for this compound. There are no comparable data on the non-chlorinated compound. It is notable that single and repeated inhalation studies on another chloro-fluoroalkene, $CF_2=CClF$, (HOOD et al., 1956) did not reveal liver damage in rats, rabbits, guinea pigs, or dogs.

G. Fluoroalcohols

It has been shown by others that the monofluorinated alcohols are highly toxic for mammals when, after oxidation to the corresponding acid, they possess the requisite number of carbon atoms which permits β-oxidation to the toxic fluoroacetate. Thus the monofluoroalcohols having an odd number of carbon atoms are lower in toxicity than those with an even number of carbon atoms. Only a few fluorinated alcohols containing more than one atom of fluorine have been investigated, and these are of an intermediate order of toxicity, as illustrated in Table 24.

Table 24. *Acute toxicity of several polyfluoroalcohols*

Structure	No. of F atoms	ALD mg/kg	ALC ppm
$HCF_2{-}CF_2{-}CH_2OH$	4	3400	2000
$HCF_2{-}CF_2{-}CHOH{-}CH_3$	4	—	3500
$HCF_2{-}CF_2{-}\overset{CH_3}{\overset{\vert}{C}}OH{-}CH_3$	4	670	1000
$CF_3{-}CF_2{-}CH_2OH$	5	2250	—
$CF_3{-}CHF{-}CF_2{-}\overset{CH_3}{\overset{\vert}{C}}H{-}CH_2OH$	6	1000	—
$HCF_2(CF_2)_3CH_2OH$	8	—	2500
$HCF_2(CF_2)_7CH_2OH$	16	7500	—

ALD is the Approximate Lethal Dose for rats, oral route.
ALC is the Approximate Lethal Concentrations for rats inhaling the compound for 4 hours.
From: Haskell Laboratory, unpublished.

In this, a moderate or low order of toxicity is evident from the oral dose (ALD) or the atmospheric level (ALC) which proved to be the lowest level causing death in rats. The compounds listed in the table range in lethal oral dosage from 670 mg/kg to 7500 mg/kg and there is a hint only that a lower oral toxicity is associated with the more highly fluorinated members, but the series is inadequate to permit this to be enunciated as a general principle. Moreover, the figures measuring inhalation toxicity do not support this hypothesis.

The fluoroalcohols have caused, after oral dosing, respiratory impairment, gastric irritation and reaction of the central nervous system. The last was evident from the narcosis, incoordination and prostration exhibited by some of the rats receiving the lower members of the series. When inhaled by rats, the salient features were the action of the fluoroalcohols upon the lungs and central nervous system. Clinical signs of toxicity demonstrated were similar to those observed in animals inhaling the polyfluoroalkanes. The action of the fluoroalcohols upon the nervous system produced, on inhalation, a response similar to that observed when the material was administered orally. A further effect observed in some rats was evidence of early change in the kidney. Higher than normal amounts of albuminoid material were frequently encountered. From studies on some fluoroalkenes there is a strong suggestion that this may be one of the first evidences of renal dysfunction, namely, the inability of the rat kidney to reabsorb albumin from the glomerular filtrate. It is well known that the leakage of albuminoid material from the kidney is normally high in the rat; however, the visual evidence cited here is not to be lightly cast aside.

H. Fluoro-aromatic compounds

Until recently fluorination of the aromatic hydrocarbon ring has yielded derivatives of benzene, naphthalene or diphenyl containing only one or two fluorine atoms. Now, however, highly fluorinated aromatic compounds have been synthesized (TATLOW, 1963). These are in an early stage of development and as yet no toxicity studies have been reported. On the other hand, mono-fluorinated aromatic compounds have been investigated for toxicity and metabolism.

In general, mono-fluorinated aromatic compounds are not highly toxic. They are managed by the body as are the non-fluoro-analogues, and with the C—F link intact. For example, mono-fluorobenzene is tolerated by rabbits receiving an oral

Table 25. *Summary of the major metabolites of benzene and halogenobenzene as % of administered dose*

Compound	Glucuronide	Ethereal sulfate	Mercapturic acid	Unchanged	Total
Benzene	11	25	1	39	76
Fluorobenzene . .	10	21	1.6	44	77
Chlorobenzene . .	25	27	20	27	99
Bromobenzene . .	40	37	21	6	104
Iodobenzene . . .	31	30	23	3	87

From: AZOUZ et al. (1952).

dose of 500 to 1000 mg/kg (AZOUZ, 1952). Because of its volatility (b.p. 85° F, vapor press. 96.6 mm Hg at 30° F), a large percentage (44—64%) of the dose is excreted unchanged in the expired air. These results indicate that fluorobenzene is handled like benzene rather than like chloro-, bromo-, and iodo-benzene. The latter are eliminated intact only to a small extent by this route. The metabolism of fluorobenzene is by oxidation with the formation of fluorinated phenolic compounds

Table 26. *The conjugation of halogen-benzoic acids by the rabbit*

Benzoic acid substituent	Dose	% Conjugation as		
	g/kg	Glycine	Glucuronic acid	Free acid
o-chloro	0.3	5	19	60
m-chloro	0.3	51	23	1
p-chloro	0.3	63	21	7
o-fluoro	0.3	43	9	34
m-fluoro	0.3—0.75	24	6	69
p-fluoro	0.3	43	9	35
p-iodo	0.4	41	46	6

From: BRAY et al. (1952).

which are then conjugated and excreted. Of a dose of 500—1000 mg fluorobenzene/kg, given orally to rabbits, some 30% of the dose is oxidized. About one-third of the oxidized fluorobenzene appears as the glucuronide and two-thirds as the ethereal sulfate. A minor metabolite is a conjugate with mercapturic acid. This latter route, viz., a mercapturic acid conjugate, accounts for about 25% of the chloro-, iodo-, and bromobenzene excretion. With benzene and fluorobenzene, it is only 1% to 2% of the administered dose. Table 25 summarizes this metabolic pattern for some mono-halogenated benzenes.

In dogs and rabbits, p-fluorotoluene and o-, m-, and p-chlorotoluene are first oxidized to the corresponding benzoic acids and are excreted partly as conjugates with glycine (WILLIAMS, 1959).

The metabolism of fluorobenzoic acids by the rabbit has been studied by BRAY et al. (1952), along with chlorobenzoic acids (Table 26). Both the fluorobenzoic acids, o-, m-, and p-isomers, and the chlorobenzoic compounds are excreted unconjugated and conjugated to various degrees. Fluorobenzoic acids are excreted free to the extent of 34% to 69% of the orally administered dose of 300 mg/kg to 750 mg/kg. These doses were not associated with any toxic effects. The conjugates excreted are mostly glycine compounds (24–43% of the dose), while a small percentage (6–9%) are the glucuronic acid compounds. The same type of toxicity order and pattern of excretion would be true for the ortho, meta, and para isomers of fluorobenzamide, since the halogenated benzamides are almost completely hydrolysed to the corresponding acid, conjugated and excreted as described above.

III. Discussion

Traditionally, most monographs or review articles dealing with the toxicology of organic fluorine compounds have almost exclusively considered monofluorinated aliphatic compounds, with fluoroacetic acid prominent among these (CHENOWETH, 1949; PETERS, 1957; SAUNDERS, 1957; PATTISON, 1959; LARGENT, 1961; and HODGE, SMITH, and CHEN, 1963). This situation is to be expected from the great amount of wartime effort assigned to these compounds as candidate chemical warfare agents. These events during World War II wrote an intriguing chapter in the annals of toxicology climaxing in the disclosure of the mechanism of action of fluoroaliphatic compounds which are metabolized to monofluoroacetic acid. The metabolic blockade resulting from the synthesis *in vivo* of fluorocitric acid was the toxic event characterizing this group of compounds. The discovery of this "Lethal Synthesis" is a classic example of the objective of toxicological investigation, aiming at mechanism of action of the toxic agent. The chemical basis for the "Lethal Synthesis" provides the basis of the discussion here in spite of the realization that the details of activity remain unknown for the majority of fluorocarbon compounds included in the present review.

Although some would reserve its use only for perfluorinated organic compounds, the name "fluorocarbon" is now generally used and is derived from the similarities that exist between the hydrocarbon and the fluorocarbon classes of compounds. Fluorine, like hydrogen, is not just another substituent which can bond with carbon. Rather, it occupies a place similar to hydrogen in that it can give rise to a whole system of organic compounds. Both hydrogen and fluorine are univalent; and while the fluorine atom is somewhat larger than hydrogen, it is small enough to occupy all four valence electrons of carbon, a feat which is accomplished only with some strain by the other halogens. The somewhat greater volume of fluorine compared to hydrogen and the greater stability of the C–F bond (rupture energy = 114 K cal) compared to the C–H bond (rupture energy = 93 K cal) provide a protective integument for a carbon chain and insure highly stable compounds among the various fluorocarbons. For example, perfluorinated alkanes such as $\underbracket{CF_2CF_2CF_2CF_2}$, CF_4, C_4F_{10}, C_2F_6 are nonflammable and have virtually no useful properties for synthesis. Their practical applications depend on physical properties and chemical inertness, for example, the use of $\underbracket{CF_2CF_2CF_2CF_2}$ as a food propellent.

Attachment of functional groups or various atoms to the carbon chain or ring already accommodating several fluorine atoms yields genera of compounds whose properties may be influenced to greater or lesser degree by the fluorine contribution to their structure. It is notable that the C—F bond is more stable than the C—Cl bond (rupture energy 72 K cal); however, in chlorofluorocarbon structures the fluorine atom stabilizes vicinal C—Cl links and also relieves the steric strain in the molecule imposed by the relatively voluminous Cl atoms.

It may be inferred from the foregoing that the biological activity of the fluorocarbons would be related to the properties of the fluorine atom and more particularly to the C—F bond. Of the latter, the high bond energy is the most notable property conferring stability and biologically, it is the pre-eminent one. On it rests the reason for the presence of biological effect or, in contrast, its absence.

The former feature is exemplified by resistance to enzymic dehalogenation of monofluoroacetic acid so that the C—F link enters the tricarboxylic acid cycle intact and passes incognito until fluorocitric acid is formed. This metabolite cannot be converted to aconitic acid by the enzyme aconitase, which it inhibits, and therefore it blocks the subsequent chain of events as when the gears of a machine reach an outsized cog. The toxicity therefore, arises from the blockage in the metabolic cycle caused by the highly stable interloper. It remains for further study to discover the relationships between the metabolic inhibitions induced by monofluorinated compounds and the pharmacologic sequelae (PATTISON, 1959).

On the other hand, in many instances, lack of biologic activity may be explained by the stable C—F bond. The fluoro-analogues of the chlorine-containing sulfur mustards may be cited as examples of this.

Owing to dehalogenation with the resultant formation of a biologically

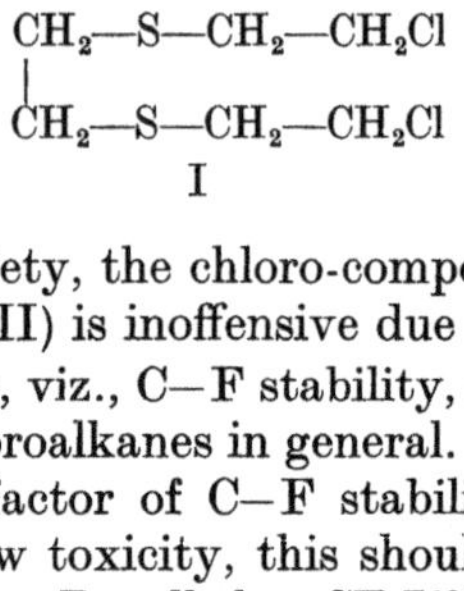
I

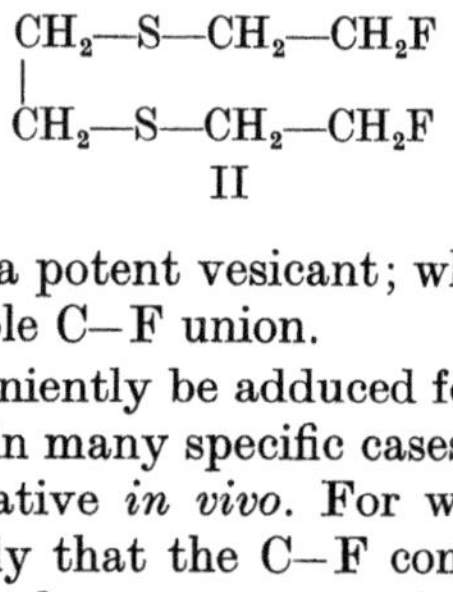
II

active organic moiety, the chloro-compound (I) is a potent vesicant; whereas the fluoro derivative (II) is inoffensive due to the stable C—F union.

The same basis, viz., C—F stability, may conveniently be adduced for the low toxicity of the fluoroalkanes in general. However, in many specific cases, it is not known how this factor of C—F stability is operative *in vivo*. For while C—F stability favors low toxicity, this should not imply that the C—F compound is biologically inactive. Recall that CF_3I^{131} may be used to trace regional blood flow in the brain, SOKOLOFF (1957). While it is known that the compound is free of toxic effects for this use, nevertheless it is obviously not biologically inert, as it can enter the circulatory paths of the brain. More often than not, with the fluorocarbons a similar situation obtains, viz., low toxicity but biological activity to varying degrees, and for reasons which remain to be elucidated. It is valuable for practical reasons of preparation, manufacture and use to cite the low toxicity of fluoroalkanes, and this in proportion to the number of fluorine atoms; it is quite another matter to be able to specify the metabolic events attaching to a particular compound. However some insight into the biologic activity of the fluorocarbons may be gained by considering a few of the salient features of the biology and chemistry of the halogenated hydrocarbons, and comparing them with the fluorocarbons.

Dehalogenation in aliphatic systems is well established for many compounds. On it is based the mechanism of action of a number of halogenated compounds (CHENOWETH and MCCARTY, 1963). Both enzymatic and non-enzymatic processes have been observed in this regard. It is noteworthy that the biologic activity is not related to the fugitive halogen but rather to the halogen-free part of the molecule. The dehalogenation of CH_3Br to form the methylating residue CH_3- is typical of this concept. It is the methyl radical which can react with sulfur-containing compounds *in vivo*, thus producing a biologically active compound. CH_3Cl is not as active as CH_3Br and CH_3F is even less active than CH_3Cl. The labile halogens of $COCl_2$ giving rise to an active $-\overset{\oplus}{\underset{|}{C}}=\overset{\ominus}{O}$ group is another example. The corresponding fluoro-compounds CH_3F and COF_2 are much lower in activity than the chloro-compounds largely due to a firm C–F bond.

Further addition of F to the molecule tends to stabilize carbon to halogen bonds. It is known that di- and tri-halogenated compounds differ markedly from the monosubstituted analogues, owing to shortened inter atomic distance and increase in steric effects from the added bulk in the former compounds. These molecular changes resulting from increasing fluorination are probably the basis for the low toxicity of the highly fluorinated anesthetics, viz., $CF_3-CHBrCl$ (halothane), $CH_3-O-CF_2-CHCl_2$, $CF_3-CHBrF$ (teflurane), $HCF_2-CF_2-CH_2Cl$, and $HCF_2-CF_2-CH_2Br$. Although dehalogenation of these may occur, it would appear to be of minor significance. The anesthetic activity of these materials may be best explained by the formation of "physical adducts" according to CHENOWETH and MCCARTY (1963), comparable to the action of nitrogen and xenon. These inert materials may become part of *in vivo* "crystal" formations in accord with PAULING's (1961) hypothesis. Another aspect of these postulated *in vivo* actions is the requirement of binding forces and a dipole moment. Completely halogenated molecules or partially halogenated, symmetrical compounds, because of the lack of the requisite dipole function would not readily form "crystals" and therefore in most cases would be poor anesthetics. CCl_4 is a notable exception, although CF_4 certainly is not. Hexafluoroethane and monochloropentafluoroethane are poor anesthetics possibly because of their symmetrical morphology. Hydrogen situated at the end of a three-carbon chain enhances chemical stability and anesthetic potency, whereas a centrally-placed hydrogen exerts the converse effect, as demonstrated by DISHART (1961).

Although highly fluorinated compounds may be poor anesthetics, they can be toxic in sufficiently high concentration. The mechanism of action in these instances may be akin to the physical adducts alluded to above; however, this remains speculative until relevant studies are conducted. Into the same category goes the mild hepatotoxic action of some of the chlorofluorocarbons. The idea that lipophilic properties of halogenated compounds influence biologic activity, as with the preceding hypotheses, must be regarded as a chance correlation, if one does exist. Any relation between this physical property and biological effects is uncertain.

Of the various fluoroalkenes covered in this review, perfluoroisobutylene is notable for its high toxicity. DANISHEVSKII and KOCHANOV (1961) claim that carbonyl fluoride, COF_2, is formed *in vivo* and that this accounts for the toxic effects. However, COF_2 is not as toxic as PFIB. The Approximate Lethal Concentration for COF_2 in four-hour rat exposures was 100 ppm (CLAYTON, 1959), whereas the comparable value for PFIB was 0.76 ppm. Carbonyl fluoride hydrolyzes rapidly to hydrogen fluoride, and the irritation observed in COF_2 rat exposures is that which would be expected from HF. Furthermore, 100 ppm of COF_2 is equivalent to 200 ppm HF which is in the lethal range of concentrations reported for HF by MACHLE et al. (1934) for rats exposed just under four hours. It seems unreasonable therefore to ascribe the toxic effects of PFIB to COF_2 liberation. PFIB reacts chemically with alcoholic hydroxyls with the loss of fluorine; herein may lie the reason for its toxicity. In contrast to the high toxicity of PFIB, a number of fluoroalkenes covered in this review are of a low order of toxicity, and tetrafluoroethylene, $CF_2{=}CF_2$; vinyl fluoride, $CH_2{=}CHF$; and vinylidene fluoride, $CH_2{=}CF_2$ may be cited in this regard. Even in this group, there are wide differences in the individual toxicities as noted in Table 22. The reasons for this extensive range are not apparent and need to be defined. The action of certain fluoroalkenes on the mammalian kidney is another area for studies on mechanism of action.

Among halogenated aromatic compounds, dehalogenation is unusual, and among the halogens the fluoro-aromatic substitution is the most stable, with rare exceptions as will be noted below. In view of the fact that most work to date has been done on monofluoro-substituted aromatics, comments here are necessarily confined to these compounds. It has been noted in a previous section that the metabolism of fluorobenzene closely resembles that of benzene. Some 40% of the administered dose of either is excreted unchanged. The remainder is converted to the corresponding phenol and then conjugated. Tables 25 and 26 show the disparity between fluorobenzene and the other aromatic halogens. The overall picture in the former is one of C—F stability, whereas the other halogenated aromatics appear to be subject to a different metabolic sequence. Regarding this difference, it is perhaps significant that the halogenated phenols display increased polarity over the non-halogenated aryl nucleus. This state may be represented by the following dipolar structure:

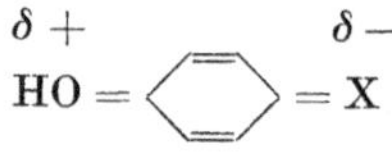

The order of activity of the halogens in this regard is I > Br > Cl > F. This is the order of their inductomeric effects, which is a measure of their capacity to collect electrons from electron rich systems and to place them in d-orbitals. The position of F at the nadir of the inductomeric sequence is possibly, in some way still to be elucidated, a factor in the *in vivo* history of the monohalogenated aromatic compounds. The potency of halogenated phenols as germicides is in the order of their inductomeric effects, viz., I > Br > Cl > F, and this may be the basis of their mode of action according to CHENOWETH and MCCARTY (1963).

A notable exception to the solidity of the C—F bond in the aromatic class is the labile F on 2,4-dinitrofluorobenzene. It would appear in this case that the strong electron attracting forces of the NO_2 substituents cause a shift of electrons away from the C—F link permitting nucleophilic attack at the electron-poor center in the molecule and the disassociation of F.

It has already been mentioned that F-substitution for Cl in the 4 position in 2-chloro-4-fluorophenoxyacetic acid is associated with a delay of *in vivo* decarboxylation of the acid. The action of the F atom in the molecule is not specifically known; however, conjecture may adduce that steric hindrance or obstructive effects are operative. Nevertheless a stable C—F union obtains in this case and its presence effects the biologic activity of the molecule. Studies of the electronic effects of fluorine in various organic molecules and their biologic significance are needed. The various electronic effects, viz., inductive, inductomeric, and tautomeric cited by CHENOWETH and MCCARTY (1963) may have opposite actions. However, these authors conclude that the negative inductive (electron attracting) forces predominate, but these are vitiated over long side chains and in ring structures. Thus, the biologic effects of F-substitution must often be relegated to steric or obstructive effects. Several examples of this have already been described. Actual mechanisms have yet to be discovered in most cases.

The relatively small atomic size of the fluorine atom is another aspect of the biologic activity of the fluorocarbons, although it should not be inferred that it is independent of the properties of the C—F bond just discussed. The two attributes would share in biologic action according to the particular situation. The similarity in atomic volume of fluorine and hydrogen may give organic fluorine molecules the requisite steric characteristics for complexing with enzymes and other cellular receptors. During the transformations of fluoroacetate to fluorocitrate, the steric requirements of the enzymes are met by the fluoro compounds. Fluorocitrate, however, is not an acceptable substrate for the enzyme aconitase and here the cycle stops. The effect of atomic volume on cellular activity is evident in the experiment of SCHANKER and JEFFREY (1961), who related the transport across the intestinal epithelium of halogenated uracils and uracil to the atomic radius of the halogen substituent. It was found the uracil and 5-fluorouracil passed across the mucosal epithelium to approximately the same extent, but the passage of 5-bromouracil was distinctly less. It was concluded that progress of the bromo-substituent was impeded by the relatively larger volume of the Br atom. Comparing the F-uracil with uracil, it was noted that the F-derivative showed a slight lag, possibly reflecting the slightly larger F atom.

In conclusion, it may be stated that investigations of mechanism of action are desirable for most of the fluoro compounds which are included in this review. A notable case in point are the fluoroalkanes which are low in toxicity, but for which it would be informative to know the mode of action, particularly at the very high concentrations requisite for biologic response, and to understand why a high degree of fluorination confers on the alkane molecule a low mammalian toxicity but nevertheless does not entirely absolve the molecule from biologic activity.

References

ADAMS, E. M., H. C. SPENCER, V. K. ROWE, D. D. MCCOLLISTER, and D. D. IRISH: Vapor toxicity of carbon tetrachloride determined by experiments on laboratory animals. Arch. industr. Hyg. **6**, 50—66 (1952).

APPLEGATE, V. C., J. H. HOWELL, and M. A. SMITH: Use of mononitrophenols containing halogens as selective sea lamprey larvicides. Science **127**, 336—337 (1958).

AZOUZ, W. M., D. V. PARKE, and R. T. WILLIAMS: Studies on detoxication. 42. Fluorobenzene. Spectrophotometric determination of the elimination of unchanged halogenobenzenes by rabbits. A comparison of the oxidation *in vivo* of fluorobenzene and benzene. Biochem. J. **50**, 702—706 (1952).

BANKS, A. A., A. CAMPBELL, and A. J. RUDGE: Toxicity and narcotic activity of fluorocarbons. Nature (Lond.) **174**, 885 (1954).

BOOTH, H. S., and E. M. BIXBY: Fluorine derivatives of chloroform. Ind. Eng. Chem. **24**, 637—641 (1932).

BRAY, H. G., R. C. CLOWES, W. V. THORPE, K. WHITE, and P. B. WOOD: The fate of certain organic acids and amides in the rabbit. 13. Chloro- and fluoro-benzoic acids and amides. Biochem. J. **50**, 583—587 (1952).

BUNKER, J. P., and C. M. BLUMENFELD: Liver necrosis after halothane anesthesia. New Engl. J. Med. **268**, 531—534 (1963).

BURN, J. H.: Pharmacological testing of anaesthetics. Proc. roy. Soc. Med. **52**, 95—98 (1959).

— H. G. EPSTEIN, and P. J. GOODFORD: The properties of the anaesthetic substance, 1,1,2-trifluoro-1,2-dichloroethane. Brit. J. Anaesth. **31**, 518—529 (1959).

BUU-HOÏ, N. P.: Les dérivés organiques du fluor d'intérêt pharmacologique. E. JUCKER, Ed. Progress in Drug Research, vol. 3, 10—74. New York: Interscience Publishers 1961.

CARPENTER, C. P., H. F. SMYTH, and U. C. POZZANI: The assay of acute vapor toxicity, and the grading and interpretation of results on 96 chemical compounds. J. industr. Hyg. **31**, 343—346 (1949).

CAUJOLLE, F.: The comparative toxicity of refrigerant liquids (Translation). (Presented at the 11th International Refrigeration Congress, August 28 — September 4, 1963.)

CHENOWETH, M. B.: Communication of the toxicity of 2,3-dichloro-1,1,1,4,4,4-hexafluorobutene-2 to the National Research Council, Subcommittee on the National Halothane Study of the Committee on Anesthesia, September 4, 1963.
— Monofluoroacetic acid and related compounds. Pharmacol. Rev. **1**, 383—424 (1949).
—, and L. P. MCCARTY: On the mechanism of the pharmacophoric effect of halogenation. Pharmacol. Rev. **15**, 673—707 (1963).
CLAYTON, J. W.: Inhalation toxicity of decafluorobutane. Unpublished report from Haskell Laboratory (1958).
— Inhalation toxicity of carbonyl fluoride. Unpublished report from Haskell Laboratory (1959).
— M. A. DELAPLANE, and D. B. HOOD: Toxicity studies with octafluorocyclobutane. Amer. industr. Hyg. Ass. J. **21**, 382—388 (1960).
— J. R. BARNES, D. B. HOOD, H. SHERMAN, and S. D. MORRISON: Toxicity studies on 1,1,2,2-tetrachloro-1,2-difluoroethane ("Freon-112") and 1,1,1,2-tetrachloro-2,2-difluoroethane. Paper presented at the Meeting of the Society of Toxicology, Williamsburg, Va., March 11, 1964.
— D. B. HOOD, M. S. NICK, and R. S. WARITZ: Inhalation studies on chloropentafluoroethane ("Freon-115"). In press (1965).
COHEN, E. N., J. W. BELLVILLE, H. BUDZIKIEWICZ, and D. H. WILLIAMS: Impurity in halothane anesthetic. Science **141**, 899 (1963).
— H. W. BREWER, J. W. BELLVILLE, and R. SHER: The chemistry and toxicology of dichlorohexafluorobutene. In press (1964).
COMSTOCK, C. C., F. P. MCGRATH, S. D. GOLDBERG, and L. H. LAWSON: An investigation of the toxicity of proposed fire extinguishing fluids. II. The Approximate Lethal Concentration to rats by inhalation for fifteen minutes. Chemical Corps Medical Division Report No. 23, 1—47 (1950).
—, and F. W. OBERST: Comparative inhalation toxicities of four halogenated hydrocarbons to rats and mice in the presence of gasoline fires. Arch. industr. Hyg. **7**, 157—167 (1953).
— J. KERSCHNER, and F. W. OBERST: Toxicology of inhaled trifluoromonobromomethane and difluorodibromomethane vapors from subacute and chronic exposures of rats and dogs. Chemical Corps Medical Laboratories Report No. 180 (1953).
—, and F. W. OBERST: Comparative inhalation toxicities of carbon tetrachloride, monochloromonobromomethane, difluorodibromomethane, and trifluoromonobromomethane to rats and mice in the presence of gasoline fires. Chemical Corps Medical Laboratories Research Report No. 107, 1—19 (1952).
COOK, W. A.: Maximum allowable concentrations of industrial atmospheric contaminants. Industr. Med. **14**, 936—946 (1945).
DANISHEVSKII, S. L., and M. M. KOCHANOV: On the toxicology of some fluoroorganic compounds. Gig. Tr. prof. Zabol. **5**, 3—8 (1961).
DISHART, K. T.: The synthesis and evaluation of some new fluorinated inhalation anesthetics. Presented at the Meeting of the American Chemical Society, Chicago (1961).
DOWNING, R. C., and D. MADINABEITIA: The toxicity of fluorinated hydrocarbon aerosol propellants. Aerosol Age **5**, 25—31 (1960).
EDGERTON, L. J., and M. B. HOFFMAN: Fluorine substitution affects decarboxylation of 2,4-dichlorophenoxyacetic acid in application. Science **134**, 341—342 (1961).
ENSOR, E. M.: The toxicology of some fluorinated cyclohexanes. Porton Technical Paper No. 738, 1—19, (1960).
FERGUSON, J.: The discovery of the anaesthetic halothane-an example of industrial research. Chem. & Ind. **1964**, 818—824.
GAGE, J. C.: The acute toxicities of chlorobromoethane, trifluorobromomethane, difluorodibromomethane, and tetrafluorodibromoethane. Report IHR/54, Imperial Chemical Industries Ltd., Industrial Hygiene Research Labs. 1—10 (1954).
— Toxicological report on "Arcton 66." Unpublished report of Imperial Chemical Industries Ltd. 1957. 1 page.
GIBSON, J. A.: Fluothane toxicity; pathological studies of mouse liver and kidney. Canad. Anaesth. Soc. J. **6**, 148—152 (1959).
GREENBERG, L. A., and D. LESTER: Toxicity of the tetrachlorodifluoroethanes. Arch. industr. Hyg. **2**, 345—347 (1950).
HALEY, F. C., and G. M. WYANT: The effect of halothane on the liver of dogs exposed to mild hypoxia. Canad. Anaesth. Soc. J. **6**, 271—276 (1959).
HAMILTON, J. M.: The organic fluorochemicals industry. Advances in fluorine chemistry, Vol. III, 117—180. Washington, D. C.: Butterworth, Inc. Publishers 1963.
HENNE, A. L.: Fluorinated derivatives of methane. J. Amer. chem. Soc. **59**, 1400—1401 (1937).
HODGE, H. C., F. A. SMITH, and P. S. CHEN: Fluorine chemistry. J. H. SIMONS, Ed., Vol. III. Biological effects of organic fluorides. New York, N. Y.: Academic Press 1963.

HOOD, D. B., M. E. HARRINGTON, J. R. BARNES, K. E. RANTA, and D. M. GAY: The toxicity of chlorotrifluoroethylene. Presented at the AIHA Meeting, Philadelphia (1956).
JONES, W. M., G. MARGOLIS, and C. R. STEPHEN: Hepatotoxicity of inhalation anesthetic drugs. Anesthesiology **19**, 715—723 (1958).
KARPOV, B. C.: The chronic toxicity of Freon-22. Tr. Leningr. Sanit.-Gigien. Med. Inst. **75**, 231—240 (1963).
KOCHANOV, M. M.: Data on the toxicology of chlorotrifluoroethylene. Gig. Tr. prof. Zabol. **2**, 25—31 (1958).
KUBLER, H.: Physiological properties of propellants. J. Soc. Cosm. Chem. **14**, 341—351 (1963).
KYLIN, B., H. REICHARD, I. SUMEGI, and S. YLLNER: Hepatotoxicity of inhaled trichloroethylene, tetrachloroethylene and chloroform. Single exposure. Acta pharmacol. Kbh. **20**, 16—26 (1963).
LARGENT, E. J.: Fluorosis; the health aspect of fluorine compounds. Columbus: Ohio State University Press 1961.
LE BEAU, P., and A. DAMIENS: Chimie Minerale sur le Tetrafluorure de Carbone. C. R. Acad. Sci. (Paris) **182**, 1340—1342 (1926).
LEHMANN, F.: Über Konstitution und Wirkung. Untersuchungen an aromatischen Fluorverbindungen. Naunyn-Schmiedebergs Arch. exp. Path. Pharmak. **130**, 250—255 (1928).
LESTER, D., and L. A. GREENBERG: Acute and chronic toxicity of some halogenated derivatives of methane and ethane. Arch. industr. Hyg. **2**, 335—344 (1950).
LIMPEROS, G.: Toxicity of vinyl fluoride monomer. Unpublished report from Haskell Laboratory (1956).
MACHLE, W., F. THAMANN, K. KITZMILLER, and J. CHOLAK: The effects of the inhalation of hydrogen fluoride. I. The response following exposure to high concentration. J. industr. Hyg. **16**, 129—145 (1934).
MATSON, A. F., and R. E. DUFOUR: The life hazards and nature of the products formed when chlorobromomethane extinguisher liquid is applied to fires. Underwriters' Laboratories Bulletin of Research, 42 (August, 1948).
— — The life hazards and nature of the products formed when monobromomonochlorodifluoromethane ("Freon-12B1"), dibromodifluoromethane ("Freon-12B2"), monobromotrifluoromethane ("Freon-13B1"), or dibromotetrafluoroethane ("Freon-114B2") extinguishing agents are applied to fires. Underwriters' Laboratories Report NC-445 (1945).
MIDGLEY, T., and A. L. HENNE: Organic fluorides as refrigerants. Industr. Eng. Chem. **22**, 542—545 (1930).
NUCKOLLS, A. H.: The comparative life, fire, and explosion hazards of common refrigerants. Miscellaneous Hazards. Underwriters' Laboratories No. 2375 (1933).
— R. E. DUFOUR, and A. J. PERKINS: The comparative life, fire, and explosion hazards of tetrafluoromonochloroethane ("Freon-124"). Miscellaneous Hazards. Underwriters' Laboratories Report No. 3135 (1940).
— — — The comparative life, fire, and explosion hazards of trifluorotrichloroethane ("Freon-113"). Miscellaneous Hazards. Underwriters' Laboratories Report No. 3072 (1941).
ODOU, B. L.: Personal communication (1963).
PATTISON, F. L. M.: Toxic aliphatic fluorine compounds. (Elsevier Monograph.) Elsevier Publishing Company, New York, N. Y. 1959.
PAULET, G.: Toxicological and physiological studies with bromotrifluoromethane (CF_3Br). Arch. Mal. prof. **23**, 341—347 (1962).
PAULING, L.: A molecular theory of general anesthesia. Science **134**, 15—21 (1961).
PETERS, R. A.: Lethal synthesis [Croonian Lecture] Proc. roy. Soc. (London) B **139**, 143 (1952).
— Mechanism of the toxicity of the active constituent of *Dichapetalum cymosum* and related compounds. Advanc. Enzymol. 18, 113—160 (1957).
QUEVAUVILLER, A.: Hygiene and safety of propellants in medicated aerosols. Prod. probl. Pharm. **20**, 14—29 (1965).
— M. SCHRENZEL et VU NGOC HUYEN: Local tolerance of skin, mucous membranes, sores, and burns of animals to chlorofluorinated hydrocarbons. Therapie **19**, 247—263 (1964).
— M. CHAIGNEAU et M. SCHRENZEL: Experimental studies with mice on the tolerance of the lung to chlorofluorinated hydrocarbon. Ann. pharm. franç. **24**, 727—734 (1953).
RAVENTOS, J.: The action of fluothane — a new volatile anaesthetic. Brit. J. Pharmacol. **11**, 394—410 (1956).
ROBBINS, B. H.: Preliminary studies of the anesthetic activity of the fluorinated hydrocarbons. J. Pharmacol. exp. Ther. **86**, 197—204 (1946).
RUFF, O., and R. KEIM: Die Reaktionsprodukte der verschiedenen Kohlearten mit Fluor. I. Das Kohlenstoff-4-Fluorid (Tetrafluoromethan). Z. Anorg. Allgem. Chem. **192**, 249—256 (1930).
SARANGI, B. K., L. E. MORRIS, and J. R. HOUSEHOLDER: Observations on an azeotrope of "Fluomar" and "Freon-113". Anesthesia Anal. Curr. Res. **41**, 702—706 (1962).

SAUNDERS, B. C.: Phosphorus and fluorine. The chemistry and toxic action of their organic compounds. Cambridge University Press Cambridge, Engl. 1957.

SAYERS, R. R., W. P. YANT, J. CHORNYAK, and H. W. SHOAF: Toxicity of dichloro-difluoro methane: a new refrigerant. U.S. Bureau of Mines Report No. 3013 (MAY 1930).

SCHANKER, L. S., and J. J. JEFFREY: Active transport of foreign pyrimidines across the intestinal epithelium. Nature (Lond.) **190**, 727—728 (1961).

SCHOLZ, J.: New toxicologic investigations of Freons used as propellants for aerosols and sprays. Fortschr. Biol. Aerosolforsch. **4**, 420—429 (1957—1961).

—, and W. WEIGAND: Toxicological studies on bromotrifluoromethane. Zbl. Arbeitsmed. **14**, 129—131 (1964).

SIEGEL, J.: Personal communication from U.S. Navy Toxicology Unit (1964).

SOKOLOFF, L.: New research techniques of neuroanatomy. W. WINDLE, Ed. Chas. C. Thomas, Springfield, Ill.: 1957.

SPENCER, H. C., V. K. ROWE, E. M. ADAMS, D. D. MCCOLLISTER, and D. D. IRISH: Vapor toxicity of ethylene dichloride determined by experiments on laboratory animals. Arch. industr. Hyg. **4**, 482—493 (1951).

STANSLY, P. G., and D. S. RAMSEY: Some properties of fluorocarbon-treated animal tissue. Proc. Soc. exp. Biol. (N. Y.) **103**, 20—22 (1960).

STEPHEN, C. R., and D. M. LITTLE JR.: Halothane (Fluothane). Baltimore, Md.: Williams and Wilkins 1961.

— G. MARGOLIS, L. W. FABIAN, and M. BOURGEOIS-GAVARDIN: Laboratory observations with fluothane. Anesthesiology **19**, 770—781 (1958).

STRUCK, H. C., and E. B. PLATTNER: A study of the pharmacological properties of certain saturated fluorocarbons. J. Pharmacol. exp. Ther. **68**, 217—219 (1940).

SUCKLING, C. W.: Some chemical and physical factors in the development of "Fluothane." Brit. J. Anaesth. **29**, 466—472 (1957).

TATLOW, T. C.: The aromatic fluorocarbons and their derivatives. Endeavour **22**, 89 (1963).

TREON, J. F., F. P. CLEVELAND, E. E. LARSON, J. CAPPEL, and E. WERT: Toxicity and air concentration of "F-13B1" and its decomposition products. Kettering Laboratory Report (July 10, 1957).

VIRTUE, R. W., K. W. PAYNE, L. J. CARANNA, G. S. GORDON, and R. R. REMBER: Observations during experimental and clinical use of Fluothane. Anesthesiology **19**, 478—487 (1958).

VON OETTINGEN, W. F.: The halogenated hydrocarbons; toxicity and potential dangers. U.S. Public Health Service Publication No. 414 (1955).

WILLIAMS, R. T.: Detoxication Mechanisms. 2nd Ed. New York: John Wiley & Sons 1959.

YALE, H. L.: The trifluoromethyl group in medicinal chemistry. J. med. pharm. Chem. **1**, 121—133 (1959).

YANT, W. P., H. H. SCHRENK, and F. A. PATTY: Toxicity of dichlorotetrafluoroethane. U.S. Bureau of Mines Report of Investigations. R. I. 3185, 1—10 (1932).

ZAPP, J. A.: The toxicological basis of threshold limit values. 3. Physiological criteria. Amer. industr. Hyg. Ass. J. **20**, 350—356 (1959).

— G. LIMPEROS, and K. C. BRINKER: Toxicity of pyrolysis products of "Teflon" tetrafluoroethylene resin. Presented at the AIHA Meeting, Buffalo, New York (1955).

ZHEMERDEI, A. I.: Data on the toxicology of tetrafluoroethylene. Tr. Leningrad Sanit. Giglen. Med. Inst. **44**, 164—175 (1958).

Chapter 10

The Fluorinated Anesthetics

By

John C. Krantz jr. and Frieda G. Rudo

With 5 Figures

Experimental work with fluorinated anesthetics

I. General introduction

Certain hydrocarbons such as ethylene and cyclopropane elicit surgical anesthesia when inhaled in sufficient concentrations. The saturated hydrocarbons of the aliphatic series do not evoke anesthesia. Anesthetic properties are conferred upon the lower members of this series of hydrocarbons by halogenation with either chlorine or bromine. For example, chloroform and ethyl chloride have been used as anesthetics for more than a century. It therefore appeared prudent to determine the effect of halogenation of hydrocarbons and ethers with fluorine in order to determine what effect the presence of fluorine in the molecule would exert on the anesthetic properties of these compounds. The wisdom of this effort has been justified by the investigations of the last two decades, leading to the production of the most useful anesthetic agents containing fluorine. This chapter portrays this signal advance in the field of anesthesiology.

The compounds considered in this chapter are fluorine containing hydrocarbons and ethers (with or without other halogens) which elicit anesthesia or have been tested for anesthetic properties. To facilitate the organization of the material the chapter is divided in two parts: in the first part the experimental work in the field of fluorinated anesthetics is arranged in historical sequence and only mention is made of those compounds now used clinically. These are discussed in detail in part II along with extensive pharmacologic studies of these agents.

II. Historical development of fluorinated hydrocarbons and ethers

A. Early studies of fluorinated hydrocarbons

The first organic compound of fluorine prepared was the gas CF_4 (Partington 1925). It was synthesized accidentally in an unsuccessful attempt to isolate elemental fluorine in a carbon vessel. Tetrafluoromethane has no anesthetic properties. Today the number of fluorine-containing hydrocarbons and ethers is legion.

When the fluorinated members of the lower aliphatic hydrocarbons became available, most of the studies on these compounds were concerned with their use as refrigerants (Booth and Bixby, 1932). Struck and Plattner (1940) investigated the possible anesthetic properties of C_4F_{10}, C_5F_{10} and C_6F_{12}. Mice exposed

Table 1. *The concentrations of various halogenated hydrocarbons necessary to produce anesthesia and respiratory arrest in 50% of the mice exposed*

Also the time necessary for induction of anesthesia as well as times necessary for recovery of pain sensation and ability to walk after exposure to the LD_{50} for 10 minutes are given.

Formula	BP°	AD_{50} vol.%	LD_{50} vol.%	LD_{50}/AD_{50}	No. Mice	Time A.	Time P.	Time W.	Remarks
Fluorine substituted hydrocarbons and ethers									
CF_3CH_3	-46	50—60			5				conv. on recovery
$CF_3CH{=}CH_2$	-24	60			13				conv. on recovery
$CF_3CH_2CH_3$	-12	50			5				
$CF_3CH_2CF_3$	- 0.5	11	44	4	14	30″	30″	90″	
$CH_3CF_2CF_2CH_3$	17	20	60	3	18	30″	10″	90″	
$CH_3CF_2CH{=}CH_2$	24	8.3	25	3	26	20″	20″	2′—3′	
$CH_3CF_2CH_2CH_3$	30.8	6	12	2	24	1′	20″	60″	
$CF_3CH_2CF_2CH_3$	40	5			9		30″	60″	
$CF_3CH_2OCH_3$	30	8	16	2	20	20″	2′	4′	
$CF_3CH_2OC_2H_5$	50.3	4	8	2	16	30″	20″	60″	
$CHF_2CH_2OC_2H_5$	65	4	9	2.2	24	1′	2′	5′—20′	
Bromine substituted fluoro hydrocarbons									
CF_3CH_2Br	26.5	2.8	11.7	4.2	74	15″	75″	3′	
$CF_3CHBrCH_3$	48.6	1.7	7.6	4.5	22	15″	60″	2′—3′	
CHF_2CH_2Br	57	1.3	4.6	3.5	90	45″	2′	8′	
$CF_3CH_2CH_2Br$	62	1.5	4.5	3	24	45″	45″	90″	D.D.
CF_2ClCH_2Br	68	.8	3.7	4.6	72	20″	5′	10′	
CF_3CHBr_2	73	.4	2	5	44	20″	4′	10′	
$CH_3CF_2CH_2Br$	75.4	1.25	5.8	4.6	36	20″	3′	10′	
$CF_2ClCHBrCH_3$	89	.56	2.2	4	26	15″	7′	10′—20′	
$CF_3CHBrCH_2Br$	116	.1	.67	6.7	52	45″	10′	20′	D.D.
Chlorine and iodine substituted fluoroethane									
CF_2ClCH_3	—9.6	25			12				conv. on recovery
CF_3CH_2Cl	6.1	8	25	3	23				conv. on recovery
CF_3CHCl_2	28.7	2.7	7.7	2.8	24	30″	70″	90″	
$CFCl_2CH_3$	31.7	2.5	5	2	26	75″	75″	90″	
CHF_2CH_2Cl	36	2.15	7.5	3.5	56	45″	3′	5′	
CF_2ClCH_2Cl	46.8	1.3	4.3		8	60″	4′	7′	D.D.
CF_3CH_2I	55	1.25	5	4	30	15″	2′	5′	
Chlorine substituted fluoropropane									
$CF_2ClCH_2CH_3$	25—26	8	16	2	10	30″	30″	90″	
$CF_3CH_2CH_2Cl$	45	3	9.7	3.2	20	20″	30″	60″	D.D.
$CF_3CCl_2CH_3$	48.1	4	10	2.5	32	20″	20″	60″	
$CHF_2CHClCH_3$	52	1.7	7.6	4.5	30	15″	3′	7′	
$CH_3CF_2CH_2Cl$	55	2.15	8.4	4	50	20″	45″	4′	
$CFCl_2CH_2CH_3$	66.7	1.5	5.3	3.5	30	20″	90″	2′—3′	
$CF_2ClCHClCH_3$	69.5	.96	4.1	4.3	66	20″	3′	6′	
$CF_3CH_2CHCl_2$	71	.56	2.4	4.3	36	45″	90″	5′	D.D.
$CF_3CHClCH_2Cl$	75.5	.4—.5	2.2	4.5	20	30″	3′	7′	
$CF_2ClCH_2CH_2Cl$	80.8	0.9	2.25	2.5	30	45″	45″	3′	D.D.
$CF_2ClCHClCFCl_2$	85	0.6	1.8	3	30	90″	2′	6′	D.D.

Table 1. (continued)

Formula	BP°	AD_{50} vol.%	LD_{50} vol.%	$\frac{LD_{50}}{AD_{50}}$	No. Mice	Time A.	Time P.	Time W.	Remarks
Chlorine substituted fluorobutane									
C_4HClF_6	34								convulsions
$CH_3CF_2CFClCH_3$	53	3.4	11.8	3.5	26	30″	90″	4′	
$CH_3CFClCH_2CH_3$	67	1.8	6	3.3	44	30″	1′	5′	
$CH_2CF_2CHClCH_3$	71.4	.74	3.7	5	34	30″	90″	3′	
$C_4H_7F_2Cl$	89	1	4	4	28	45″	2′	6′	
$CH_3CF_2CH_2CHCl_2$	117	0.35	1.3	3.7	32	90″	5′	10′	D.D.
$CH_3CF_2CHClCH_2Cl$	120	0.2	1	5	40	60″	5′	15′	
$C_4H_5F_2Cl_3$	137	0.12	0.7	5.8	44	2′	8′	15′	
Diethyl ether and chloroform for comparison									
$C_2H_5OC_2H_5$	35	3.2	11.2	3.5	38	45″	3′	5′	
$CHCl_3$	61.2	0.78	2.6	3.3	26	45″	2′—3′	5′	

conv. on recovery = convulsions during the recovery period.
D.D. = delayed death, within 24—48 hours after anesthesia.
A = Time necessary for induction of anesthesia of mice when exposed to LD_{50} concentration.
P = Time necessary for recovery of pain sensation after exposure to the LD_{50} concentration for 10 minutes.
W = Time necessary for the return of normal walking after exposure to the LD_{50} concentration for 10 minutes.
From Robbins (1946).

to these compounds did undergo complete anesthesia and upon stimulation exhibited convulsive seizures. Henne et al. (1939) described the synthesis of aliphatic compounds (methane to heptane) which contained a CF_2 group. The difluorides in this series are odorless gases or liquids which have no apparent physiological effect. These authors discuss the synthesis of difluorides and their physical-chemical characteristics. They also investigated the chlorination of these fluorohydrocarbons.

The first comprehensive study of fluorinated hydrocarbons and ethers as anesthetics was reported by Robbins (1946). Dr. C. T. McBee and his associates at Purdue University provided Robbins with 46 fluorinated and mixed halogenated (containing fluorine as one of the halogens) hydrocarbons. Preliminary studies were conducted on mice and those compounds that showed promise as anesthetics were tested on dogs. Unfortunately a paucity of supply of many of the compounds thwarted extensive investigation. Besides, methods of purification of fluorinated ethers and hydrocarbons were in their incipiency at this time and one is inclined to believe that many of the compounds did not enjoy the highest degree of chemical purity.

The compounds screened for anesthetic activity on mice by Robbins are shown in Table 1.

In an extension of these studies Robbins determined the effect of varying the type and number of secondary halogen substituents. His results are set forth in Table 2.

From the observations in these screening tests Robbins selected 18 compounds exhibiting the highest LD_{50}/AD_{50} ratios and tested them for their anesthetic activity on dogs. The results of these studies are shown in Table 3.

From these experiments on dogs Robbins drew the following conclusions.

"1. All of the eighteen compounds produced anesthesia in dogs.

Table 2. *The effect of varying the type and number of secondary halogen substituents upon the concentration of the agents necessary for anesthesia and respiratory arrest*

Formula	Boiling point	AD_{50} %	LD_{50} %	LD_{50}/AD_{50}
		Trifluoroethanes		
CF_3CH_3	−46°	50		
CF_3CH_2Cl	6.1	8	25	3
CF_3CH_2Br	26.5	2.8	11.7	4.2
CF_3CH_2I	55	1.25	5	4
CF_3CHCl_2	28	2.7	7.7	2.8
CF_3CHBr_2	73	0.4	2	5
		Trifluoropropanes		
$CF_3CH_2CH_3$	−12	50		
$CF_3CH_2CH_2Cl$	45	3	9.7	3.2
$CF_3CH_2CH_2Br$	62	1.5	4.5	3
$CF_3CHClCH_2Cl$	75	0.4—0.5	2.2	4.5
$CF_3CHBrCH_2Br$	116	0.1	0.67	6.7
		Difluoropropanes		
$CH_3CF_2CH_2Cl$	55	2.15	8.6	4
$CH_3CF_2CH_2Br$	75	1.25	5.8	4.6
$CF_2ClCHClCH_3$	69.5	0.96	4.1	4.3
$CF_2ClCHBrCH_3$	89	0.56	2.2	4

From ROBBINS (1946).

2. These agents produced a fall in blood pressure which became more marked in the deeper levels of anesthesia.

3. Abnormalities of the cardiac rhythm as shown by electrocardioscopic examination were very frequently produced, and ventricular fibrillation was observed in four instances.

4. Dogs under nine of the eighteen compounds showed hyper-activity of the skeletal muscles, and this was more marked during the deeper levels of anesthesia.

5. The results obtained with four of these compounds, $CF_3CHBrCH_3$, CF_3CHBr_2, $CF_3CHClCH_2Cl$ and $CHF_2CHClCH_3$, are such that we feel further investigations of them as possible anesthetic agents are indicated."

It is unfortunate that ROBBINS did not pursue further this provocative study. The reason was likely due to a limited supply of the fluorinated compounds and the difficulties and expense involved in their synthesis. At the close of World War II, it was revealed that many fluorinated hydrocarbons and ethers had been prepared in various defense projects. Synthesis had become simplified and expense materially reduced. Thus, many investigators in the field of anesthetics became interested in extending their studies to include the fluorinated compounds. Extensive work in this area during the decade beginning in 1953 culminated in three excellent fluorinated anesthetics: fluroxene, halothane and methoxyflurane.

B. Further studies of fluorinated hydrocarbons and ethers

Prompted by ROBBINS' work, the anesthetic properties of 24 fluorinated ethers and hydrocarbons, with and without halogens in the molecule were investigated by LU et al. (1953).

The wide variety of compounds studied and the results obtained by the screening procedure are shown in Tables 4 and 5.

Table 3. *Effect of various halogenated hydrocarbons upon the blood pressure and rhythm of the heart during anesthesia by these agents*

Compound	Expt. No.	Blood pressure					Cardiac arrhythmia	Remarks
		Control	III_2	III_3	III_4	IV[1]		
CF_3CH_2Br	1	125	100	80	70		None	Skeletal movement III_4
	2	140		125	70		V. ex.; v. tach.	Tremor stages III_3 and IV
	3	120		80		55	V. ex.	Tremor stages III_3 and IV
	4	130		110	70	40	V. ex.; nodal	Rigid stage IV
CHF_2CH_2Br	1	130		120	100		V. ex.; nodal	Rigid; convulsion
CF_3CH_2I	1	130		105		70	Nodal; v. ex.	
	2	125		100	75	65	V. ex.	
CF_2ClCH_2Br	1	120	115	100	85		A.V. dis.; nodal	
	2	100	90	90	60—40		4:1 block; nodal v. fib.	
	3	120		90	60		V. ex.; v. tach.; nodal	
	4	120	100	90	60—40	30	Nodal; v. tach.	
$CFCl_2CH_3$	1	150	90		55		Nodal	Rigid
$CH_2ClCF_2CH_3$	1	115		85	70		None	
	2	100	90	80	60		Nodal	
	3	130	50		60		A. V. block	
	4	110	100	30	20		V. tach.; nodal	
$CClF_2CHClCH_3$	1	140	90	75	40		Low voltage Stage III_{2-4}	
	2	90	70	60	55		None	
	3	120		70	40		None	
	4	100	70	70			None	
$CF_3CH_2CHCl_2$	1	130	120	110			None	
	2	120					V. fib. stage II	
	3	120					Nodal; v. ex.; v. fib. stage II	
	4		100	90	80		Low voltage	
	5				70		None	
$CF_2ClCH{=}CH_2$	1	130	90	85			Nodal; v. ex.	Tremor
$CF_3CH_2OC_2H_5$	1	150	150	140			None	Rigid with convulsions on stimulation
$CH_3CF_2CFClCH_3$	1	140	105	50			Nodal	Tremor; rigid
	2						V. tach.; v. fib.	V. fib. during induction
	3	135	50	40			Nodal	
$CH_3CF_2CF_2CH_3$	1	130	60			50	Nodal; v. ex.; A.V. dis.	Tremor; convulsion

Table 3. (continued)

Compound	Expt. No.	Blood pressure					Cardiac arrhythmia	Remarks
		Control	III_2	III_3	III_4	IV[1]		
$CF_3CHBrCH_3$	1	140		125	80	45	None	Rapid rise in Bp. when anesthesia stopped
	2	110	95	85	75	45	None	Rapid rise in Bp. when anesthesia stopped
	3	140		90	70—80	20	None	Rapid rise in Bp. when anesthesia stopped
	4	130		90	80	40	None	Rapid rise in Bp. when anesthesia stopped
	5	120	100	90	80	50	None	Rapid rise in Bp. when anesthesia stopped
CF_3CHBr_2	1	100	85	80	100	75	None	
	2	120	100	100		65	None	
$CF_3CHClCH_2Cl$	1	115		100	85 to 100	60	None	
	2	115	90	105	70	20	None	
$CHF_2CHClCH_3$	1	125		120	95	40	None	
	2	115	100	100	85	70	None	
$CF_2ClCHBrCH_3$	1	130		75	60	40	Low voltage stage III_4	Tremor on recovery
	2	160		105	75	70	M.F. v. ex. induction	Tremor on recovery
	3	130		65	75		A.V. nodal; irregular	
$CH_2BrCF_2CH_3$	1	95		65	25		S.A. inhibition stage I	
	2	150		100	60		V. ex., stage I; low voltage	Leg movement, stage III_4

[1] Classification after SEEVERS et al. (1934).

V. ex. = ventricular extra systole; v. tach. = ventricular tachycardia; nodal = auriculoventricular nodal rhythm; A.V. dis. = auriculoventricular dissociation; A.V. block = auriculoventricular block.

From ROBBINS (1946).

1. Trifluoroethyl vinyl ether (Fluroxene, Fluoromar®)

An examination of Table 4 indicates that these compounds containing fluorine atoms and other halogens were not suitable as anesthetic agents. Most of them produced marked respiratory irritation, muscular rigidity and violent incoordinated muscular activity of the extremities.

By unsaturating these mixed substituted halogenated hydrocarbons containing fluorine, anesthetic properties appeared to manifest themselves in certain of the compounds, namely, 1,2-dichloro-perfluoro-propylene-1 in Table 4. This compound elicited anesthetic action, but produced marked changes in the electrocardiogram.

By removal of the other halogens from the fluorinated hydrocarbons, anesthetic properties appeared to diminish, and although certain of these agents produced anesthesia, the induction was stormy, accompanied by marked struggle and extensor rigidity.

Table 4. *Mixed halogenated hydrocarbons*

Name	Formula	Animal	Dose or concentration	Anesthesia	Remarks
			Saturated		
Trifluoro-mono-iodo-methane	CIF_3	1 dog	50%	No	Coughing, choking, retching and convulsion after 30 seconds' inhalation
1,3-dichloro-perfluoro-propane	$CF_2ClCF_2CF_2Cl$	1 dog	12 ml (divided)	No	Muscular rigidity, tremors of the extremities, slight sedation
		1 dog	10 ml (divided)		
1,2,2,3-tetrachloro-perfluoro-propane	$CF_2ClCCl_2CF_2Cl$	1 dog	3.5 ml (divided)	No	Muscular rigidity, opisthotonos, pulmonary edema, tremors, incoordination, later marked depression; died within 24 hours
2,3-dibromo-1,1,1-trifluoro-2-methyl-propane	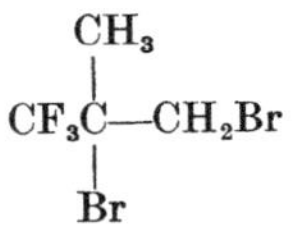	2 rats	2 ml	Yes	Postanesthetic analgesia, pulmonary edema, rapid recovery
1,2-dibromo-2-chloro-perfluoro-propane	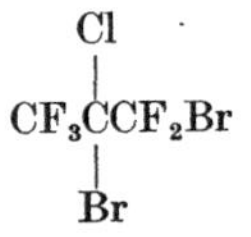	2 rats	1 ml	No	Violent respiratory depression and failure, convulsion; both died
1,2-dichloro-perfluoro-cyclo-pentene	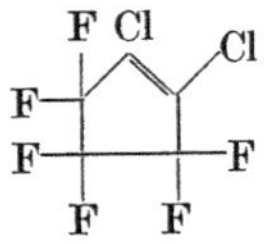	2 rats	2 ml	No	Extreme depression, analgesia, respiratory depression and failure; both died within 18 hours
1,2-dibromo-perfluoro-propane	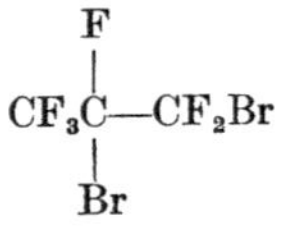	3 rats	2 ml	No	Marked salivation, prolonged convulsions lasting until death

Table 4 (continued)

Name	Formula	Animal	Dose or concentration	Anesthesia	Remarks
			Unsaturated		
1,2-dichloro-perfluoro-propylene-1	$CF_3\overset{\overset{Cl}{\vert}}{C}=CFCl$	4 dogs	Av. 6 ml (divided)	Yes	Induction quiet, recovery uneventful, like ethyl ether, heart slowed although no fall of blood pressure, EKG changes: inversion of T-wave, bradycardia, prolongation of Q—R interval
2-chloro-perfluoro-propylene	$CF_3\overset{\overset{Cl}{\vert}}{C}=CF_2$	1 dog	75%	No	Marked struggle and gasping, respiratory arrest, revived by artificial respiration
1,1,2-trichloro-3,3,3-trifluoro-propylene	$CF_3CCl=CCl_2$	1 dog	3.5 ml (divided)	No	Muscular rigidity, opisthotonos, pulmonary edema, incoordination, marked depression later; died within few hours
2,3-dichloro-perfluoro-butene-2	$CF_3\overset{\overset{Cl}{\vert}}{C}=\overset{\overset{Cl}{\vert}}{C}CF_3$	4 rats	2 ml	Yes	2 rats had convulsions at the point of anesthesia; all rats had postanesthetic analgesia, died within 18 hours
1,2-dichloro-3,3,3-trifluoro-propylene	$CF_3\overset{\overset{Cl}{\vert}}{C}=CHCl$	2 rats	2 ml	No	Depression, slight analgesia, respiratory depression, failure; one animal could not be revived, the other recovered quickly
1,1-difluoro-perchloro-propylene-2	$CF_2Cl\overset{\overset{Cl}{\vert}}{C}=CCl_2$	2 rats 1 rat	2 ml 3 ml	No Yes (light)	Depression, analgesia, pulmonary edema, irritation to eyes, convulsions and death within one hour
1-methyl-1-trifluoro-methyl-cyclopropane	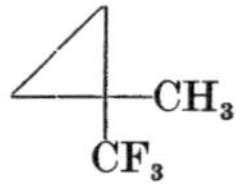	1 dog	7 ml (divided)	Yes	Induction rapid and smooth, some extensor rigidity in front legs and some tremors in hind legs, relaxation fair, recovery rapid and uneventful
Trifluoroisobutene	$CF_3\underset{\underset{CH_3}{\vert}}{C}=CH_2$	3 dogs	75%	Yes	Marked struggle, extensor rigidity, tremors throughout body and extremities, relaxation poor, stertorous respiration, recovery prompt, extreme salivation
Perfluoro-2-butine	$CF_3C\equiv CCF_3$	1 dog	75%	No	Animal died within a few hours of pulmonary edema
Perfluoropropylene	$CF_3CF=CF_2$	2 dogs	50% 75%	No No	No demonstrable effect; tremors, respiratory irritation
1,1,1-trifluoropropylene	$CF_3CH=CH_2$	2 dogs	50%	No	Tremors, incoordination

From Lu et al. (1953).

Table 5. *Fluorinated ethers*

Name	Formula	Animal	Dose or concentration	Anesthesia	Remarks
Perfluorodiethyl ether	$C_2F_5—O—C_2F_5$	1 dog	75%	No	No deleterious effects
		2 rats	air in jar displaced by compound	No	No deleterious effects
2,2,3,3,3-pentafluoropropyl methyl ether	$CF_3CF_2CH_2—O—CH_3$	1 dog	6 ml	No	Labored respiration, cardiac irregularities, slow recovery
		1 dog	10 ml	Yes	Extensor rigidity of hind legs, tremors throughout body, respiratory depression, slow recovery
2,2,2-trifluoroethyl methyl ether	$CF_3CH_2—O—CH_3$	1 dog	10 ml	No	Rigidity of extremities, marked salivation and irritation to mucous membranes
		1 dog	10 ml	No	Tremors of extremities, marked salivation and irritation to mucous membranes
		1 dog	12 ml	Yes	No tremors or rigidity, marked salivation and irritation to mucous membranes
2,2,3,3,4,4,4-heptafluorobutyl methyl ether	$CF_3CF_2CF_2CH_2—O—CH_3$	1 rat	2 ml	Yes	Threatened respiratory arrest, quick recovery
		1 rat	2 ml	No	Pulmonary edema, deep depression, respiratory failure, convulsions, death
2,2,2-trifluoroethyl vinyl ether	$CF_3CH_2—O—CH=CH_2$	2 rats	1 ml	Yes	No untoward symptoms
		6 dogs	av. 5.5 ml (divided)	Yes	Good relaxation, little struggle during induction, rapid recovery, no abnormal changes of EKG, average anesthetic index in 4 dogs = 2.5
2,2,3,3,3-pentafluoropropyl vinyl ether	$CF_3CF_2CH_2—O—CH=CH_2$	2 rats	3 ml	No	Irritation of eyes, peripheral vasodilatation, pulmonary edema, opisthotonos, threatened respiratory collapse, quick recovery

From Lu et al. (1953).

The most promising results were obtained by the fluorination of ethers, as shown in Table 5. Four out of six of these compounds exhibited anesthetic properties. Most amazing was the fact that perfluorodiethyl ether was completely devoid of any pharmacologic effect, even in concentrations of 75%.

The best responses obtained in this series were those elicited by trifluoroethyl vinyl ether, the analogue of ethyl vinyl ether studied by KRANTZ et al. (1947). The promising anesthetic properties of trifluoroethyl vinyl ether prompted KRANTZ and his associates to study the compound in detail and explore its finer pharmacologic profile (see p. 544).

2. Halothane, Fluothane®

In 1956 RAVENTOS introduced the mixed halogenated hydrocarbon 1,1,1-trifluoro-2,2-bromochlorethane, $CF_3CHBrCl$, as an anesthetic agent. The use of halothane as a clinical anesthetic agent was accepted with rapidity in England, Canada and the United States (see p. 552).

C. Recent studies of other fluorinated hydrocarbons and ethers

1. Methoxyflurane, Penthrane®

VAN POZNAK and ARTUSIO (1960a) screened a number of fluorinated and mixed halogenated hydrocarbons on dogs for anesthetic activity. During the period of inhalation, electrocardiograms, electroencephalograms, blood pressure and oxygen saturation of the blood were determined. In addition, ease of induction, speed of recovery and response to pain stimuli were observed. The results of their studies are shown in Table 6.

They considered $CF_3CHClCH_2Cl$ to be a satisfactory anesthetic agent. The most promising of the compounds tested for anesthetic activity was CF_3CFClH. This compound like halothane evoked a reversible depressor response. They state from their studies that it appears, "... a nonflammable gaseous anesthetic agent of approximately 40% potency can probably be synthesized for future study."

By the foregoing procedure VAN POZNAK and ARTUSIO (1960b) studied a series of fluorinated ethers. Results of these studies are shown in Table 7.

From this series of fluorinated ethers methoxyflurane was made available clinically and rapidly gained a limited degree of acceptance (p. 553).

2. Halogenated propanes containing fluorine

FABIAN et al. (1960) studied a series of mixed halogenated propanes on various laboratory animals. Their studies demonstrated that the most satisfactory anesthetic agents among the compounds investigated were 1-chloro-2,2,3,3-tetrafluoropropane and 1-bromo-2,2,3,3-tetrafluoropropane (halopropane). The chloro derivative has been tested clinically and the bromo compound appeared to be suitable for human anesthesia.

The properties of the chloro derivative are reported by FABIAN et al. as follows:

The chloro-substituted compound 1-chloro-2,2,3,3-tetrafluoropropane ($CHF_2CF_2CH_2Cl$), which has received clinical investigation, has the following physical and chemical properties: molecular weight, 150.5; boiling point, 54° C; vapor pressure, 192 mm of mercury; liquid density, 1.43 at 20° C; specific volume, 0.692; flammability in air, not flammable; flammability in oxygen, greater than 17% concentration; stability to hot alkali, complete; exposure to ultraviolet radiation, no decomposition.

Table 6. *Anesthetic effects of fluorohydrocarbons on dogs*

	Name of drug	Formula	Dogs	Dose %	Anesthesia: Anesthesia	Anesthesia: EEG	Anesthesia: EKG	Remarks
A	Dichlorodifluoromethane	CCl_2F_2	3 2	50 15	Unsatisfactory	Grand mal	S-T ↓	Convulsions; Satisfactory anesthesia if combined with thiopental or succinylcholine
B	Tetrafluorodichloroethane	CF_2ClCF_2Cl	1 1	50 25	Unsatisfactory	Grand mal	Obscured tachycardia	Severe convulsions limiting respiration. Rapid recovery, no ill effects
C	Trifluoromethane	CHF_3	2	80	No	No record	No record	No loss of consciousness. Analgesia questionable
D	Difluoromonochloromethane	CHF_2Cl	1	25	Partial	Excitation with some slow waves	S-T ↓ tachycardia	Running and twitching movements. No response to pain. Rapid and complete recovery
			1	50	Partial	Obscured by muscle potentials	S-T ↓ tachycardia	Light surgical anesthesia with some twitching movements
			1	70	Partial	Obscured by mus. pot.	S-T ↓ tachycardia	Respiration depression. Death by hypoxia
			1	25 50 70	Partial	Combined fast and slow activity	S-T ↓ tachycardia	With assisted and controlled ventilation, 70% produced light surgical anesthesia. No untoward effects. Rapid uneventful recovery
			1 1	70 50	Good	Moderate depression	S-T ↓	Light surgical anesthesia. Rapid recovery when ventilated with O_2
			2	25	No	Slow and fast waves combined	S-T ↓	Twitching and running movements unless paralyzed. Rapid recovery
			1	40	Partial	Obscured	Obscured	Running and twitching movements

Table 6 (Continued)

E	Difluoroethane	CH_3CHF_2	3	50	Good	Light surgical anesthesia	No change	Tried by several volunteers. Good analgesia. Impending loss of consciousness. Explosive
F	Pentafluoroethane	CF_3CF_2H	1	80	Excitement	No record	No record	True surgical anesthesia not attained after five minutes; complete recovery in one minute
G	1,1,1,2-Tetrafluoro-2-chloroethane	CF_3CFClH	6	40—70	Good	Light surgical anesthesia	S-T ↓	Rapid induction and emergence. Rare vomiting. Full ventilation. BP fall at higher concentrations. No ventricular fibrillation after Epinephrine i.v. at 2,4, and 8 γ/kg
H	1,1,1,2-Tetrafluoro-2-bromoethane	CF_3CFHBr	1	50	Yes	No record	No record	Very rapid and smooth induction. Respiratory depression. Good heart action. Rapid complete recovery on ventilation with O_2
			1	25	Yes	Moderate depression	No record	Rapid induction. Moderate surgical anesthesia. Good relaxation. No respiratory depression. Rapid recovery with no untoward effects
			1	10	Yes	Motion artefact	Normal	Prolonged induction. Very light surgical anesthesia. Rapid uneventful recovery
I	1,1,1-Trifluoro-2-bromoethane	CF_3CH_2Br	1	bubble vaporizer	No	Grand mal	S-T ↓ T inverted VPC's	Convulsions; respiratory depression; flammable. Rapid complete recovery. Much salivation
J	1,1,1-Trifluoro-2,3-dichloropropane	$CF_3CHClCH_2Cl$	1	bubble vaporizer	Good	Moderate depression	No change	Satisfactory anesthesia. Rapid recovery
			5		Good	—	—	Five short surgical procedures. Entirely satisfactory. Complete recovery
			1		Good	Fast activity low voltage	No abnormality	Good anesthesia. Rapid recovery
			1		Good	Fast activity low voltage	S-T ↓	Good anesthesia. Rapid recovery

Table 6 (Continued)

	Name of drug	Formula	Dogs	Dose	Anesthesia			Remarks
				%	Anesthesia	EEG	EKG	
K	1,1,1-Trifluoro-2-bromo-propene	CF_3—CBr=CH_2	1	closed circle	Yes	Low voltage fast activity	Normal sinus rhythm, S-T segment depression	Excellent anesthesia. Rapid uneventful recovery
L	1,1,1,3,3,3-Hexafluoro-2-chloropropane	CF_3—CHCl—CF_3	1	40	Initially satisfactory	Low voltage fast activity	S-T segment depression, normal rhythm	Canister became very hot; dog vomited, defecated, recovered very slowly from anesthesia, died. Agent probably unstable with alkali
M	Bromodifluoromethane	CF_2BrH	1	50	Initially satisfactory	No record	No record	Canister rapidly became hot; gasping respiration, rapid recovery; dog vomited, defecated, appeared very ill; apparently well in one day

From VAN POZNAK and ARTUSIO (1960a).

Table 7. *Anesthetic effects of fluorinated ethers on dogs*

Compound	Flammability	Number of dogs	Anesthesia satisfactory	Required time for Induction (min)	Maintenance (min)	Emergence (min)	EKG Lead II	EEG	Intravenous epinephrine	Remarks
CH_3—O—CF_2—CHFCl BP 70° C	yes	2	yes	5	15	5	S-T ↓ NSR	Plane 1–2 6/sec 200 μv, plane 2 20/sec 20 μv, 21–23/sec 100 μv, plane 3 flat with some high frequency low amplitude	VPC's T-wave changes	Good surgical anesthesia
CH_3—O—CF_2—$CHCl_2$ BP 104° C	no	10	yes	10	10 to 120	10—40	S-T ↓ NSR	Plane 1 16–20/sec 10 μv, plane 3 14/sec 10 μv, 2–3/sec 50 μv	Sinus tachycardia, lead II T-wave changed from inverted to upright for 10 sec, occasional VPC's	Full even ventilation in light planes, good surgical relaxation
CH_3—O—CF_2—CHClBr BP 124° C	no	2	yes	10	71—81	20—40	S-T ↓ NSR	Plane 1 22/sec 10 μv, plane 3 16–18/sec 20 μv	AV block, VPC's	Extensor rigidity at moderate depth could be abolished by lightening or deepening, otherwise satisfactory
CHClF—O—CFH_2 BP 54° C	no	1	no	4	7	died	Nodal rhythm then death	No record	Not tried	Rapid induction, apnea, no pulse or EKG, death; attempted resuscitation unsuccessful
CH_2Cl—O—CF_2—CHClF BP 111° C	no	1	no	10	14	3	Bradycardia S-T ↓ NSR	20/sec 10 μv on 10/sec 20 μv	Not tried	Anesthesia with twitching, shivering, jerking movements
CF_2Cl—O—CF_2CHFCl 80% $CFCl_2$—O—CF_2—CHF_2 20% BP 64—65° C	no	1	no	1.5	3	3.5	No record	No record	Not tried	Rigidity, twitching, shivering
CH_2Cl—O—CF_2CF_2H BP 77° C	no	2	yes	3	30	5	S-T ↓ NSR	Plane 2 13/sec 20 μv	Few VPC's	Satisfactory anesthesia, delayed deaths 24 and 48 hours after anesthesia

From VAN POZNAK and ARTUSIO (1960b)

Laboratory experiments on mice demonstrated the anesthetic activity of 1-chloro-2,2,3,3-tetrafluoropropane at concentrations of 1.5%. Anesthesia in dogs with the agent was uneventful.

FABIAN and his associates used the chlorine derivative of this fluorinated propane on 29 patients and were favorably impressed with the anesthesia it produced. They state "In summarizing the data accumulated in this series, the apparent advantages offered by $CHF_2CF_2CH_2Cl$ are as follows: (1) The compound is nonflammable and nonexplosive in concentrations of less than 20% in oxygen and nonflammable in any concentration in air. It is stable chemically. (2) The drug acts rapidly and is eliminated rapidly. (3) Hypotension occurs to a very slight extent during anesthetic planes required for producing the necessary muscle relaxation. (4) There is an extremely low incidence of postanesthetic nausea or vomiting. (5) Studies of excretion of sulfobromophthalein dye did not show significant interference with this phase of liver function 24 hours after anesthesia. (6) Profound muscle relaxation is provided in light planes of anesthesia."

Halopropane ($CHF_2CF_2CH_2Br$) was studied in animals by this group. Further clinical investigations are under way with halopropane.

Halopropane appears to be more promising than the chloro derivative, which has been noted by FABIAN to produce some cardiac arrhythmias in man.

VIRTUE et al. (1963) in laboratory and clinical studies of halopropane anesthesia in man noted no significant changes in cardiac output, venous pressure, oxygen uptake, carbon dioxide output and respiratory minute volume. Some hypotension developed with this agent. Induction and recovery times were of considerable duration.

3. Mixed halogenated ethers and a hydrocarbon

BURNS et al. (1961 a) screened several mixed halogenated fluorine compounds on mice for their anesthetic activity. These compound were:

(2-Chloro-1,1,2-trifluoroethyl) methyl ether boiling point, 69°	$CHClF \cdot CF_2 \cdot O \cdot CH_3$
(2-Chloro-1,1,2-trifluoroethyl) ethyl ether boiling point, 88°	$CHClF \cdot CF_2 \cdot O \cdot C_2H_5$
(2-Chloro-1,1,2-trifluoroethyl) iso-propyl ether boiling point, 100°	$CHClF \cdot CF_2 \cdot O \cdot CH(CH_3)_2$
(2-Chloro-1,1,2-trifluoroethyl) n-propyl ether boiling point, 109°	$CHClF \cdot CF_2 \cdot O \cdot CH_2CH_2CH_3$
1,2-difluoro-1,1,2-trichloroethane boiling point, 72°	$CFCl_2 \cdot CFHCl$

From these studies it was concluded that the most satisfactory agent in the group that warranted further study was 1,2-difluoro-1,1,2-trichloroethane. This type of screening for anesthetic activity in mice is not conclusive in indicating the value or lack of value of an agent for anesthetic purposes. It is hoped that further studies will be conducted on a variety of laboratory animals to determine definitely the potential value of this series of compounds as anesthetics.

4. Cyclic fluorinated hydrocarbon

BURNS et al. (1961 b) examined the anesthetic properties of C_6F_6. Hexafluorobenzene produced anesthesia in 15 mice. The results obtained by this group are listed below.

Effects on mice (summary of experiments):

1. 0.2% v/v hexafluorobenzene produced light anesthesia in one mouse for thirty minutes.
2. 1.6–2.4% produced deep anesthesia for thirty minutes in one mouse with complete, but slow, recovery.
3. 4.4% produced respiratory arrest followed by death in one mouse. Exposure was for twenty minutes.
4. 1.25% produced light anesthesia for thirty minutes with rapid recovery (four mice used).
5. 3.5% produced very deep anesthesia in two mice for thirty minutes, with slow recovery.
6. Six mice were lightly anesthetised for twenty minutes on two consecutive days, with rapid recoveries.

The results show that hexafluorobenzene is an anesthetic in relatively low concentrations.

Hexafluorobenzene is a highly stable compound; it does not react with soda lime and it is nonflammable in air. BURNS states that this work is of interest since some of their unpublished results show that six-membered ring compounds are extremely toxic to mice. This study is very limited in the number of experiments and the fact that only one species of laboratory animal was used. Further studies on dogs and monkeys may yield valuable information.

BURNS et al., in 1964 examined the anesthetic properties of fourteen fluorinated ring compounds, some with other halogens, in mice. They were as follows:

six-membered ring compounds
- pentafluorobenzene
- monomethylnonafluorocyclohexene
- monoethoxynonafluorocyclohexene
- decafluorocyclohexene
- perfluoromethylcyclohexane
- perfluorodimethylcyclohexane
- perfluorobromobenzene
- perfluorotoluene
- 1-(1′,1′,1′-trifluoroethoxy)nonafluorocyclohexene

other ring compounds
- 3,3,4,4,5,5-hexafluorotetrahydropyran(3,3,4,4,5,5-hexafluoroepoxyhexane)
- octofluorocyclopentene
- monomethoxyheptafluorocyclopentene
- 1,H:3,H-octafluorocyclopentane
- 1,H:2,H-hexafluorocyclobutane.

None of the foregoing compounds showed sufficient promise as anesthetics to justify further work. Pentafluorobenzene and hexafluorotetrahydropyran produced no obvious toxic symptoms. The remainder of the compounds produced variable degrees of undesirable side effects and toxicity. All the compounds were flammable to some degree in oxygen and air. The authors emphasize that six-membered fluorinated ring compounds need not be necessarily toxic as previously considered. These authors noted that different results are frequently observed with these compounds when highly purified.

5. Teflurane

ARTUSIO and VAN POZNAK (1961a) reinvestigated the anesthetic properties of teflurane, CF_3CFHBr, which they had previously studied in 1958. Teflurane, 1,1,1,2-tetrafluoro-2-bromoethane, is a nonflammable, nonexplosive, base-stable gas which boils at 8°. Using an anesthetic concentration of 25% in oxygen, anesthesia occurred within 3 minutes. Intravenous epinephrine 5—40 mcg/kg failed to induce fibrillation in any of the dogs studied. In a study on 30 patients, induction was achieved with 50% concentration of teflurane and maintenance with 25%. Surgical anesthesia was reached within 5 minutes. In deep planes of anesthesia blood pressure decreased on an average of 15% from control levels. Recovery in patients was rapid, occurring in 5 to 10 minutes. Sulfobromophthalein retention was elevated in the patients; however, it returned to normal values within 10 days. In 1963 ARTUSIO and VAN POZNAK reported on further clinical explorations with teflurane and refer to this agent as the "nonflammable cyclopropane". Teflurane was the product of their search for a nonflammable, gaseous anesthetic agent with a potency of about 40% concentration in the inspired air. The future of this compound will be determined by the clinical trials.

6. Roflurane

ARTUSIO and VAN POZNAK (1961b) in an attempt to combine the desirable features of methoxyflurane and teflurane, synthesized roflurane. Roflurane, 1,1,2-trifluoro-2-bromoethyl methyl ether, is a nonflammable, volatile liquid which boils at 88.8° and is stable in the presence of fixed alkali. Roflurane elicits excellent anesthesia in animals and man. In dogs this agent produces more rapid induction and recovery than does methoxyflurane. No significant changes in respiration or circulation were noted by these authors in dogs undergoing anesthesia with roflurane. Sulfobromophthalein retention was within normal limits after multiple anesthesias with this compound. Liver biopsies did not reveal any pathological changes. Respirations were normal and secretions minimal. Blood pressure declined with increasing depths of anesthesia but was less depressed than with methoxyflurane under comparable anesthetic levels. Muscle relaxation could be achieved with roflurane alone. Since this preliminary study these authors have not reported further on roflurane even though the compound looked so promising.

7. Heavily halogenated fluorohydrocarbons

BURNS et al. (1962) examined six heavily halogenated aliphatic compounds, and their results are summarized in Table 8.

Five of the six compounds showed anesthetic properties, however none is recommended for further trials. Pentafluoroethane was pharmacologically inert.

8. Fluoro-iodo hydrocarbon

Although chlorine and bromine-containing fluorohydrocarbons are used as anesthetic agents, those containing iodine have not been employed. However, trifluoroethyl iodide (2,2,2-trifluoroethyl iodide) was among the compounds screened by ROBBINS (1946). He observed the anesthetic activity of the compound in 3 dogs. Anesthesia was accompanied by hypotension, nodal rhythm and some ventricular extrasystoles. KRANTZ et al. (1963) studied the compound in detail as an anesthetic agent and extrapolated the results to man.

The results of their studies are summarized in the following statements.

Trifluoroethyl iodide is a nonflammable, volatile liquid eliciting anesthetic activity when administered by inhalation to various species of laboratory animals.

The potency of trifluoroethyl iodide is comparable to that of halothane, and the anesthetic index is double that of halothane.

In the dog, trifluoroethyl iodide produced no functional hepatic impairment, as shown by the sulfobromophthalein test.

Table 8. *Summary of investigations on heavily halogenated aliphatic compounds*

Substance, purity and stability to soda lime, inflammability	Effects on mouse
Pentafluoroethane 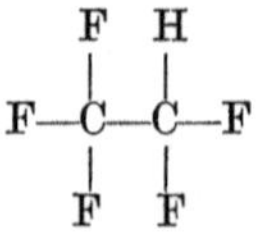 (Halothane with Cl and Br replaced by F) BP —50° C Pure and stable to soda lime Non-inflammable in air or oxygen	13%, 62%, 93% failed to produce anesthesia (7 mice)
2,2,3,3,3-pentafluoropropyl bromide 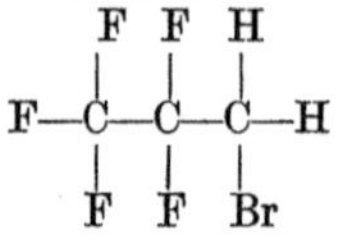 (Contains CF_3 as halothane, but has three carbon atoms) BP 45° C Pure and stable to soda lime Inflammable in oxygen, probably not in air	3% for six minutes produced deep anesthesia in one mouse Slow recovery 1% for six minutes produced deep anesthesia in one mouse Slow recovery 1.5% for seven minutes produced light anesthesia in one mouse Rapid recovery 1% for seven minutes produced fairly deep anesthesia in two separate mice Sudden recovery one and a half minutes later
2,2,3,3,3-pentafluoropropyl chloride 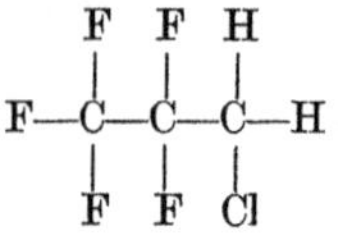 BP 27° C Purity = 99% Some evidence of reaction with soda lime Inflammable in oxygen, probably not in air	1% produced no anesthesia in one mouse 2.5% produced light anesthesia in one mouse Rapid recovery 5% produced light anesthesia in the same mouse 30% produced deep anesthesia with rapid recovery in two separate mice
1,1,2-trifluoro-1-bromo-2-chloroethane 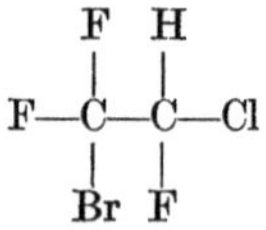 (Halothane with Br replacing the F of the CF_3 group) BP 50° C Pure and stable to soda lime Non-inflammable in air	5.8% for four minutes killed one mouse 3.5% for seventeen minutes killed one mouse 1.6% for thirty minutes produced light anesthesia in seven minutes Rapid recovery in one mouse 2.2% for thirty minutes produced deep anesthesia (induced in one minute) Slow recovery in one mouse
1,1,1-trifluoro-2,2-dichloroethane 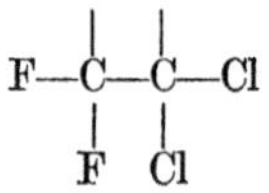 (Halothane with Br replaced by another Cl) BP 27° C Pure and stable to soda lime Inflammability not tested, but expected to be non-inflammable	14% for four minutes killed one mouse after extremely quiet and rapid induction 4% for ten minutes produced rapid, deep anesthesia Rapid recovery in one mouse 3% for forty minutes produced deep anesthesia (almost respiratory arrest) Slow, but apparently good recovery in one mouse

Table 8 (continued)

Substance, purity and stability to soda lime, inflammability	Effects on mouse
Chlorotrifluoroethylene 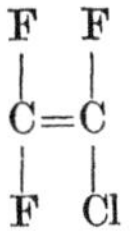 BP —27° C Pure and stable to soda lime Inflammable in oxygen	14% produced no anesthesia, but mouse died within twenty-four hours 63% produced anesthesia in one minute Mouse sluggish even after ninety minutes post-recovery Died within twenty-four hours 48% produced anesthesia in one minute Fairly rapid recovery Died within twenty-four hours

From BURNS et al. (1962).

The depression of oxygen uptake under trifluoroethyl iodide anesthesia is in keeping with our observations on other halogenated hydrocarbons.

The blood pressure in dogs was not significantly lowered with this agent. The electroencephalograms in dogs and monkeys showed no unusual distrubances. The dog's heart did not show any significant changes during anesthesia with trifluoroethyl iodide; however, nodal rhythm and extraventricular systoles were seen in the monkey's heart.

Trifluoroethyl iodide does not appear to be decomposed by body tissues. No increase in protein-bound-iodine or iodide in serum was observed after trifluoroethyl iodide anesthesia. Trifluoroethyl iodide is stable in the presence of moist soda lime.

The animal experiments indicated that trifluoroethyl iodide might prove to be a useful addition as another volatile anesthetic agent in the armamentarium of the anesthesiologist. Its physical and pharmacologic properties suggested that careful trial in human anesthesia was indicated.

On December 5, 1961, at 9:30 A.M., trifluoroethyl iodide was administered by KRANTZ in a closed system to a healthy volunteer, Dr. WILLIAM H. L. DORNETTE. The subject was carried to the first plane of surgical anesthesia within 20 minutes, using a total dose of 11 ml of trifluoroethyl iodide. The induction was without excitation. The electrocardiogram and blood pressure remained unchanged. The recovery was rapid and uneventful. There was a marked postanesthetic analgesia. There were no untoward postanesthetic sequelae.

DORNETTE used trifluoroethyl iodide in a series of patients but later abandoned its use owing to the frequency of occurrence of cardiac arrhythmias. It does appear that the study of other iodine-fluorine bearing hydrocarbons and ethers might be a fruitful field of investigation in a search for new anesthetic agents.

III. Summary tables of hydrocarbons and ethers containing fluorine

In Tables 9 and 10 below are summarized work done with a large number of fluorine-containing hydrocarbons and ethers during the course of investigations into the anesthetic properties of these compounds.

Table 9. *Fluorinated hydrocarbons*

Formula	B.P. °C	Anesth. conc.	Author	Nature of physiological action
			Methanes	
CHF_3	—84.4	80%	VAN POZNAK and ARTUSIO JR., 1960a	No loss of consciousness; analgesia questionable
		50—89%	KRANTZ et al., 1961b	No anesthesia; cyanosis at higher concentrations
CF_4	—128	50—90%	KRANTZ, 1960a	No anesthesia, inert
$CHBrF_2$	—14.5	50%	VAN POZNAK and ARTUSIO JR., 1960a	Initially satisfactory anesthesia, canister rapidly became hot, dog ill, vomited, well in 24 hours
$CHClF_2$	—41	25—70%	VAN POZNAK and ARTUSIO JR., 1960a	Partial and light anesthesia; twitching movements; rapid and complete recovery
$CClF_3$	—81.1	40—80%	KRANTZ et al., 1961b	No anesthesia; cyanosis at higher concentrations
CCl_2F_2	—28	15% 50%	VAN POZNAK and ARTUSIO JR., 1960a	Convulsions, satisfactory ansthesia if combined with thiopental or succinylcholine
CF_3I	—22.5	50%	LU et al., 1953	No anesthesia, retching and convulsions after 30 seconds inhalation in dog
			Ethanes	
CH_3CHF_2	—26	50%	VAN POZNAK and ARTUSIO JR., 1960a	Good anesthesia and analgesia; explosive; dogs and man
CF_3CH_3	—46	50—60%	ROBBINS, 1946	Anesthesia, convulsions on recovery in mice
CF_3CHF_2	—50	90%	BURNS et al., 1962	No anesthesia
CF_3CH_2Cl	6.1	8%	ROBBINS, 1946	Anesthesia, convulsions on recovery in mice
CF_3CH_2Br	26.5	2.8%	ROBBINS, 1946	Anesthesia, tremors, ventricular extrasystoles in dogs
			VAN POZNAK and ARTUSIO JR., 1960a	Convulsions, respiratory depression, rapid, complete recovery, much salivation
CF_3CH_2I	55	1.25%	ROBBINS, 1946	Anesthesia, nodal ventricular extrasystoles in dogs
			KRANTZ et al., 1961b	Potent, good anesthetic, cardiac arrhythmias in man
CF_3CF_2I	13	10%	KRANTZ et al., 1961b	Anesthesia in mice not dogs, uneventful recovery, arrhythmias in dogs and monkeys

Table 9 (continued)

Formula	B.P. °C	Anesth. conc.	Author	Nature of physiological action
CHF_2CH_2Br	57	1.3%	ROBBINS, 1946	Anesthesia in mice, convulsions and rigidity in dogs
CHF_2CH_2Cl	36	2.15%	ROBBINS, 1946	Anesthesia in mice
$CFCl_2CH_3$	31.7	2.5%	ROBBINS, 1946	Anesthesia in mice, rigidity and anesthesia in dogs
CF_3CHCl_2	28.7	2.7%	ROBBINS, 1946	Anesthesia in mice
		14%	BURNS et al., 1962	Toxic, mice
		4%	BURNS et al., 1962	Rapid and deep anesthesia rapid recovery in mice
		3%	BURNS et al., 1962	Deep anesthesia, slow but good recovery, mice
CF_3CHBr_2	73	0.4%	ROBBINS, 1946	Good anesthesia, no cardiac change; dogs
			RAVENTOS and SPINKS, 1958	Marked fall in B.P.; dogs
CF_3CHFCl		40—70%	VAN POZNAK and ARTUSIO JR., 1960a	Good anesthesia, rapid induction; blood pressure fall at higher concentrations, no ventricular fibrillation after epinephrine
CF_3CHFBr (Teflurane)	8	25%	VAN POZNAK and ARTUSIO JR., 1960a	Good anesthesia, rapid recovery; ventilation good, no untoward effects
CF_3CHFI	39	0.24 ml/min	KRANTZ et al., 1962a	Anesthesia, good relaxation; no irritation, mice; marked arrhythmias, no anesthesia in monkeys
$CF_3CHBrCl$ (Halothane)	50.2	0.4 to 1.5%	RAVENTOS, 1956	Excellent anesthesia; muscle relaxation; man
CF_2ClCH_3	—9.6	25%	ROBBINS, 1946	Anesthesia, convulsions on recovery (mice)
CF_2ClCH_2Br	68	0.8%	ROBBINS, 1946	Anesthesia, cardiac arrhythmias in dogs
CF_2ClCH_2Cl	46.8	1.3%	ROBBINS, 1946	Anesthesia; delayed death (mice)
CF_2BrCF_2Br	47	6%	KRANTZ et al., 1961b	Tremors, convulsions, respiratory arrest, death
			RAVENTOS and SPINKS, 1958	Convulsions
$CF_2BrCHClF$	50	1.6 to 5.8%	RAVENTOS and SPINKS, 1958	Blood pressure depressant in dogs
			BURNS et al., 1962	Anesthesia, slow recovery mice
			KRANTZ et al., 1961b	Irritation and delayed toxicity in rats
$CFCl_2CHFCl$	72	0.7 to 3.7%	BURNS et al., 1961a	Anesthesia, uneventful induction and recovery; mice

Table 9 (continued)

Formula	B.P. °C	Anesth. conc.	Author	Nature of physiological action
CCl_3CF_3	42.2	6%	KRANTZ et al., 1961b	Anesthesia, no excitation, respiratory arrest
			RAVENTOS and SPINKS, 1958	Delayed deaths
CF_2ClCF_2Cl	3.6	25% 50%	VAN POZNAK and ARTUSIO JR., 1960a	Unsatisfactory anesthesia, severe convulsions, rapid recovery with no ill effects
$CCl_2{=}CClF$	71		BURGISON et al., 1955	Sensitizes myocardium to epinephrine
$CHCl{=}CF_2$	—17.7		BURGISON et al., 1955	Sensitizes myocardium to epinephrine
$CF_2{=}CH_2$	—82		BURGISON et al., 1955	Myocardium not sensitized epinephrine
$CF_2{=}CF_2$	—76		BURGISON et al., 1955	Incapable of sensitizing myocardium to epinephrine
$CF_2{=}CFCl$	—27	14%	BURNS et al., 1962	No anesthesia, delayed death, mice
		63%		Anesthesia, delayed death
		48%		Anesthesia, rapid recovery, delayed death
			BURGISON et al., 1955	Sensitizes myocardium to epinephrine
		Propanes		
$CH_3CF_2CH_2Cl$	55	2.15%	ROBBINS, 1946	Anesthesia in mice
$CH_3CF_2CH_2Br$	75.4	1.25%	ROBBINS, 1946	Anesthesia in mice
$CFCl_2CH_2CF_3$	66.7	1.5%	ROBBINS, 1946	Anesthesia in mice
$CHF_2CHClCH_3$	52	1.7%	ROBBINS, 1946	Good anesthesia, no cardiac changes, dogs
$CHF_2CF_2CH_2Br$ (Halopropane)	74	1.0 to 2.5%	FABIAN et al., 1960	Good anesthesia, some cardiac arrhythmias in man
$CHF_2CF_2CH_2Cl$	54	1.5%	FABIAN et al., 1960	Excellent muscle relaxation, good anesthesia in man
$CF_2ClCCl_2CF_2Cl$	112	3.5 ml	LU et al., 1953	No anesthesia, muscular rigidity, opisthotonos, marked depression, death in dog
$CF_2ClCF_2CF_2Cl$	36	12 ml 10 ml	LU et al., 1953	No anesthesia, muscular rigidity, tremors, slight sedation in dog
$CF_2ClCH_2CH_3$	25	8%	ROBBINS, 1946	Anesthesia in mice
$CF_2ClCHClCH_3$	69.5	0.96%	ROBBINS, 1946	Anesthesia in mice
$CF_2ClCHClCFCl_2$	85	0.6%	ROBBINS, 1946	Anesthesia; delayed death in mice
$CF_2ClCH_2CH_2Cl$	80.8	0.9%	ROBBINS, 1946	Anesthesia, delayed death in mice

Table 9 (continued)

Formula	B.P. °C	Anesth. conc.	Author	Nature of physiological action
$CF_2ClCHBrCH_3$	89	0.56%	ROBBINS, 1946	Anesthesia, tremors on recovery in dog
$CF_3CH_2CH_3$	—12	50%	ROBBINS, 1946	Anesthesia in mice
$CF_3CF_2CH_2Br$	45	1—3%	BURNS et al., 1962	Anesthesia, rapid recovery in mice
$CF_3CF_2CH_2Cl$	27	2.5—30%	BURNS et al., 1962	Light anesthesia, rapid recovery in mice, reacts with soda lime
$CF_3CHClCH_2Cl$	75.5	0.4	ROBBINS, 1946	Good anesthesia, no cardiac arrhythmias in dogs
			VAN POZNAK and ARTUSIO JR., 1960a	Good anesthesia, rapid recovery, no EKG change, dog and man
$CF_3CH_2CF_3$	0.5	11%	ROBBINS, 1946	Anesthesia in mice
Cl CF_3CCF_2Br Br	104	1 ml	LU et al., 1953	Violent respiratory depression, convulsions, no anesthesia, 2 rats died
F $CF_3C—CF_2Br$ Br	71	2 ml	LU et al., 1953	Marked salivation, no anesthesia, prolonged convulsions, death in rats
$CF_3CH_2CH_2Cl$	45	3%	ROBBINS, 1946	Anesthesia, delayed death in mice
$CF_3CH_2CHCl_2$	71	0.56%	ROBBINS, 1946	Anesthesia, delayed death
$CF_3CH_2CH_2Br$	62	1.5%	ROBBINS, 1946	Anesthesia, delayed death in mice
$CF_3CHBrCH_2Br$	116	0.1%	ROBBINS, 1946	Anesthesia, delayed death in mice
$CF_3CCl_2CH_3$	48.1	4%	ROBBINS, 1946	Anesthesia in mice
$CF_3CHBrCH_3$	48.6	1.7%	ROBBINS, 1946	Good anesthesia, no cardiac changes, rapid rise in blood pressure when anesthesia stopped in dogs
$CF_3CCl{=}CCl_2$	88.3	3.5 ml	LU et al., 1953	No anesthesia, muscular rigidity, opisthotonos, incoordination, marked depression later, death in one dog
$CF_3CBr{=}CH_2$	33.5		VAN POZNAK and ARTUSIO JR., 1960a	Excellent anesthesia, rapid uneventful recovery
Cl $CF_3C{=}CFCl$	47.3	6 ml	LU et al., 1953	Anesthesia, recovery uneventful, EKG changes in dogs
Cl $CF_3C{=}CF_2$	6.8	75%	Lu et al., 1953	No anesthesia, marked struggle and gasping, respiratory arrest in dog

Table 9 (continued)

Formula	B.P. °C	Anesth. conc.	Author	Nature of physiological action
$CF_3C(Cl){=}CHCl$	53.7	2 ml	Lu et al., 1953	No anesthesia, slight analgesia, depression in rats, one died
$CF_2ClC(Cl){=}CCl_2$	128	3 ml	Lu et al., 1953	Light anesthesia, depression, pulmonary edema, convulsion and death in rats
$CF_3CF{=}CF_2$	—29	50% 75%	Lu et al., 1953	No anesthesia, tremors, respiratory irritation in dogs
$CF_3CH{=}CH_2$	—18	50%	Lu et al., 1953	No anesthesia, tremors, incoordination in dogs
$CF_3CH{=}CH_2$	—24	60%	Robbins, 1946	Anesthesia, convulsions on recovery in mice
Butanes				
C_4HClF_6	34		Robbins, 1946	No anesthesia, convulsions in mice
$CH_3CF_2CFClCH_3$	53	3.4%	Robbins, 1946	Anesthesia, tremors, rigidity, cardiac arrhythmias in dogs
$CH_3CF_2CF_2CH_3$	17	20%	Robbins, 1946	Anesthesia, tremor, convulsions, cardiac arrhythmias in dogs
$CH_3CF_2CH{=}CH_2$	24	8.3%	Robbins, 1946	Anesthesia in mice
$C_4H_5F_2Cl_3$	137	0.12%	Robbins, 1946	Anesthesia in mice
$C_4H_7F_2Cl$	89	1.0%	Robbins, 1946	Anesthesia in mice
$CF_3CH_2CF_2CH_3$	40	5%	Robbins, 1946	Anesthesia in mice
$CH_3CFClCH_2CH_3$	67	1.8%	Robbins, 1946	Anesthesia in mice
$CH_3CF_2CHClCH_2Cl$	120	0.2%	Robbins, 1946	Anesthesia in mice
$CH_3CF_2CH_2CH_3$	30.8	6%	Robbins, 1946	Anesthesia in mice
$CH_3CF_2CH_2CHCl_2$	117	0.35%	Robbins, 1946	Anesthesia, delayed death in mice
$CH_3CF_2CHClCH_3$	71.4	0.74%	Robbins, 1946	Anesthesia in mice
$CF_3C{\equiv}CCF_3$	—25	75%	Lu et al., 1953	No anesthesia, death from pulmonary edema in dog
$CF_3C(CH_3){=}CH_2$	6.4	75%	Lu et al., 1953	Anesthesia, marked struggle and rigidity, tremors, poor relaxation extreme salivation in dogs
$CF_3C(Cl){=}C(Cl)CF_3$	67.8		Lu et al., 1953	Convulsions at point of anesthesia, postanesthetic analgesia, death in rats
C_4F_{10}	4		Struck and Plattner, 1940	Anesthesia; on stimulation, convulsive seizures
$CF_3C(CH_3)(Br){-}CH_2Br$	131	2 ml	Lu et al., 1953	Postanesthetic analgesia, pulmonary edema, rapid recovery in rats

Table 9 (continued)

Formula	B.P. °C	Anesth. conc.	Author	Nature of physiological action
		Miscellaneous		
C_6F_6	80	0.2%	BURNS et al., 1961b	Light anesthesia in mice
		1.6 to 2.4%		Deep anesthesia in mice
		4.4%		Respiratory arrest in mice
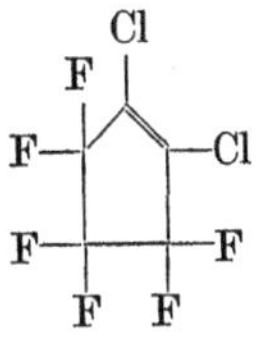	90.7	2 ml	LU et al., 1953	No anesthesia, extreme depression, analgesia, death in rats
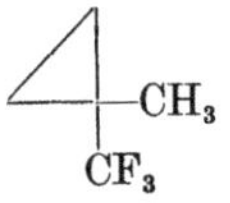	38	7 ml	LU et al., 1953	One dog, rapid and smooth induction, anesthesia, rapid and uneventful recovery, tremors and rigidity in dog
C_5F_{12}	30		MULLINS, 1954	No anesthesia in mice
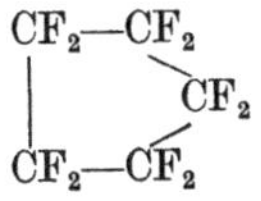	23.5		STRUCK and PLATTNER, 1940	Mice underwent complete anesthesia; on stimulation exhibited convulsive seizures
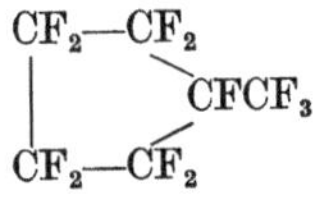	51		STRUCK and PLATTNER, 1940	Mice underwent complete anesthesia; on stimulation exhibited convulsive seizures
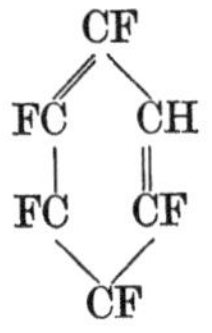	85	0.5 to 2.8%	BURNS et al., 1964	Good anesthesia in mice; all survived
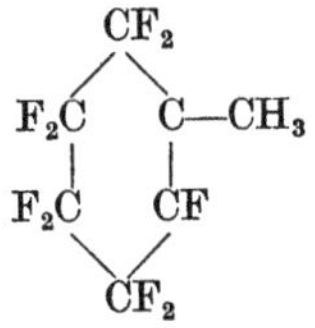	90.7	0.8 to 3.4%	BURNS et al., 1964	No anesthesia; all mice died
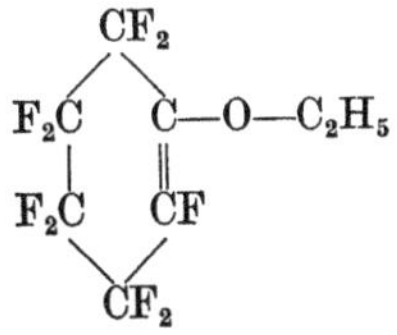	106	0.1 to 0.6%	BURNS et al., 1964	Poor anesthesia; one out of two mice died
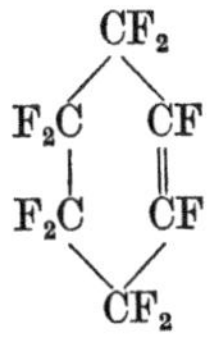	54	0.8 to 1.5%	BURNS et al., 1964	No anesthesia; all mice dead in 20 min

Table 9 (continued)

Formula	B.P. °C	Anesth. conc.	Author	Nature of physiological action
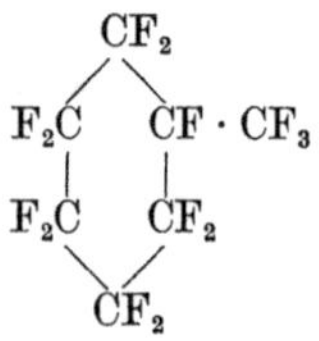	75	1.2 to 25%	BURNS et al., 1964	No anesthesia or deaths in 4 mice
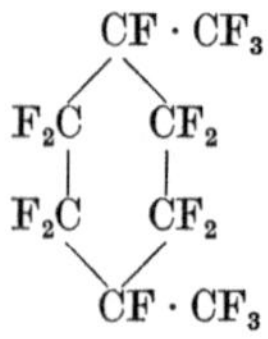	100.2 to 100.5	3.3 to 4%	BURNS et al., 1964	No anesthesia; all mice survived
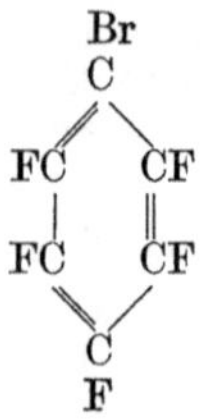	134 to 135	1.8 to 2.4%	BURNS et al., 1964	No anesthesia; all mice survived
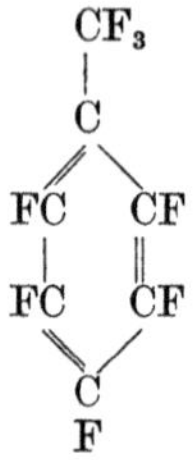	103	0.5 to 0.9%	BURNS et al., 1964	All mice died in six hours, after 10 minutes exposure to drug
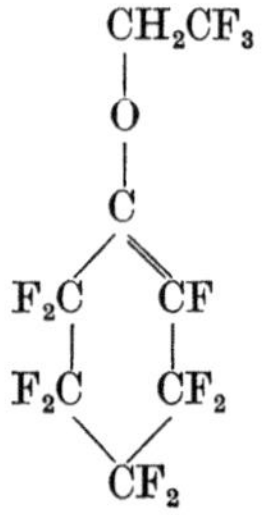	120	1.9 to 2.8%	BURNS et al., 1964	Killed all mice in 3 hours after 15 minutes exposure
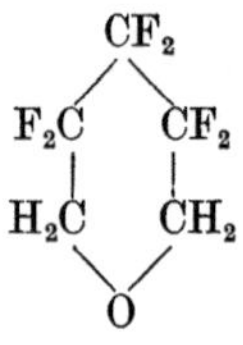	102	0.3% 0.5 to 1.6% 3.0%	BURNS et al., 1964	No anesthesia Anesthesia, all mice survived Respiratory arrest
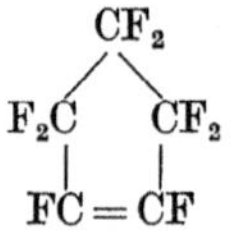	25	3.0 to 7.3%	BURNS et al., 1964	Convulsive movements; death in 6 minutes in 3 mice

Tabelle 9 (continued)

Formula	B.P. °C	Anesth. conc.	Author	Nature of physiological action
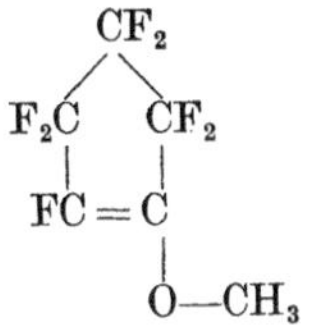	104	1.2 to 2.3%	BURNS et al., 1964	Slow induction and recovery; one out of 3 mice died
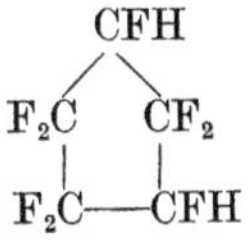	65.5	0.9 to 1.8%	BURNS et al., 1964	Anesthesia, slow recovery in 5 mice; all survived
		1.8 to 3.4%		All 5 died; all showed some convulsions during induction and respiratory depression
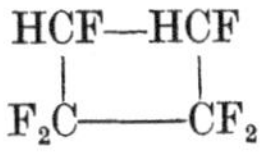	63	1.9 to 6.0%	BURNS et al., 1964	2 mice; anesthesia, slow recovery, irregular respiration, both survived

Table 10. *Fluorinated ethers*

Formula	B.P. °C	Anesth. conc.	Author	Nature of physiological action
		Methyl, ethyl and other ethers		
$HFCl—O—CH_2F$	54		VAN POZNAK and ARTUSIO JR., 1960b	Rapid induction, apnea, no pulse or EKG, death, dog
$H_3—O—CH_2CF_3$	30	8%	ROBBINS, 1946	Anesthesia in mice
		10 ml	LU et al., 1953	Tremors, marked salivation, irritation to mucous membranes in dogs
$H_3—O—CF_2CHFBr$ (Roflurane)	88.8		RUDO and KRANTZ, 1963b (emulsion)	Rapid, good anesthesia, no excitation, excellent relaxation, man
			ARTUSIO JR. and VAN POZNAK, 1961b (inhalation)	
$H_3—O—CF_2CHFI$	118		KRANTZ et al., 1962a	Anesthesia, good relaxation, sensitizes myocardium to epinephrine
$H_3—O—CF_2CHClBr$	124		VAN POZNAK and ARTUSIO JR., 1960b	Satisfactory anesthesia, extensor rigidity at moderate depth could be abolished by lightening or deepening plane
$H_3—O—CF_2CHFCl$	70		VAN POZNAK and ARTUSIO JR., 1960b	Good surgical anesthesia in dogs
	64	1.9 to 3.1%	BURNS et al., 1961a	Jerky twitching movements, 2 deaths in mice
$H_3—O—CF_2CHCl_2$ (Methoxyflurane)	104		VAN POZNAK and ARTUSIO JR., 1960b	Good anesthesia, good relaxation in man

Table 10. (continued)

Formula	B.P. °C	Anesth. conc.	Author	Nature of physiological action
			KRANTZ et al., 1961a, 1962b (emulsion)	Good anesthesia in about 60 patients
$CH_2Cl—O—CF_2CHFCl$	111		VAN POZNAK and ARTUSIO JR., 1960b	Anesthesia unsatisfactory, twitching, jerking move- ments in one dog
$CF_2Cl—O—CF_2CHFCl$ 80% } $CFCl_2—O—CF_2CHF_2$ 20%	64—65		VAN POZNAK and ARTUSIO JR., 1960b	Unsatisfactory anesthesia, gidity, twitching and sh ering, dogs
$CH_2Cl—O—CF_2CHF_2$	77		VAN POZNAK and ARTUSIO JR., 1960b	Satisfactory anesthesia, layed deaths in dogs
$CF_3CF_2CH_2—O—CH_3$	48	6 ml 10 ml	LU et al., 1953	Labored respiration, slow covery, tremors and exten rigidity in dogs
$CF_3CF_2CF_2CH_2—O—CH_3$	70.7	2 ml	LU et al., 1953	Threatened resp. arrest, de depression, convul., dea in rats
		Diethyl ethers		
$CF_3CH_2—O—CH_2CH_3$	50.3	4%	ROBBINS, 1946	Anesthesia, no cardiac chang rigid with convulsions stimulation in dogs
$CHF_2CH_2—O—CH_2CH_3$	65	4%	ROBBINS, 1946	Anesthesia in mice
$CF_3CH_2—O—CH{=}CH_2$ (Fluroxene)	43.2	1.2 to 8%	LU et al., 1953	Good anesthesia, no untowa symptoms, good relaxatic rapid recovery in man
$CF_3CF_2—O—CF_2CF_3$	1	75%	LU et al., 1953	No anesthesia, inert, dog
$CF_3CH_2—O—CH_2CF_3$ (Indoklon)	63.9		KRANTZ et al., 1957	Convulsant in man, no u toward effects
$CHClFCF_2—O—CH(CH_3)_2$	100	1.7 to 2.4%	BURNS et al., 1961a	Anesthesia, jerking move- ments, death in mice
$CHClFCF_2—O—CH_2CH_2CH_3$	109	1.0 to 1.3%	BURNS et al., 1961a	Anesthesia, jerking movements in mice
$CHClFCF_2—O—CH_2CH_3$	88	1.9 to 3.1%	BURNS et al., 1961a	Anesthesia, delayed death, twitching in mice
$CF_3CF_2CH_2—O—CH{=}CH_2$	57.8	3 ml	LU et al., 1953	No anesthesia, irritation eyes, pulmonary edema, opisthotonos in rats

IV. Structure-activity relationships in fluorinated anesthetics

A. Physicochemical properties and anesthetic activity

Anesthetic activity cannot be predicted from molecular structure. Structure alone does not predetermine activity as is exemplified by the wide variety of unrelated molecules which are now used to produce general anesthesia. There has been some elucidation of physicochemical properties related to biological activity of the general anesthetics. This will be considered in this section. For simplicity, the physicochemical properties will be considered individually, although it is clear that the net balance among molecular weight, boiling point, vapor pressure, oil-water coefficient, blood-gas coefficient, *etc.* determines the final activity of the compound *in vivo.*

1. Vapor pressure

A striking correlation between molecular properties and narcotic potency was pointed out by FERGUSON (1939). He set forth a hypothesis on the mechanism of action of volatile anesthetic agents which was in essence an expression of their potency or narcotic activity. FERGUSON's theory states that substances which are present at equal thermodynamic activities in a given medium have the same degree of biological action. In other words, the biological activity of these compounds is proportional to their thermodynamic activity. He divided the partial pressure in mm Hg of an agent necessary to produce an anesthetic equilibrium by its saturated vapor pressure in mm Hg at the temperature of the experiment, arriving at a value which SUCKLING (1957) called "relative saturation for anesthesia." The relative saturation reflects the number of free active molecules of a compound in a system available to exert a specific biological effect. The relative saturation for anesthesia of a number of volatile anesthetic agents ranges from 0.01–0.07 and varies by a factor of 7. When this is expressed in volumes per cent of anesthetic required to maintain anesthesia the range of concentration is 0.5–100% and varies by a factor of 200. The relative saturation for anesthesia denotes the biological potency of a compound. The higher the ratio the more free active molecules required to exert an anesthetic effect. Compounds with low ratios are more potent, needing fewer free molecules to produce the same level of narcosis.

Table 11. *Anesthesia of mice*

Substance	Boiling point	Vapor pressure at 20° C p_s mm Hg	Anesthetic concentration per cent by volume	Partial pressure producing anesthesia p_a mm Hg	Relative saturation for anesthesia p_a/p_s
$CF_3 \cdot CHBr_2$	73	104	0.4	3	0.03
$CF_3 \cdot CH_2Cl$	6	1400	8.0	60	0.04
$CF_3 \cdot CH_2Br$	26	600	2.8	21	0.04
$CF_3 \cdot CHCl_2$	29	550	2.7	21	0.04
$CFCl_2 \cdot CH_3$	32	470	2.5	19	0.04
$CHF_2 \cdot CH_2Cl$	36	420	2.2	17	0.04
$CF_2Cl \cdot CH_2Cl$	47	280	1.3	10	0.04
$CF_3 \cdot CH_2I$	55	200	1.3	10	0.05
$CHF_2 \cdot CH_2Br$	57	190	1.3	10	0.05
$CF_2Cl \cdot CH_2Br$	68	130	0.8	6	0.05
$CF_2Cl \cdot CH_3$	—10	2300	25	190	0.08

Anesthetic concentrations by volume from ROBBINS (1946).

SUCKLING (1957) discusses some of the physical and chemical factors involved in the development of halothane and was principally influenced by FERGUSON in choosing compounds for screening possessing adequate anesthetic potency. Table 11 and 12 express the relative saturation for anesthesia of compounds taken from SUCKLING's work. Data listed in Table 11 were calculated from work reported by ROBBINS (1946), while Table 12 lists data obtained by RAVENTOS and SUCKLING.

Table 12. *Anesthesia of mice*

Substance	Boiling point	Vapor pressure at 20° C p_s mm Hg	Anesthetic concentration per cent by volume	Partial pressure producing anesthesia p_a mm Hg	Relative saturation for anesthesia p_a/p_s
$CF_3 \cdot CHBrCl$	50	243	0.9	7	0.03
$CF_3 \cdot CHBr_2$	73	104	0.6	5	0.05
$CF_2Cl \cdot CHCl_2$	72	110	0.8	6	0.05
$CF_3 \cdot CHBr \cdot CH_3$	49	260	2.2	17	0.07
$CF_2Br \cdot CF_2Br$	46	290	4.1	31	0.11
$CF_3 \cdot CCl_3$	47	280	4.6	35	0.13
$CF_2Cl \cdot CFCl_2$	48	270	5.6	43	0.16

From SUCKLING (1957).

The determination of thermodynamic activity of anesthetic agents is a useful tool for comparing potency in a homologous series. This correlation does not apply for unrelated compounds such as nitrous oxide and chloroform, that have the same thermodynamic ratio, 0.01; the former is a very weak anesthetic and the latter a potent one. See Table 13.

Table 13

	Vol. % for anesth.	Partial pressure/ saturated pressure
Nitrous oxide	100.0	0.01
Acetylene	65.0	0.01
Methyl ether	12.0	0.02
Ethyl chloride	5.0	0.02
Ethyl ether	3.4	0.03
Ethyl bromide	1.9	0.02
Chloroform	0.5	0.01
Fluothane	0.9	0.03

Taken from ADRIANI (1962).

2. Molecular weight

As the molecular weight of the general anesthetics such as saturated straight chain halogenated hydrocarbons, cyclic hydrocarbons and halogenated ethers increases, their potency and toxicity increase and their margin of safety decreases. Fluothane with a molecular weight of 197 has the highest molecular weight and greatest potency of the widely used clinical anesthetics. The molecular weight cannot be considered separately, since with its increase usually occurs a concomitant increase in boiling point and oil solubility. The degree of potency attributed to the former property and that to the latter factors is not known. The molecular concept does not always hold; KRANTZ et al. (1959) found methylchloroform less potent than chloroform even though its molecular weight is higher.

A series of halogenated ethers studied in our laboratories demonstrates increased potency as a function of molecular weight among these multihalogenated anesthetic agents. The relationship is indicated in Table 14. The halogens confer potency on the molecule in this group in the following order: I > Br > Cl > F.

It is interesting to note in this series of compounds the boiling point increases with an increase in molecular weight. This is not the case in the series of compounds listed in Table 25 where the boiling point and molecular weight vary inversely.

Table 14. *Relation of increasing molecular weight to narcotic activity in a series of halogenated methyl ethyl ethers, listed in order of increasing potency* (CASCORBI et al., 1962)

Potency increases	Ethers	MW	B.P. °C
↓	CH_3—O—CF_2CHF_2	132	36.6
	CH_3—O—CF_2CHFCl	148	70.6
	CH_3—O—CF_2CHFBr	193	88.8
	CH_3—O—CF_2CHFI	240	118.0

3. Boiling point

The boiling point usually varies with the molecular weight, as is seen in Table 14 and compounds with high boiling points are generally more potent anesthetics.

ROBBINS (1946) noted that compounds with low boiling points evoked convulsive movements in mice and dogs during the recovery period from anesthesia. He also observed that the length of the induction phase varied only slightly with compounds of different boiling points. The recovery times closely paralleled the boiling points of the compounds; those with the highest boiling points showed the longest recovery time. This was also observed by RUDO et al. (1963a) while studying the induction and recovery time of 2.5% concentrations of methoxyflurane (104°), roflurane (88.8°), and halothane (50.2°) in mice. Each bar in Fig. 1 represents the mean value obtained from 20 mice. The induction times for these three agents under identical conditions ranged from 0.71 to 0.91 minute. There was only 0.2 minute difference in induction time among the three agents although their boiling points differed by 54°. The recovery times for these three anesthetics varied directly with the boiling points. The agent with the highest boiling point exhibited the longest recovery time. The Ostwald coefficients play a major role in the clearance of these compounds via the lungs. The Ostwald coefficent for halothane is 2.35, for methoxyflurane 11—12 (LOWE, 1963) and roflurane lies somewhere between these values. These coefficients parallel the boiling points and are the major factor affecting the recovery time.

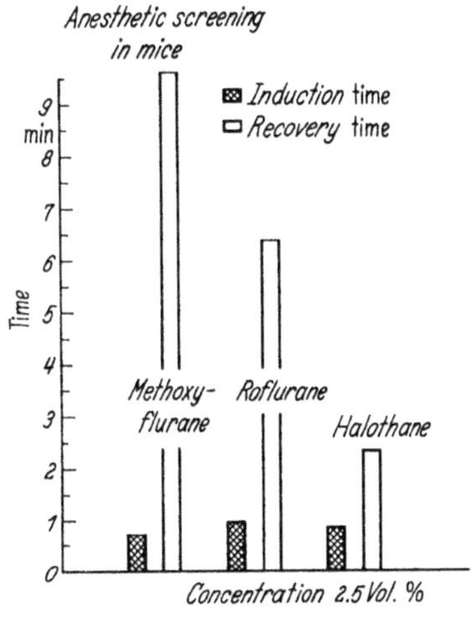

Fig. 1. A correlation of boiling point with induction and recovery times in mice using 2.5 % methoxyflurane, roflurane and halothane. (From RUDO et al., 1963a.)

4. Oil-water coefficient

The relative solubility of volatile anesthetic agents in oil and water is important in determining their distribution *in vivo*. MEYER and OVERTON correlated oil-water, coefficients with narcotic potency. They felt these two properties were mutually dependent; the greater the oil-water coefficient the more potent the compound. They postulated the high solubility of anesthetics in the lipids of the brain was the mechanism by which these agents produced narcosis. Chloroform has an oil-water coefficient of 100 while halothane, which is more potent, has a ratio of 330. This theory applies to many of the clinically used agents. However, many compounds with high oil-water coefficients are not anesthetics; methane has a high oil-water coefficient yet is ineffective as an anesthetic. The MEYER-OVERTON theory describes the distribution in body tissues and not the mechanism of action of volatile anesthetics. Generally as the molecular weight of a compound increases the lipid solubility and the oil-water partition coefficient increase. Halogenation of hydrocarbons and ethers increases their molecular weight and their oil solubility.

Table 15, taken from ROOT and HOFMANN (1963), lists the oil-water coefficients for anesthetic compounds arranged in order of potency.

Table 15. *Oil-water ratio of inert and anesthetic gases arranged in order of potency*

Gas	Oil-water ratio	Temp. (°C)
Helium	1.7	37
Nitrogen	5.2	37
Xenon	20.0	37
Sulfur hexafluoride	200.	20
Nitrous oxide	3.2	37
Ethylene	14.4	37
Cyclopropane	35.0	37
Divinyl ether	41.3	37
Trifluoroethyl vinyl ether	90.	23
Ethyl ether	3.2	37
Chloroform	110.	37
Halothane	330.	23
Methoxyflurane	440.	25

From ROOT and HOFMANN (1963).

The authors are not in agreement with the order of potency of the compounds listed in Table 15. They have observed that trifluoroethyl vinyl ether and divinyl ether are more potent than ethyl ether.

5. The blood-gas coefficient

The blood-gas solubility coefficient (Ostwald solubility coefficient) is one of the most important factors in determining the uptake and elimination of anesthetic agents. The Ostwald coefficient or lambda (λ) is defined as the ratio of distribution of a gas or vapor in equal volumes of a gaseous and a liquid phase equilibrated at a given temperature at one atmosphere pressure. The Ostwald coefficient for ethyl ether at 37° C is 15. This indicates 15 parts of ether will dissolve in 100 ml of blood when 1 part dissolves in 100 ml of the overlying gaseous phase.

Table 16. (ROOT and HOFMANN, 1963) lists the blood-gas partition coefficients of some commonly used anesthetics. An Ostwald coefficient of 5 is listed for trifluoroethyl vinyl ether; this is not in agreement with direct blood determinations of this coefficient by LOWE (1963) which yielded a value of 1.55.

LARSON et al. (1962) reported a study on uptake and excretion of several anesthetic agents in man. They found nitrous oxide and cyclopropane to have the same uptake and excretion curves and almost identical Ostwald coefficients; that for N_2O was 0.466 and was 0.456 for cyclopropane. The boiling point of the former is $-88.5°$ and the latter $-34°$. Their oil-water coefficients are quite different. The blood-gas solubility coefficients are the important determining factor in the rate of uptake and excretion of these agents *via* the lungs. Employing LARSON's

Table 16. *Coefficients of solubility of anesthestic gases and vapors at 37° C and correlation with induction times*

Anesthetic	Blood-gas	Water-gas	Induction time (min)	Recovery time (min)
Xenon	—	0.097	3—5	3—5
Ethylene	0.140	0.089	3—4	3—4
Nitrous oxide	0.473	0.40	3—4	3—4
Cyclopropane	0.457	0.20	3—5	10—12
Acetylene	0.842	0.850	3—5	3—5
Divinyl ether	—	1.32	3—5	3—5
Ethyl chloride	1.43	0.973	3—5	3—5
Halothane	2.6 (23° C)	0.87 (23° C)	3—5	Variable
Ethyl vinyl ether	—	0.8	4—5	4—5
Trifluoroethyl vinyl ether	5.0	—	5—6	15—20
Chloroform	7.3	4.6	5—10	Variable
Trichloroethylene	8.0	1.55	20—30	Variable
Ethyl ether	15.0	15.5	20—30	Variable

From Root and Hofmann (1963).

formula, the per cent clearance in each passage through the lungs for any anesthetic agent can be calculated. In the example following, the values used are for a 70 kg man with a ventilation of 4 liters per minute and a blood flow to the lungs of 5 liters per minute. The final formula becomes:

$$\text{Per cent clearance} = \frac{\dot{V}_A \times 100}{\dot{V}_A + \lambda \dot{Q}_c}$$

$\dot{V}_A$ = Alveolar ventilation per minute
$\dot{Q}_c$ = Pulmonary capillary flow per minute
λ = Ostwald coefficient.

The main variable in this formula is λ (lambda), the Ostwald coefficient for the anesthetic agent. Ethyl ether has an Ostwald coefficient of 15.08 and its per cent clearance equals 5; it is retained in the tissues for a comparatively long period after anesthesia. Halothane has an Ostwald coefficient of 2.3 and its clearance equals 26%.

Chemical methods for determining blood levels and Ostwald coefficients of anesthetics have often been inadequate or lacking. The advent of gas chromatograph techniques has simplified the determinations of blood levels and tissue concentrations of these fluorinated anesthetics as well as other agents. Accuracy is good and impurities can readily be detected (Glover and Hodgson, 1961). Lowe (1964) has recently developed a simple new technique for rapid determination of volatile organic anesthetics in blood, using the gas chromatograph. This will be a useful tool in the research laboratory as well as in the clinic.

The scope of this chapter does not permit discussion of all the physicochemical factors, lung factors and circulation factors which influence the duration and quality of anesthetic activity. For detailed information concerning these parameters the reader is referred to a comprehensive volume on the uptake and distribution of anesthetic agents, edited by Papper and Kitz (1963).

B. Halogenation and anesthetic potency

1. Fluorine

Fluorine is the most active of the halogen elements. The element was discovered by Ampère of France in 1810. The name was derived from fluorspar, calcium fluoride, which was used as a flux, hence *fluo* meaning "to flow." As an acceptor of electrons the activity of fluorine far exceeds that of oxygen. For example, substances such as alcohol, ether, cork and turpentine ignite spontaneously in an atmosphere of fluorine. Again, the strong chemical avidity of fluorine is noted in its combination with the noble gas xenon to form XeF_4.

The addition of fluorine atoms to a halogenated hydrocarbon or ether increases the stability of the compound.

Alkyl fluorides are reported to lose hydrogen fluoride readily. Many monofluoro compounds are toxic in the body not because they hydrolyze but because the FCH_2CO-group enters the Krebs cycle intact. Alkyl hydrocarbons substituted with CF_2 groups are more stable but do undergo some degree of degradation. Compounds substituted with a trifluoro group are very stable and are extremely refractory to chemical modification *in vivo*. The accumulation of fluorine on one carbon atom increases the stability of both the C–F bond and C–X bonds on the adjacent carbon (HINE and GHIRARDELLI, 1958).

The place occupied by fluorine in MENDELÉEFF's periodic arrangement (atomic number 9) makes it the first representative of the halogen group. From this standpoint fluorine shares with chlorine, bromine and iodine the property of being strongly electronegative. According to the electronic theory, their degree of electronegativity varies in the direction $F > Cl > Br > I$.

In respect to covalent atomic radii fluorine has the lowest place among the halogens. PAULING and HUGGINS (1934) using crystalographic techniques to observe the relative atomic radii of the various halogens linked by simple valence, obtained values increasing as follows in Table 17:

Table 17

Element	Atomic radii, in Å
Hydrogen	0.29
Fluorine	0.64
Chlorine	0.99
Bromine	1.14
Iodine	1.33

Table 18. *Characteristics of carbon-halogen bonds*

Bond (in aliphatic series)	Internuclear distance (in Å)	Breaking energy (in kg/cal)
C—H	1.14	93
C—F	1.45	114
C—Cl	1.74	72
C—Br	1.90	59
C—I	2.12	45

From BUU-HOÏ (1961).

From the standpoint of covalent atomic radii therefore, fluorine is much less different from hydrogen than the other halogens.

The characteristics of the carbon-fluorine chemical bond are determinants for the biological activity and disposition of the fluorinated organic molecule. Fluorine is found to have in some respects a "normal" position among the halogens, but in other respects an exceptional one. For instance, in the case of internuclear distances in C–X bonds, there is continuous progression when going from hydrogen (C–H) to iodine (C–I); on the other hand, in the breaking energy of C–X bonds, the figure for fluorine is much higher than for either hydrogen or the other halogens as shown in Table 18.

Fluorine and boiling points. A liquid boils when its molecules possess sufficient kinetic energy to overcome the intermolecular forces. When fluorine is introduced into a halogenated hydrocarbon molecule, the intramolecular binding forces are increased, and intermolecular forces become weaker than are found in the corresponding nonfluorinated halogenated hydrocarbon. Therefore, the heat energy required for vaporization is less than that for the nonfluorinated halogenated hydrocarbons. The effect of introducing the fluorine atom then, is to reduce the boiling point markedly. The reduction in boiling point concomitant with the replacement of hydrogen by fluorine in the chloro-, bromo-, and iodomethanes is evident from the data in Table 19.

Table 19. *Effect of fluorine on the lowering of boiling points*

$CH_3 \cdot Cl$	—23.7°	$CF_3 \cdot Cl$	—82°
$CH_3 \cdot Br$	+ 4.5°	$CF_3 \cdot Br$	—59°
$CH_3 \cdot I$	+42.5°	$CF_3 \cdot I$	—22.5°

Thus one is permitted to introduce other halogen elements such as chlorine and bromine into the molecule and keep the boiling point low and the vapor pressure sufficiently high to utilize these agents as volatile anesthetics.

Fluorine and degree of ionization. The strongly negative activity of the fluorine atom and its avidity for the electron to complete its outer orbit of eight electrons is shown in its effect upon the dissociation constant of acetic acid following fluorination. Table 20 is illustrative of the strong nuclear force of the fluorine atom in removing the electron from the hydrogen atom, although it is not directly attached to it, to form a hydrogen ion.

Table 20. *Fluorine and ionization constants*

$CH_3 \cdot COOH$	1.8×10^{-5}
$CH_2F \cdot COOH$	2.2×10^{-3}
$CHF_2 \cdot COOH$	5.7×10^{-2}
$CF_3 \cdot COOH$	5.9×10^{-1}

Fluorine and biological activity. Hydrocarbons and ethers substituted with fluorine alone are usually devoid of anesthetic activity. For example CHF_3 is inert whereas $CHCl_3$ is a very potent anesthetic agent. The effect of fluorination on a series of ethers is seen in Table 21.

Table 21. *The nature of the physiological activity of a series of fluorine-substituted ethers*

Formula	Name	Activity
$CH_3—O—CH_2CF_3$	Trifluoroethyl methyl ether	Anesthesia in mice, not dogs
$CHF_2—O—CH_2CF_3$	Pentafluoroethyl methyl ether	Convulsant, anesthetic
$CF_3CH_2—O—CH{=}CH_2$	Trifluoroethyl vinyl ether	Good anesthetic
$CF_3CH_2—O—CH_2CH_3$	Trifluorodiethyl ether	Weak anesthetic
$CF_3CH_2—O—CH_2CF_3$	Hexafluorodiethyl ether	Convulsant
$CF_3CF_2—O—CF_2CF_3$	Perfluorodiethyl ether	Inert

Complete substitution of hydrogen with fluorine as in perfluorodiethyl ether produces a biologically inert compound. Artusio (1963) noted in his screening program that some hydrogen was necessary for a central nervous system depressant effect. In compounds with no hydrogen the excitant properties are so marked that any depressive effect may be masked. Trifluorodiethyl ether is a weak anesthetic and trifluoroethyl vinyl ether, fluroxene, is a good anesthetic used clinically. Unsaturation increases potency of these ethers as it does in non-halogenated ethers. Trifluoroethyl methyl ether produces anesthesia in mice (Robbins, 1946) but not in dogs (Lu et al., 1953).

Addition of fluorine to CH_2Cl_2 forming CF_2Cl_2 produces a less active compound chemically and physiologically. When two fluorine atoms are attached to the same carbon atom to which chlorine is linked, the narcotic activity and toxicity conferred by the chlorine atom are reduced (ARTUSIO, 1963).

The fluorinated analog of Trilene®, $CCl_2{=}CHCl$, is chlorotrifluoro ethylene $CF_2{=}CFCl$, which is flammable and has no anesthetic properties (BURNS et al., 1961c). One would predict that chlorotrifluoro ethylene would be a nonflammable anesthetic, but this is not the case. It is strange but in this example, fluorination increases flammability.

The authors have observed that many halogenated hydrocarbons and ethers having five or six mixed halogens substituted on the terminal carbon atoms usually produce convulsions. Some of these compounds are listed in Table 22.

Table 22. *Relationship between substitution on terminal carbon atoms and physiologic activity*

CHF_2—O—CH_2CF_3	Anesthetic, convulsant
CF_2Cl—O—CF_2CFCl_2	Convulsant, delayed death
CCl_3—O—CF_2CFCl_2	Anesthetic, convulsant
CF_3CH_2—O—$CFClCF_3$	Convulsant, delayed death
CF_3CH_2—O—CCl_2CF_3	Convulsant
CF_3CH_2—O—CCl_2CF_2Cl	Severe convulsant
CF_3CHF_2	Mixed excitation and depression
CF_2BrCF_2Br	Convulsant, death
$CF_2BrCFClBr$	Convulsant

From the screening experiments presented by ROBBINS (1946) and by LU et al. (1953), certain generalizations become apparent. Firstly, the fluorination of a hydrocarbon or ether appears to reduce its anesthetic potency, although there are noteworthy exceptions; for example, trifluoroethyl vinyl ether is a more potent anesthetic than ethyl vinyl ether. Secondly, fire hazard is materially reduced or eliminated by fluorination of hydrocarbons or ethers. Thirdly, certain fluorinated ethers are marked central nervous system stimulants, such as hexafluorodiethyl ether (Indoklon®) used as a substitute for electroshock therapy in the treatment of mentally ill patients (KRANTZ et al., 1957). Fourthly, the fluorine to carbon bond in any of the anesthetics studied is not ruptured liberating fluorine ions. The conclusions of VAN POZNAK and ARTUSIO (1960a, 1960b) are interesting as they elucidate further structural-activity relationships. The compounds containing one carbon atom were frequently excitant, but also evoked some depressant activity. Complete substitution of hydrogen by halogen elements was associated with convulsant activity. Several of the two carbon atom compounds appeared to evoke satisfactory anesthetic action.

2. Chlorine

Chlorination of fluorocarbons increases their biological potency. It may accomplish this by increasing the molecular weight or by making the compound more lipophilic, thus increasing its specificity for the highly lipoidal nerve tissue. Halogenation reduces the volatility of the compound influencing the relative partial pressure which develops. Potency of these compounds is increased as the lenght of the carbon chain increases.

Addition of chlorine to a fluorinated compound usually enhances its anesthetic activity, as as is seen in Table 23.

Table 23. *Halogenated hydrocarbons of the ethane series listed in order of increasing anesthetic potency* (ARTUSIO, 1963)

	Ethanes	
Potency increases ↓	$CF_2H—CH_3$	Flammable
	$CF_3—CH_3$	Flammable
	$CF_3—CHF_2$	Mixed excitation and depression
	$CF_3—CHFCl$	Anesthetic
	$CF_3—CHFBr$	Anesthetic
	$CF_3—CHClBr$	Anesthetic

3. Bromine

LUCAS (1928) studied the fate of bromine substituted hydrocarbons used as anesthetics in rabbits. He observed that these bromine derivatives were decomposed in the body producing pathological changes in the liver and the lungs. LUCAS postulated that the tissue toxicity could be due to the intact molecule; he felt, however, it was more likely due to the decomposition products. LUCAS' compounds were brominated hydrocarbons without fluorine and were unstable *in vivo*. When bromine is added to fluorocarbons the fluorine stabilizes the bromine on the adjacent carbon and the compounds become more stable chemically and less toxic.

ROBBINS (1946) made several generalizations concerning his investigations of fluorohydrocarbons. Bromine substituted fluorohydrocarbons had a greater margin of safety than ether or chloroform. The introduction of a second halogen atom to fluorinated hydrocarbon significantly increased its potency as an anesthetic. A bromine atom increased anesthetic potency two to four times more than a chlorine atom in this series of compounds. Fluorinated hydrocarbons substituted with di-bromo or di-chloro were more active anesthetics than their mono-substituted analogs.

The authors have observed an interesting relationship in two brominated fluorocarbons, roflurane (CH_3–O–CF_2CHFBr) and teflurane (CF_3CFHBr). Each is a good anesthetic agent, although of the two, roflurane is more potent. Each contains the radical –CHFBr. One wonders what structure-activity relationship exists in an asymmetric carbon atom of this type. There appears suggestive evidence that there is a correlation between an asymmetric carbon atom and anesthetic properties in these and other compounds. Halothane has an asymmetric carbon atom as have some of the compounds listed in Tables 9 and 10, all of which produce anesthesia.

Table 24. *Relation of asymmetric carbon atom to anesthetic activity*

Compound	Activity
CF_3*CHFCl*	Anesthetic
CF_3*CHFBr*	Anesthetic (teflurane)
CF_3*CHClBr*	Anesthetic (halothane)
CH_3—O—CF_2*CHFCl*	Anesthetic (halomar)
CH_3—O—CF_2*CHFBr*	Anesthetic (roflurane)
CH_3CH_2—O—CF_2*CHFCl*	Anesthetic
CH_2ClCH_2—O—CF_2*CHFCl*	Anesthetic

In their anesthetic screening the authors have observed that many compounds containing an asymmetric terminal carbon atom, as seen in Table 24, usually produce anesthesia. This is especially true when the other end carbon atom is not heavily halogenated.

Are the anesthetic effects of –CHFBr, –CHFCl and –CHClBr radicals owing to increased molecular volume, van der Waal's constants, polarizability, or thermodynamic activity? More investigations in this field are needed to elucidate further this problem.

4. Iodine

Iodine is the heaviest of the halogens with an atomic weight of 126.9. MATHEWSON (1961) stated iodine is of no value in conferring anesthetic properties to a compound, alkyl iodides do not possess narcotic properties and are largely non-volatile. KRANTZ et al. (1963) are not in accord with MATHEWSON. They observed the addition of iodine to trifluoroethane markedly increased its anesthetic activity. If one fluorinates in a step-wise fashion the terminal carbon atom, preparing mono-, di-, and trifluoroethyl iodides respectively, the iodine-carbon bond is strengthened in proportion to the degree of fluorination. HINE and GHIRARDELLI (1958) demonstrated this by measuring the rate constant for the second order reactions between sodium phenoxide and iodoethane, 1-fluoro-2-iodoethane, 1,1-difluoro-2-iodoethane, and 1,1,1-trifluoro-2-iodoethane. The rate constant for the first reaction proved to be 17,450 times greater than that for the latter reaction, *i.e.* the carbon-iodine bond was far stronger in 1,1,1-trifluoro-2-iodoethane than it was in iodoethane.

Such studies show the possibility of utilizing the anesthesia-promoting effect of the iodine in iodine-containing volatile anesthetics, by employing the adjacent carbon-fluorine bond to firmly fix the iodine in the molecule.

Exploring this field further KRANTZ et al. prepared pentafluoroethyl iodide. This interesting compound containing no hydrogen atom in the molecule, evoked anesthesia in mice and rats but not in monkeys, even at 50% concentration. The most marked effect of pentafluoroethyl iodide in the monkey was its capacity to provoke severe cardiac arrhythmias upon the inhalation of the agent for less than one minute.

CASCORBI et al. (1962) studied a series of iodinated fluorohydrocarbons; their anesthetic activity, formulas and boiling points are listed in Table 25.

Table 25. *A series of fluoroiodoethanes.* (CASCORBI et al., 1962)

Formula	Name	Mol.Wt.	B.P. °C	Physiological activity
CF_3CF_2I	Pentafluoroethyl iodide	246	13	Anesthesia in mice, not dogs; Marked arrhythmias
CF_3CHFI	Tetrafluoroethyl iodide	228	39	Anesthesia; no irritation; Arrhythmias
CF_3CH_2I	Trifluoroethyl iodide	210	55	Potent anesthetic; some arrhythmias

Trifluoroethyl iodide has been used in man (p. 519). It potency is in the range of halothane. Clinical investigation was discontinued because of the occurrence of cardiac arrhythmias in light levels of anesthesia.

C. Effects of saturated and unsaturated molecules

ABREU (1941) studied a series of bromine and chlorine substituted ethenes, propenes, and n-butenes. He concluded that compounds with the halogen on the unsaturated carbon showed decreased irritation, decreased tissue damage, decreased toxicity and increased anesthetic potency. Monohalogenated compounds are flammable in anesthetic concentrations but less so than their nonhalogenated parent compound. Monohalogens of the ethane series are decomposed in the body more slowly than those of methane. The di-, tri- and tetrahalogens are virtually nonreactive and stable in the body. They exert their anesthetic activity as intact molecules. ABREU observed that compounds of the type R—C—C—Br invariably liberated more inorganic bromide than those of the type R—C=C—Br or R—C(Br)=C. None of ABREU's compounds were fluorinated but it is interesting to note that unsaturation of the halogen substituted hydrocarbon made the compounds more stable and less toxic.

Among the nonhalogenated compounds divinyl oxide is more potent than ethyl ether and ethylene is more potent than ethane. Unsaturation in these compounds enhances potency.

BURGISON et al. (1955) investigated the effect of unsaturated fluorocarbons on myocardial sensitization. An interesting relationship was shown between the hydrogen-carbon and the fluorine-carbon bond in these studies. It was established many years ago that hydrocarbons sensitize the heart to arrhythmias upon the injection of catecholamines or when endogenous catecholamines are released into the circulation. Among the anesthetics, cyclopropane is the classical offender

Table 26. *Summary of myocardial sensitization*

Name of compound	Number of animals[1] in which sensitization of myocardium occurred and number used
Tetrafluoroethylene	0/4
Tetrafluoroethylene (cats)	0/2
Difluoroethlene	0/8
Difluoroethylene (cats)	0/2
Trifluorochlor-ethylene (Genetron-265)	4/4
Monochloro-difluoroethylene	4/4
Trichloro-monofluoroethylene	2/2
Cis-dichloroethylene	4/4
Trans-dichloroethylene	5/5

[1] Dogs unless otherwise stated.
From BURGISON et al. (1955).

Dogs under difluorethylene anesthesia showed no cardiac arrhythmias when injected intravenously with a challenging dose of epinephrine. However, under anesthesia with monochloro-difluoroethylene a challenging dose of epinephrine evoked cardiac arrhythmias similar to those elicited by epinephrine under cyclopropane anesthesia.

(SEEVERS et al., 1934). BURGISON et al. showed that the sensitization prevailed with numerous straight chain hydrocarbons, other cyclic hydrocarbons and spiropentane. Ethylene was a striking exception; in a series of dogs and cats under ethylene anesthesia the hearts of none of the animals was sensitized to a challenging dose of epinephrine. Of interest also was the fact that deuteroethylene behaved in the same manner as did ethylene.

They then became interested in the effect of fluorine substitution in the ethylene molecule, and several fluoroethylenes and mixed halogen fluoroethylenes were synthesized and studied. The effect of these agents upon cardiac sensitization is shown in Table 26.

It is clear from the data in the table that the fluorine-carbon bond resembles the hydrogen-carbon bond of ethylene, in that the fluorinated ethylenes to not sensitize the myocardium. This property, however, does not obtain with the chlorine-carbon bond.

Their explanation of this phenomenon is set forth as follows. First, there exists a difference between carbon-carbon linkage in ethane, which is not an anesthetic and does sensitize the heart to epinephrine, and that in the ethylene molecule. In the latter molecule two pairs of electrons are shared between the two carbon atoms drawing them closer together with a distance of 1.33 Å in contrast to a 1.54 Å distance in ethane with one pair of shared electrons. Furthermore, fluorine with an atomic number of 9 fits close to the carbonatom nucleus and therefore resembles more closely a hydrogen-carbon bond than does the chlorine-carbon bond. Chlorine with an atomic number of 17 is more readily separated from its linkage to carbon than is fluorine. The chlorine-carbon bond presents a larger molecular volume in a substituted ethylene than does the fluorine-carbon bond. This molecular volume is likely concerned with the passage of molecules through cellular membranes. Ethylene is a very flat, two-dimensional type of molecule with a small molecular volume. This property is shared by the substituted fluoroethylenes, but not by chloroethylene. Indeed, ethane and methane, which produce sensitization, are more three-dimensional than is ethylene. Thus, the unique property of fluorine among the halogen elements, is demonstrated and the similarity of the fluorine-carbon bond to the hydrogen-carbon bond is evidenced in this biologic behavior.

Certain characteristics of the carbon-halogen bond have been indicated in Table 18. From these data, it is clear that the fluorine-carbon bond is shorter than those of the other halogens, exemplifying again the greater affinity of the fluorine atom for an electron.

D. Comparison of fluorinated hydrocarbons and ethers

In general it appears that halogenated hydrocarbons depress the oxygen consumption in animals more than do the ethers. Observations by the authors with several compounds have indicated that halogenated hydrocarbons depress the oxygen consumption (metabolic rate) of animals during anesthesia much more than do the ethers. The following decreases in oxygen consumption in monkeys were reported: trifluoroethyl vinyl ether, 10.2%; ethyl ether, 16.3% (Park et al., 1957); halothane, 37.7% (Krantz et al., 1958); trichloroethane, 26.7% (Krantz et al., 1959); and trifluoroethyl iodide, 43% (Krantz et al., 1963). According to Nunn and Matthews (1959) halothane depresses the oxygen uptake 17% in humans, a depression comparable with normal sleep. This does not agree with the results of the authors in monkeys; it may be due to a species difference.

As mentioned in the preceding section, mixed halogenated hydrocarbons sensitize the heart to epinephrine; fluorinated ethers generally do not evoke this sensitization.

Most halogenated hydrocarbons apparently cause some degree of liver damage whereas the halogenated ethers are not hepatotoxic; Fluoromar® is not hepatotoxic (Krantz et al., 1953). Little et al. (1958) found halothane produced no greater depression of hepatic function than did cyclopropane or ether. According to Jones et al. (1958) chloroform was the most toxic agent in their series to the livers of mice, ether the least toxic, and divinyl ether caused necrosis. The effects of halothane on the liver are further discussed in on page 548.

Clinical impressions seem to indicate halogenated ethers produce a more prolonged analgesia sequential to anesthesia than do the halogenated hydrocarbons. Ethers produce less hepatotoxicity and little or no arrhythmias with or without epinephrine. Ethers evoke better muscular relaxation.

E. Summary of structure-activity observations

The following summary of structure-activity observations lists general trends noted by investigators in the field. They are proposed to explain responses seen with varying structures. The authors wish to emphasize that there are exceptions to each of these statements.

1. Halogenation of hydrocarbons and ethers increases potency in the following order F < Cl < Br < I.
2. Unsaturation increases potency.
3. Fluorination usually decreases potency, boiling point, flammability and increases stability. The carbon-fluorine bond is more stable than the other halogen-carbon bonds; in addition, the fluorine-carbon bond confers stability on halogens substituted on the adjacent carbon atom.
4. Methyl ethyl ethers appear to be more potent than diethyl ethers.
5. As a class halogenated hydrocarbons are more likely to sensitize the myocardium to epinephrine, produce hepatotoxicity and depress the oxygen uptake more than halogenated ethers.
6. Increased potency in a homologous series is usually accompanied by increased oil-water coefficient, molecular weight and boiling point.
7. One or more hydrogen atoms in the molecule are necessary for effective central nervous system depression.
8. Complete hydrogen substitution by fluorine usually produces a physiologically inert compound. Five or six mixed halogens substituted on the end carbon atoms often produce a convulsant.
9. Mixed halogenated methanes tend to be more excitant than substituted ethanes.
10. Compounds containing an asymmetric end carbon seem to produce good anesthesia (*e.g.* –CHFCl, –CHFBr and –CHClBr).
11. Cyclic halogenated compounds tend to be toxic.
12. Double ethers, with few exceptions, tend to be convulsants.
13. Compounds substituted with dibromines and dichlorines tend to be more potent than their monosubstituted analogs. The dibromine compounds are more potent than the dichlorine ones.
14. Varying boiling points do not seem to markedly affect induction time in animals; however, they do influence recovery time. The higher the boiling point, the longer the recovery time.
15. Bromine substituted fluorocarbons have a greater margin of safety than ether or chloroform.

F. Mechanism of action of volatile anesthetics

The mechanism of the action of the volatile anesthetics has been the subject of study for many years. Its importance as a biological phenomenon cannot be overestimated. Lillie (1916) stated, "The problem of the general nature of anesthesia is a fact inseparable from the wider problem of the nature and conditions of irritability in general." Besides, many of the keys to the nature of consciousness and perhaps behavior patterns might be elucidated if this problem were completely understood.

Since the action of fluorinated anesthetics appears to follow the same pattern of activity as do the other volatile anesthetics, a summary of our current knowledge on their mechanism of action follows.

At the turn of the century Hans Horst Meyer (1899) and E. Overton (1901) expressed their theory of narcosis in the following postulates:

1. All chemically indifferent substances which are soluble in fats and fat-like bodies must exert a narcotic action on living protoplasm, insofar as they can become distributed in it.

2. The effect must manifest itself first, and most markedly, in those cells in which fatty or lipoid substances predominate in the chemical structure and presumably in which they form essential participants of the cell function; *viz.*, in the nerve cells.

3. The relative efficiency of such narcotic agents must be dependent upon their mechanical affinity for lipoid substances on the one hand, and for the remaining body constituents, *i.e.*, principally water, on the other hand. Their efficiency is therefore dependent upon their partition coefficient which determines their distribution in a mixture of water and lipoid substances.

4. MEYER calculated that the molar concentration of chemically inert substances required to produce narcosis, even though they vary in potency, is a fixed value of 0.06 M per L.

One is inclined to call these time-honored postulates a statement of narcotic distribution in the body rather than a theory of narcosis. However, when viewed with respect to our knowledge of cellular respiration many years ago, they were a definite contribution and have stood the test of time.

FERGUSON (1939) pointed out that the significance of data on narcosis is much greater when concentrations of the drugs administered are expressed on a thermodynamic scale rather than in volumes per cent. Thermodynamic activity is a measure of those molecules of a given substance which are not involved in nonspecific interactions with other molecules of the same substance or with solvent molecules; it is a measure of those molecules which are free to exert a specific biological effect. FERGUSON further noted that the various theories of narcosis presented in the past were not completely independent, but actually had some features in common. The physical properties of anesthetics which were measured, *e.g.* vapor pressure, solubility, surface tension, oil-water coefficient, adsorbability and others and to which anesthesia was attributed in whole or in part, were actually measures of the tendency of a substance to distribute itself between two phases. Further, when equilibrium was established, the chemical potential became the same in each phase; hence, the anesthetic concentration in a narcotized cell could be estimated by measuring the thermodynamic activity in some more readily accessible phase in equilibrium with the cell contents. BRINK and POSTERNAK (1948) contend that the work required per mole in the transfer of the anesthetic from the pure liquid to the narcotized cell is the same for all substances which produce equal degrees of narcosis at equal thermodynamic activities. They speculate that anesthetics probably produce their effect in regions of the cell in which their molecules fit much as they fit into their own pure liquid.

MULLINS (1954) extended Ferguson's theory of thermodynamic activity to include molecular volume. Mullins stated "Narcosis by chemically inert molecules appears to take place when a constant fraction of the total volume of some nonaqueous phase in the cell is occupied by narcotic molecules. If the narcotic behaves ideally in this nonaqueous phase, the thermodynamic activity of the narcotic multiplied by its molal volume is a constant, about 1 ml/mole."

WULF and FEATHERSTONE (1957) consider these concepts consistent with their hypothesis, namely, that the increasing potency of clinical anesthetic agents parallels in general their van der Waal's constants. Based upon these data they explain the anesthetic activity of the inert gas xenon. They point out that its anesthetic potency should be equivalent to that of nitrous oxide and ethylene since their van der Waal's constants are essentially the same. Xenon, nitrous oxide, and ethylene do exhibit about the same degree of anesthetic potency.

Other investigators have attempted to correlate the physical properties of the anesthetic gases with their biological activity. MILLER (1961) proposed the theory of "gas hydrates." The gas hydrates are clathrate compounds of a gas encaged in a distorted ice matrix. Helium, hydrogen, and neon do not exhibit anesthetic properties – they form no gas hydrates. Many anesthetic gases do form gas hydrates. MILLER found a correlation between the pressure of the anesthetic required for surgical anesthesia and the dissociation pressure of the corresponding gas hydrate at 0° C; he contends that the anesthetic gas will increase the number of hydrates present in neuronal tissue. This forms a sort of "ice cover" at a membrane or protein surface. The ice cover probably lowers conductance, "stiffens up" the lipid membrane, "plugs up" the pores in the membrane and thus reduces transmision of neuronal impulses at synapses.

PAULING (1961) proposed a challenging hypothesis of anesthetic activity. This hypothesis, "the hydrate microcrystal theory," involves the interaction of the nonhydrogen-bonding anesthetic with water molecules in the brain. PAULING proposes that hydrate microcrystals, similar in structure to known hydrate crystals of chloroform, xenon, and other anesthetics may entrap ions and electrically charged side chains of protein molecules. This in turn decreases the energy of the electrical oscillations of the brain. Thus consciousness is lost. The striking correlation between the anesthetic partial pressure of the agent and the partial pressure necessary to form hydrate crystals lends a measure of support to the hypothesis.

The investigations of CLEMENTS and WILSON (1962) showed that inert gases can interact significantly with lipoprotein membranes of living cells. Their presence may change the effective dielectric constant and permeability of cell membranes, and ion transport may also undergo alteration. Mitochondrial membranes may be affected and thus enzymic activity, *viz.*, oxidative phosphorylation, may be affected by a gaseous anesthetic. It thus appears that although the anesthetic is not metabolized and leaves the target cells as an intact molecule, its presence, through "gas hydrates," "microcrystals," or adsorption on lipoprotein membranes may produce profound cellular alterations.

These interesting studies of the physical properties of anesthetic agents have contributed useful information to our knowledge. But the key to the problem lies in a knowledge of what distortion of enzymic activity is provoked by their presence which causes a hiatus in consciousness.

Many studies have been designed to pinpoint the specific enzyme system which is responsible for anesthetic action and the concomitant loss of consciousness. Numerous anesthetic agents have been shown to depress the oxygen uptake of brain brei. They exert little or no effect upon anaerobic glycolysis. It appears that in the process of "main line" oxidation, anesthetic agents interfere with a sensitive flavoprotein which connects the phosphonucleotide dehydrogenase system with the cytochromes. The depression is reversible.

It has become apparent that there are many ways in which anesthetic agents can exert their action at an enzyme level and produce unconsciousness. Further, all agents which evoke anesthesia do not affect the same target enzyme system. BRODY and BAIN (1951) demonstrated that certain barbiturates, in anesthetic concentrations, uncoupled oxidation from phosphorylation in the mitochondrial fraction of rat's brain. HULME and KRANTZ (1955) showed that ether produces the same effect in anesthetic concentrations. Since the high energy phosphate bonds of adenosine triphosphate (ATP) are necessary for the synthesis of acetylcholine, a diminution of ATP would result in a paucity of acetylcholine necessary for neuronal transmission. However, xenon, which produces anesthesia when inhaled, was shown by LEVY and FEATHERSTONE (1954) to be incapable of uncoupling oxidation from phosphorylation. On this enzyme system nitrous oxide was also inert. Nevertheless, nitrous oxide was shown to inhibit anaerobic glycolysis and also to depress certain facets of the hydrogen transport system.

Thus it is clear that the precise mechanism of anesthesia at an enzyme level has not been demonstrated. The enzymic activities responsible for consciousness appear so complex and intricately interdependent that an agent influencing one facet of the system concomitantly affects the harmonious function of the whole. Moreover, it seems likely that the various anesthetic agents in use affect enzymic activity of brain at different links in the complex chain of consciousness.

In summary, our present knowledge permits the following generalizations:

1. The Overton-Meyer theory is useful as a statement of anesthetic distribution in the body.
2. Anesthetic agents in the central nervous system attack the "main line" oxidation in cells of this system; target enzymes for different anesthetics are not always the same.
3. Anesthetics have been shown to act on a flavoprotein connecting the phosphonucleotide dehydrogenases with the cytochromes. Certain agents uncouple oxidation from phosphorylation.
4. The enzymic inhibitions are reversible processes.
5. The physical properties of the anesthetic vapor, by virtue of "gas hydrate" or "microcrystal" formation or adsorption on lipoprotein membranes, may be responsible for enzymic changes, diminution of synaptic transmission, and other alterations of neuronal activity resulting in anesthesia.

The new era of fluorinated anesthetics has produced many potent, stable and nonflammable agents. Fluorine does not appear to increase the potency of a compound *per se;* it decreases flammability and is responsible for the stability of associated halogens in the molecule. It is clear that the possibilities of synthesis in this field are numerous and it is likely that many agents, either ethers or hydrocarbons containing fluorine and other halogens will be extensively studied as anesthetic agents in the future.

The pharmacologic and clinical studies of fluorinated anesthetics

I. Trifluoroethyl vinyl ether (Fluroxene)

A. Physical properties

Fluroxene $CF_3 \cdot CH_2-O-CH=CH_2$ is a clear, colorless liquid emitting a mild unobjectionable, characteristic odor. The specific gravity is 1.13, the boiling point 43.2°, and the oil-water coefficient 90. The organically bound fluorine is stable to soda lime and the molecule is unaltered by the metabolic processes of the body. Although fluroxene is flammable its lower limit of flammability is 4.2% and it is not readily ignited.

B. Blood levels

DUNDEE et al. (1957) determined the arterial blood levels of fluroxene in a series of 22 patients. Their data are listed in Table 27 and as would be expected, progressive depression of the nervous system accompanied increasing blood concentrations of the drug.

Table 27. *Arterial blood trifluoroethylvinyl ether levels*[1]

Depth of anesthesia	Number of readings	Blood trifluoroethylvinyl ether level (mg%)		
		Average	Standard deviation	Range
Surgical Anesthesia[2]				
Plane 1	12	14.6 ± 0.77	2.65	10.8—20.0
Plane 2	17	20.4 ± 1.35	5.57	12.1—31.5
Plane 3	19	28.5 ± 1.08	4.69	18.7—34.7
Plane 4	7	38.7 ± 2.88	7.62	33.0—50.0
Apnea[3]	6	49.3 ± 1.62	6.56	40.3—61.0

[1] Atropine only as preoperative medication.
[2] Thirteen readings where it was impossible to decide the exact depth of anesthesia are included in two planes, *e.g.*, a blood level obtained at the junction of plane 3 and 4 would be included above in both planes.
[3] Four of these cases had minimal respiratory excursions in plane 4 of surgical anesthesia. Spontaneous apnea was not allowed to occur, but the gas concentration of trifluoroethylvinyl ether was maintained for five minutes with controlled respiration.

From Dundee et al. (1957).

C. Pharmacologic studies

Fluroxene was studied pharmacologically by Krantz et al. (1953). The following statements summarize their studies.

1. Fluroxene elicits anesthetic activity when administered by inhalation to various species of laboratory animals.
2. The potency of fluroxene is approximately equal to that of ethyl ether in the dog.
3. In the dog, fluroxene produced no functional hepatic impairment, as shown by the sulfobromophthalein test. In these experiments in the rat and dog, anesthesias with fluroxene produced no histopathologic changes in the liver or kidneys.
4. Neither the monkey's heart nor the dog's heart showed any significant electrocardiographic changes under anesthesia with fluroxene. Likewise electroencephalograms in the dog and monkey under ethyl ether anesthesia and fluroxene were not dissimilar.
5. The blood pressure of the dog was not significantly lowered by anesthesia with fluroxene.
6. Fluroxene has a mild non-objectionable odor. In anesthetic concentrations the fluroxene vapor is nonirritating and does not stimulate respirations in light levels of surgical anesthesia. The lack of stimulation on the respiration makes this agent especially useful in thoracic surgery (Dornette, 1963).
7. This fluorinated ether does not appear to be decomposed readily by hydrolysis. Metabolic processes of the body do not liberate fluoride from the molecule.
8. This fluorinated ether presents less of a fire and explosion hazard than similar non-fluorinated ethers.
9. Fluroxene compares favorably with ethyl ether, ethyl vinyl ether and isopropyl vinyl ether as an inhalation anesthetic in the dog, monkey and rat.

D. Clinical experience

The first human anesthesia with a fluorinated anesthetic was with fluroxene. On April 10, 1953 at 2 p.m. Krantz anesthetized Dr. Max S. Sadove, an anesthesiologist in the Research and Educational Hospital of the University of Illinois. The clinical studies with fluroxene have revealed that it is a stable compound with a boiling point and vapor pressure within the intermediate range, allowing simplicity of vaporization and administration. Induction is rapid and as a rule pleasant and free of appreciable excitement. This feature is especially helpful in pediatric cases. Rapid change of planes of anesthesia is possible with fluroxene. Laryngospasm is minimal and bronchospasm has not been reported.

There is absence of cardiovascular depression in lighter planes of anesthesia. The depression that may occur in deeper planes of anesthesia is rapidly reversible when the level of fluroxene anesthesia is lightened. Pulse is regular, with some tendency toward bradycardia in deeper planes of anesthesia. Under fluroxene anesthesia there is stability of cardiac rhythm. Nodal rhythm is the only significant change reported.

Recovery is rapid with early return of reflexes. Postoperatively, there is minimal nausea, emesis and excitement, with no effect on the hepatic or renal system.

Fluroxene is compatible with all other anesthetic agents, intravenous muscle relaxants, vasopressors, oxytocics, and soda lime. It is adaptable for use with all techniques of inhalation anesthesia. Fluroxene may be employed singly or in combination with any of the other general anesthetic agents (Dornette, 1956, 1963; Dornette et al., 1962).

Comparative studies with fluroxene and other agents are discussed on page 556.

E. Fluroxene azeotrope

The azeotropic mixture of fluroxene and Genetron 113 contains 51.2% of fluroxene and boils at 40.5° C. Its specific gravity at 25° C is 1.28. Fluroxene and Genetron 113 form an azeotropic mixture that has been shown to exhibit satisfactory anesthesia in the rat, dog and monkey (Krantz et al., 1960b). A single case of anesthesia for surgical purposes in man is recorded. Clinical studies with this azeotrope were conducted by Morris (1961).

It appears that this azeotrope is not as satisfactory clinically as is fluroxene. The lower limit of flammability has been raised to 6.2%. Genetron 113 is essentially inert pharmacologically; its presence diminishes the anesthetic potency of fluroxene.

II. Halothane, fluothane

A. Physical properties

Halothane, $CF_3CHBrCl$ is a clear, colorless mobile liquid with a characteristic odor which resembles that of chloroform. The liquid boils at 50.2° C. Its vapors are completely nonflammable. The oil-water coefficient is 330 which is indicative of its powerful anesthetic activity.

B. Absorption, distribution and excretion

1. Mice and rats

Duncan and Raventos (1959) made the following observations on absorption, distribution and exhalation of halothane in mice:

1. Halothane is rapidly absorbed during induction.
2. The concentration of halothane in arterial blood reaches equilibrium in a very short period of time and after this remains constant.
3. Halothane accumulates rapidly in the fat compartments. The concentrations of halothane in the liver and brain increase slowly.
4. They estimated it would take 20 to 30 hours of 1.5% halothane anesthesia to saturate the adipose tissue.

5. The brain does not absorb large amounts of halothane.

6. Halothane is cleared rapidly from the lungs, producing a short recovery time.

Figures 2 and 3 express the concentration of halothane in the tissues and blood of rats.

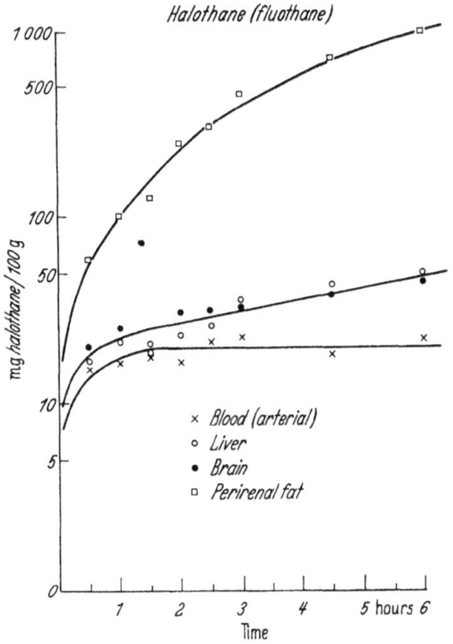

Fig. 2

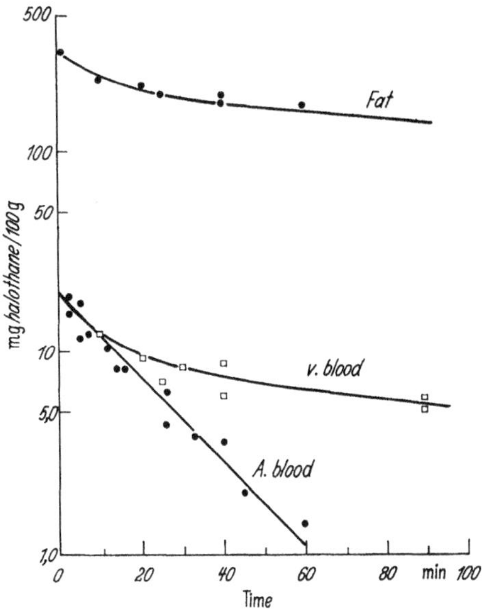

Fig. 3

Fig. 2. Mean concentrations of halothane in the tissues of rats anesthetized with 1.5 volumes per cent of halothane. (From Duncan and Raventos 1959.)

Fig. 3. Concentrations of halothane in the arterial and venous blood and perirenal fat of rats during recovery after 3 hours of anesthesia with 1.5 volumes per cent of halothane. Each point represents one animal. (From Duncan and Raventos 1959.)

2. Tissue distribution

Larson et al. (1962) determined the partition coefficient for halothane in various body tissues. The Ostwald coefficient for halothane is 2.3 and 26% is cleared in one passage through the lungs. This fact accounts for the fast recovery of patients from this anesthetic. The tissue/blood coefficients for halothane measured at 37° C were: 2.6 brain, 2.6 liver, 1.6 kidney, 3.5 muscle and 60 for the fat tissues. This study indicates that halothane is more soluble in tissue compartments than in whole blood. This may well be one of the reasons for the fast induction with this agent.

3. Excretion

Halothane, like the other volatile anesthetics is excreted unchanged by the lungs in the exhaled air. Although this method of excretion prevails with most of the volatile anesthetics, recent evidence indicates that a limited degree of biotransformation takes place in the body. For example van Dyke et al. (1963) using C^{14} labeled halothane and other compounds, showed that when these agents were inhaled by rats $C^{14}O_2$ was exhaled; with $CHCl_3$ it was from 4 to 5%; with CCl_4 it was 11%; the precise per cent with halothane was not determined.

4. Placental transfer of halothane

Many depressant drugs, such as the barbiturates and ether have been shown to cross the placental barrier. SHERIDAN and ROBSON (1959) showed that halothane shares this property. They used halothane anesthesia in vaginal deliveries and determined the concentration of the agent in the blood from a hand vein of the mother and in the blood from a cord segment of the infant at the time of delivery. Their results are shown in Table 28. Halothane could be demonstrated in the umbilical blood after only 2 minutes of inhalation of the anesthetic by the mother.

Table 28. *Maternal and fetal blood halothane levels in mg per cent with increasing durations of anesthesia*

Duration of anesthesia (minutes)	Average concentration of halothane administerd (%)	Blood halothane (Mg per cent)	
		Maternal	Fetal
2	3.0	7.8	5.6
3	1.5	8.0	4.2
5	2.0	5.7	2.2
6	2.0	4.0	0
9	1.5	3.6	2.8
9	2.0	10.5	4.2

Adapted from SHERIDAN and ROBSON (1959).

C. Pharmacologic studies

RAVENTOS (1956) showed that halothane vapor when inhaled caused rapid and deep anesthesia in a variety of laboratory animals. The agent enters and leaves the body unchanged. Its principal pharmacologic action, aside from anesthesia, was hypotension. The degree of hypotension appears to be a function of the depth of anesthesia. Anesthesia with halothane does not evoke cardiac arrhythmias, but the myocardium is sensitized to challenging doses of epinephrine. The only pathologic lesion noted by RAVENTOS following anesthesia with halothane was mild dilatation of the proximal tubules of the kidney. There was no impairment of renal function. In 1958 KRANTZ et al. observed a mean decrease of 47% in the oxygen uptake of the monkey under halothane anesthesia. This is comparable to chloroform anesthesia. The oxygen uptake of rat heart ventricular slices *in vitro* also exhibited diminished oxygen uptake when exposed to anesthetic concentrations of halothane.

1. Effect on the liver

JONES et al. (1958) evaluated the relative hepatotoxicity of several inhalation anesthetic drugs and observed chloroform to be the most toxic and ethyl ether the least toxic; halothane produced liver cell injury which was manifested as a fatty infiltration without necrosis.

VIRTUE and PAYNE (1958) observed a postoperative death after halothane anesthesia due to liver toxicity. BARTON (1959) reported two cases of jaundice after halothane anesthesia.

No effect was seen on the liver histopathology of dogs exposed to halothane for three hours while adequately ventilated. Also, no adverse effects were noted when this agent was administered in an atmosphere slightly deficient in oxygen (HALEY and WYANT, 1959).

Green et al. (1959) investigated the effects on the liver of dogs of two doses (dose for analgesia and for surgical anesthesia) of halothane, chloroform and diethyl ether. Chloroform in both concentrations produced structural and functional hepatic changes which were more severe than those observed with halothane and ethyl ether. Livers of most dogs returned to normal within nine days.

Since halogenated hydrocarbons are notorious for their hepatotoxic action, Stephen et al. (1958) carried out studies on dogs and monkeys by anesthetizing them for 3 hours daily on 5 consecutive days with halothane, chloroform and ether, respectively. The livers from the dogs receiving halothane showed lobular fatty alteration and glycogen depletion. The livers from the dogs anesthetized with chloroform showed broad zones of necrosis about the central zone lobule, surrounded by severe fatty infiltration. Chronic ether anesthesia produced minimal glycogen depletion and fatty change about the central lobule.

Cohen et al. (1963) isolated a halogenated butene from commercially available halothane. The compound was found in all halothane bottles tested, freshly opened or not. The average concentration in a freshly opened bottle was 0.01% and under clinical conditions when stored in a "copper kettle" for five days the concentration of this butene increased as much as tenfold in some instances. The butene identified was 2,3-dichloro-1,1,1,4,4,4-hexafluorobutene-2 which was partially studied by Lu et al. (1953). They noted that this compound produced convulsions in two out of four rats at the point of anesthesia and all four rats had postanesthetic analgesia and died within 18 hours.

Halothane, when refluxed in the presence of copper filings in an oxygen atmosphere, yielded an increased concentration of the butene. Heat further accelerated this reaction. In the absence of either copper or oxygen the concentration of the compound did not increase.

A feasible chemical mechanism of formation of the compound from halothane offered by Cohen et al. was:

$$CF_3CHClBr \xrightarrow{Cu} CuBr + CF_3CHClCHClCF_3 \xrightarrow{O_2} CF_3\overset{\overset{\textstyle Cl}{|}}{C} = \overset{\overset{\textstyle Cl}{|}}{C}CF_3 + H_2O$$

The wide use of copper vaporizers in this country as opposed to nickel-plated or glass vaporizers in many other countries may be a significant factor in the formation of this compound. The relative toxicity of this butene has not been established. To what extent 2,3-dichloro-1,1,1,4,4,4-hexafluorobutene-2 is implicated in the hepatotoxic problems observed in a limited number of halothane anesthesias remains a subject for further investigation.

The question of toxic contaminants in halothane is also discussed in this volume in Chapter 9 by Clayton.

Brody and Sweet (1963) noted in their report that three out of four selected cases under study with halothane anesthesia died of massive hepatic necrosis. Liver biopsies from two of these patients were normal preoperatively. Morris (1963) reported, "Severe liver damage was demonstrated in patients receiving carbon dioxide during halothane and methoxyflurane anesthesia. No damage seen was similar to that observed after chloroform administration. Among the significant results of this study is the lack of liver damage following Fluoromar, indicating that it is the only halogenated drug not capable of producing hepatic damage." In a recent review on halothane and hepatic necrosis Vandam (1963) indicated that the relationship between halothane and liver changes has by no means been proved; further controlled studies are needed to conclusively solve this serious problem.

Table 29. *Mean effect of 1.5% fluothane on the circulation as altered by autonomic denervation*[1]

	Drug used and system blocked							
	No drug; no system blocked (6 subjects)		Arfonad, phenylephrine; sympathetic and parasympathetic systems (7 subjects)		Atropine; parasympathetic system (3 subjects)		High spinal, phenylephrine; sympathetic system (2 subjects)	
	Control	Fluothane	Control	Fluothane	Control	Fluothane	Control	Fluothane
Cardiac output (liters/min)	6.3	4.0 —31% ± 18%	7.0	3.9 —44% ± 9%	7.3	6.1 —15% ± 11%	6.9	4.2 —39% ± 10%
Mean arterial pressure (mm Hg)	96	72 —25% ± 15%	107	60 —44% ± 4%	125	83 —32% ± 17%	95	58 —36% ± 17%
Total peripheral resistance (dynes sec cm^{-5})	1300	1540 +18% ± 15%	1360	1350 —1% ± 14%	1520	1120 —20% ± 15%	1200	1280 +6% ± 11%
Heart rate per min	61	60 —2% ± 13%	85	71 —17% ± 13%	115	102 —12% ± 9%	68	68 0% ± 8%
Stroke volume (ml)	100	65 —35% ± 13%	80	54 —30% ± 13%	63	60 —5% ± 4%	98	60 —40% ± 3%
Venous pressure (cm H_2O)	5.0	9.4 +4.4 ± 3 cm	1.0	2.0 +1 ± 1 cm	—0.8	0.5 +1 ± 1 cm	2	3 +1 (1 subj.)
Stroke work (kg m)	0.162	0.078 —51% ± 17%	0.140	0.052 —62% ± 9%	0.120	0.080 —33% ± 18%	0.151	0.056 —63% ± 13%

[1] All subjects were artificially ventilated with 75% nitrous oxide except one awake in the first column control, and one with compressed air in the fourth column. Fluothane data are also expressed as mean percentage change from control with standard deviation of this change.

From STEPHEN and LITTLE (1961).

A total of 12 hepatic deaths (mostly in cholecystectomies) have been reported in the literature incriminating halothane as the causative agent. As yet there is no clear cause and effect relationship between liver damage and halothane. However, at present halothane is not recommended for use in patients with known liver or biliary tract disease or for obstetrical use.

2. Effect on heart and blood pressure

WYANT et al. (1960) hold the view that the hypotension seen with azeotropic halothane-ether is due to peripheral vasodilatation; however, their work does not indicate the mechanism of the hypotension. It appears that the hypotension involves several components. The first of these is decreased cardiac output. This results from direct myocardial depression. The second facet is decreased peripheral resistance evoked by a depressant action on the vasomotor center and a relaxant action on the walls of the blood vessels. The third factor is a selective autonomic ganglionic blockade as suggested by RAVENTOS (1956). BURN et al. (1957) were unable to demonstrate any strong ganglionic blocking action produced by halothane. If autonomic ganglionic blockade is a factor in the hypotension of the anesthetic syndrome of halothane, it appears to be of minor significance.

JOHNSTONE (1956) demonstrated that halothane evokes a direct action on the conduction system of the heart. He showed that this was cholinergic in character and could be adequately blocked by atropine. Bradycardia is often observed during halothane anesthesia; frequently this is masked by atropine pre-medication. DUNDEE and BLACK (1960) suggest that the changes in the heart rate may be either due to vagal stimulation or depression of sympathoadrenal activity.

Table 29 illustrates the mean effect of 1.5% Fluothane on the circulation as altered by autonomic denervation (STEPHEN and LITTLE 1961).

3. Effect on cerebrospinal pressure

Cerebrospinal fluid pressure, arterial pressure and venous pressure measurements before and during halothane anesthesia were made by MARX et al. (1962) in ten elderly patients. There were two types of increase in cerebrospinal pressure. First, during intubation there was a sharp increase in the cerebrospinal pressure while venous pressure lagged behind and the changes in arterial blood pressure were variable. During maintenance anesthesia the increased cerebrospinal pressure corresponded to the increased venous blood pressure, while at this time the arterial blood pressure decreased concomitantly. The changes noted were proportional to the different concentrations of halothane used.

4. Effect on central nervous system

DAVIS et al. (1961) noted the effects of 0.25, 0.5, 1 and 2% halothane anesthesia on the evoked responses in the posterioventrolateral nucleus of the thalamus and the periaqueductal reticular formation of the midbrain tegmentum in fifteen cats. Halothane depressed both these regions more than these authors had observed in earlier studies with diethyl ether, divinyl ether, trichlorethylene and chloroform. The authors stated "These findings add support to the concept that a reversible depression of the midbrain reticular activating system is of primary importance in the production of the general anesthetic state. They further add to the growing body of evidence suggesting the lemniscal pathways are not immune to the influence of the commonly used general anesthetics as originally thought. The apparent paradox of significant depression of a region conventionally linked with transmission and primitive perception of pain (the thalamus) by halothane, an agent which is a poor analgesic clinically, has no obvious explanation at this time."

D. Clinical experiences

Using concentrations in the inspired air of 2 to 2.5% (which must be meticulously controlled by an especially designed vaporizer) smooth, easy and rapid induction may be achieved. Surgical anesthesia may be produced within 5 to 7 minutes.

ABAJIAN et al. (1959) used halothane in 5000 cases. They reported no evidence of hepatic, renal or "undue" myocardial toxicity. They concur in the previous statements of ease of induction. Relaxation appears to be good under halothane anesthesia and skeletal muscle relaxants do not appear to be necessary. Numerous other reports in the literature confirm the value of halothane as an anesthetic agent and support the observations of the foregoing investigators (MOYERS and PITTINGER, 1959).

DOBKIN (1959) reported no significant changes in acid-base balance during halothane anesthesia in 90 patients.

D'ARCY et al. (1959) reported on their clinical experiences with halothane in over 2,000 patients. They stressed the importance of technique of administration because halothane is a potent agent and the vapor concentration must be controlled accurately. D'ARCY et al. noted:

1. There was no direct relationship between the electroencephalogram and the depth of anesthesia with halothane anesthesia.
2. Halothane has very weak analgesic properties.
3. Halothane potentiates the ganglionic blocking properties of tubocurarine and severe hypotension may follow its administration.
4. The autonomic effect of halothane is important. They observed evidence of parasympathetic depression such as decreased secretions. The vagotonic action of halothane stressed the need for premedication to protect against detrimental cardiovascular effects.
5. They attributed the muscular relaxation to the central effect of the agent.
6. They observed epinephrine was potentially dangerous in patients anesthetized with halothane because of the likelihood of producing cardiac arrhythmias.
7. The degree of hypotension was directly related to the concentration of halothane used and the mechanism of hypotension was not clear.
8. Halothane is non-irritant to the respiratory tract. It increases the respiratory rate and decreases the tidal volume. The overall effect is one of slightly decreased minute volume therefore, producing a slight decrease in alveolar ventilation.
9. Some decrease in oxygen uptake was noted which is directly proportional to the depth of anesthesia.
10. Halothane decreases uterine tone and therefore is contraindicated for use in obstetrical cases.

E. Azeotrope (Halothane and ethyl ether)

BOIVIN et al. (1958) used a stable azeotrope compound made of 31.7 parts by volume of ethyl ether and 68.3% halothane. This azeotrope has a boiling point of 51.5° C and was observed to be stable after four months. These authors felt the halothane-ether azeotropic compound compares favorably with the best anesthetics already known.

Dobkin (1959) used an azeotropic mixture of halothane and ethyl ether on fifty patients undergoing surgery. He observed no change in acid-base balance, electrolyte balance, blood sugar or blood urea nitrogen. Dobkin was able to maintain a smooth, stable level of anesthesia with this mixture and feels it warrants extensive clinical trial as an alternative to halothane.

III. Methoxyflurane, Penthrane®

A. Physical properties

Methoxyflurane, $CH_3-O-CF_2CCl_2H$ is a clear, colorless liquid having a characteristic fruity odor. The boiling point is 104.65° C at 760 mm of mercury, the freezing point is −35° C, the specific gravity is 1.4224 at 25° C, the oil-water coefficient is 440 and the blood-gas coefficient 11–12 (Lowe, 1963). Methoxyflurane is completely stable in the presence of alkali, air, light or moisture and can be safely employed in a closed circuit.

The concentration of methoxyflurane in anesthetic mixtures is limited to a maximum of about 4% at 23° C by the vapor pressure of methoxyflurane and by the efficiency of the vaporizer.

B. Distribution and excretion

1. Tissue levels

The distribution and excretion of methoxyflurane was studied by Chenoweth et al. (1962b). The levels of the compound in various tissues during deep and light anesthesia in two dogs are shown in Table 30.

Table 30. *Tissue content of methoxyflurane (± 50 ppm) after 2.5 hours' anesthesia*

	Dog A (Light) ppm	Dog B (Deep) ppm
Arterial	257	510
Brain	500	720
Adrenal cortex	1400	3300
Adrenal medulla	1500	2100
Fat	360	4750
Right ventricle	260	580
Skeletal muscle	160	190
Lung	140	190
Liver	330	820
Spleen	150	200
Kidney	250	590
Urine	trace	trace
Bile	400	360
Thyroid	1040	490
Pancreas	300	290

Adapted from Chenoweth et al. (1962b).

It is interesting to note that the highest concentration of the anesthetic was observed in the adrenal cortex and the lowest in the lungs.

Methoxyflurane is unaltered by the body. The major organ of excretion is the lung. Methoxyflurane persists on the breath for many hours owing to the slow elimination of the drug absorbed by the adipose tissues (oil-water coefficient 440). Chenoweth found only trace amounts of methoxyflurane in the urine; therefore, renal excretion is apparently not an avenue of elimination of the anesthetic.

2. Blood levels

Methoxyflurane is a potent anesthetic agent as indicated by the comparative low blood levels required to produce anesthesia. These data observed by CHENOWETH et al. (1962b) are shown in Fig. 4.

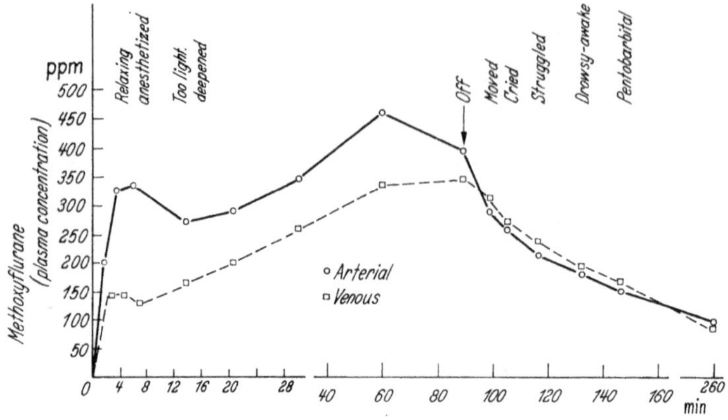

Fig. 4. Levels of methoxyflurane in arterial and venous blood of a dog. (From CHENOWETH et al., 1960.)

C. Pharmacologic studies

CHENOWETH et al. (1962b) studied extensively the pharmacologic responses to methoxyflurane. In dogs anesthesia was induced in 10 minutes and muscular relaxation was excellent. The emergence time from anesthesias of 30 to 150 minutes was 60 to 120 minutes. Induction was slow but anesthesia could rapidly be induced with thiopental sodium or halothane and then supplemented with methoxyflurane.

1. Effect on electroencephalogram

Electroencephalographic studies on humans as well as dogs demonstrate in light levels of anesthesia fast, regular, low-voltage activity and as anesthesia is deepened there is a slight shift of the spectrum to slower frequencies and slightly greater amplitude. This change is a subtle one, however, and is not nearly as marked as the change seen with diethyl ether, cyclopropane, or thiopental.

2. Effect on respiration

The respiratory response to methoxyflurane, although somewhat similar to that of ether, gave no indication of respiratory stimulation as observed with ether. Minute volume was slightly increased during light anesthesia, but depressed during deep anesthesia.

3. Effect on blood pressure

The blood pressure is lowered by anesthesia with methoxyflurane. The depressor response is progressive with the depth of anesthesia. The mechanism of the depressor response has not been delineated. Since atropine was found to diminish the depressor response, it appears that vagal stimulation is one of its components. The pulse rate is generally decreased under methoxyflurane anesthesia. Ventricular arrhythmias were not encountered, neither were they induced by challenging doses of epinephrine. Although this is not agreed upon by all investigators, this appears to be a constant finding with the halogenated ethers in contradistinction to the halogenated hydrocarbons.

4. Effect on blood elements

There was no evidence of damage to the elements of blood or change in the coagulation time by methoxyflurane anesthesia.

5. Effect on liver

Methoxyflurane appears to have about the same effect upon liver function as does ether. Of all the various tests for liver function, the sulfobromphthalein test appeared to be the most sensitive. The effect on this test of anesthesia with methoxyflurane was studied in patients by ARTUSIO et al. (1960). His data are shown in Fig. 5.

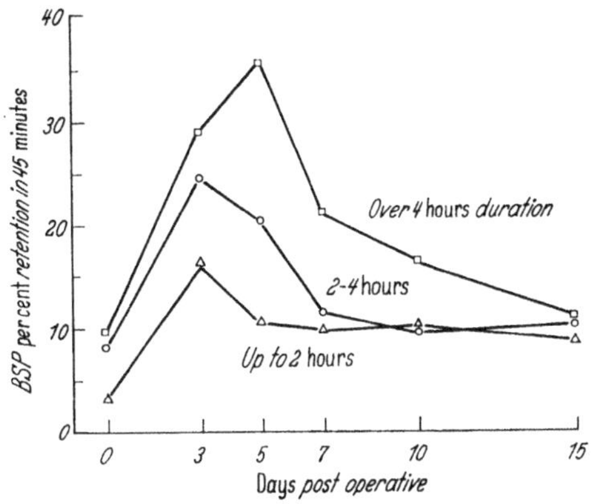

Fig. 5. Postoperative sulfobromphthalein retention of 40 patients according to the duration of the anesthesia. (From ARTUSIO et al., 1960.)

Methoxyflurane is a potent volatile anesthetic, as first suggested by VAN POZNAK and ARTUSIO (1960b). It has been widely used and their work amply confirmed. It appears that slow induction, slow emergence and hypotension during anesthesia are its principal drawbacks.

IV. Emulsions of fluorinated ethers

A. Methoxyflurane

KRANTZ et al. (1961a and 1962b) demonstrated, using methoxyflurane and its brominated analog, that a volatile anesthetic agent in an emulsion of the oil-in-water type, injected into animals and man evokes a satisfactory anesthesia. The agents are excreted by the lungs in the exhaled air. Should further experience show the feasibility of this procedure, many high boiling anesthetics may be made available, which at present are not used owing to their low degree of volatility. Simplicity and accuracy of dosage administered are features of this technique of administration.

Methoxyflurane emulsion has been used successfully on a series of patients requiring surgery. Anesthesia was induced directly with the emulsion and with Surital® sodium in some cases. The procedure was compatible with the usual preoperative medications. Rebreathing of the exhaled methoxyflurane was employed for varying periods of time. The quantities of emulsion required were amazingly small compared with our animal data. The average was approximately 3 ml per kilogram per hour of a 3.5% methoxyflurane emulsion. The anesthetic syndrome compared favorably with that evoked by methoxyflurane given by inhalation. Blood chemistry and other clinical observations were within normal limits for the postanesthetic periods.

B. Roflurane

RUDO and KRANTZ (1963b) reported on the anesthetic properties of roflurane when administered intravenously in an oil-in-water emulsion. A 0.6 molar roflurane emulsion was used in 127 dogs and 9 patients. In all cases induction was rapid, relaxation excellent, analgesia good and recovery rapid. No untoward side effects such as vomiting or increased secretions were noticed. Blood pressure was normal during light planes of anesthesia and declined with deeper planes. The hypotensive response was always less than that observed with methoxyflurane as was also noted by ARTUSIO and VAN POZNAK (1961b) in their studies of these two anesthetics by inhalation. The ECG during roflurane anesthesia was normal and 10 mcg/kg of epinephrine did not produce cardiac arrhythmias. Liver, lung and kidney biopsies were unremarkable. No hemolysis was observed in dogs or man after anesthesia with the roflurane emulsion. No significant changes in plasma lipid concentration were observed in dogs after one hour of anesthesia with roflurane emulsion.

The animal experiments indicate that roflurane emulsion anesthesia may prove to be a useful addition to the list of present anesthetic agents. However, the authors feel this agent is better suited for induction and short term anesthesias.

V. Comparative studies of fluorinated anesthetics

CHENOWETH and HAKE (1962a) wrote a comprehensive review of comparative studies of the clinically used anesthetics.

A. Halothane and fluroxene

VIRTUE et al. (1962) conducted an interesting comparison of the respiratory and hemodynamic effects of halothane and fluroxene anesthesia on 10 normal sujects. Their data confirm many of the observations that have been recorded by various investigators.

Table 31. *Hemodynamic studies (halothane and fluroxene)*

Agent	Cardiac output l/min	Pulse	Venous pressure[1] mm Hg	Blood pressure[1] mm Hg	Total systemic resistance dynes sec cm^{-5}
Control	4.94 ± .16	65 ± 5.0	7.7 ± .70	119 ± 9.3A	1440 ± 187
Fluroxene	5.42 ± .46	79 ± 7.0	9.4 ± .86	108 ± 7.8	1160 ± 96
Halothane	5.17 ± .50	80 ± 6.7	9.0 ± .77	89 ± 4.8B	1098 ± 101

[1] Systolic pressure.
± Refers to standard error of the mean; $p < 0.01$ A—B. (The probability that the difference between A (blood pressure in the control group) and B (blood pressure of the group anesthetized with halothane) might have arisen as an accident of sampling is less than 0.01.)
From VIRTUE et al. (1962).

The data in Table 32 indicate that under anesthesia with halothane the oxygen uptake is depressed significantly. This does not prevail with fluroxene. The same type of diminution of oxygen uptake under halothane anesthesia was shown by KRANTZ et al. (1958) using monkeys.

It appears that no consistent changes in cardiac output occurred under anesthesia with either agent. However, it is clear from the data in Table 31, that halothane anesthesia is accompanied by a significant degree of hypotension. The authors commented favorably on the rapidity of the awakening of the subjects from fluroxene anesthesia.

Table 32. *Ventilation studies (halothane and fluroxene)*

	Calculated O_2 uptake ml/min	Predicted O_2 uptake ml/min	Respiratory rate	Tidal volume ml	R.Q.	Basal metabolic rate	CO_2 Output ml/min	Minute Volume Liters
ontrol	250 ± 16.2	238	13 ± 1.1 C	353 ± 45 F	.71 ± .03	5.9 ± 4.3	173 ± 12.8 J	5.66 ± .40
luroxene	279 ± 13.3 A		24 ± 2.1 D	285 ± 50	.61 ± .03	14.4 ± 3.6	158 ± 7.9 K	6.15 ± .42
alothane	212 ± 15.6 B		34 ± 2.6 E	183 ± 21 G	.58 ± .05	—10.7 ± 3.2	120 ± 9.3 L	5.90 ± .23

± Refers to standard error of the mean; $p < 0.001$ A—B, C—D, C—E, F—G, J—L, K—L; p 0.01 D—E. (The probability that the difference between A (calculated O_2 uptake in the group anesthetized with trifluoroethyl vinyl ether) and B (calculated O_2 uptake in the group anesthetized with halothane) might have arisen as an accident of sampling is less than 0.001.)

From VIRTUE et al. (1962).

B. Halothane and chloroform

Since halothane and chloroform are halogenated aliphatic hydrocarbons and each is a potent anesthetic, interesting studies have been conducted comparing their respective anesthetic syndromes. References has been made previously to the work of STEPHEN et al. (1958) (p. 549) comparing their hepatotoxic effects.

BAMFORTH et al. (1960) compared the two anesthetics using the double blind technic. A series of 100 patients were anesthetized with halothane or chloroform supplemental to nitrous oxide-oxygen anesthesia. The anesthesiologist was not informed as to the agent employed. His only criterion was his observation of the anesthetic syndrome. Their conclusion was that the changes in blood pressure, pulse rate, respiration and complications during anesthesia were similar in the two groups of patients. They state, "We believe that halothane bears a strong clinical resemblance to chloroform."

DOBKIN et al. (1961a) compared halothane and chloroform in dogs using crossover experiments and accurately measuring the concentrations of the two drugs. In this study halothane appeared to be the better agent.

JONES et al. (1958) compared halothane and chloroform anesthesia in patients in which most of the variables were eliminated. The chloroform was administered by means of the halothane-type vaporizer in carefully controlled concentrations. There were 29 patients who received chloroform and 32 halothane. The anesthetic syndromes were strikingly similar. Chloroform evoked a lesser degree of hypotension and less coughing during induction. Halothane anesthesia elicited nausea and vomiting postoperatively in fewer patients than did chloroform.

Indeed, these studies indicate a definite similarity between the anesthetic syndromes of halothane and chloroform. This is especially true with regard to ease of induction, hypotensive effect and sensitization of the myocardium to epinephrine. On the other hand, it appears from experiments in animals and human anesthesias, that of the two agents, halothane evokes a lesser degree of hepatotoxicity.

C. Halothane and methoxyflurane

DOBKIN and FEDORUK (1961b) compared methoxyflurane and halothane in crossover experiments in dogs. Halothane produced a greater degree of hypotension and decreased cardiac output than did methoxyflurane. Methoxyflurane depressed pulmonary ventilation more deeply than did halothane.

D. Fluroxene and hexafluorodiethyl ether

In screening studies of compounds related to fluroxene (trifluoroethyl vinyl ether) KRANTZ et al. (1957) observed that hexafluorodiethyl ether was a potent convulsive agent when inhaled by various laboratory animals. Their studies prompted them to use the compound as a substitute for electroshock therapy in the treatment of mental illness.

Hexafluorodiethyl ether, $CF_3 \cdot CH_2{-}O{-}CH_2 \cdot CF_3$, known as Indoklon, is a clear, colorless volatile liquid. The boiling point is 63.9° and the specific gravity 1.41 $\frac{20°}{20°}$. It is insoluble in water, but soluble in alcohol, ether and oils.

Indoklon is administered by inhalation in an especially designed anesthetic mask. It may also be given intravenously dissolved in alcohol, water and Carbowax 300. The inhalation of 0.5 to 1 ml of the drug in the form of a vapor induces a grand mal type of seizure within 30 seconds. There is a very short period of apnea which automatically terminates the inhalation of the drug. Unconsciousness supervenes prior to the convulsive seizure. Recovery is prompt and uneventful.

This type of convulsive therapy has been used by KURLAND et al. (1959) in approximately 300 patients embracing over 2500 convulsions. Its therapeutic value appears to be tantamount to that of electroconvulsive therapy. It was observed that the majority of patients experienced less apprehension and the inhalation of a vapor was less threatening than the concept of an electric shock. The untoward effects observed appeared to be similar to those frequently encountered after electroconvulsive therapy but symptoms disappear rapidly.

Since hexafluorodiethyl ether and trifluoroethyl vinyl ether are closely related chemically and the former is a convulsant and the latter an anesthetic, LING and KRANTZ (1960) studied their effects upon cerebral metabolism. Their first experiments were performed on guinea pig whole brain using the Warburg technic. Each flask contained hexafluorodiethyl ether 0.1% (v/v) or 0.35% (v/v) of trifluoroethyl vinyl ether. Their data are shown in Table 33.

Table 33. *Effect of hexafluorodiethyl ether and trifluoroethyl vinyl ether on guinea pig whole brain oxygen utilization*

Substrate (0.01 M)	Mean Q_{O_2} ± S.E. mean		
	Control	Hexafluorodiethyl ether — treated	Trifluoroethyl vinyl ether — treated
None	2.44 ± 0.240 (16)	2.46 ± 0.279 (20)	2.16 ± 0.269 (20)[1]
Glucose	2.63 ± 0.361 (16)	2.75 ± 0.399 (20)	2.16 ± 0.380 (20)[1]
Pyruvate	2.72 ± 0.281 (18)	2.87 ± 0.324 (20)	2.28 ± 0.301 (20)[1]
Fumarate	2.80 ± 0.161 (20)	2.88 ± 0.185 (20)	2.43 ± 0.214 (15)[1]
Succinate	4.54 ± 0.636 (18)	4.21 ± 0.783 (18)	4.05 ± 0.799 (20)

[1] Mean values differ significantly from those of the controls at a probability level of > 0.05 based on the Student's t test.

Figures in parentheses refer to the number of determinations.

From LING and KRANTZ (1960).

In considering the possibility of specificity of action of either agent on different areas of the brain, subsequent studies were conducted to determine whether or not this occurred. These data are shown in Table 34.

The data in Tables 33 and 34 show that hexafluorodiethyl ether exerted no significant effect on whole brain oxidative metabolism while trifluoroethyl vinyl ether depressed such activity in the absence of succinate substrate. Further, the effect on isolated areas of the brain did not necessarily parallel that on the whole brain. Thus hexafluorodiethyl ether inhibited cerebral tissue respiration when fumarate was present, but stimulated medullary oxygen uptake in pyruvate-containing medium. Trifluoroethyl vinyl ether increased the respiration of hypothalamic-thalamic and cerebellar tissue.

Table 34. *Effect of hexafluorodiethyl ether and trifluoroethyl vinyl ether on oxygen utilization of four areas of the guinea pig brain*

Area	Substrate (0.01 M)	Mean Q_{O_2} ± S.E. mean		
		Control	Hexafluorodiethyl ether — treated	Trifluoroethyl vinyl ether — treated
Cerebrum	None	3.20 ± 0.451 (10)	2.82 ± 0.493 (10)	3.54 ± 0.598 (10)
	Glucose	3.59 ± 0.236 (12)	3.53 ± 0.305 (10)	3.45 ± 0.268 (10)
	Pyruvate	3.54 ± 0.247 (8)	3.64 ± 0.318 (10)	3.53 ± 0.287 (10)
	Fumarate	3.73 ± 0.842 (10)	2.77 ± 0.843 (10)[1]	4.24 ± 0.905 (10)
	Succinate	5.85 ± 0.529 (8)	5.74 ± 0.780 (10)	6.20 ± 0.840 (10)
Hypothalamus-thalamus	None	2.61 ± 0.266 (8)	2.43 ± 0.302 (10)	3.08 ± 0.310 (10)[1]
	Glucose	2.59 ± 0.192 (8)	2.62 ± 0.265 (10)	2.93 ± 0.244 (8)[1]
	Pyruvate	2.65 ± 0.113 (8)	2.71 ± 0.187 (10)	2.73 ± 0.143 (10)
	Fumarate	2.35 ± 0.230 (10)	2.14 ± 0.270 (10)	2.76 ± 0.253 (10)[1]
	Succinate	4.90 ± 0.916 (10)	4.30 ± 1.030 (8)	5.82 ± 1.178 (10)
Cerebellum	None	1.84 ± 0.309 (10)	1.80 ± 0.358 (10)	2.39 ± 0.429 (10)[1]
	Glucose	2.42 ± 0.377 (8)	2.87 ± 0.433 (10)	2.23 ± 0.400 (10)
	Pyruvate	2.39 ± 0.477 (12)	2.14 ± 0.472 (10)	2.86 ± 0.475 (10)[1]
	Fumarate	1.55 ± 0.236 (8)	1.51 ± 0.250 (8)	1.78 ± 0.285 (10)
	Succinate	4.21 ± 0.756 (10)	4.60 ± 1.028 (10)	3.46 ± 0.924 (10)
Medulla	None	1.33 ± 0.214 (12)	1.15 ± 0.267 (10)	1.26 ± 0.273 (10)
	Glucose	1.20 ± 0.502 (12)	0.90 ± 0.522 (10)	1.59 ± 0.568 (10)
	Pyruvate	1.33 ± 0.139 (10)	1.53 ± 0.184 (8)[1]	1.29 ± 0.179 (10)
	Fumarate	0.79 ± 0.146 (10)	0.89 ± 0.182 (10)	0.74 ± 0.178 (10)
	Succinate	4.43 ± 0.430 (12)	4.56 ± 0.202 (8)	4.29 ± 0.799 (8)

[1] Mean values differ significantly from those of the control at a probability level of < 0.05 based on the Student's t test.

Figures in parentheses refer to the number of determinations.

From Ling and Krantz (1960).

These investigators also studied hexafluorodiethyl ether and trifluoroethyl vinyl ether on the salamander *Triturus viridescens*. These animals are devoid of a cerebral cortex and have been used as a natural decorticated test animal for the study of the locus of action for convulsive agents (Peters et al., 1958). The exposure of 10 salamanders to hexafluorodiethyl ether vapor failed to produce convulsions. The response was principally that of depression. Six other salamanders were each injected intra-abdominally with this agent (0.10 to 0.40 ml). One of the 6 animals given 0.30 ml showed a transient tonic-clonic convulsion followed by depression while the remaining 5 were only depressed. Exposure of 5 salamanders to trifluoroethyl vinyl ether vapor induced hyperexcitability, including hyperreflexia, followed by marked depression. Five additional animals were each given pentylenetetrazole (1 mg per gram body weight) intra-abdominally, and responded with tonic-clonic seizure. It is of special interest that in these test animals hexafluorodiethyl ether failed to evoke the characteristic convulsive response. Furthermore, trifluoroethyl vinyl ether elicited marked depression, sequential to a period of excitation not observed in higher animals.

These investigators extended their work on the mechanism of the hexafluorodiethyl ether convulsive seizure to the effect on cerebral electrolytes and water distribution. The studies were made on rats and the data are shown in Table 35 (LING and KRANTZ, 1963).

Table 35. *The effect of Indoklon seizures on brain Na^+, K^+, and water*

Fraction	Mean value
Control (10 rats)	
Serum Na^+	151.7 ± 4.34 mEq/L
Serum K^+	6.8 ± 0.44 mEq/L
Brain Na^+	244.5 ± 17.84 μEq/g dry wt
Brain K^+	427.0 ± 24.30 μEq/g dry wt
Brain H_2O A	3.5 ± 0.03 (g/g dry wt) —or—
Brain H_2O B	77.8 ± 0.16% (g H_2O/total brain dry wt)
Indoklon (14 rats)	
Serum Na^+	153.7 ± 4.92 mEq/L
Serum K^+	8.1 ± 0.16 mEq/L[1]
Brain Na^+	389.3 ± 41.11 μEq/g dry wt[1]
Brain K^+	206.8 ± 18.36 μEq/g dry wt[1]
Brain H_2O A	3.5 ± 0.04 g/g dry wt —or—
Brain H_2O B	77.9 ± 0.22% (g H_2O/total brain dry wt)

[1] Significant: based on t test for paired means with the differences from control being at least at the 1% level of probability.
From LING and KRANTZ (1963).

It is clear from the data in Table 35 that Indoklon seizures in the rat were accompanied by a decrease in brain potassium and a concomitant increase in serum potassium. Also there is observed a significant increase in brain sodium and no significant changes in serum sodium or brain water content.

VI. Conclusion

Activity in this field at present is tremendous. Newer methods of synthesis will introduce new fluorinated anesthetics and decrease the cost of the available agents. The introduction of the fluorinated ethers and hydrocarbons as anesthetics has given an impetus for research to obtain that anesthetic that will approach perfection. This field is being explored by many investigators. Newer concepts of the mechanism of action of anesthetics are being proposed. A more adequate knowledge of absorption, distribution and excretion of anesthetic agents is being acquired. Not the least among the advantages that have accrued from these studies is the fact that the explosion and/or fire hazard has been removed from anesthesia by the use of these agents.

Acknowledgements

The authors are indebted to Dr. LOUISE SPEERS, Project Leader, Chemical Research of the Air Reduction, Inc., Murray Hill, New Jersey, for her critical review of this chapter. They are also indebted to Dr. ARTHUR H. NEELEY of the Ohio Chemical and Surgical Equipment Company, Madison, Wisconsin, for his many helpful suggestions. Most of the compounds studied in this laboratory and reviewed in this chapter were synthesized by the chemical staff of the Air Reduction Company.

References

ABAJIAN, J. JR., E. H. BRAZELL, G. A. DENTE, and E. L. MILLS: Experiences with 5000 cases of anesthesia with halothane. J. Amer. med. Ass. **171**, 535—540 (1959).

ABREU, B. E.: Unsaturated mono halogenated hydrocarbons as general anesthetic agents. Anesthesiology **2**, 393—397 (1941).

ADRIANI, J.: The chemistry and physics of anesthesia, page 583. Springfield, Illinois: Charles C. Thomas Co. 1962.

ARTUSIO, J. F. JR., Ed.: Halogenated anesthetics. Philadelphia, Pa.: F. A. Davis Co. 1963.

—, and A. VAN POZNAK: Laboratory and clinical investigation of teflurane, 1,1,1,2-tetrafluoro-2-bromoethane. Fed. Proc. **20** (1), 312 (1961a).

— — Laboratory and clinical studies with 1,1,2-trifluoro-2-bromoethyl methyl ether. Fed. Proc. **20** (1), 312 (1961b).

— — R. E. HUNT, F. M. TIERS, and M. ALEXANDER: A clinical evaluation of methoxyflurane in man. Anesthesiology **21**, 512—517 (1960).

BAMFORTH, B. J., K. L. SIEBECKER, J. E. STEINHAUS, and O. S. ORTH: A clinical comparison of chloroform and halothane by a blind study technique. Anesthesiology **21**, 273—380 (1960).

BARTON, J. D. M.: Letter to the editor. Lancet **1**, 1097 (1959).

BOIVIN, P. A., F. HUDON, and A. JACQUES: Properties of the fluothane-ether anaesthetic. Canad. Anaesth. Soc. J. **5**, 409—413 (1958).

BOOTH, H. S., and E. M. BIXBY: Fluorine derivatives of chloroform. Ind. and Eng. Chem. **24**, 637—641 (1932).

BRINK, F., and J. M. POSTERNAK: Thermodynamic analysis of the relative effectiveness of narcotics. J. cellular comp. Physiol. **32**, 211—233 (1948).

BRODY, G. L., and R. B. SWEET: Halothane anesthesia as a possible cause of massive hepatic necrosis. Anesthesiology **24**, 29—37 (1963).

BRODY, T. M., and J. A. BAIN: Barbiturates and oxidative phosphorylation. Proc. Soc. exp. Biol. (N. Y.) **77**, 50—53 (1951).

BURGISON, R. M., W. E. O'MALLEY, C. K. HEISSE, J. W. FORREST, and J. C. KRANTZ JR.: Anesthesia XLVI. Fluorinated ethylenes and cardiac arrhythmias induced by epinephrine. J. Pharmacol. exp. Ther. **114**, 470—472 (1955).

BURN, J. H., H. G. EPSTEIN, G. A. FEIGAN, and W. D. M. PATON: Some pharmacological actions of fluothane. Brit. med. J. **2**, 479—490 (1957).

BURNS, T. H. S., J. M. HALL, A. BRACKEN, and G. GOULDSTONE: An investigation of new fluorine compounds in anaesthesia (4). Anesthesia **16**, 440—444 (1961a).

— — — — An investigation of new fluorine compounds in anaesthesia (3). Anaesthesia **16**, 333—339 (1961b).

— — — — Fluorine compounds in anaesthesia (5). Examination of six heavily halogenated aliphatic compounds. Anaesthesia **17**, 337—343 (1962).

— — — — Fluorine compounds in anesthesia (6). Anesthesia **19**, 167—176 (1964).

— — — — and D. S. NEWLAND: An investigation of new fluorine compounds in anesthesia (1). Anesthesia **16**, 440—444 (January 1961c).

BUU-HOÏ, N. P.: Les derives organiques de fluor d'interet pharmacologic. Fortschr. Arzneimittelforsch. **3**, 9—74 (1961).

CASCORBI, H. F., J. C. KRANTZ JR., and F. G. RUDO: Unpublished data (1962).

CHENOWETH, M. B., and C. L. HAKE: The smaller halogenated aliphatic hydrocarbons. Ann. Rev. Pharmacol. **2**, 363—398 (1962a).

— D. N. ROBERTSON, D. S. ERLEY, and R. GOLHKE: Blood and tissue levels of ether, chloroform, halothane and methoxyflurane in dogs. Anesthesiology **23**, 101—106 (1962b).

CLEMENTS, J. H., and K. M. WILSON: Narcotic agents and interfacial films. Proc. nat. Acad. Sci. (Wash.) **48**, 1008—1014 (1962).

COHEN, E. N., J. W. BELLVILLE, H. BUDZIKIEWICZ, and D. H. WILLIAMS: Impurity in halothane anesthetic. Science **141**, 899 (1963).

D'ARCY, E. J., M. H. HOLMDAHL, and J. P. PAYNE: The pharmacology of halothane in man: A review. Brit. J. Anaesth. **31**, 424—432 (1959).

DAVIS, H. S., V. E. QUITMEYER, and W. F. COLLINS: The effect of halothane (fluothane) on the thalamus and midbrain reticular formation. Anesthesiology **16**, 32—49 (1961).

DOBKIN, A. B.: Anaesthesia with the azeotropic mixture of halothane and diethyl ether. Brit. J. Anaesth. **31**, 53—65 (1959).
—, and S. FEDORUK: Comparison of the cardiovascular, respiratory and metabolic effects of methoxyflurane and halothane in dogs. Anesthesiology **22**, 355—362 (1961 b).
— J. H. HARLAND, and S. FEDORUK: Chloroform and halothane in a precision system comparison of some cardiovascular, respiratory and metabolic effects in dogs. Brit. J. Anaesth. **33**, 239—257 (1961 a).
DORNETTE, W. H. L.: Fluroxene. *In:* J. F. ARTUSIO JR., Ed., Halogenated anesthetics. Philadelphia, Pennsylvania: F. A. Davis Company 1963.
— Trifluoroethylvinyl ether (Fluoromar). A preliminary report on clinical experiences and animal experiment. Calif. Med. **85**, 311 (1956).
— G. L. MILLER, W. E. SHEFFIELD, R. J. CAVALLARO, and M. F. POE: Clinical experiences with trifluoroethylvinyl ether anesthesia. Anesth. Analg. Curr. Res. **41**, 605—614 (1962).
DUNCAN, W. A. M., and J. RAVENTOS: The pharmacokinetics of halothane (fluothane) anesthesia. Brit. J. Anaesth. **31**, 302—315 (1959).
DUNDEE, J. W., and G. W. BLACK: A review of cardiovascular effects of halothane. Anaesthesia **15**, 349—356 (1960).
— H. W. LINDE, and R. D. DRIPPS: Observations on trifluoroethyl vinyl ether. Anesthesiology **18**, 66—72 (1957).
FABIAN, L. W., H. DE WITT, and M. A. CARNES: Laboratory and clinical investigation of some newly synthesized fluorocarbon anesthetics. Anesth. Analg. Curr. Res. **39**, 456—462 (1960).
FEATHERSTONE, R. M., and C. A. MUEHLBAECHER: The current role of inert gases in the search for anesthesia mechanisms. Pharmacol. Rev. **15**, 97—121 (1963).
FERGUSON, J.: The use of chemical potentials as indices of toxicity. Proc. roy. Soc. B. **127**, 387—404 (1939).
GLOVER, J. H., and H. W. HODGSON: An investigation of new fluorine compounds in anaesthesia (2). Anesthesia **16**, 19—23 (1961).
GREEN, H. D., S. H. NGAI, M. H. SULAK, J. B. CROW, and H. C. SLOCUM: Effects of anesthetic agents on hepatic structure and function in dogs. Anesthesiology **20**, 776—784 (1959).
HALEY, F. C., and G. M. WYANT: The effect of halothane on the liver of dogs exposed to mild hypoxia. Canad. Anaesth. Soc. J. **6**, 271—276 (1959).
HENNE, A. L., M. W. RENOLL, and H. M. LEICESTER: Aliphatic difluorides. J. Amer. chem. Soc. **61**, 938—940 (1939).
HINE, J., and R. G. GHIRARDELLI: The Sn 2 reactivity of β-fluoroethyl iodides. J. Organic Chem. **23**, 1550—1552 (1958).
HULME, N., and J. C. KRANTZ JR.: Ether on oxidative phosphorylation in the brain. Anesthesiology **16**, 627—631 (1955).
JOHNSTONE, M.: The human cardiovascular response to fluothane anesthesia. Brit. J. Anaesth. **28**, 392—410 (1956).
JONES, W. M., G. MARGOLIS, and C. R. STEPHEN: Hepatotoxicity of inhalation anesthetic drugs. Anesthesiology **19**, 715—723 (1958).
KRANTZ JR., J. C.: Unpublished data (1960 a).
— C. J. CARR, G. G. LU, and F. K. BELL: Anesthesia XL. The anesthetic action of trifluoroethyl vinyl ether. J. Pharmacol. exp. Ther. **108**, 488—495 (1953).
— — R. D. MUSSER, and M. J. SAUERWALD: Anesthesia XXVIII. The anesthetic action of ethyl vinyl ether. J. Pharmacol. exp. Ther. **90**, 88—94 (1947).
— —, and J. F. VITCHA: Anesthesia XXXI. A study of cyclic and noncyclic hydrocarbons on cardiac automaticity. J. Pharmacol. exp. Ther. **94**, 315—318 (1948).
— H. F. CASCORBI, M. HELRICH, R. M. BURGISON, M. I. GOLD, and F. G. RUDO: A note on the intravenous use of anesthetic emulsions in animals and man with special reference to methoxyflurane. Anesthesiology **22**, 491—492 (1961 a).
— —, and F. G. RUDO: Unpublished data (1961 b).
— — — Unpublished data (1962 a).
— — — The intravenous administration of methoxyflurane emulsions in animals and man. Anesth. Analg. Curr. Res. **41**, 257—262 (1962 b).
— J. S. L. LING, and V. F. KOZLER: Anesthesia LXI. The anesthetic properties of the azeotropic mixture of trifluoroethyl vinyl ether (fluoromar) and 1,1,2-trifluoro-2,2,1-trichloroethane (genetron 113). J. Pharmacol. exp. Ther. **130**, 492—496 (1960 b).
— G. G. LU, L. SPEERS, F. G. RUDO, and H. F. CASCORBI: Anesthesia LXV. The anesthetic properties of 2,2,2-trifluoroethyl iodide. Anesth. Analg. Curr. Res. **42**, 12—18 (1963).
— C. S. PARK, and J. S. L. LING: Anesthesia LX. The anesthetic properties of 1,1,1-trichloroethane. Anesthesiology **20**, 635—640 (1959).
— — E. B. TRUITT JR., and A. S. C. LING: Anesthesia LVII. A further study of the anesthetic properties of 1,1,1-trifluoro 2,2-bromochlorethane (fluothane). Anesthesiology **19**, 38—44 (1958).

KRANTZ JR., J. C., E. B. TRUITT JR., A. S. C. LING, and L. SPEERS: Anesthesia LV. The pharmacologic response to hexafluorodiethyl ether. J. Pharmacol. exp. Ther. **121**, 362—368 (1957).
KURLAND, A. A., T. E. HANLON, A. J. ESQUIBEL, J. C. KRANTZ JR., and C. S. SHEETS: A comparative study of hexafluorodiethyl ether (Indoklon) and electro-convulsive therapy. J. nerv. ment. Dis. **129**, 95—98 (1959).
LARSON, C. P. JR., E. I. EGER II, and J. W. SEVERINGHAUS: The solubility of halothane in blood and tissue homogenates. Anesthesiology **23**, 349—355 (1962).
LEVY, L., and R. M. FEATHERSTONE: Oxidative phosphorylation with xenon and nitrous oxide. J. Pharmacol. exp. Ther. **110**, 221—225 (1954).
LILLIE, R. S.: The theory of anesthesia. Biol. Bull. **30**, 311—366 (1916).
LING, A. S. C., and J. C. KRANTZ JR.: Anesthesia LXII. The effect of hexafluorodiethyl ether and trifluoroethyl vinyl ether on cerebral metabolism. Anesthesiology **21**, 518—521 (1960).
— — The effect of bis-(2,2,2-trifluoroethyl) ether on brain electrolytes and water distribution in the rat. Biochem. Pharmacol. **12**, 394—395 (1963).
LITTLE, D. M., G. M. BARBOUR, and J. B. GIVEN: The effects of fluothane, cyclopropane and ether anesthesias on liver function. Surg. Gynec. Obstet. **107**, 712—718 (1958).
LOWE, H. J.: Determination of volatile compounds in blood and tissues. Scientific exhibit section of anesthesiology. AMA 112th annual meeting (1963).
— Flame ionization, Determination of volatile organic anesthetics in blood, gases and tissues. Anesthesiology **25**, 808, 194 (1964).
LU, G. G., J. S. L. LING, and J. C. KRANTZ JR.: Anesthesia XLI. The anesthetic properties of certain fluorinated hydrocarbons and ethers. Anesthesiology **14**, 466—472 (1953).
LUCAS, G. H. W.: Study of the fate and toxicity of bromine and chlorine containing anesthetics. J. Pharmacol. exp. Ther. **34**, 223—237 (1928).
MARX, G. F.: Placental transfer and drugs used in anesthesia. Anesthesiology **22**, 294—313 (1961).
— I. C. ANDREWS, and L. R. ORKIN: Cerebrospinal fluid pressures during halothane anaesthesia. Canad. Anaesth. Soc. J. **9**, 239—245 (1962).
MATHEWSON, H. S.: Structural forms of anesthetic compounds. Springfield Illinois: Charles C. Thomas 1961.
MEYER, H. H.: Zur Theorie der Alkoholnarkose. Naunyn-Schmiedebergs Arch. exp. Path. Pharmak. **42**, 109—118 (1899).
MILLER, S. L.: Theory of gaseous anesthetics. Proc. nat. Acad. Sci. (Wash.) **47**, 1515—1524 (1961).
MORRIS, L. E.: Personal communication (1961).
— Liver function with fluorinated anesthetics. Surv. Anesth. **7**, 372 (1963).
MOYERS, T., and C. P. PITTINGER: Changes in blood pressure and pulse rate during fluothane anesthesia: A comparative clinical study. Anesthesiology **20**, 605—607 (1959).
MULLINS, L. J.: Some physical mechanisms in narcosis. Chem. Rev. **54**, 289—323 (1954).
NUNN, J. F., and R. L. MATTHEWS: Gaseous exchange during halothane anesthesia: The steady respiratory state. Brit. J. Anaesth. **31**, 330—340 (1959).
OVERTON, E.: Studien über die Narkose. Jena 1901.
PAPPER, E. M., and R. J. KITZ, Ed.: Uptake and distribution of anesthetic agents. New York, Toronto, London: McGraw-Hill Book Company 1963.
PARK, C. S., E. B. TRUITT JR., and J. C. KRANTZ JR.: Anesthesia LI. A comparative study of ethyl vinyl and trifluoroethyl vinyl ethers. Anesthesiology **18**, 250—256 (1957).
PARTINGTON, J. R.: A Text-Book of Inorganic Chemistry, 2nd Edition, page 416. London: MacMillan and Co., Ltd. 1925.
PAULING, L.: Molecular theory of general anesthesia. Science **134**, 15—21 (1961).
—, and M. L. HUGGINS: Covalent radii of atoms and interatomic distances in crystals containing electro-pair bonds. Z. Kristallogr. **87**, 205—238 (1934).
PETERS, J. J., A. R. VONDERAHE, and T. H. POWERS: Comparative effects of some convulsant drugs on behavior and electrical activity of nervous and muscular system of the salamander. J. Pharmacol. exp. Ther. **103**, 28—34 (1958).
RAVENTOS, J.: The action of fluothane — a new volatile anesthetic. Brit. J. Pharmacol. **11**, 394—410 (1956).
—, and A. SPINKS: The development of halothane, Part II. Manchester Univ. med. School Gaz. **37**, 55—59 (1958).
ROBBINS, B. H.: Preliminary studies of the anesthetic activity of fluorinated hydrocarbons. J. Pharmacol. exp. Ther. **86**, 197—204 (1946).
ROOT, W. S., and F. G. HOFMANN, Ed.: Physiological pharmacology, Vol. 1. New York and London: Academic Press 1963.
RUDO, F. G., H. F. CASCORBI, and R. S. ROZMAN: Unpublished data (1963a).
—, and J. C. KRANTZ JR.: Induction anesthesia with intravenous emulsions. Fed. Proc. **22**, 187 (1963b).

SEEVERS, M. H., W. J. MEEK, E. A. ROVENSTINE, and J. A. STILES: A study of cyclopropane anesthesia with special reference to gas concentrations, respiration and electrocardiographic changes. J. Pharmacol. exp. Ther. **51**, 1—17 (1934).
SEVERINGHAUS, J. W., and S. C. CULLEN: Depression of myocardium and body oxygen consumption with fluothane. Anesthesiology **19**, 165—177 (1958).
SHERIDAN, C. A., and J. G. ROBSON: Fluothane in obstetrical anesthesia. Canad. Anaesth. Soc. J. **6**, 365—374 (1959).
STEPHEN, C. R., and D. M. LITTLE JR.: Halothane (fluothane). Baltimore, Maryland: The Williams & Wilkins Company 1961.
— G. MARGOLIS, L. W. FABIAN, and M. BOURGEOIS-GAVARDIN: Laboratory observations with fluothane. Anesthesiology **19**, 770—781 (1958).
STRUCK, H. C., and E. B. PLATTNER: A study of the pharmacological properties of certain saturated fluorocarbons. J. Pharmacol. exp. Ther. **68**, 217—219 (1940).
SUCKLING, C. W.: Some chemical and physical factors in the development of fluothane. Brit. J. Anesth. **29**, 466—472 (1957).
VANDAM, L. D.: Halothane and hepatic necrosis. Editorial Views. Anesthesiology **24**, 109 (1963).
VAN DYKE, R. A., M. B. CHENOWETH, and A. VAN POZNAK: Metabolism of volatile anesthetics. I. Conversion *in vivo* of several anesthetics to $^{14}CO_2$ and chloride. Biochem. Pharmacol. **13**, 1239—1247 (1964).
VAN POZNAK, A., and J. F. ARTUSIO JR.: Anesthetic properties of a series of fluorinated compounds. I. Fluorinated hydrocarbons. Toxicol. appl. Pharmacol. **2**, 363—373 (1960a).
— — Anesthetic properties of a series of fluorinated compounds. II. Fluorinated ethers. Toxicol. appl. Pharmacol. **2**, 374—378 (1960b).
VIRTUE, R. W., and K. W. PAYNE: Postoperative death after fluothane (case report). Anesthesiology **19**, 562—563 (1958).
— J. H. K. VOGEL, P. PRESS, and R. F. GROVER: Respiratory and hemodynamic measurements during anesthesia. Use of trifluoroethyl vinyl ether and halothane. J. Amer. med. Ass. **179**, 224—225 (1962).
— R. V. YOUNG, L. O. LUND, J. H. K. VOGEL, and R. F. GROVER: Halopropane anesthesia in man. Anesthesiology **24**, 217—221 (1963).
WYANT, G. M., J. E. MERRIMAN, J. H. HARLAND, and H. V. DONALDSON: The cardiovascular effects of azeotropic halothane-ether. Canad. Anaesth. Soc. J. **7**, 91—99 (1960).
WULF, R. J., and R. M. FEATHERSTONE: A correlation of van der Waals constants with anesthetic potency. Anesthesiology **18**, 97—105 (1957).

Author Index

Page numbers in *italics* refer to the bibliography

Subject Index

(Compiled by the Sub-Editor with the collaboration of the individual contributors)

GPSR Compliance

The European Union's (EU) General Product Safety Regulation (GPSR) is a set of rules that requires consumer products to be safe and our obligations to ensure this.

If you have any concerns about our products, you can contact us on ProductSafety@springernature.com

In case Publisher is established outside the EU, the EU authorized representative is:

Springer Nature Customer Service Center GmbH
Europaplatz 3
69115 Heidelberg, Germany

Batch number: 10844661

Printed by Printforce, the Netherlands